Physical Medicine and Rehabilitation Patient-Centered Care

Mastering the Competencies

Physical Medicine and Rehabilitation Patient-Centered Care
Mastering the Competencies

EDITORS

Adrian Cristian, MD, MHCM
Vice-Chairman and Residency Program Director
Department of Physical Medicine and Rehabilitation
Kingsbrook Jewish Medical Center
Brooklyn, New York

Sorush Batmangelich, EdD, MHPE
President
BATM Medical Education Consultants
Buffalo Grove, Illinois
Founding Director of Medical Education
American Academy of Physical Medicine and Rehabilitation
Founding Director of Education
American Congress of Rehabilitation Medicine
Past Assistant Professor
Department of Physical Medicine and Rehabilitation
Rush University Medical Center
Chicago, Illinois

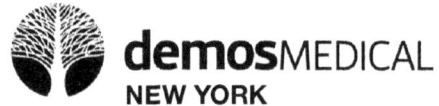

NEW YORK

Visit our website at www.demosmedical.com

ISBN: 9781936287833
e-book ISBN: 9781617051333

Acquisitions Editor: Beth Barry
Compositor: Integra Software Services Pvt. Ltd.

© 2015 Demos Medical Publishing, LLC. All rights reserved. This book is protected by copyright. No part of it may be reproduced, stored in a retrieval system, or transmitted in any form or by any means, electronic, mechanical, photocopying, recording, or otherwise, without the prior written permission of the publisher.

Medicine is an ever-changing science. Research and clinical experience are continually expanding our knowledge, in particular our understanding of proper treatment and drug therapy. The authors, editors, and publisher have made every effort to ensure that all information in this book is in accordance with the state of knowledge at the time of production of the book. Nevertheless, the authors, editors, and publisher are not responsible for errors or omissions or for any consequences from application of the information in this book and make no warranty, expressed or implied, with respect to the contents of the publication. Every reader should examine carefully the package inserts accompanying each drug and should carefully check whether the dosage schedules mentioned therein or the contraindications stated by the manufacturer differ from the statements made in this book. Such examination is particularly important with drugs that are either rarely used or have been newly released on the market.

Library of Congress Cataloging-in-Publication Data

Physical medicine and rehabilitation: competency-based practice / editors, Adrian Cristian, Sorush Batmangelich.
   p. ; cm.
 Includes bibliographical references and index.
 ISBN 978-1-936287-83-3 (alk. paper)—ISBN 978-1-61705-133-3 (e-book)
 I. Cristian, Adrian, 1964- editor. II. Batmangelich, Sorush, editor.
 [DNLM: 1. Competency-Based Education. 2. Physical and Rehabilitation Medicine—education. WB 460]
 R733
 610—dc23

                                                                           2014012511

Special discounts on bulk quantities of Demos Medical Publishing books are available to corporations, professional associations, pharmaceutical companies, health care organizations, and other qualifying groups. For details, please contact:

Special Sales Department
Demos Medical Publishing, LLC
11 West 42nd Street, 15th Floor
New York, NY 10036
Phone: 800-532-8663 or 212-683-0072
Fax: 212-941-7842
E-mail: specialsales@demosmedical.com

Printed in the United States of America by Bradford & Bigelow.
14 15 16 17 / 5 4 3 2 1

This book is dedicated to:

My loving wife and best friend, Eliane, for her encouragement, patience, humor and understanding,
My children, Alec and Chloe, who have added immeasurable joy, meaning, and fun to my life,
My mother, Steluta Cristian, who has taught me compassion for others,
My sister, Dr. Daniela Spector, for her boundless optimism,
The memory of Cali Cristian, Rasela Cru, Joseph Katz, and Camille Katz for their wisdom and support,
And my patients, mentors, and residents from whom I have learned that as physicians, we are always both students and teachers.

AC

It's with great joy that I dedicate this book to my wife, Marilyn; my son, Ramsey; and my dear parents. In addition, I wish to acknowledge a handful of wonderful professors and teachers, who served as my mentors and role models, both in the United States and abroad, in medicine, medical education, and adult learning—your wisdom, encouragement, and generosity helped me to shape a rich, satisfying, and ever-expanding career. On behalf of all our authors, editors, contributors, I want to say thanks to an entire generation of physiatrist educators. We are grateful to you as mentors and leaders. You influenced us, taught us, and encouraged us. Your wisdom and values provide a solid foundation for this book and the future of professional education and life-long learning in Physical Medicine and Rehabilitation.

SB

Contents

Contributors   *ix*
Preface   *xiii*

PART I: BASIC PRINCIPLES

1. The Use of Milestones in Physical Medicine and Rehabilitation Residency Education   *3*
   Karen P. Barr
   Teresa L. Massagli

2. The Use of Narrative Medicine and Reflection for Practice-Based Learning and Improvement   *9*
   Alice Fornari
   Adam B. Stein

3. Conscious, Compassionate Communication in Rehabilitation Medicine   *16*
   Susan Eisner

4. Application of Principles of Professional Education for Physicians   *31*
   Sorush Batmangelich

5. Ethical Considerations in the Practice of Rehabilitation Medicine—A Contextual Framework for Addressing Ethical Issues in Rehabilitation Medicine   *54*
   Sarita Patel
   William Donovan
   Adrian Cristian

6. Professionalism   *66*
   Frantz Duffoo
   Adrian Cristian

7. Systems-Based Practice in Rehabilitation Medicine   *71*
   Adrian Cristian

8. Essentials of Leadership in the Field of Physical Medicine and Rehabilitation—A Personal Perspective   *82*
   Kristjan T. Ragnarsson

PART II: CORE CLINICAL COMPETENCIES

9. Upper Extremity Limb Loss   *89*
   Nicole Sasson

10. Lower Extremity Amputation   *99*
    Gail Latlief
    Christine Elnitsky
    Robert Kent

11. Cardiopulmonary Rehabilitation   *112*
    Matthew Bartels

12. Cancer Rehabilitation   *130*
    Adrian Cristian
    Julie Silver
    Frances Atupulazi
    Yan Li

13. Stroke   *144*
    Michelle Stern
    Antigone Arygriou
    Roshni Durgam
    Jennifer Gomez
    Hejab Imteyaz
    Rakhi Sutaria

14. Moderate and Severe Traumatic Brain Injury   *165*
    Ajit B. Pai
    Isaac Darko
    William Robbins

15. Mild Traumatic Brain Injury   *177*
    Foluke A. Akinyemi
    Shane McNamee

16. Spinal Cord Injury   *190*
    Thomas N. Bryce
    Vincent Huang

17. **Parkinson Disease** 200
    Mohammed Zaman
    Neil Patel
    Marc Ross
    Miksha Patel

18. **Neuromuscular Diseases** 211
    C. David Lin
    Grigory Sirkin
    Marwa A. Ahmed

19. **Multiple Sclerosis** 223
    Chauncy Eakins
    Debra Brathwaite*
    Adrian Cristian

20. **Osteoarthritis** 235
    Christine Hinke
    Travis R. von Tobel
    Brandon Von Tobel

21. **Rehabilitation Following Total Knee Arthroplasty and Total Hip Arthroplasty** 248
    Basem Aziz
    Neil Patel
    Miksha Patel

22. **Spasticity** 257
    Navdeep Singh Jassal
    Dayna McCarthy
    Jennifer Schoenfeld
    Matthew Shatzer

23. **Musculoskeletal Disorders: Upper Extremity** 268
    Jonah Green
    Monica Habib
    Rachel Mallari
    Tova Plaut

24. **Lumbar Spine Disorders** 278
    Hamilton Chen
    Danielle Perret Karimi

25. **Rheumatoid Arthritis** 288
    Dallas Kingsbury
    David Bressler

26. **Fibromyalgia** 303
    Lauren R. Eichenbaum
    Geet Paul
    Stephen Nickl
    David Bressler

27. **Cervical Radiculopathy** 314
    Samuel P. Thampi
    Travis R. von Tobel
    Monica Habib

28. **Sports Medicine: Preparticipation Evaluation** 322
    Kiran Vadada
    Mahmud Ibrahim
    Joseph Herrera

29. **Entrapment Neuropathies** 329
    Todd R. Lefkowitz

30. **Pediatric Traumatic Brain Injury** 339
    Rajashree Srinivasan

31. **Juvenile Idiopathic Arthritis** 353
    Rajashree Srinivasan
    Callenda Hacker
    Nora Cubillos

Answers 367
Index 381

*Deceased.

Contributors

Marwa A. Ahmed, MD, MS
Spine and Sports Medicine of New York
Bronx, New York

Foluke A. Akinyemi, MD
PM&R Service
Fayetteville VA Medical Center
Fayetteville, North Carolina

Antigone Argyriou, MD
Department of Physical Medicine and Rehabilitation
Albert Einstein Medical College
Montefiore Medical Center
New York, New York

Frances Atupulazi, MD
Department of Rehabilitation Medicine
Kingsbrook Jewish Medical Center
Brooklyn, New York

Basem Aziz, MD
Department of Rehabilitation Medicine
Kingsbrook Jewish Medical Center
Brooklyn, New York

Karen P. Barr, MD
Associate Professor of Rehabilitation Medicine
University of Washington
Seattle, Washington

Matthew Bartels, MD, MPH
Professor and Chairman
The Arthur S. Abramson Department of Physical Medicine and Rehabilitation
Albert Einstein College of Medicine
Montefiore Medical Center
Bronx, New York

Debra Brathwaite, MD*
Department of Rehabilitation Medicine
Kingsbrook Jewish Medical Center
Brooklyn, New York

Sorush Batmangelich, EdD, MHPE
President
BATM Medical Education Consultants
Buffalo Grove, Illinois
Founding Director of Medical Education
American Academy of Physical Medicine and Rehabilitation
Founding Director of Education
American Congress of Rehabilitation Medicine
Past Assistant Professor
Department of Physical Medicine and Rehabilitation
Rush University Medical Center
Chicago, Illinois

David Bressler, MD
Assistant Professor
Department of Physical Medicine and Rehabilitation
Ichan School of Medicine at Mount Sinai
New York, New York

Thomas N. Bryce, MD
Associate Professor
Icahn School of Medicine at Mount Sinai
New York, New York

Hamilton Chen, MD
Pain Medicine Fellow
Department of Anesthesiology and Perioperative Care
University of California, Irvine
Irvine, California

Adrian Cristian, MD, MHCH
Vice-Chairman and Residency Program Director
Department of Physical Medicine and Rehabilitation
Kingsbrook Jewish Medical Center
Brooklyn, New York

---
*Deceased.

Nora Cubillos, MD
Physical Medicine and Rehabilitation
Baylor Health Care System
Dallas, Texas

Isaac Darko, MD
PM&R Service
Department of Veterans Affairs
Hunter Holmes McGuire VA Medical Center
Richmond, Virginia

William Donovan, MD
Emeritus Professor of PM&R
UT Health
Past Medical Director
TIRR/Memorial Hermann
Houston, Texas

Frantz Duffoo, MD
Associate Chairman and Residency Program Director
Department of Medicine
Kingsbrook Jewish Medical Center
Brooklyn, New York

Roshni Durgam, MD
Department of Physical Medicine and Rehabilitation
Albert Einstein Medical College
Montefiore Medical Center
New York, New York

Chauncy Eakins, MD
Department of Rehabilitation Medicine
Kingsbrook Jewish Medical Center
Brooklyn, New York

Lauren R. Eichenbaum, MD
Department of Rehabilitation Medicine
Stanford School of Medicine
Stanford, California

Susan Eisner, MPH, CASAC
President, Visionary Health Solutions
Professional Trainer and Speaker
Executive, Corporate and Personal Coach
Kings Park, New York

Christine Elnitsky, PhD, RN
Associate Professor
The University of North Carolina at Charlotte
College of Health and Human Services
Health Services Research PhD Program and School of Nursing
Charlotte, North Carolina

Alice Fornari, EdD, RD
Associate Professor of Science Education, Population Health and Family Medicine
Associate Dean of Educational Skills Development
Hofstra North Shore-Long Island Jewish School of Medicine
Hempstead, New York

Jennifer Gomez, MD
Department of Physical Medicine and Rehabilitation
Albert Einstein Medical College
Montefiore Medical Center
New York, New York

Jonah Green, MD
Chairman
Department of Physical Medicine and Rehabilitation
Woodhull Medical and Mental Health Center
Brooklyn, New York

Monica Habib, MD
Department of Rehabilitation Medicine
Kingsbrook Rehabilitation Institute
Brooklyn, New York

Callenda Hacker, MD
Physical Medicine and Rehabilitaiton
Baylor Health Care System
Dallas, Texas

Joseph Herrera, DO
Director of Sports Medicine
Interventional Spine and Sports Medicine
Department of Rehabilitation Medicine
Icahn School of Medicine at Mount Sinai
New York, New York

Christine Hinke, MD
Site Chair
Department of Physical Medicine and Rehabilitation
Mount Sinai Beth Israel
New York, New York

Vincent Huang, MD
SCI Fellow
Department of Rehabilitation Medicine
Icahn School of Medicine at Mount Sinai
New York, New York

Mahmud Ibrahim, MD
Fellow
Interventional Spine and Sports Medicine
Icahn School of Medicine at Mount Sinai
New York, New York

Hejab Imteyaz, MD
Department of Physical Medicine and Rehabilitation
Albert Einstein Medical College
Montefiore Medical Center
New York, New York

Navdeep Singh Jassal, MD
Department of Physical Medicine and Rehabilitation
Hofstra North Shore-Long Island Jewish School of Medicine
Great Neck, New York

Danielle Perret Karimi, MD
Associate Dean for Graduate Medical Education
Director, Fellowship Program in Pain Medicine
Director, Residency Program in PM&R
HS Associate Clinical Professor
Departments of Anesthesiology and Perioperative
    Care and PM&R
The University of California, Irvine
Irvine, California

Robert Kent, DO, MHA, MPH
Pain Spine Sports Physiatry
The Kent Clinic
Orlando, Florida

Dallas Kingsbury, MD
Department of Physical Medicine and Rehabilitation
Mount Sinai Hospital
New York, New York

Gail Latlief, DO
Residency Program Director
Physical Medicine and Rehabilitation
University of South Florida College of Medicine
James A. Haley Veterans Hospital
Tampa, Florida

Todd R. Lefkowitz, DO, DABPMR, CAQSM
New York Methodist Hospital
Medical Director, Comprehensive Back and
    Neck Pain Center
Brooklyn, New York

Yan Li, MBBS
Department of Physical Medicine and Rehabilitation
Kingsbrook Jewish Medical Center
Brooklyn, New York

C. David Lin, MD
Associate Professor of Clinical Rehabilitation Medicine
Weill Cornell Medical College
New York, New York

Rachel Mallari, MS, OTR/L
Adjunct Faculty
Department of Occupational Therapy
LaGuardia Community College
Long Island City, New York

Teresa L. Massagli, MD
Professor of Rehabilitation Medicine and Pediatrics
University of Washington
Seattle, Washington

Dayna McCarthy, DO
Department of Physical Medicine and Rehabilitation
Hofstra North Shore-Long Island Jewish
School of Medicine
Great Neck, New York

Shane McNamee, MD
Associate Chief of Staff
Clinical Informatics
Hunter Holmes McGuire VAMC
Richmond, Virginia

Stephen Nickl, MD
Department of Physical Medicine and Rehabilitation
Mount Sinai Hospital
New York, New York

Ajit B. Pai, MD
Chief, PM&R Service
Department of Veterans Affairs
Hunter Holmes McGuire VA Medical Center
Richmond, Virginia

Miksha Patel, MD
Department of Rehabilitation Medicine
Kingsbrook Jewish Medical Center
Brooklyn, New York

Neil Patel, MD
Department of Rehabilitation Medicine
Kingsbrook Jewish Medical Center
Brooklyn, New York

Sarita Patel, MD
Director, Pain and Palliative Medicine
Department of Internal Medicine
Kingsbrook Jewish Medical Center
Brooklyn, New York

Geet Paul, MD
Department of Physical Medicine and Rehabilitation
Mount Sinai Hospital
New York, New York

Tova Plaut, BA
Medical Student
NYIT-College of Osteopathic Medicine
Old Westbury, New York

Kristjan T. Ragnarsson, MD
Lucy G. Moses Professor and Chairman
Department of Rehabilitation Medicine
Icahn School of Medicine at Mount Sinai
New York, New York

William Robbins, MD
Department of PM&R
Virginia Commonwealth University
Richmond, Virginia

Marc Ross, MD
Chairman
Department of Rehabilitation Medicine
Kingsbrook Jewish Medical Center
Brooklyn, New York

Nicole Sasson, MD
Chief
Physical Medicine and Rehabilitation
VA NY Harbor Healthcare System
Clinical Associate Professor of Rehabilitation Medicine
New York University School of Medicine
New York, New York

Jennifer Schoenfeld, DO
Department of Physical Medicine and Rehabilitation
Hofstra North Shore-Long Island Jewish School of Medicine
Great Neck, New York

Matthew Shatzer, DO
Residency Program Director and Assistant Professor
Department of Physical Medicine and Rehabilitation
Hofstra North Shore-Long Island Jewish School of Medicine
Great Neck, New York

Julie Silver, MD
Associate Professor
Department of Physical Medicine and Rehabilitation
Harvard Medical School
Boston, Massachusetts

Rajashree Srinivasan, MD
Associate Medical Director
Our Children's House
Baylor Health Care System
Dallas, Texas

Adam B. Stein, MD
Professor and Chair
Department of Physical Medicine and Rehabilitation
Hofstra North Shore-Long Island Jewish School of Medicine
Great Neck, New York

Michelle Stern, MD
Associate Professor
Clinical Physical Medicine and Rehabilitation
Albert Einstein Medical College
Chair
Department of Physical Medicine and Rehabilitation
Jacobi Medical Center
Bronx, New York

Rakhi Sutaria, MD
Department of Physical Medicine and Rehabilitation
Albert Einstein Medical College
Montefiore Medical Center
New York, New York

Grigory Syrkin, MD
Cancer Rehabilitation Fellow
Sillerman Center for Rehabilitation
Memorial Sloan-Kettering Cancer Center
New York, New York

Samuel Thampi, MD
Department of Physical Medicine and Rehabilitation,
Kingsbrook Jewish Medical center
Brooklyn, New York

Travis R. von Tobel, MD
Department of Rehabilitation Medicine
Kingsbrook Rehabilitation Institute
Brooklyn, New York

Brandon Von Tobel, MD, MBE
Chief Financial Officer
ImaCor Inc.
Garden City, New York

Kiran Vadada MD
Fellow
Interventional Spine and Sports Medicine
Icahn School of Medicine at Mount Sinai
New York, New York

Mohammed Zaman, MD
Kingsbrook Jewish Medical Center
Department of Rehabilitation Medicine
Kingsbrook Jewish Medical Center
Brooklyn, New York

Preface

Although a number of excellent textbooks on physical medicine and rehabilitation are available, this comprehensive, self-directed textbook is the first to establish a standard in practice, education, and training with the introduction of a coordinated competency-based approach to shape the future of physiatric patient care.

In Part I, foundations for the core competencies are provided with some basic principles for application toward competency-centric practice entwined with professional education strategies.

Part II focuses on the major physiatric areas of practice with information specific to each area organized in the context of the six Accreditation Council of Graduate Medical Education (ACGME)/American Board of Medical Specialties (ABMS) core competencies and quality metrics. Each practice chapter includes goals and objectives for the six competencies, a case study with open-ended discussion questions, and self-examination questions and answers for self-assessment. Throughout, the text is supported with valuable clinical tips, how-to and where-to guides, key points, tables, charts, and references for further study.

The book can be used independently to build essential skills for patient-centered care or as part of a physical medicine and rehabilitation resident training curriculum as a useful adjunct during clinical rotations.

Many clinicians, academics, educators, residents, and fellows have contributed to this book. Self-assessment questions for most of the chapters have been developed and organized with an answer key and references supporting the correct answers. The authors recommend first taking the self-assessment examination as a pretest before reading the chapter to discover strengths and limitations in knowledge, skills, and attitudes. After reading the chapter, the reader may want to again review the self-assessment questions for outcome and understanding.

We hope that this book will help trainees in physical medicine and rehabilitation improve their skills as practitioners, learners, and educators and better prepare for the ongoing process of professional development throughout their medical careers.

Adrian Cristian, MD, MHCM
Sorush Batmangelich, EdD, MHPE

Physical Medicine and Rehabilitation Patient-Centered Care
Mastering the Competencies

I: Basic Principles

Karen P. Barr
Teresa L. Massagli

1: The Use of Milestones in Physical Medicine and Rehabilitation Residency Education

COMPETENCY-BASED MEDICAL EDUCATION

The Accreditation Council of Graduate Medical Education (ACGME) is a private nonprofit organization that sets the standards for and evaluates and accredits allopathic residency and fellowship programs in the United States. In 2002, the ACGME Outcome Project identified and endorsed six general competencies to assess resident competence: medical knowledge, patient care (PC), practice-based learning and improvement (PBLI), professionalism, interpersonal and communication skills, and systems-based practice (1). Although the goal of the Outcome Project was to increase accountability for individual resident competence, no national definitions of the competencies were developed, nor were uniform sets of assessments adopted (2). Residents were presumed to be competent because they had successfully completed the process of training in their residency program. To address these problems, the ACGME adopted a new accreditation system. As of July 2014, all residency programs will need to ensure that individual residents are achieving progressive milestones of competence during residency. The milestone narratives enhance transparency of residency education for residents, faculty, and ultimately the public (3).

THE PHYSICAL MEDICINE AND REHABILITATION MILESTONES

The Physical Medicine and Rehabilitation (PM&R) milestones were developed by a group of physician educators with periodic input from the field of PM&R in the years 2010 to 2012. Milestone narratives were developed for each of the six competencies. The milestones do not represent the entire scope of each competency but were constructed to capture the most important knowledge, skills, and attitudes residents should be developing in each of the six competencies. The six general competencies are part of the core program requirements that are revised by the ACGME approximately every 10 years. The milestones are not part of the core requirements and may be revised more frequently, depending on changes in the practice of PM&R and on whether national data analysis shows they demonstrate true progression of skill development. Currently, the ACGME requires PM&R residency programs to report seven PC milestones, one medical knowledge milestone, two interpersonal and communication milestones, and three milestones each in professionalism, PBLI, and systems-based practice. There are nine additional medical knowledge milestones that programs may use for developing curriculum, structuring clinical rotations, and evaluating residents. These nine medical knowledge milestones are for spinal cord disorders, brain disorders, stroke, amputation, neuromuscular disorders, musculoskeletal disorders, pain, pediatrics, and spasticity.

Each milestone set has five levels of observable behaviors arrayed from less to more advanced. The PM&R milestone levels are not postgraduate year (PGY) level specific because PM&R programs structure the timing of clinical experiences in diverse ways. However, each resident is expected to demonstrate progress over time. Level 1 represents the knowledge, skills, and attitudes of an entry-level resident. For some PM&R programs, entry-level residents are PGY1, and for others, they are PGY2. Because the milestones are PM&R specific, PGY1 residents may not have opportunities for learning or performing Level 1 milestones; in this case, the program would "score" that milestone as "has not achieved Level 1." Levels 2 and 3 represent progressively more advanced skills. Level 4 is the target for a graduating resident, and Level 5 represents an aspirational goal that might be achieved by a few residents in some milestones. Level 4 is a *target*, not a requirement for resident graduation. The milestones are a framework for evaluation that the program director will use to determine if a resident is competent to enter practice without direct supervision (3). The milestones are also not intended to be used to accelerate completion of residency because their reliability and validity have not been established for use in high-stakes decisions. They do not represent the entirety of the dimensions of competence, and programs may have other additional requirements for scholarly work or clinical training that are not encompassed by the milestones. Finally, the duration of training that allows a resident to become eligible for Board certification is specified by the American Board of PM&R, not by the ACGME.

To be able to evaluate each resident using the milestones, programs will need an integrated mix of assessment tools. Table 1.1 summarizes the milestones, gives an example of some of the narratives in each milestone, and suggests what assessment tools may be helpful to determine an individual resident's milestone attainment. For each milestone, several tools could be used together to assess a level, and the best tool varies depending on what is being measured. Choosing the best method of assessment depends on several different variables. Criteria for good assessment include the following:

- *Validity*: Coherence, or does the method really assess the described behavior?
- *Reliability*: Reproducibility or consistency, so are measurements consistent across evaluators or repeatable over time?
- *Educational effect*: Does preparing to do well on the assessment motivate and educate the resident in the most relevant way?
- *Feasibility*: Is the assessment method practical, realistic, sensible, efficient, and affordable given the circumstances and context?
- *Acceptability*: Will faculty use it, and will residents and faculty find it credible and trust the results?
- *Equivalence*: Will different versions of an assessment yield equivalent scores or decisions?
- *Catalytic effect*: Does the assessment provide results and feedback in a fashion that creates, enhances, and supports education? (4)

On the surface, choosing the best method may seem daunting, but by closely reading the milestones, it often becomes obvious what tools could evaluate the skills, and then each program, and, in some cases, individual faculty within a program, can determine what method is feasible for their situation, the timing of when to evaluate each milestone, and how progress will be measured.

In addition to evaluation tools, sometimes additional opportunities will need to be created or adjusted to meet certain milestones, such as committee work or learning plans. For example, with PBLI milestone 3 (PBLI3), quality improvement (QI), residents are expected to understand basic QI principles and identify specific care processes that need improvement (Level 2) and then demonstrate active involvement in processes aimed at improving

TABLE 1.1 Methods to Assess Milestones

MILESTONE (CORE COMPETENCIES IN BOLD)	EXAMPLE OF PORTION OF A MILESTONE	POSSIBLE WAYS TO ASSESS
Patient Care (PC)		
PC1: History appropriate for age and impairment	"Documents and presents in a complete and organized manner"	Direct observation and workroom discussion Chart review OSCEs
PC2: Physiatric physical examination	"Identifies and correctly interprets atypical physical findings"	Direct observation and discussion OSCEs
PC3: Diagnostic valuation	"Orders appropriate diagnostic studies"	Case discussion Chart review Written and oral examinations
PC4: Medical management	"Manages patients with complex medical comorbidities"	Direct observation (counseling patients and families) Case discussion Chart review
PC5: Rehabilitation/functional management	"Prescribes commonly used prostheses"	Case discussion Chart review Written and oral examinations
PC6: Procedural skills	"Performs injections with direct supervision"	Direct observation Simulations
PC7: Electrodiagnostic procedures	"Identifies sites of EMG needle insertion in muscles commonly studied"	Direct observation Case discussion Chart review Written tests OSCEs

(continued)

TABLE 1.1 Methods to Assess Milestones (*continued*)

MILESTONE (CORE COMPETENCIES IN BOLD)	EXAMPLE OF PORTION OF A MILESTONE	POSSIBLE WAYS TO ASSESS
Medical Knowledge (MK)	"Predicts functional outcome and prognosis"	Case discussion Oral examinations Written tests
Systems-Based Practice (SBP)		
SBP1: Systems thinking	"Has learned to coordinate care across a variety of settings"	Observation of patient case management Case discussion
SBP2: Team approach	"Leads the interdisciplinary team"	Observation of patient case management
SBP3: Patient safety	"Identifies health system factors that increase risk for errors"	Patient safety committee work Participation in practice improvement project Observation of patient case management
Practice-Based Learning and Improvement (PBLI)		
PBLI1: Self-directed learning and teaching	"Develops and follows a learning plan"	Written learning plan Individual mentoring discussions Lecture attendance and participation Presentations
PBLI2: Evidence from scientific studies	"Effectively appraises evidence for its validity and applicability to individual patient care"	Journal club participation Presentations of case reports
PBLI3: Quality improvement (QI)	"Demonstrates active involvement in processes aimed at improving patient care"	QI committee work Practice improvement projects
Professionalism (PROF)		
Prof 1: Compassion, integrity, and respect for others	"Exhibits compassion, integrity, and respect in challenging interaction with patients and families"	Direct observation Patient surveys 360° evaluations
Prof 2: Ethical principles	"Analyzes common ethical issues and seeks guidance when appropriate"	Case discussions Observation of patient case management
Prof 3: Professional behaviors and accountability	"Demonstrates that the responsibility of patient care supersedes self-interest"	Observation of patient case management Discussions with mentor
Interpersonal and Communication Skills (ICS)		
ICS 1: Relationship management	"Effectively educates and counsels patients and families"	Patient survey 360° evaluations Direct observation OSCEs
ICS 2: Information gathering and sharing	"Ensures medical records are accurate and complete"	Chart review Observation of case management

the care of patients (Level 3). These levels would best be assessed by residents learning about the QI process, and then participating in a QI project. To reach Level 4, the graduation target, they would then be expected to identify opportunities for process improvement in everyday work.

For PC milestones, the cornerstone of evaluation will be evaluation in the workplace. However, for certain skills, this could be supplemented by more standardized evaluation methods. For example, to determine if a resident has reached Level 2 for PC milestone 6 (PC6), procedural skills, a group activity to assess this level could be standardized that showed the three skills that must be observed:

- "Demonstrates basic understanding of which injections should be used to treat specific conditions." This could be assessed by a written or oral examination.
- "Educates patients regarding procedure-specific information and treatment options on a basic level." This could be assessed by an observed standardized clinical encounter (OSCE) or by direct observation using a tool such as the Resident Observation and Competency Assessment (ROCA) (5).
- "Performs injections with direct supervision." This could be assessed with an injection model, or on an actual patient, using methods ranging from the ROCA to a detailed checklist to make sure that the observation is standardized (6).

To determine if a resident has reached Level 3 on this milestone, the resident needs to show that he or she:

- "Makes appropriate choices regarding medication options, dosing, and guidance methods"
- "Obtains informed consent, confirming patient understanding and inviting questions"
- "Modifies procedure to accommodate the patient's impairment and minimizes discomfort"

A single observation would not be sufficient to show that a resident had reached this level. Multiple clinical encounters should be observed to see how the resident can adapt his or her basic skills, which were evaluated in the Level 2 milestone, to specific clinical situations.

To obtain a Level 4 in this milestone, which is the target for graduation, a resident must demonstrate 2 skills:

- "Performs injections without attending intervention," which would best be observed at the bedside.
- "Demonstrates thorough understanding of situations when injections are indicated and contraindicated, taking into account level of evidence, cost effectiveness, and long-term outcomes," which could be assessed by discussions in the workroom as clinical decisions are made, or perhaps by a presentation that addresses the level of evidence and long-term outcomes in a population of patients.

Other PC milestones, such as PC4 medical management, would be difficult to assess by written tests or standardized situations and would be better to assess with direct observation of the resident's work with patients. This type of assessment, called workplace-based assessment, is considered particularly valuable for complex skills such as medical management, because it is the only way of assessing what a resident actually does in the context of PC. This milestone (PC4) requires skills such as "manages patients with complex medical comorbidities and secondary conditions" and "develops and implements a comprehensive treatment plan." To be able to reach these milestones, an integration of many separate skills, such as medical knowledge, physical examination skills, clinical reasoning, and communication skills, is needed. Measuring these skills in the way that they are actually used is considered more valid than breaking them into isolated micro skills, and hoping that the sum of these equals good patient care (7).

One concern about workplace-based assessment of complex skills is a lack of reliability of the evaluation because it is not standardized in the way that an OSCE can be and often does not lend itself to detailed checklists. However, this can be addressed by appropriate sampling across different contexts and by having different assessors (7). Recent studies that use direct observation of skills in the workplace have shown that these tools are reliable using multiple assessors. Using multiple assessors helps control for individual biases and idiosyncrasies (8,9).

Assessments based on direct observation of a resident by faculty are only as good as the observation. Residents can improve the observation experience by being knowledgeable about the content of the milestones, so they will be aware of what needs to be observed, and alerting the attending when the skill is going to be performed, so that it can be observed and evaluated. For example, residents can ask their attending physicians to observe a portion of the physical examination, so that they can receive feedback about PC2, the physiatric physical examination milestone. Programs can promote this behavior by making available easy-to-complete observation forms that include space for narrative feedback, so that the observation is both evaluative and formative. Programs need to promote consensus that direct observation of specific skills is important and worth the time and effort it takes to complete. The completion of these observations could even be a requirement of the clinical rotation.

Faculty can improve the workplace assessment by improving their skills in observation. Expertise in performance assessment can be developed, much as clinical expertise is developed, with targeted effort and experience. Skills include expert content knowledge of the area under assessment, practicing assessment in the clinical setting, receiving feedback and incorporating feedback on assessments, and recognizing bias (10). Programs can support this by providing training in direct observation, which has been shown to decrease interrater variability, improve rater confidence, and lead to more stringent assessment (11). Less experienced raters are more likely to literally describe behaviors observed in clinical encounters, whereas experienced raters are able to make inferences from their observations and pay more attention to situation-specific features, which may lead to richer and more formative feedback (12).

Workplace-based assessments can also be completed by other health care professionals on the team. Multisource feedback (often called 360 evaluations) can be very helpful in evaluation of the milestones, particularly those that involve skills such as team work and communications (see Table 1.1).

THE CLINICAL COMPETENCY COMMITTEE

Each PM&R residency program will need to ensure that its curriculum addresses the milestones so that individual resident progress can be documented. Residency programs will also need a system to determine if residents have successfully passed a rotation (i.e., what level of milestone attainment and other requirements constitute successful completion of a rotation). The programs will report individual resident milestone levels to the ACGME twice a year.

Determining what level in the milestones each resident has obtained and if the resident is making sufficient progress is a high-stakes decision. The ACGME common program requirements specify that each program director must appoint a clinical competency committee (CCC) to review all resident evaluations semiannually, prepare the milestone evaluations of each resident, and advise the program director about resident progress, including promotion, remediation, or dismissal (3,13,14). The benefit of a CCC is that it bases resident evaluation on the insight and views of a group of faculty members, not just on those of the program director. Multiple assessors and multiple tools used across multiple samples enhance the reliability and validity of the assessment process (4,7).

The CCC is to consist of at least three members of the physician faculty who have experience observing and evaluating the residents. Other nonphysician educators can be included as well. The ACGME does not specify the role of the program director (PD) on the CCC, but the PD may serve better in a supporting role, rather than as leader of the committee. The PD has many roles including resident advocate and confidant; this may help the CCC understand resident situations or develop plans for remediation, but may also adversely influence the deliberation and decision-making process.

The work of the CCC will initially be difficult. Twice each year, the committee must review all evaluations for each resident and make a consensus decision about milestone ratings for each resident. Programs use many types of evaluations to assess the competencies, including global faculty evaluations, direct observation such as the ROCA, written and oral examinations, conference participation, procedure logs, 360 evaluations, procedure checklists, and chart-stimulated oral examinations (5,6,15,16). The CCC will need to discuss the milestone narratives and reach common agreement on their meaning. While the CCC faculty should have firsthand knowledge of many of the residents, each faculty must leave personal bias aside, review all evaluations available, assess the quality of each evaluation, aggregate the data, and then select the narrative within the milestones that best fits the resident. The milestone reporting form has half-step levels between 1 and 2, 2 and 3, 3 and 4, and 4 and 5. Selection of a whole number indicates that a resident substantially demonstrates the narratives in that level as well as those in lower levels. Selection of the half step in between levels indicates that the resident has substantially demonstrated the milestones below the whole number as well as some milestones in higher levels (17). In order to assign a level to the single medical knowledge milestone, the CCC should consider the experiences of the resident to date, evaluations in any of the nine appendix medical knowledge milestones, and performance on milestones in other competency domains that address medical management, self-directed learning, and the use of evidence-based medicine (17).

Subsequent to CCC meetings, residents should receive feedback about their progress on the milestones and other aspects of the curriculum. This feedback can include specific areas of strengths or weaknesses, readiness for promotion, a plan for remediation, or even termination of training. Use of the milestones at frequent intervals during training should help identify problems early and avoid the situation of recognizing late in residency that an individual is not prepared to enter practice without supervision. Although not specified by the ACGME, the CCC can also contribute to faculty and program development by identifying problems with evaluation tools or in the quality of narratives provided in global or 360 evaluations.

After all programs submit milestone ratings for each resident, the ACGME will construct a Milestones Evaluation Report that will be available to programs. The program can identify gaps in its curriculum and can compare individual resident performance to other residents in the same year who have had similar learning experiences. The PM&R Review Committee of ACGME will also conduct an annual review of each program's aggregate and de-identified milestone performance as part of the annual evaluation of each program. The Review Committee will be assessing progress of the resident cohort over time and help to identify areas for program improvement (3).

In summary, the milestones outline for residents, faculty, and the public some competency-specific knowledge skills and attitudes that PM&R residents in any PM&R residency program should achieve during their residency education. Successful use of the milestones requires direct observation of clinical skills in the workplace and other assessment measures; residents cannot be assumed to have achieved milestones because they have spent a certain amount of time in training. Detailed feedback to the residents is essential, and both residents and faculty must embrace this so that programs can clearly identify problem areas early in the resident's progress and development. This spotlights not only areas in which individual residents need to improve, but also areas in which the program can improve its curriculum.

REFERENCES

1. Taradejna C. ACGME history. Accreditation Council of Graduate Medical Education website. http://www.acgme.org/acgmeweb/tabid/122/About/ACGMEHistory.aspx. Published May 2007. Accessed January 5, 2014.
2. Swing SR, Beeson MS, Carraccio C, et al. Educational milestone development in the first 7 specialties to enter the next accreditation system. *J Grad Med Educ.* 2013;5:98–106.
3. Frequently Asked Questions About the Next Accreditation System. Accreditation Council of Graduate Medical Education website. http://www.acgme.org/acgmeweb/Portals/0/PDFs/NAS/NASFAQs.pdf. Updated July 25, 2013. Accessed January 5, 2014.
4. Norcini J, Anderson B, Bollela V, et al. Criteria for good assessment: consensus statement and recommendations from the Ottawa 2010 conference. *Med Teach.* 2011;33:206–214.
5. Musick DW, Bockenek W, Massagli TL, et al. Reliability of the PM&R Resident Observation and Competency Assessment (ROCA) tool: a multi-institution study. *Am J Phys Med Rehabil.* 2010;89:235–244.

6. Escaldi SV, Cuccurullo SJ, Terzella M, et al. Assessing competency in spasticity management: a method of development and assessment. *Am J Phys Med Rehabil.* 2012;91:243–253.
7. Van der Vleuten CPM, Schuwirth LWT. Assessing professional competence: from methods to programmes. *Med Educ.* 2005;36:309–317.
8. Wilkinson JR, Crossley JG, Wragg A, et al. Implementing workplace based assessment across the medical specialties in the United Kingdom. *Med Educ.* 2008;42:364–373.
9. Moonen-van Loon JMW, Overeem K, Donkers HHLM, et al. Composite reliability of a workplace-based assessment toolbox for postgraduate medical education. *Adv Health Sci Educ Theory Pract.* 2013;18(5):1087–1102.
10. Berendock C, Stalmeijer RE, Shuwirth LWT. Expertise in performance assessment: assessors' perspectives. *Adv Health Sci Educ Theory Pract.* 2013;18:559–571.
11. Holmboe ES, Hawkins RE, Huot SJ. Effects of training in direct observation of medical residents' clinical competence. *Ann Intern Med.* 2004;140:874–881.
12. Govaerts MJB, Schuwirth LWT, Van der Vleuten CPM, et al. Workplace based assessment: effects of rater expertise. *Adv Health Sci Educ Theory Pract.* 2011;16:151–165.
13. ACGME Common Program Requirements. Accreditation Council of Graduate Medical Education website. http://www.acgme.org/acgmeweb/Portals/0/PFAssets/ProgramRequirements/CPRs2013.pdf. Published February 11, 2007. Revised June 9, 2013. Accessed January 5, 2014.
14. Frequently Asked Questions: Clinical Competency Committee and Program Evaluation Committee, Common Program Requirements, ACGME. Accreditation Council of Graduate Medical Education website. http://www.acgme.org/acgmeweb/Portals/0/PDFs/FAQ/CCC_PEC_FAQs.pdf. Published July 19, 2013. Accessed January 5, 2014.
15. Pasquina PF, Kelly S, Hawkins RE. Assessing clinical competence in PM&R residency programs. *Am J Phys Med Rehabil.* 2003;82:473–478.
16. Massagli TL, Carline JD. Reliability of a 360-degree evaluation to assess resident competence. *Am J Phys Med Rehabil.* 2007;86:845–852.
17. The Physical Medicine and Rehabilitation Milestone Project: a joint initiative of the Accreditation Council of Graduate Medical Education and the American Board of Physical Medicine and Rehabilitation. Accreditation Council of Graduate Medical Education website. http://www.acgme.org/acgmeweb/Portals/0/PDFs/Milestones/PMRMilestones.pdf. Published December 2013. Accessed January 5, 2014.

Alice Fornari
Adam B. Stein

2: The Use of Narrative Medicine and Reflection for Practice-Based Learning and Improvement

THEORETICAL FRAMEWORK FOR LEARNING THROUGH REFLECTIVE PRACTICE

Carl Rogers (1) has distilled the writings of John Dewey on reflection to four criteria. These will frame the background of the work we describe to connect reflection as a skill contributing to competency-based resident education:

1. "Reflection is a meaning-making process that moves learners from one experience into the next, each time with a deeper understanding of its relationships with and connections to other experiences and ideas. It is the thread that makes continuity of learning possible."
2. "Reflection is a systematic, rigorous, disciplined way of thinking, with its roots in scientific inquiry."
3. "Reflection needs to happen in community, in interaction with others."
4. "Reflection requires attitudes that value the personal and intellectual growth of one's self and others." (1)

Continuing medical education (CME) and continuing professional development (CPD) are the hallmarks of practice-based learning and improvement (PBLI). This chapter aligns PBLI, a core ACGME (Accreditation Council of Graduate Medical Education) competency for our trainees, to the skill of reflective practice. This skill is a natural educational strategy to achieve the goals of self-assessment and lifelong learning, which are core to the PBLI competency. Developing these skills naturalistically crosses the ACGME competency of professionalism, as well. An outcome we value when using reflection as pedagogy with trainees is the fostering and maintenance of appropriate humanistic qualities in the physicians. An added bonus to follow is the development of their professional identity over the course of their training and beyond. In addition, comfort with reflective practice as a skill set will allow our trainees to display behaviors that demonstrate responsibility and accountability to patients, themselves, and the larger society they practice among. This will strengthen their ability to advocate and be responsive to patient needs and ultimately improve quality of care.

Donald Schön (2) was an influential thinker in developing the theory and practice of reflective professional learning in the 20th century. Schön believed that people and organizations should be flexible and incorporate their life experiences and lessons learned throughout their life. His theory is supportive of reflective practice as a skill set for physicians to use their experiences to loop back and apply to future experiences. Schön (2) describes 2 types of reflection: reflection-in-action and reflection-on-action. "*Reflection-in-action* helps us as we complete a task. This process allows us to reshape what we are working on, *while* we are working on it. We reflect *on* action, *thinking back* on what we have done in order to discover how our knowing-in-action may have contributed to an unexpected outcome."

Epstein et al. (3,4) define self-assessment: "Self-assessment is the process of integrating data about our own performance and comparing it to an explicit standard," and further states that "the power of self-assessment lies in two major domains—the integration of high quality external and internal data to assess current performance and promote future learning, and the capacity for ongoing self-monitoring during everyday clinical practice." When this definition frames the conversation, one can use diverse pedagogical activities, and more specifically critical reflection, to increase one's capacity to achieve this skill. This allows self-assessment to be a reflective assessment process that is integral to learning and practice. Critical and deliberate reflection on data that learners have available to them is key to the interpretation phase required for self-assessment.

Self-assessment (4) remains an essential tool for enabling physicians to discover the discomfort of a performance gap, which may lead to changing concepts and mental models or changing work-flow processes. Guided self-assessment should be incorporated at the earliest stages of medical training as an essential professional skill. We can align reflective practice strategies as a form of guided self-assessment if they are designed with that intention.

To continue the dialogue in this chapter we must put forth a common definition of reflection to help us tighten up our understanding of this powerful small word. Reflection is intended to indicate a conscious and deliberate reinvestment of mental energy aimed at exploring and elaborating one's understanding of a circumstance one has faced or is facing currently (5). This requires exploring "why" questions to add to this understanding. This reinvestment of mental energy supports achieving true expert status in one's pursuit of personal and career goals but does not necessarily judge competence. Eva and Regehr (6) state self-reflective exercises that are formative can facilitate performance improvement through a greater understanding of the world, and apply this to future performance improvement through professional development strategies. Aronson (7) has framed reflection as "critical reflection," the process of analyzing, questioning, and reframing experience in, or to make an assessment of it, for the purpose of learning (reflective learning) and/or to improve practice (reflective practice).

Reflection and reflective writing have become familiar terms and practices with a goal of instilling, and perhaps increasing, empathetic interactions with patients and to also improve communication skills with both patients and colleagues (8). Generally, trainees are asked to reflect on an experience. This conceptual framework of using experience as a core learning tool began with John Dewey, who states "reconstruction or reorganization of experience" is the very heart of education (9). His theory on experience is expanded on by Carl Rogers (1), who states: "An experience is not an experience unless it involves interaction between self and another person and/or the larger environment." For our learners' place in the medical environment as their larger world, this experience can be a patient interaction, an ethical issue, a short story, or an interaction with a colleague. Wear (8) argues that the use of reflection in medical education requires more thoughtfulness and precision. She proposes that reflection not be approached as a singular event nor as a nebulous method but be part of a larger ongoing process in the education of physicians in the medical environment.

Wear (8) focuses on important questions to ask as we think about preparing reflective practice strategies in our education environment.

1. Is reflection merely mulling over an experience?
2. Is it a stream of consciousness?
3. How do portfolios (of reflections) serve as evidence of reflective practice (and perhaps meeting core ACGME competencies)?
4. How can the authenticity of a learner's experiences be encouraged and sustained in an environment of formulaic approaches and growing demands for documented outcomes and demonstrated competencies?
5. How overly regulated exercises in reflection might inadvertently serve as tools for surveillance and regulation rather than opportunities for revelation and transformation? (8)

Moon (10) identifies four key elements of reflection to assure medical educators are asking learners to truly reflect:

1. Reflect on experience and interrogate the experience.
2. Reflection has as a purpose the identification and deconstruction of an issue arising from an experience.
3. Reflection is a complicated mental processing of issues for which there is no obvious solution and requires bringing together previous experiences (and knowledge) to make sense of an experience and attend to one's feelings.
4. Reflecting allows the processing of an experience with a goal of *transformative action*. This will result in doing or saying something differently the next time one is in a similar situation and can result in changed thinking or a new attitude that influences these subsequent interactions (10).

Ultimately, this *transformative action* will result in a deepened commitment and renewed desire to continue investigating an experience. *Transformative action*, using reflective practice, recognizes the need for action, risk-taking, and doing things differently next time by re-forming decisions and actions. This type of action moves the act of reflective practice from a solitary act to one involving a community of others.

At the most basic level, writing of an experience enables the writer to perceive and undergo the experience. Reading and writing can be used to accelerate and deepen the clinical lessons learned in the shared work of providing health care. Early visionaries in the field of reflective writing, including Rita Charon, suggested that incorporating singular stories of patients and doctors into one's medical education and practice might aid doctors in recognizing patients' lived experiences and might support doctors' awareness of the meaning of their own experiences (11). This greater understanding among health care providers could possibly improve the effectiveness of health care (12). The teaching and learning of reflection is to equip learners with the language skills to represent and recognize complex events. Learners learn to read while they practice writing. For example sessions may begin with a close reading of selected literature. This is accomplished in small groups, and there is opportunity to read and listen to others with the goal of multiple interpretations of the writing. A requirement is nonjudgmental listening. In this model of close reading and reflective writing, the teacher is not to judge but rather read and tell what is heard. This reflective process aligns with the mission of medical education in teamwork, peer learning, trust building, and caring for others.

It is common to use personal narratives as starting points for collective reflection. Space is created to tell and write about one's experiences. Sharing of the stories among peers creates a common ground: shared core values of kindness, human connection, and commitment to social justice. In addition, fears, frustrations, and shame are shared. These stories have the power to show learners the future they are trying to create, name their core values, and identify threats to these core values (13).

A humanities teaching strategy that has been less often incorporated in medical education is the communal viewing of artistic paintings to increase sensitivity, team building, and collaboration among medical trainees. Reilly et al. (14) described a facilitated session using Visual Teaching Strategies (VTS) at a faculty/house staff retreat held at a museum. VTS uses 3 questions: (a) *What's going on in this picture?* (b) *What do you see that makes you say that?"* and (c) *What else can you find?* This technique and facilitation of discussion honors ambiguity and multiple viewpoints as valuable. The evidence asked for is from the art itself.

It is common to use artwork depicting physicians participating in clinical encounters with patients. The goal is to select images the participants can interpret without specialized artistic knowledge; the analysis is a group process. There is a shared observation process that fosters critical, creative, and flexible thinking. The authors' experience with residents is very positive and concludes that incorporating humanities in medical education can positively influence empathy, awareness, and sensitivity to the art of medicine. Specifically, they see the impact on team building as they are challenged to form a cohesive idea about art, and this skill can be transferred to patient care teams.

A larger question addressed by Mann (15) goes beyond our understanding of reflection as a tool to deepen learning, to how and when the act of reflection might influence professional practice and benefit patients. Here is an education and research effort to theorize how the use of reflection can improve diagnostic accuracy and minimize error. Another area of research investigates how mindfulness impacts knowing when problems require a new approach to prevent errors (16). This certainly requires self-assessment and self-monitoring skills to identify the need for reflective analytical reasoning, which allows reframing of a challenging problem. Mamede et al. (17) report that reflection was associated with increased accuracy of diagnoses in challenging complex cases, but was not additive in common cases.

One way to understand the influence of house staff training is through narrative accounts of their experiences (18). The narratives generated by young learners and physicians in training provide an understanding of the interplay among resident interactions with patients, their own personal issues, and the struggles during the stages of professional development. The authors suggest that to gain self-awareness through writing narratives, reflective writing should be incorporated into curricula time in training programs. Equally as important, the faculty facilitators must have advanced facilitation skills and be self-aware through their own reflective process. The goal is an educational model that encourages being reflective so that a trainee can understand how one's experiences influence learning and professional development. This can only naturally lead to graduating physicians who are more compassionate and fully developed to practice medicine.

There is growing evidence that reflection improves learning and performance in essential competencies. These competencies include professionalism, clinical reasoning, continuous practice improvement skills, and better management of complex health systems and patients. There are diverse pedagogical approaches and educational goals when planning curriculum to foster reflective learning and practice (7).

Aronson (7) describes 12 tips for teaching reflection. Elaboration of these tips can be found in her article and guide both learner and faculty development efforts, which will support successful experiences.

1. Define reflection vs. critical reflection
2. Decide on learning goals for the reflective exercise
3. Choose an appropriate instructional method for the reflection
4. Decide whether you will use a structured or unstructured approach and create a prompt
5. Make a plan for dealing with ethical and emotional concerns
6. Create a mechanism to follow up on learners' plans
7. Create a conducive learning environment
8. Teach learners about reflection before asking them to do it
9. Provide feedback and follow up
10. Assess the reflection
11. Make this exercise part of a larger curriculum to encourage reflection
12. Reflect on the process of teaching reflection (7)

Aronson (7) concludes, "With a greater understanding of the conceptual frameworks underlying critical reflection and greater advanced planning, medical educators will be able to create exercises and longitudinal curricula that not only enables greater learning from the experience being reflected upon but also develop reflective skills for life-long learning."

PRACTICAL APPROACHES FOR IMPLEMENTATION OF NARRATIVE MEDICINE

There are a variety of techniques that can be implemented to utilize narrative reflection for the purpose of PBLI that have been alluded to in the preceding part of this chapter. Prior to beginning any program though, it is important that learners obtain background information about why they are being asked to participate in this type of activity. They need to understand what may be gained, and some of the theoretical principles upon which narrative medicine rests. This may be easily accomplished through a brief didactic session, which can include examples of the writings of past program participants. They may also be assigned selected readings on the subject, followed by an interactive moderated discussion to ensure that the readings have been completed and understood. This is an opportunity to introduce the growing body of evidence on the use of reflection as a skill that can support competency-based education. In addition, opportunities for making narratives public and scholarly as publications can also be shared with learners.

Perhaps the simplest type of narrative medicine is based on one's experiences, often referred to as critical incidents (19). Residents, or other learners, may be asked to regularly write about an experience that has made a powerful impression upon them. While this most often occurs in relation to a clinical setting, it need not. They may choose to write about an educational activity, a research-based experience, or an experience that is encountered in an administrative setting. In this example of narrative medicine, there need not be a prompt and residents are free to write about whatever it is that has made an impression on them, an experience that they are choosing to think about in greater depth. While traditional journaling is most commonly thought of as a private activity, this model limits the potential for the transformative action described by Moon (10). Sharing of the narrative allows for discussion, alternative viewpoints, probing questions, and transformative learning from experiences; these ultimately impact future decisions. Sharing may be accomplished in many ways today beyond the traditional face to face in small group settings. For example, the residents may be instructed to e-mail their narratives to a designated faculty member with an interest in this educational strategy. For those inclined, there can be electronic discussion boards set up to facilitate dialogue. Using technology, an electronic back-and-forth conversation can occur. Alternatively, protected time may be set aside during the program's didactic sessions for this type of activity, where the residents voluntarily share their narratives with their peers. Moderated discussion then ensues, with an appointed moderator who has experience in facilitating such sessions.

An example of a narrative written within these parameters subsequently follows:

There's No Place Like Home

Nisha Patel, MD

Tapping on her ruby slippers three times, Dorothy in *The Wizard of Oz* chants, "There's no place like home." Even in 1939, a young girl from Kansas enlightened movie-going audiences with this special message. For her, as many others, *home* is a place that evokes a feeling of peace and serenity, a sense of comfort and understanding, a sanctuary to be unfettered in one's own skin. For a physiatrist, *home* is a place of function where we conduct our daily activities with potential barriers that could possibly impede one's quality of life.

"Every day is a journey and the journey itself is home." (20)

From my experiences of the home visits I have gone on during my residency, I came to see how these two different definitions of *home* merged. It was not long before I came to realize the importance and necessity of these visits. In October 2009, I conducted a home visit with a previously discharged patient from the acute rehabilitation facility. The patient was a 71-year-old male with T12 paraplegia, which resulted from an epidural steroid injection. Then, in June 2010, I had the opportunity to make a home visit and see a 32-year-old male with T6 paraplegia, which resulted from a fall from scaffolding at work, and whom I initially encountered at an outpatient visit. Lastly, in September 2010, I went on two separate occasions to follow up with a 56-year-old female with incomplete tetraplegia from a skiing accident who had spent a total of six months in various hospitals. In all three cases, I realized the greatest challenge is the transition home because it marks the next phase in their healing process.

Most of us take for granted the ease with which we perform the simplest day-to-day tasks that do not require contemplation or consideration, such as preparing meals or dressing. However, for anyone who has endured an injury, every day can present itself with new obstacles and may require a planned effort to carry out these same tasks. This is prevalent immediately after an acute hospital course, in which going home means adjusting to a new reality. With time and the proper modifications and equipment, he or she can be at *home* again. Therefore, in this field, consideration of a patient's social history, particularly their place of residence, is necessary. In fact, it is even more critical to witness and visualize that patient's home environment firsthand. Therefore, the appropriate recommendations can be made to restore the patient to his or her optimal functional level.

"Home . . . is the place where we tear off that mask of guarded and suspicious coldness which the world forces us to wear in self-defense, and where we pour out the unreserved communications of full and confiding hearts." (21)

Just as important as the physical structure of a home, it is equally vital to address the emotional aspects. Meaningful recovery can be achieved through the hard work and support of family members, home attendants, visiting nurses, and therapists. The three patients I visited were in a period of adjustment and it was evident that their homes became shelters from the world. In discussion with their loved ones, they were having a difficult time maintaining their spirits and adjusting to the changes and new challenges associated with their injuries. It is crucial to meet with their support structure and educate them on appropriate medical issues such as bowel, bladder, and skin care. Also, it is paramount to offer counseling and create a comfortable and encouraging environment. After all, great strides in rehabilitation are achieved through the dedication and efforts of a team working together.

Fast forward to present day and the message is still the same. With the right resources and tools, a physiatrist can play a key role in translating this vision for their patient. So say it with me: "There's no place like home, there's no place like home, THERE'S NO PLACE LIKE HOME." (22)

One can certainly see a variety of lessons, insights, and confidences that this resident gained through her home visits. The use of reflective narrative has reinforced these key learning points including those relating to physical and emotional adaptation to disability, consideration of the importance of a support structure for the disabled individual, and an appreciation of the realities of day-to-day living with such a disability. One can easily imagine that Dr. Patel, who following residency completed a fellowship in Brain Injury Medicine, regularly considers such issues as she plans for her patient's transitions from inpatient rehabilitation with an eye toward a host of critical issues.

Another technique that may be utilized for narrative reflection is the prompted narrative. The prompt may be a phrase, a photograph, a painting, a video, or a piece of music. The prompt is designed to stimulate the learner to write in response to the given prompt based on his or her experiences. The prompt is not disclosed by the moderator ahead of time, and the narrative response is written by all members of the group to the same prompt, for example, a group of Physical Medicine and Rehabilitation (PM&R) residents, immediately after the prompt is given. Time for writing needs to be relatively short to ensure that there is adequate time in the session reserved for sharing of the narratives. In addition, a shorter writing time helps those less inclined to write spontaneously to participate, knowing length is not an expectation. The sharing among peers is often what allows for the transformative action, not just of the person writing the narrative, but for all members of the group. To ensure that this type of narrative medicine session succeeds, there are several parameters that are suggested. First, members of the group need to know that the contents of their shared narratives will remain confidential. The moderator should state this at the outset and the learners should actively pledge to protect confidentiality. Second, the group's membership should be clearly defined. For example, if this activity will include only the PM&R residents, it cannot include medical students who are rotating on and off the service for a brief period of time. Third, sharing must be voluntary and no peer pressure or moderator pressure should be applied to cajole a particular individual to share his or her narrative. As in all group activities, some group members will be more

TABLE 2.1 Steps in Establishing a Narrative Medicine Group

1. Define group membership and identify moderator.
2. Moderator provides didactic information regarding theoretical basis and rationale for use of narrative medicine for this group. Allow for moderated discussion.
3. Supplement didactic information with additional readings identifying benefits of narrative medicine.
4. Establish a schedule and physical setting for group meetings.
5. Lead group members in pledging to maintain confidentiality for material disclosed in group.
6. Identify a method of generating narratives by group participants (e.g., prompted reflection).
7. Limit time for writing to ensure adequate time for sharing of narratives and discussion of shared material.
8. Engage a volunteer from the group to "break the ice" and read, verbatim, their narrative.
9. Allow for moderated discussion among group participants with a goal of identifying important themes, challenges, and conflicts.
10. Attempt to cover multiple narratives during a single session.
11. Consider providing a forum for group participants who did not share their narratives during the completed session to do so (e.g., electronic submission to moderator, and blog).
12. Thank participants, plan next session.

vocal, while others will be more reticent to initially share. Over time, however, when the sanctity of the group is demonstrated, all members will eventually participate. The person who volunteers to read his or her narrative should do so exactly as written, without verbal editing. Once the narrative is read, the moderator elicits feedback from the members of the group that will hopefully lead to impactful discussion, ultimately resulting in, in best cases, truly transformative action.

An excellent example of the power of prompted narrative reflection is subsequently demonstrated Table 2.1. In this case, a group of PM&R residents was asked to write in response to the prompt "Doctor-Centered Care":

On Doctor-Centered Care

Melissa Fleming, MD

"My rotations in the medical ICU were the toughest part of intern year. Days in the unit were always busy, with a long list of tasks and frequent rounds. Interns took call every fourth night, working at least 24 consecutive hours. The intern was often the sole doctor in the unit overnight, as the senior resident and attending were dealing with consults and codes in the rest of the hospital. Having the grave responsibility of caring for critically ill patients only a few months after graduating from medical school was terrifying and required a great deal of focus and attention to detail.

One night, there was an elderly, demented woman in the step down side of the unit. This woman was ready to be transferred to the medical floor and we were just waiting for a bed to open up; she had no pressing medical issues that needed my attention. She was, however, very scared. The unit, with its constant lights and alarms and commotion, is a distressing place for anyone, let alone a frail person with dementia. Although it was the middle of the night and the woman was in a room by herself (a relative luxury in the hospital), she was not sleeping. Instead, she was screaming "help!" repeatedly—it was the only word she used. Various staff members had attempted to calm her and whenever someone went into the room, she would stop yelling. However, as soon as they left and she was alone again, her cries would instantly resume.

Her screams were distracting and upsetting to hear. I finally could not take it anymore and went into her room myself. "What do you want?" I asked impatiently. Trying to tame my frustration, I said, "I'm here now and I can help you. What do you want?" She was silent, looking at me with fearful eyes. I offered to reposition her, or get her a drink or a pillow but she remained silent, just staring at me. I recognized that what she really needed was simple human comfort, someone to hold her hand. But no one on the unit had the time to sit next to her when there were so many other tasks to attend to. After a few moments of her silent staring, I turned around and walked out of the room. Immediately, the loud cries of "help!" started again. I felt helpless. I wanted her out of the unit. Not just because she would have been better off being somewhere quieter, where the lights could be turned off and she could naturally fall asleep, but mostly because I could not listen to her screams anymore. I just needed her to shut up. In retrospect, I should have taken the time to push for a bed for her on the floor. But in that moment, I ordered a one-time dose of Haldol. Within minutes, she was sedated, and most importantly, quiet. Up until that point in my training, I never thought I'd be the kind of doctor to chemically restrain someone like that. It's a decision that has haunted me ever since."

After Dr. Fleming read her narrative, one of her colleagues commented to the group that he wondered how it had come to pass that when notified by the nursing staff that one of his patients is having a potentially acute medical issue, his immediate internal reaction had become "You must be kidding me." This led to a spontaneous discussion about how the residents' experiences during training had subtly evolved into a variety of behaviors that they were not proud of, behaviors that were often lacking in humanity and patient centeredness, behaviors that were very much at odds with ideals that had led them to pursue medicine as a career. Once this realization was verbalized and discussed, this group of residents was able to propose an improvement in their patient centeredness by functioning as a more cohesive team, and aspired to support each other through the demands of residency training, rather than criticizing one another for perceived lapses, such as failure to complete nonurgent items on a sign-out list. This simple one-hour session thus led to the potential for transformative action that Moon (10) identifies as one of the most important benefits of reflective medical practice.

Artwork may be used to prompt reflection in medical practice. An example of a work of art used is presented in Figure 2.1.

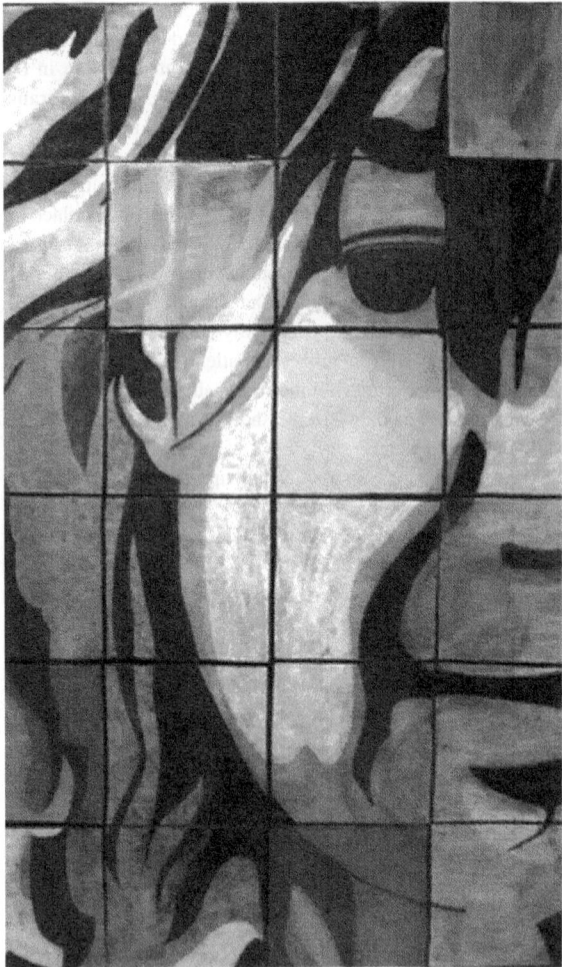

FIGURE 2.1 Self-Portrait by Eliette Markhbein

In this setting, a group of PM&R residents was asked to write in response to the artist's rendering. No other directions were given. One resident, in his first month of PM&R residency, wrote the following over the course of the next 10 minutes:

"Images and feelings of jumbled, jagged, and worry come to mind when I see this contemporary piece before me. I feel the artist is delineating a somber mood with dark pictures, darkened hues and depressive tones. I feel that things are out of place; however, I can't help but feel that each picture in every box is like a phase in one's life, ultimately creating a mosaic of one's life. One interesting aspect of this piece is the touch of warm colors amongst a sea of achromatic pictures, possibly representative of bright moments in what is seemingly dark in its entirety.

As I spend more time looking at this piece, I am reminded of a young patient that I encountered in clinic. She was a woman in her early 20s who suffered a traumatic spinal cord injury from a car accident. Fully independent before this injury, she now requires the care of her mother for some of her activities of daily living and personal care. What really struck me was the pain she was in, not from the injury, but from the difficulty she had with her mother who was caring for her.

Her mother was overbearing, aggressive and anxious; always pushing her daughter to work harder to recover. I remember sensing great tension in the room whenever her mother spoke, but I could also see in the mother's eyes that all she wanted is what is best for her daughter. However, the mother doesn't understand that she is slowly tearing her daughter apart by setting such high expectations for therapy and recovery. Midway through the patient encounter, both parents were asked to leave the room. With her mother gone, our patient was able to share with us how she was suffering to the point where she had thoughts of hurting herself. Her smiles were to ease others around her but inside, she was breaking apart.

Just like in the art piece, our patient was living in a dark, depressive mood where things seem jumbled and broken. However, one warm moment during our conversation was the realization of how much her mother loves her as she has been her advocate since her injury. I was given the opportunity to see how traumatic injury can have a large impact on family dynamics. As difficult as it is for the patient herself to cope with the injury, it can be just as difficult for the people around them."

By Kevin Trinh, MD

The use of this artistic rendering, painted by a woman who had sustained a traumatic brain injury, allowed the young resident to think more deeply about a complicated patient encounter and consider issues of adjustment, dependency, depression, and family dynamics. A discussion ensued about how well these issues had been addressed and whether the treating physicians had adequately advised the young woman. Ultimately, the fact that these issues were simply brought forward and discussed with the patient was taken as a significantly positive step, thus reinforcing the importance of these central themes in physiatric practice.

In conclusion, this overview provides the theoretical principles and framework, as well as practical examples, of how to implement reflective activities into the education of our trainees. The reflective practices we are sharing in this chapter support reflection-*on*-action as described by Schön (2), a four-step thinking-back process for trainees to capture critical moments in their training. This reflection-*on*-action process is very similar to the reflective process applied to our formal educational sessions with trainees (2). Our goal is for a formal narrative medicine program to facilitate the achievement of competence in PBLI as part of residency training.

Future questions connecting reflection to PBLI should address whether or not sharing one's reflections with peers, faculty, or mentors is beneficial to elicit full advantage from this educational strategy and, most important, the mechanism for feedback to the learner and will this feedback move the learner further along in his or her ability to self-assess from prior experiences. Ultimately, we would hope to know that developing the habit of self-reflection in one context (i.e., residency training) tends to transfer readily to maintain the skill/habit in other future contexts over one's career development (6).

Further questions can be asked specific to the connection of the ACGME competency of professionalism to reflective practice as a skill to assess this competency: (a) Will learning through reflection counteract the loss of empathy and compassion that occurs during medical training? (b) Can reflective practice positively influence one's practice of medicine and ultimately impact the quality of patient care? Scholarship that seeks to answer these questions is encouraged.

SELF-EXAMINATION QUESTIONS
(Answers begin on p. 367)

1. Name setting(s) where use of narrative has been useful in medical education.
   A. Patients with chronic illness
   B. Medical student or resident small group learning to reflect on critical incidents
   C. Promotion of interprofessional skills and teamwork
   D. All of the above

2. A narrative prompt
   A. Should be open-ended
   B. Should ask writers only to write about medically related experiences
   C. Should be explained before writers respond
   D. Should have unlimited time for response for maximum effectiveness

3. In responding to a narrative prompt
   A. Writers should explain why they chose what they wrote about
   B. Facilitators should force all group members to read their responses
   C. All group members should exhibit the same courtesy they would want if they themselves are reading their material
   D. Facilitators should determine the best responses at the end of the session

4. Often a poem or a short story can be coupled with a narrative prompt. Which answer is the best?
   A. The poem should be well known to the group
   B. The story should be about a medical encounter
   C. The prose or poetry should be short enough to leave time for responding to the facilitator's prompt
   D. The poem or short story should be read to the group rather than distributed for participants to read

5. Describe how art observation can enhance the "art of observation" of the patient during a clinical examination.

6. What is the difference between reflection and critical reflection?

7. Why does small group sharing (after writing) enhance learning from one's experiences as a clinician?

8. How does reflective practice support self-assessment as a skill set for physicians throughout their practice of medicine?

9. Identify the ultimate goal of a narrative medicine program and discuss how this goal may result from such a program.

ACKNOWLEDGMENTS

The authors gratefully acknowledge the contributions of Nisha Patel, MD, Melissa Fleming, MD, Kevin Trinh, MD, and Eliette Markhbein, who have generously shared their personal reflections to enhance this work. Ms. Samantha Tyler contributed clerical support in the preparation of this manuscript.

REFERENCES

1. Rogers C. Defining reflection: another look at John Dewey on reflective writing. *Teach Coll Rec.* 2006;104:842–866.
2. Schön DA. Teaching artistry through reflection-in-action. In: *Educating the Reflective Practitioner.* San Francisco, CA: Jossey-Bass Publishers; 1987:22–40.
3. Epstein RM, Siegel DJ, Silberman J. Self-monitoring in clinical practice: a challenge for medical educators. *J Contin Educ Health Prof.* 2008;28:5–13.
4. Duffy FD, Holmboe ES. Self-assessment in lifelong learning and improving performance in practice. *JAMA* 2006;296(9):1137–1139.
5. Mann K, Gordon J, MacLeod A. Reflection and reflective practice in health professions education: a systematic review. *Adv Health Sci Educ.* 2009;14:595–621.
6. Eva KW, Regehr G. "I'll never play professional football" and other fallacies of self-assessment. *J Contin Educ Health Prof.* 2008;28(1):14–19.
7. Aronson L. Twelve tips for teaching reflection at all levels of medical education. *Med Teach.* 2011;33:200–201.
8. Wear D, Zarconi J, Garden R, et al. Reflection in/and writing: pedagogy and practice in medical education. *Acad Med.* May 2012;87:603–609.
9. Dewey J. *Democracy and Education.* New York, NY: Free Press; 1944.
10. Moon JA. Reflection in learning and professional development: theory and practice. London: Kogan Page; 1999.
11. Charon R. Our heads touch: telling and listening to stories of self-reflective writing. *Acad Med.* September 2012;87(9):1154–1156.
12. Charon R, Herman N. A sense of story, or why teach reflective writing. *Acad Med.* January 2012;87(1):5–7.
13. Batalden M, Gaufberg E. Two kinds of intelligence. *Acad Med.* 2012;87:1157–1158.
14. Reilly JM, Ring J, Duke L. Visual thinking strategies: a new role for art in medical education. *Fam Med.* 2005;37(4):250–252.
15. Mann KV. Reflection: understanding its influence or practice. *Med Educ.* 2008;42:449–451.
16. Epstein R. Mindful practice in action. *Fam Syst Health.* 2003;21:1–9.
17. Mamede S, Schmidt HG, Riker R. Effects of reflective practice on the accuracy of medical diagnoses. *Med Educ.* 2008;42:468–475.
18. Brady DW, Corbie-Smith G, Branch WT. "What's important to you?" The use of narratives to promote self-reflection and to understand the experiences of medical residents. *Ann Intern Med.* August 2002;137:220–223.
19. Branch WT. Use of critical incident reports in medical education. *J Gen Intern Med.* 2005;20(11):1063–1067.
20. Basho M, and translated by Sam Hamill. *Narrow Road to the Interior and Other Writings.* Boston: Shambhala Publications; 1998.
21. Robertson FW. Sermons by Reverend Frederick W. Robertson: *Narrow Road to the Interior and Other Writings.* 3rd Series. London: Kegan Paul, Trench, Trubner & Co.; 1904.
22. Wolf EA, Fleming V, Baum IF, Ryerson F, Langley N. The Wizard of Oz: Screenplay. Culver City (CA): Metro-Goldwyn-Mayer; 1939.

Susan Eisner

3: Conscious, Compassionate Communication in Rehabilitation Medicine

GOAL

To demonstrate interpersonal and communication skills that result in effective information exchange and collaboration with patients, their families, and other health professionals.

OBJECTIVES

1. Exhibit effective communication with patients, families, other health professional team members, and the public across socioeconomic and cultural backgrounds.
2. Demonstrate how to educate and counsel patients and family members.
3. Demonstrate conscious, compassionate, caring, and respectful behavior.
4. Be more self-aware of their inner beliefs and attitudes regarding communication, and modify those that need to change to enhance their ability to function well independently as well as to be part of a team.
5. Be more personally self-aware of, and in tune with, their personal needs and emotions overall, as well as those of others.

Effective communication in medicine is the foundation upon which positive patient outcomes are built and is the basis for successful relationships between physicians and other team members, patients, families, and others indirectly involved in patient care, such as administrators and related agencies. In fact, it's crucial in *any* relationship, professional or personal. It's so important in medicine that it's mandated by the Accreditation Council of Graduate Medical Education (ACGME) to be one of six core competency areas in residency training.

Unfortunately, many challenges in medicine preclude successful communication—lack of interpersonal skills, stressful working conditions, short appointment times, language barriers, and more (to be discussed in more detail). Poor communication is a main cause of medical errors and can cause disastrous results. The Joint Commission shows that communication (oral, written, electronic, among staff, with/among physicians, with administration, and with patient or family) problems from 2010 to 2012 was the root cause of 68% of reported sentinel events. From 2004 to 2012 it was the root cause of 71% of medication errors. It surpassed other common root causes such as patient assessment and care planning (1).

The goal of this chapter is to promote human connection by teaching communication that is *conscious*—done with forethought and skill. This will be done by identifying the components of communication and describing tools that physiatrists can use to improve their communication skills. Practically speaking, the aim is to connect in many ways: giving information, solving problems, conveying feelings, persuading, alleviating distress, reassuring, and forming and maintaining relationships (2). The ultimate goal is improved health outcomes and safety for patients.

Keep in mind that learning to communicate well, when approached positively, can be viewed as a personal adventure and an exercise in self-growth—with great outcomes. As physicians and others become more aware of their own opinions, emotions, and needs, and get better at expressing these and hearing those of others, relationships improve. The result is greater kindness, tolerance, compassion, and empathy toward oneself and others. Mutual understanding and trust grow. Self-esteem and happiness rise. Professionally, goals, success, and work satisfaction are achieved, and the fulfillment of one's life's purpose—in this case, for physicians to give of themselves and heal others—becomes so much more attainable.

IMPORTANT NOTE TO READERS: If communication skills training or even a mentor doesn't help you change, seek additional help such as therapy and communication skills coaching, especially if job jeopardy exists, due to, for example, anger issues. Old habits die hard. A neutral outside professional can make a significant difference.

CHALLENGES TO EFFECTIVE COMMUNICATION

There are many challenges to achieving good communication, some more obvious than others. This section delineates these and offers possible solutions and suggestions for resolving such challenges.

Communication Skills Are Not Taught Early Enough

Unfortunately, human beings are not born with communication skills manuals. Nor do children typically learn the skills in school. Not until adulthood are people taught how to connect well with others—in chapters like this. Instead we fumble along through life and learn to communicate by default—for better or worse, from society, culture, and role models—parents, teachers, professors—who learned from their own role models—and not always to great effect. These chains can be broken, however, and new skills learned.

Medicine Is a Stressful Profession

Effective communication is a major component of any personal, emotional, and physical wellness program, as great stress occurs when relationships don't go well. The system of medicine itself compounds the problem further.

> Increasing, indeed seemingly endless, demands are being placed on physicians and other health care professionals that do not contribute to a culture of collegiality and effective communication. There are significant, and at times seemingly deliberate, barriers to communication at all levels of patient care. Accordingly, physicians are frequently required to deal with frustrating communication problems. Stress, exhaustion, professional dissatisfaction and even depression are additional impediments to effective communication among colleagues. (3)

Therefore, in addition to learning better communication skills, stress management is also critical. Physicians should do their best, even if done in smaller time snippets, to exercise; rest sufficiently; meditate; eat healthily; use support in friends, family, therapists, and clergy persons; go on vacation; and so on, to increase their resilience, keep calm, and foster communication.

Keeping Up With the Changing Culture in Medicine

Traditional culture in medicine promotes the individual physician as the "in-charge" professional of patient care. It also fosters a strong, distinct hierarchy between levels of professionals starting with doctors, followed by nurses, technicians, secretaries, and so on, and finally by patients and families. The culture is now changing to one of more teamwork, with a physician leader, but where all members are seen as equally vital to the team regardless of status, and collaboration is more the guiding concept. Effective July 1, 2013, the ACGME will make public its new Next Accreditation System, with revised Common Program Requirements. In Section VI.F. on Teamwork, a core requirement, it stresses, "Residents must care for patients in an environment that maximizes effective communication. This must include the opportunity to work as a member of effective interprofessional teams that are appropriate to the delivery of care in the specialty" (4). Good communication within medicine is thus now more important than ever.

A Personal Resistance to Change

Changes in the profession require those in the profession to change. But many people lack insight about themselves, and when made aware of their communication shortcomings, become resistant to change and self-reflection. They may also believe they already communicate well and even that the conflicts they get into are due to the poor communication skills of others. This is often seen in medicine, where, for example, a doctor may blame a nurse, physical therapist, or social worker for the difficult conversations he or she has with them. *A good rule of thumb to remember: "We take ourselves with us wherever we go."* If one finds oneself having communication problems in several relationships, including personal ones, the conclusion should be: "*I must be part of the problem, as I'm the common denominator in all these relationships.*"

Breaking old communication patterns and forming new ones takes work, as well as:

- A strong desire to do so.
- The willingness to become CONSCIOUS of oneself, by becoming self-introspective and self-honest.
- The willingness to closely examine one's own communication skills and style, and how well it works (or doesn't).
- The willingness to seek feedback from others about one's communication style, and seeing this as credible and invaluable input for changing oneself.
- The ability to get past one's own resistance to improving personal communication skills.

Ingrained Beliefs That Impede Change

Another typically overlooked block to personal change is deeply ingrained—often subconscious—attitudes and beliefs, in this case about communication, which may need to be altered. If they don't align with skills being taught, the skills won't "stick," as what's in the subconscious mind will "win out." The following are a few examples:

- Male physicians taught to value all teammates equally and speak to them respectfully may be condescending to female doctors, if they believe women shouldn't be in medicine.
- Doctors taught to speak up and ask direct questions who were taught as children that "children should be seen and not heard," or to not have eye contact with elders, may withhold valid opinions.

Self-Reflective Exercise: Beliefs

To uncover your personal beliefs about communication, try this:

Do this with eyes open, or, privately, close your eyes. Take a few deep breaths. In your mind, go back in time from today, to medical school, college, high school, and so on, to childhood. Say aloud to yourself the beliefs and attitudes you learned or developed on your own about communication: "It's good to ask patients what problems they foresee in doing their treatment plan"; "Yelling at others makes them do what I want"; "My opinions don't matter." Do they work for you? If not, create healthier ones like: "People learn best when spoken to respectfully," and "My opinions do matter and are worth expressing."

Issues That Arise During the Doctor–Patient Visit

Certain factors, some uncontrollable, inhibit communication: too short appointment visits—a tough problem to address—cultural and language differences, unclear accents, and medical jargon. *Pragmatic solutions for these issues include:*

- Facilities should provide cultural sensitivity training to staff.
- For language barriers, patients should have personal or on-staff interpreters.
- Doctors with thick accents can hire communication coaches to help them speak clearly.
- Age-appropriate lay language and printed materials should be used with patients.

Other issues during a visit are anxious or upset patients, or those afraid to ask questions, as "the doctor is always right." In addition, doctors who don't involve patients and families in their care, who have a poor "bedside manner," or who lack empathy create more barriers.

The impact from all these problems on patient care is high. Patients unclear about treatment plans can't follow them. Results are poor resolution of physical symptoms, function, pain control, and physiological measures such as blood pressure, as well as poor emotional health outcomes. Frustration ensues for all. Patients may not return to these physicians and may sully their reputations. And the ultimate injury is lawsuits.

Issues Between Physicians, Colleagues, Nurses, and Other Staff

In Physical and Rehabilitation Medicine, patients' disabilities affect many parts of their lives, making a well-functioning team critical. Physiatrists, nurses, social workers, dieticians, psychologists, occupational and physical therapists, speech therapists, case managers, and the patient and family are all involved (5).

Often team members won't speak up, especially in risky, controversial, and emotional conversations. The one thing skilled people do is find a way to get all relevant information from themselves and others out into the open. "At the core of every successful conversation lies the free flow of relevant information. People openly and honestly express their opinions, share their feelings, and articulate their theories. They willingly and capably share their views, even when their ideas are controversial or unpopular" (6).

Team communication can fail on many levels. Many physicians won't confront and resolve concerns with each other. When peers fail to—or are incompetent to—do their share, for example, resentments build up. Doctors may stay silent and allow resentments to simmer for years, thinking they're avoiding stress by avoiding these conversations—when in fact they're magnifying it. In fact, doctors who more quickly and effectively confront performance problems with peers experience improved quality of work life and relationships (7).

Conflicts also exist between professions; these are commonly seen between doctors and nurses. Medical culture also fosters those of higher status to poorly treat those below. Rebelling ensues. A nurse who cowered from a screaming doctor now yells back. Worse, he or she may watch that physician commit a grave patient error and say nothing out of fear or revenge—a passive–aggressive move, clearly not for the good of the patient. In addition, patients who see staff argue may lose confidence in their providers or facility, and leave.

Change can occur. A hospital's pilot program to build physician–nurse leadership partnerships led to breakthrough improvements in patient safety and quality, and forged better physician–nurse collaboration and job satisfaction, after which they came to appreciate each other's pressures and challenges (8).

Electronic Communication Erodes Connection

Texts and e-mails are eliminating in-person conversations. Daniel Moore, MD, PMR Chairman at the Brody School of Medicine, says, "Electronic media is king. The tweet, text, email, twitter, and Facebook page are all popular with billions of dollars being consumed. But, face to face communication is still the ultimate way to communicate. Electronic communication is efficient, but often the reader inserts their own context and emotion into the message" (9). Feelings can get hurt. Emotional e-mails or texts should be avoided, and discussion of those issues should occur by phone or in person where tone and body language are clearer. Many people purposely use electronic means to avoid confrontation. Avoid this—it creates more problems than it solves. Also avoid texting and phone use in meetings. It signals no interest in the group, and is disrespectful to the speaker and attendees.

COMPONENTS OF COMMUNICATION: INTRODUCTION

There are various components of communication that will be discussed in the following four sections. Part I includes basic ground rules, attitudes, and beliefs that maximize the effectiveness of communication. Part II covers concepts that are "internal" and not necessarily consciously thought about such as emotions, needs, and empathy, or behaviors that are more "ingrained" or based on personality, such as communication styles and preferences. Part III addresses practical areas in which behaviors are obvious to others and can be changed by the learning of new skills. These are body language, listening, and speaking. Here, examples will be given that apply to communication with colleagues, patients, and families. Part IV offers additional skills to be used specifically with patients.

COMPONENTS OF COMMUNICATION—PART I: GROUND RULES

> **Ground Rules, Attitudes, and Beliefs—When Communicating With *Anyone***
>
> - It starts from the top down. Leadership must communicate well and act as role models.
> - *YOU TAKE YOURSELF WITH YOU WHEREVER YOU GO.*
> - Know yourself and work on yourself.

(continued)

- ALWAYS look within yourself for *your* part in any conflict, and verbally own it. It takes two to tango.
- You are ALWAYS responsible for your own behavior.
- Respect for self and for others is critical.
- Honesty and transparency are key.
- All members of the team are equally important.
- Learn to empathize and put yourself in someone else's shoes.
- Conflict is good when handled well, as it promotes learning and change.
- Avoid "triangulation," or putting a third party in the middle of your conflict.
- Don't assume negative motives behind people's behavior. Give them the benefit of the doubt.
- Deal directly if at all possible, and quickly, with those with whom you have an issue.
- Apologize when you are wrong, and gracefully accept apologies from others.

Additional Ground Rules, Attitudes, and Beliefs—When Communicating With *Patients and Families*

- Patients, and families, are the center of the patient care team.
- Many of today's patients are better informed about health care matters (due to the Internet).
- Patients deserve clear information about their symptoms, tests, diagnosis, treatment plan, prognosis, ans so on.
- Patients and their designated family members should be involved in decisions regarding treatment plans.
- Patients should be encouraged to participate, ask questions, and speak up.

COMPONENTS OF COMMUNICATION—PART II: EMOTIONS, NEEDS, EMPATHY, COMMUNICATION STYLES, AND COMMUNICATION PREFERENCES

Emotions

Emotions are the life blood of human existence. They let us feel fully alive. On a continuum, they go from expansive and freeing (e.g., joy, love, and bliss) to constricting (e.g., sadness, fear, and anger). Humans can feel a full range of emotions, and doing so greatly enhances their lives.

Emotions are simply expressed with the words "I feel" plus an emotion: "I feel sad," "I feel angry," "I feel elated." This may seem ridiculously obvious, but it's one of the hardest things to do—to feel and identify a specific emotion felt in a given moment, and to say it simply without superfluous words.

NOTE: People often start sentences with "I feel..." but in fact are not expressing emotions. "I feel that doctors and nurses should collaborate more" is an opinion. "I feel frustrated that doctors and nurses don't collaborate more" expresses an emotion. This is an important distinction.

It's best to fully feel emotions—when done, they come and pass. But often, due to past painful experiences and wanting to avoid that pain and vulnerability again, people deaden their feelings—with compulsive behaviors like drinking or overeating, busyness, or intellectualizing emotions. This just buries the feelings, which have an uncanny way of surfacing sideways later—in illness, anger outbursts, and self-destruction.

Understandable to a degree, medical schools promote suppressing emotions. Emotional attachment to patients is undesirable, and emotions are inconvenient if a patient dies but there's no time to cry. But those emotions won't just disappear, and should be expressed at some point soon after. Physicians might thus "retrain" themselves to feel their feelings, and "compartmentalize" them, or feel and express them when appropriate. So if a patient dies, having dinner with a friend that evening and discussing it and crying is much better than, say, getting drunk. Getting it out of one's body is a *much* healthier alternative.

Remember, good communication necessitates one to feel and express emotions. Compassion for patients, others, and oneself also requires being able to feel. Yes, doctors may not want to "fall apart" in front of patients. But they can do it behind closed doors, or away from work. This will do wonders to maintain their humanity, a major push in medicine today. It will also enhance their personal relationships, because numbing out in medicine will spill over into nonprofessional relationships and cause problems there.

Self-Reflective Exercise: Emotions

To feel your emotions—and we typically feel several at once or in succession, often opposing—try this:

1. In the midst of any situation, quietly take a few deep breaths, and ask, "How do I feel right now?" Try to identify several emotions (disappointed, scared). Let yourself feel each of them fully till they pass.
2. Or later, after a situation, close your eyes if you can, take a few deep breaths, and re-envision the situation in your mind. Ask yourself, "What emotions did I feel then?" Try to let yourself feel these.
3. When anticipating an upcoming difficult situation, sit quietly and take a few deep breaths. Envision the situation in your mind and how it may go. Ask yourself, "What emotions do I feel now as I anticipate this situation?" Fear or dread may arise, but with practice of that situation, calmness and ease may also arise.

Needs

Humans have different levels of needs. Basic needs, for example, are food, clothing, and shelter. Higher-level needs are for time off from work, time with family, good health, and so on. Even deeper needs are to be heard, loved, respected, or connected to others (10). A problem is that many people don't know their own needs, though they know the needs of others, especially if they're caretakers like doctors or nurses.

"People pleasers" are also acutely aware of others' needs. As this term implies, they have a strong desire to meet those needs and please others, often to their own detriment, because in the process they put their own needs aside, if they're even aware of them at all. This is an ineffective attempt to raise their own self-esteem and feel better about themselves by making others feel happy with them. So clearly it is very important to become aware of and express one's needs, or they may not get met.

> **Self-Reflective Exercise: Needs**
>
> *To become more aware of your needs and those of others:* Do this with eyes open, or privately, close your eyes. Take a few deep breaths. Ask yourself:
>
> 1. "What needs do I have?" Then scan through your life and ask, "Are my needs being met?" Identify where they are and aren't. Ask, "What emotions arise as I think about this?"
> 2. "What needs do I or do I not meet in others—patients, colleagues, family, friends? Why or why not?" Discuss your answers to these questions with others. Then try to adjust your life so your needs get met and you meet those of others. This can be difficult to do. If you're really stuck, consider a therapist or mentor.

Empathy

Empathy is listening with one's heart. It's "the power of understanding and imaginatively entering into another person's feelings" (11). It's critical in communication, especially for physicians and professionals who deal with patients. It goes beyond compassion, letting one put oneself into another's shoes to sense his or her emotions and needs. Empathy also helps people genuinely connect with the human race, and gets people out of themselves. Because it lets one separate from the other, it allows one to also stay aware of one's own emotions and needs as well as those of others, even in situations that are difficult to handle.

An example of this is an empathetic physician who sees an emotional patient, and realizes he or she simply needs to be heard and reassured. If the doctor feels overwhelmed, as he or she focuses on the patient's needs, he or she will become calmer and listen vs. telling the patient to calm down. The more empathy is practiced, the more rational and caring "responses" one will have vs. knee-jerk "reactions" that may worsen the situation.

> **Self-Reflective Exercise: Empathy**
>
> *To practice empathy, try this:*
>   Do this quietly with eyes open, or close your eyes. Take a few deep breaths. Think of someone you feel tense with or with whom you had a conflict. Imagine literally standing in their shoes. Become them. If you feel safe, step inside their body. Be still and tune into them—to what they feel or experience in life in general, or specifically in the conflict you had. What emotions are they feeling? See if you can feel them too. What are their thoughts and needs? What is their life like for them? Then ask, "What emotions do I feel being them or being in them?" Any compassion? If you're angry at them, see it from their angle.

Communication Styles

There are basic communication styles that people use, each implying a certain level of underlying self-esteem. They tend to be more "automatic" than "chosen" ways of communicating. While no one always uses only one style, most people can categorize themselves as primarily being one of the following:

Passive—Passive people are quieter and don't say much, though they may if asked, and have lower self-esteem. They may be "people pleasers" who avoid rocking the boat. They may not think highly of themselves or of what they have to say, or that it will matter. Others' opinions matter more. They may not want to bother others. But quietness isn't always from passivity. It could be a person who has good self-esteem who won't speak up in that moment, or whose culture fosters not speaking up to elders, but whose self-esteem is fine.

Aggressive—Aggressive people are some combination of loud, pushy, angry, a bully, domineering, demanding, threatening, condescending, uses foul language, ans so on. They may not listen well. They engender fear and dislike. Contrary to popular belief, their self-esteem is low, not high. They may really dislike themselves, and use aggression to cover this up and to compensate for their low self-esteem.

Passive-Aggressive—Passive-aggressive people have low self-esteem, and express their anger through vengeful behaviors rather than directly stating their anger. This typically occurs unexpectedly, making it particularly virulent. For example, they may act pleasantly toward someone in person, but then get back at the person by not relaying an important message out of anger. Or they might agree to be on a committee but dislike the chairman, and then not attend the meetings. Passive-aggressive people also use sarcasm—a nasty mix of humor and anger that can be very hurtful.

Assertive—Assertive people speak up and are clear, direct, and to the point. They listen well. People often confuse assertiveness and aggressiveness. Assertive people "assert" themselves and pull no punches, but aren't pushy. They have high self-esteem. They value what they feel and say—and value what others feel and say. They set boundaries. Though some find it intimidating, assertiveness is the style to strive for.

> **Self-Reflective Exercise: Determining My Communication Style**
>
> *Ask yourself these questions:*
>   "Which of the above communication styles fit you most closely most of the time?"
>   "Regarding my style, what aspects about how I communicate do I already know I'd like to improve?" "What do I think about the importance of my questions, feelings, needs, and opinions?"
>   "How do I come across to others, and how do they experience me?" "How well do I listen to others?"

(continued)

> "How do I typically respond to others' requests of me—with a yes or no?" "Have I ever been told I'm unapproachable?"
>
> "Do people like and respect me? Why or why not?" "Do people trust me? Why or why not?"
>
> "What feedback have others given me about how I communicate?"
>
> Then ask a few people in your professional and personal life who'll be honest with you to spend 30 to 60 minutes or lunch with you. Say you need their help—you want to improve your communication skills, and want their honest feedback about how they experience you or how they've observed you with others. Use the above questions as is, or personalize them: "How well do I listen to you?" Reassure them you'll never use this against them. And you'll keep their name confidential if they so desire. Then thank them profusely!

Communication Preferences

People also have preferred ways of communicating, and one aspect of this is how they prefer to give and receive information. One might see generalizations of this with certain specialties of physicians, or simply among individuals in various specialties. It is helpful to learn about how one's "audience" prefers to share information, and to calibrate a message to that person's or group's preferences. Those preferences may reflect personality traits of a physician, how they best learn, who they were trained by, how much time they have or typically allot for conversations, and so on.

To learn the preferences of colleagues, physicians can observe them as they work—at rounds, meetings, when leading a seminar, and so on, or when interacting with themselves or with others, such as a nurse or a family member. Physicians can also ask their colleagues directly what type of information they want at various times and in what format; then, after giving them the information, they can ask for feedback as to whether they gave what the colleague needed.

Some physicians, especially when faced with challenging cases, use a "group thinking" approach and prefer to seek opinions and input from other doctors they trust while making decisions. They have colleagues they've worked with over the years, in the same specialty or not, with whom they regularly cross-consult. Others may exhibit a more independent approach to their work.

Personality may motivate some physicians to go through conversations slowly, while others exchange information and get to the point quickly. The amount and type of information shared also varies among physicians. Some are detail oriented and want specific facts about a case. Others may be more bigger-picture oriented and prefer a general synopsis. Some may want only current medical facts, whereas others want to know the context and circumstances behind a situation as well. Some physicians want to know the social aspects of a patient—how involved family members are and if they function well together. Others focus on a patient's personal emotional situation when looking at the causes of their illness or injury. Teaching and training styles may also reflect a more lecture-type style when information is more likely to be given, or a more interactive approach where trainees are expected to provide much of the information.

COMPONENTS OF COMMUNICATION—PART III: BODY LANGUAGE, LISTENING, AND SPEAKING

Body Language

Body language can speak volumes without a word being said, and is an important aspect of communication. During communication, how people act, how they express emotion, how close they stand to each other, the tone of their voice, where they focus their gaze, how relaxed or tense they are, how well they speak and listen, and other things they do all reflect their cultural norms, how interested they are, how connected they feel, how well they handle conflicts, how comfortable or confident they feel, and much more.

Body language incongruent with other aspects of communication can also be revealing. Someone avoiding eye contact may be withholding information or lying. A big smile but a lack of warmth and distancing demeanor may indicate that a person looks happy but isn't and won't say why. An angry person may cross his or her arms and look defensive but when asked about this, he or she may say, "No, I'm not mad!" Astute listeners and observers pick up on these miscues. It's important that body language matches how one speaks and listens.

> ### Body Language
>
> *Examples of Body Language*
>
> - Eye contact.
> - Providing undivided attention to someone, or not—by doing something else while he or she is talking to you.
> - Facial expressions and gestures.
> - Physical stance and position: arms crossed, hands in pockets, pointing an accusing finger, hands on hips.
> - Distance or closeness to another: being in someone's personal space.
> - Vocal sounds like "Hmmm" or "Uh huh."
> - Voice volume, voice clarity, voice pace.
> - Voice tone: angry, soothing, forceful.
> - Touch: doing a physical examination, treating a patient, shaking hands, touching someone's shoulder, hugs, sex.
>
> *How to's on Body Language—With Colleagues and Others*
>
> - Make eye contact with a person, but avoid staring or looking at the person too intensely. In the United States, eye contact is respectful, and fosters a feeling of connection.
> - Indicate you're listening with "Uh huh," "I hear you," and nodding your head up and down.
> - Avoid multitasking and give your undivided attention in conversations, in person, or by phone. Stop what you're doing and look at the person. Writing chart notes or being online makes you not fully present.

(continued)

> - Smile. You'll relax, and so will those around you.
> - Use "open" body language to show interest in what someone is telling you. Keep your arms at rest at your side or in your lap vs. crossed on your chest, which could indicate emotional distance or even anger.
> - Keep a comfortable distance from people. Avoid getting "in their face" or being too close in their space.
> - Use a normal voice volume. You can express anger without yelling. Softness makes people strain to hear you.
> - Speak clearly, at a normal speed vs. mumbling or racing. Slowness makes others wait with baited breath.
> - Be conscious of your tone of voice. If strong emotions arise, express them calmly, not nastily.
> - Shaking a patient's hand, a hug to a colleague you haven't seen for weeks, and a caring touch on a shoulder are generally acceptable touch. Much more than that can feel inappropriate. Avoid touch below the waist. If you want to see someone's earrings, ask her if it's OK to touch them. Some people are very sensitive due to bad past experiences of inappropriate touch. Of course, sex with patients should always be avoided.
>
> **Additional How to's on Body Language—With Patients and Families**
>
> - Introduce yourself immediately when meeting a new patient or family members.
> - Smile when meeting new or established patients or families.
> - When simply talking to patients vs. examining or treating them, and when speaking with families, be on a similar eye level to not intimidate them. If they're sitting on a chair, sit on a chair as well.
> - During patient examinations and treatment, tell him what you're about to do and how you'll touch him. Ask if it's OK. Be very respectful with sexual body parts. And warn him if you'll cause pain or discomfort.
> - Consider using a chaperone when alone with female patients.
> - If you're in a teaching facility and want medical students present with a patient, get the patient's permission.

Listening

Listening is a critical part of communicating—and quite difficult to do well. Many people see themselves as good listeners, but aren't. How well do you listen? Being heard is one of the most basic and strongest of human needs. In medicine, listening takes on a whole other dimension. If not done well, it can kill someone.

Reflective or Active Listening and Open-Ended Questions

A powerful listening skill is reflective or active listening. It's paraphrasing back to someone what he or she just said, though not verbatim, including his or her content, emotions and needs (even if these weren't exactly stated). Why do this sometimes awkward strategy? It makes the person really feel heard.

The key features of active listening are as follows:

- Gathering and retaining the information correctly.
- Understanding the implications for the patient of what is being said.
- Responding to verbal and nonverbal signals and cues.
- Demonstrating that you are paying attention and trying to understand (12).

This technique uses phrases along the lines of "*What I hear you saying is…,*" "*Did I get that right?*" or "Is that correct?" For example, Parker is a patient upset about his broken leg. He's yelling and crying. "How will I manage with this big cast on my leg? I'm old, I live alone—how will I eat? Who'll feed my cat?" First, let him cry and be silent. Then say: "Mr. Parker, *I hear* how scared you are about your self-care, and you're worried about your cat. Is that right?" Mr. Parker responds, "Yeah, doc, I guess I'm really scared." You answer, "We'll find ways to ensure you won't be alone and that you'll both be cared for as your leg heals."

A good question when making a suggestion is, "*Does that work for you?*" For example, you ask Nurse Mary to tell a patient's family how to assist with home care. She says, "Are you kidding? They're very hard to talk to." You *don't* say, "Well Mary, it's your job, deal with it." You say, "*I hear* how hard it is to work with them. Just do your best," or "I'll tell the social worker you'll call her when they arrive, and to go assist you. *Would that work for you?*" She says, "Yes, thanks, that's a good idea."

Other useful phrases when giving instructions to patients or others are, "*Let me see if I got this right…*" or "Did I get that right?" It can be particularly useful during handoffs, a time when there's an increased chance of errors. For example, an outgoing resident explains to the incoming resident what a patient needs during the next shift. He says, "Mrs. Bradley needs to have her pain medication dose lowered from 30 mg every 4 hours to 20 mg every 4 hours, and you'll have to speak to the physical therapist to see when they want to schedule her first session for rehab. You also need to call her husband on his lunch break between noon and 1 p.m. if you can, because he has lots of questions about her care. OK?" You say, "So let me see if I got this right—I need to call PT and get her scheduled, to call her husband between 12 and 1 pm, and to change the dose to 20 mg, though the q 4 hours stays the same. Yes?" The resident responds, "You got it!"

Active listening also means focusing on the speaker, eliciting more information/emotions/needs, and encouraging others to talk. To do this, ask *open-ended questions* that require sentences in response, vs. *closed-ended questions* that seek one word. Ask "*What things trigger the pain*" vs. "Does it hurt when you walk?" Or ask a nurse "In what ways has the patient improved?" vs. "Is she getting better?" And ask "*What questions do you have?*" vs. "Do you have any questions?" after an explanation. Additional phrases to use to encourage speakers to share more are, "I understand, please continue…," "Go on…," and "Tell me more about…."

Verbal Read-Back Procedures

Another very effective feedback strategy is the "verbal read back" used to ensure accuracy of verbal orders, especially for medications. Giving medication orders verbally or over the phone increases the risk of patient medication errors. With read-back procedures, the person receiving an order writes it down, reads it back, and gets confirmation that it was understood correctly.

"Verbal orders—those that are spoken aloud in person or by telephone—offer more room for error than orders that are written or sent electronically. Interpreting speech is inherently problematic because of different accents, dialects, and pronunciations. Background noise, interruptions, and unfamiliar drug names and terminology often compound the problem. Once received, a verbal order must be transcribed as a written order, which adds complexity and risk to the ordering process. The only real record of a verbal order is in the memories of those involved (13)."

"When the recipient records a verbal order, the prescriber assumes that the recipient understood correctly. No one except the prescriber, however, can verify that the recipient heard the message correctly. If a nurse receives a verbal order and subsequently calls it to the pharmacy, there is even more room for error. The pharmacist must rely on the accuracy of the nurse's written transcription of the order and the pronunciation when it is read to the pharmacist. Sound-alike drug names also affect the accuracy of verbal orders (13)." In addition, numbers can easily be misheard, and medication errors can also occur when a patient's laboratory values are verbally communicated and misheard by the recipient, because incorrect doses are then given to fix the misheard value (13).

Some strategies to enhance the read-back procedure are as follows:

"Limiting verbal communication of prescription or medication orders to urgent situations in which immediate written or electronic communication is not feasible. For example, verbal orders can be disallowed when the prescriber is present and the patient's chart is available. Verbal orders can be restricted to situations where it is difficult or impossible for hard copy or electronic order transmission, such as during a sterile procedure" (14).

"For prescribers, enunciating verbal orders clearly. For order recipients, it means writing down the complete order or entering it into a computer, reading it back, and receiving confirmation from the individual who gave the order. As an extra check, either the prescriber or the listener can spell unfamiliar drug names, using "D as in David," "B as in Bravo," and so forth. Pronouncing each numerical digit separately can also help avoid confusion—saying, for example, "one six" instead of "sixteen," which is often heard as "sixty" " (14).

"Dysfunctional" Listening Behaviors and Their "Functional" Solutions

The following are some things that make someone a poor listener, and strategies to overcome them:

- *Getting distracted*: Avoid multitasking when someone is speaking to you, even on the phone.
- *Being preoccupied*: If something else is on your mind but you have to listen, force yourself. If it can wait, honestly say you're preoccupied and ask if you can speak later.
- *Planning a response*: Rather than waiting to jump in and respond, just listen—you'll get your turn.
- *Tuning others out*: If you can't handle someone's honesty or the subject matter is too "close to home," say that: "You may have a valid point, but I can't hear it right now. Can we discuss this later?"
- *Getting defensive*: If you get negative feedback about yourself, or if it's said angrily, listen to the words, not the tone. Those who know us best usually see us accurately.
- *Deflecting*: If confronted and you disagree, try "I need time to think about what you've said" vs. deflecting the comments with "No, you're the problem" or "You don't know what you're talking about."
- *Feeling attacked, criticized, blamed, or shamed*: Honestly say, "I'm feeling attacked (blamed, etc.) and I don't want to attack back. Can we tone this down or speak later?"
- *Invalidating others*: Some comments, perhaps well meaning, minimize or invalidate others' feelings. People feel what they feel whether others think they should or not. Instead, acknowledge others:
  - Say: "I hear how (angry, sad, scared, etc.) you are" vs. "You shouldn't feel that way."
  - Say: "I hear how uncomfortable you are" vs. "It's not that bad—get over it."
  - Say: "I really validate how you feel. And remember, you're not alone—others feel that way too" vs. "You're not the only person who ever felt that way."
- *Cutting people off*: Let people finish speaking vs. finishing their sentences or interrupting. To a wordy person say, "I'd like to respond to what you're saying."
- *Judging*: Stay open minded to another's viewpoint vs. judging what the person has to say.
- *Giving unsolicited advice*: Unless your role is to treat/advise, and someone tells you his or her problem, avoid jumping in to "fix" it. Ask the person if he or she wants your advice. If not, just listen.
- *Analyzing*: Sometimes people "stay up in their heads" when listening, remaining emotionally detached and analytical. Instead, feel the emotions you're having and share those, or how you relate to what is said.
- *Refusing to respond out of anger*: If you're enraged and unilaterally end a conversation—you walk away or yell out "This conversation is over!" or you give the "silent treatment" and don't respond for days or even years—realize these are controlling, manipulative, destructive behaviors. Instead, say, "I'm angry now and I need to walk away so I don't say anything I'll regret. Let's pick this up tomorrow, OK?"

(continued)

Speaking

Courtesy

A very obvious but underused strategy is common courtesy. "Please," "Thank you," or "Excuse me" are often omitted, especially in crises. Those who demand vs. request things, and don't offer thanks elicit a desire to not cooperate. Try, "Please find me when the Medical Director calls," "Thanks for handling that family so well," and "Thanks for coming for your visit." Remember, patients can go elsewhere.

Praise

Praise also greatly improves morale, motivation, and relationships. Include positive results of the new behavior. A chairman may say to his secretary: "Thanks for no longer being late and arriving on time. The office now runs more smoothly." A physiatrist might tell a patient who wouldn't do at-home physical therapy exercises but now does: "It's great you're doing your exercises at home. You'll be able to walk much sooner because of your effort."

Additional tips on offering praise are as follows:

- Do it as soon as possible: Timing is important. Don't delay praise.
- Be as sincere as possible, or your words will seem hollow.
- Be specific regarding details of the achievement.
- Offer the praise in person, face to face, whenever possible.
- Stay positive—don't undercut praise with a concluding note of criticism.

"I" Statements

"I" statements, vs. "You" statements, are critical in effective communication. Typical ones are as listed:

- "I feel_____" (a one-word emotion: confident, excited)
- "I need_____" (a need: to be given clear information about my condition, to be treated with respect)
- "I'd like, want_____" (a desire: my doctor to spend more time with me, a week off next month for vacation)
- "I think_____" (a thought, opinion: my physical therapist is very skilled, the secretary is incompetent)

"I" statements keep people focused on themselves and their emotions vs. blaming another's behavior. They prevent defensiveness in the listener and create vulnerability in the speaker. But they're hard to remember to use, especially in conflicts, where the urge is to blame. Feel the energy difference in the following:

- "I'm not being heard" vs. "You're not listening to me."
- "I'm uncomfortable with how you're speaking to me" vs. "You don't know how to talk to people."
- "I feel unappreciated." vs. "You never say thank you."
- "I'm concerned about problems with your work." vs. "You're incompetent."
- "I feel angry" vs. "You make me angry."

NOTE: The phrase "You make me angry" makes another responsible for one's feelings. But people don't make others feel a certain way (though they can push their buttons)—they're responsible for their own feelings. People's emotions are often due more to their history and personality than a current situation. And different people react differently to the same circumstance. For example, a chairman might say to three residents, "I need to talk to you about something regarding your patient." A sensitive resident feels scared of being fired. An angry resident gets mad that the chairman dares to question his competence. An open-minded resident feels confident, knows there may or may not be a problem, and is open to praise or constructive criticism.

Catch Phrases to Help Resolve Conflicts

Discussing and resolving conflicts makes many people uncomfortable. It can be helpful to use certain phrases that signal a desire to work out the issue, and interest in the other person's point of view:

Useful Catch Phrases

When anticipating an awkward or difficult conversation, ask for time to talk with phrases like:

- "Do you have a minute? I'd like to talk to you about something...."
- "Can we pick a time later today to talk about what happened between us this morning?"

To signal your desire for you both to work it out together, try:

- "Can we talk about how we can both resolve this?"
- "Our getting along is important to me—would you agree? Can we find a mutually satisfying solution?"

To signal your willingness to see your side of the problem and to work on it, say these powerful words:

- "Help me to understand this from your point of view."
- "What am I doing that upsets you?"
- "How can I do that differently so it will work for you?"

DESC Communication Model

DESC, a simple communication model using "I" statements created by Sharon Cox, RN, MSN, CNAA (15), is frequently used in medical and other industries to help resolve conflicts and to facilitate expression of emotions and needs in a way that is easy to hear. It should be practiced often, following the basic format, though not necessarily verbatim.

NOTE: In a conversation, any of the four DESC components can also be used alone, or less than four can be used. Each component is an excellent way to express that particular concept. DESC stands for:

Describe Situation: "When you_____." (describe a situation)
Explain Impact: "I feel_____." (an emotion) and/or: "The impact on me is_____." (describe effects)

***State* Needs/Wants**: "I need/am asking you to ____. Can you do that? Does that work for you?"
Consequences: *Use if necessary*: "If this doesn't change, I'll have to ____" or "The results will be ____" (16).

Some prefer to memorize the key words in this model for a structure to follow, and it's easy to remember:

D When you...
E I feel/felt ... and the impact on me was...
S I want/need...
C If not, I'll...

The DESC model can also be varied:

- After *D*escribing and *E*xplaining, ask: "Can you tell me why that happened?"
- After *D*escribing and *E*xplaining the effects and *S*tating your need, ask: "Can you tell me how you feel about what I'm saying?"

Here are some examples:

A nurse keeps texting or beeping a resident who doesn't respond. He asks to speak privately with her later:

D—"Nancy, I had a patient emergency. When you text or beep me 3 times in 15 minutes,
E—I feel frustrated and rushed to finish what I'm doing and it distracts me.
S—If you have something important and I don't respond after say two attempts to reach me, assume I can't get back to you. Please call the secretary or a nurse on the unit and ask them to relay your message to me or if necessary, call the chief resident and let her take care of the problem. Would that work for you?" If Nancy finds this acceptable, she'd say: "OK, fine, I'll try that. If it doesn't work I'll let you know." And you say, "Great, let's see how that goes, thanks." And the conversation ends. If Nancy refuses to call someone else, has no other solution, and insists you respond immediately, you say:
C—"Since you're not willing to try this, I'll bring this up to my Residency Program Director. Maybe she can discuss it with your Nursing Director and they can help solve this problem."

A patient with a broken ankle hasn't elevated her leg at home and the swelling is not going down. You say:

D—"Miss Batista, when you don't elevate your leg throughout the day at home as I've asked you to,
E—I feel concerned about your healing. Can you tell me why this is happening?"
She says, "I can't lift it up myself. My husband is angry that I had this accident so he won't help me."
S—"I see. Well, I need for you and your husband to work this out because he's your only caretaker. How about I have the social worker call him and set up an appointment for the two of you to see her tomorrow? It would be good for him to also talk about how he's feeling. Would that be OK with you?
C—Because if the leg is not elevated it will take longer to heal and you'll be in more pain."
She agrees, and the appointment with the social worker is scheduled.

A patient needs a painkiller and wants you to prescribe an opioid medication. You're reluctant to do this out of concern for his safety given his aberrant and unsafe use with this type of medication in the past. You say:

D—"Mr. James, from our conversations, I understand you'd like me to prescribe oxycodone for your pain.
E—I feel reluctant to do this and concerned for your health and safety since in the past you were not able to take it as prescribed. As we have discussed in the past, this type of medication can have significant negative effects on your health if not taken appropriately.
S—I need to treat you with a drug that lessens your pain, but doesn't pose a risk to your health. I suggest you try this other medication instead. Call me if it doesn't stop or reduce the pain. We can then discuss another option. OK?"
If Mr. James agrees, he'd say: "OK. I don't know if it will work, but I'll try it." You say, "OK, keep me posted." If not and he says, "I'd really prefer the oxycodone," you say:
C—"Yes, I hear you, but I don't think that's in your best interest. I'm sorry, I can't prescribe that. If you prefer, I can refer you to another of my colleagues for another opinion."

NOTE: The wording used in the DESC model is important. A related model, NonViolent Communication by Marshall Rosenberg, offers guidance. It consists of 4 similar components to DESC: observations, feelings, needs, and requests. Rosenberg suggests first, when "describing," to use observational, neutral phrases without judgment or evaluation, consisting of concrete things and actions. Simply say what people are doing. Avoid using inflammatory words. Neutrally say, "When you spoke loudly," not "When you screamed like a banshee." Second, state the behavior's impact on you, and how you feel when observing this action: hurt, angry, disappointed, and so on. This helps others be compassionate and change behaviors. Third, express needs connected to the feelings. And fourth, make clear, specific requests, or actions that can be done in the present moment. This is how to cooperatively and creatively ensure everyone's needs are met (17).

Giving Constructive Feedback

Another conversation people dread is telling others about their errors. These are important conversations, though, and when done well are important teaching moments that can forge a bond between the individuals and can ensure the errors don't continue. It's helpful to think of it this way: "Be tough on the problem and easy on the person." The person is not bad, or stupid. He or she just made a *mistake—something everyone does*. Again, make neutral comments about the *behavior*. Don't judge the person's *character*. "What's wrong with you? I can't believe you made that mistake, AGAIN. Just where did you go to medical school?" is not the best option. Use the DESC model instead:

A nurse tells Dr. Jones that Resident Angela ordered a wrong medication for a patient and then went home. **Opening sentence**

by Dr. Jones: Hi Angela. Got a minute? I'd like to discuss something with you privately. Angela: Sure, what is it?

D—Dr. Jones: Nurse Bonnie told me you wrote a prescription for penicillin for Mr. Morris. He's allergic to this. Bonnie realized it before she gave it to him and no harm was done. Are you aware this happened? Angela: No. She hasn't said anything to me today.

E—Dr. Jones: When I heard this, I was quite concerned for both the patient and about your judgment. Can you tell me why this happened?
Angela: I must not have checked the chart for meds allergies. I've been very fatigued as well. I'm so sorry.

S—Dr. Jones: I need for you to be very accurate when you give meds, obviously. Be sure to check the chart first. To address the reasons for your fatigue we'll set up a time to meet to look at your schedule and discuss strategies to minimize them. OK?
Angela: Yes, of course. I'll stay on my toes, Dr. Jones. I'm glad nothing happened to the patient.

C—Great. I do need you to know that if this occurs again, I'll need to write it up officially. Always check with me if you have any questions about anything. Mistakes happen, but we need to be vigilant and prevent them.
Angela: Yes, OK, I understand. I'll do my best.

Sometimes those who give feedback avoid these conversations due to their own discomfort. They may feel guilty, afraid of causing upset, or don't want to be the "bad guy." This can spiral down into a tragic situation. For example, a residency program director who has consistently avoided addressing a resident's errors may allow this less-than-competent resident to graduate because he or she doesn't want to be the person who negatively impacts the resident's career. While giving such feedback can be difficult, it is clearly that physician's responsibility to take this role seriously and engage in these discussions. Again, it's helpful to take a more objective view: "*I'm* not a bad person for correcting an error, I'm *helping* the person to not make it again, and ultimately I'm enriching the person's career."

"Dysfunctional" Speaking Behaviors and Their "Functional" Solutions

This list shows things speakers do that impede listening in others, and strategies to overcome them:

- *Not owning your part of a problem*: Say, "What I did to contribute to this conflict was…, and I'm sorry."
- *Expecting others to read your mind*: Don't make others responsible. Express your needs and opinions.
- *Sarcasm*: If you're angry with someone, express this directly vs. being sarcastic.
- *Being condescending, or shaming, blaming, and belittling*: Avoid this. Look within for why you do this.
- *Threatening others*: This is never acceptable.

(continued)

- *Giving ultimatums:* Do this only if you plan to carry them out. And rather than angrily saying "Do this or else…," use the "Consequence" part of the DESC model and deliver it calmly.
- *Cursing at others and name calling*: This is never acceptable, especially at work.
- *"Interrogating" others with rapid-fire questions*: Tone this down. It shows anger and implies a lack of trust.
- *Being the "clown" and joking too much to avoid getting serious*: Jokes can hide pain. Go inside yourself and ask what vulnerable emotions are underneath your joking, and express those instead.
- *Needing to be the center of attention and dominating a conversation*: Work on listening and let others speak.
- *Being domineering, talking over others, being demanding*: This is aggression. Consider working with a coach or therapist if you find it difficult to reverse this behavior, as your anger may be a significant problem.
- *Being vague to avoid being pinned down*: Take responsibility and make your opinion clear.
- *Being too wordy, going off on tangents, giving too much detail*: Get to the point quickly.
- *Talking fast so the listener can't respond*: Breathe between sentences and let others talk as well.
- *Lecturing or preaching*: Avoid this. Offer an opinion, and then let others decide how to resolve their issues.
- *Complaining vs. wanting to resolve an issue*: Take responsibility and find ways to solve the problem.
- *"Calling in the troops" or naming others who feel as you do to prove you're right*: Just speak for yourself.

COMPONENTS OF COMMUNICATION—PART IV: ADDITIONAL STRATEGIES FOR USE WITH PATIENTS

This section takes the communication skills and strategies discussed so far and incorporates them into specific circumstances with patients. It also adds new skills. Topics are the basics of the patient interview.

The Patient Interview

Whether during the first or subsequent visits with a patient, physicians and other clinicians need to create a connection with their patients, and be sure to involve them in the decisions regarding the management of their own care. In this light, clinicians should:

- Begin an interview in a way that helps build rapport (18):
  1. Make sure they know the patient's name, and introduce themselves to the patient.
  2. Establish an attentive (using eye contact), respectful, and nonjudgmental relationship using neutral language.
  3. Avoid taking excessive notes.
  4. Be fully transparent when discussing their findings and concerns.

- Elicit and ask about the patient's perspective on his or her illness, using open-ended questions (18):
  1. Ensure they've understood the patient's symptoms/problem by paraphrasing them back to the patient using reflective listening, and asking the patient if they've heard them accurately.
- Negotiate with their patients to reach common ground (18):
  1. Share their findings and propose/explain the management plan clearly.
  2. Ask the patient, "What questions and concerns do you have?"
  3. Answer the questions and discuss the patient's concerns.
  4. Ask, "Are you willing and able to do this?" "What obstacles may get in the way of carrying out this plan?" "How can we make this work?"
- Elicit, acknowledge, and address the patient's multitude of emotions:
  1. Use open-ended questions. Ask, "How do you feel about what I'm saying?" "What emotions are you feeling right now?"
  2. Reflect back what they've heard.
  3. Reassure the patient and indicate they understand how the patient feels (18).
- Check for understanding, feasibility, and mutual responsibility (18):
  1. Ensure the patient understands the diagnosis and treatment plan by asking the patient to reflect back to the physician what the physician said.
  2. Respect the patient's autonomy. Help the patient make a decision based on the information and advice.

Giving Information to Patients

It's important to reiterate that during the patient interview, patients must be given clear, accurate, and complete information about who their providers are, and about the following aspects of their care:

- The names of their physicians, nurses, physical therapists, social workers, and so on, whether they see these practitioners privately or when inpatient in a hospital or rehabilitation facility.
- The specifics of tests being ordered, the reason for ordering them, and the results.
- Informed consents.
- Diagnosis.
- Prognosis.
- Treatment plan procedures and strategies, including what patients can do for themselves such as at-home exercises.
- Where, when, with whom, and for how long treatment will occur.
- Side effects of treatments and medications
- How pain and emotional distress can be relieved.
- If and how families and other caretakers will be involved.
- Medical insurance paperwork, reimbursements, ans so on.

Unfortunately, many patients don't get this information. A survey of hospitalized patients and their physicians revealed fundamental gaps in patients' knowledge of their illness, with 43% of patients being unaware of their diagnosis and 90% being unaware of potential medication side effects. Physicians overestimate patients' understanding of their diagnosis and the care plan (19). In another study that interviewed hospitalized patients and their physicians, only 32% of patients correctly named at least one of their hospital physicians, and 60% correctly named their nurses. Complete agreement on the anticipated length of stay occurred only 39% of the time. A substantial portion of hospitalized patients don't understand their care plan. This may adversely affect patients' ability to provide informed consent for hospital treatments and to assume their own care after discharge (20).

How Much Sensitive Information to Reveal

Another difficult issue that physicians face is how truthful to be when telling patients information that's scary or causes strong emotion. The answer is "completely." In her writing on communication with the patient and family in palliative medicine, Leslie Fallowfield stated,

> "In efforts to protect patients from uncomfortable and distressing facts, doctors and nurses frequently censor their information in the mistaken belief that what someone does not know does not harm them. This misguided albeit well-intentioned assumption is made at all stages of the disease trajectory. Less-than honest disclosure is apparent when a patient first reports suspicious symptoms, at confirmation of the diagnosis, when the putative therapeutic benefits of treatment are discussed, at recurrence or relapse, and towards the end of life. Most attempts by doctors to protect patients from the reality of their situation often create further problems to patients, their relatives, and their friends. Furthermore, it can lead to inconsistent messages being given by other members of the multi-disciplinary team. Economy with the truth often leads to conspiracies of silence that usually build up to a heightened state of fear, anxiety, and confusion, rather than one of calmness and equanimity. The kinds of ambiguous or deliberately misleading messages received by patients may afford them short-term benefits while things continue to go well, but it has unfortunate long-term consequences. A patient with a shortened or uncertain future needs time and space to reorganize and adapt their life towards the attainment of achievable goals. Realistic hopes and aspirations can only be generated from honest disclosure. Although communicating the truth can be painful, deceit may well provoke greater problems" (21).

Delivering Bad News

What can at times make relaying sensitive information difficult is a doctor's *own* emotions. To address them, it's helpful to "anticipate" them with the "Emotions" self-reflective exercise, repeated here:

Self-Reflective Exercise: Emotions

When anticipating an upcoming difficult situation, sit quietly and take a few deep breaths. Envision the situation in your mind and how it may go. Ask yourself, "What emotions do I feel now as I anticipate this situation?" Fear or dread may arise, but with practice of that situation, calmness and ease may also arise.

As physicians become "conscious" of their emotions in these difficult situations, the emotions can be better managed. The common feelings that arise of fear, dread, anxiety, and so on, are normal, and physicians should reassure themselves of this. Telling a patient or family member about imminent death is never a pleasant task. Neither are typical conversations physiatrists face when the outcome is likely to be poor, like talking to a patient with a spinal cord injury or with a parent about a brain-injured child about the extent of the impairments and prognosis for recovery. While practice will make these discussions easier, it's important not to numb oneself to them over time. If this happens, the doctor will sound cold and lacking compassion. Maintaining one's humanity in medicine requires being able to stay connected to one's emotions.

The following strategies are helpful when preparing for and delivering bad news:

Preparing for and Delivering Bad News

- Perform deep breathing exercises or meditation for 5 minutes by yourself before speaking to a patient and/or family member.
- Be aware of your own emotions during the conversation. Quietly take deep breaths as you need to.
- Deliver bad news when you have time for the talk. Use a comfortable, pleasant private room. Sit down.
- Prepare the patient by saying you're about to tell him or her something very difficult.
- Look for nonverbal cues as the person listens to you. Be prepared for and acknowledge strong emotions.
- Straightforwardness and lack of prevarication are essential.
- Use little medical jargon.
- Give the patient ample time to express fears and worries.
- Use reflective listening to be sure the patient understands you, and encourage him or her to ask questions.
- Be informed for the session. Know about the problem, resources for the patient, and what must be done next.
- Schedule a follow-up visit even if you refer the patient elsewhere. He or she will appreciate your ongoing concern.
- People can show amazing resilience. Don't be surprised if the news upsets you more than the patient (22).
- Do 5 minutes of deep breathing afterward to get calm. If it upsets you, share your feelings with a colleague.

Calming Upset, Anxious, and Angry Patients and Families—and Staff

Another area in medicine that can challenge physicians and other staff is in calming patients who are anxious, angry, or otherwise upset or acting out. The following strategies are useful when dealing with difficult situations with patients and families.

NOTE: Many of these strategies can also be used with upset staff members:

Calming Upset, Anxious, and Angry Patients and Families—and Staff

- *Do deep breathing or meditation for 5 minutes by yourself* before speaking to them, to get calm. If you don't have 5 minutes, take several deep breaths on the elevator or while going to the situation.
- *Have a few team members respond at the scene* if the upset is significant.
- *Call security or the police* if the situation is potentially dangerous.
- *Smile and introduce yourself.* Say "I'm/we're here to help."
- *Try calming the person/group.* Say: "I hear you're upset. A good way to calm down is to take some deep breaths, OK? Let's all try it—take a slow deep breath in, now slowly breathe it out. Let's do that 3 times."
- *Set ground rules*: "OK, let's have one person speak at a time."
- *Ask someone to speak first.* Use reflective listening. Say: "Joan, tell me what the problem is."
- *Let the person speak without interruption.* Say: "Tell me more" or "What happened next?"
- *Practice empathy.* Put yourself in the patient's position. Imagine how the patient and his or her family are feeling.
- *Actively listen. Help get the patient to his or her vulnerable feelings—this in itself will calm the patient.* If they don't say the emotions directly but you hear them, reflect them back: "Joan, I hear how upset and scared you are."
- *Apologize for the problem*: "I'm so sorry this is happening."
- *Align yourself with the patient*: "Yes, I agree with you, this is a very frustrating situation."
- *Find a solution.* Ask: "How can I help?" or "What if we try this?" Involve the patient and ask, "Would do *you* think would work?"
- *Keep taking deep breaths yourself* as you need to stay calm, and stay aware of your own emotions.
- *Avoid false reassurance:* Don't say "Don't worry, all will be fine" unless you know it will. This works if you need to correct the type of meal a patient gets. It doesn't if the patient will never regain use of his or her limb.
- *Try resolving the issue.*
- *Check back later* that day or soon after to see how the situation is progressing.
- *Do 5 minutes of deep breathing afterward* to get calm. If it upsets you, share your feelings with a colleague.

Again, the above suggestions for defusing difficult patient situations can also be used with colleagues and staff, and in one's personal life. Simply substitute the patient with someone else. The strategies are identical.

REMEMBER THIS:

- *Underneath anger is fear.* The more anger, the more fear. Try to get the person to get to the source of the fear and discomfort (23). And help the patient to feel his or her fear. A mother who is very angry that her seriously injured daughter's physician hasn't visited her yet today might be terrified her daughter will die. Say: "I hear how angry you are. You must be very frightened for your daughter." Let her respond, and listen. Then offer a solution: "I'll find out when the doctor will arrive."
- *Underneath anger are also other vulnerable emotions.* To a patient angry that he or she will need to use a cane for 6 months, say: "I hear how disappointed you must be that the healing process is taking so long. It will come to an end, though, and you should have a full recovery."
- *Sometimes people just need to vent.* Especially in crises, while ambulances arrive, hospitalization occurs, and so on, vulnerable feelings get buried. It may take several days for the reality of the situation to sink in, after which the emotions surface. Expressing them and being heard is cathartic *and* promotes healing.

SUMMARY

As evidenced by the many topics in this chapter, good communication covers a large range of practical strategies and skills used in listening, speaking, and body language, as well as less obvious aspects of being aware of one's own emotions and needs and empathetic to those of others. Being fluent in these skills is critical for positive patient care outcomes and the reduction of errors, and for good relationships between health care professionals and their patients. What practitioners need is a desire to change, and a commitment to improve one's communication skills using these strategies. People who are best at dialogue understand they have to work on themselves first. "They realize that not only are they likely to benefit by improving their own approach, but also that they're the only person that they can work on anyway. As much as others may need to change, or we may *want* them to change, the only person we can continually inspire, prod and shape— with any degree of success—is the person in the mirror" (24). It's definitely worth the effort.

CASE VIGNETTES/SCENARIOS

1. Think of a situation where you as a physician don't get along with a peer physician. Write what is problematic about your relationship. What about this person bothers you? What do you do that bothers this individual? Pick an aspect of the relationship you want to work on and discuss with your peer. Using the DESC model, write out the back-and-forth dialogue you'd use, from approaching the individual, to the talk.
2. A 12-year-old child who was injured in a motor vehicle accident is expected to make a full recovery. To regain his independence at home, he needs to do more things for himself. However, his concerned mother wants to do everything for him. They come in for a visit and the child complains that his mother will not let him do more for himself. Plan to speak to the mother about this during the visit. Be empathetic. Write how you'd approach this and why. Use the DESC model, and write out the back-and-forth conversation you'd have with her.
3. Think of a leadership person you have a relationship with— chairman, professor, and so on— (or knew) whose communication skills you admire. Be specific. Write what you like about this person's skills or style. What skills does he or she use with patients and staff when speaking and listening? How do you feel in this person's presence? What traits possessed by this person can you emulate? Give examples of how you can put this into practice.
4. A 23-year-old woman is admitted to the spinal cord injury service with a newly diagnosed spinal cord injury. She has not been told about her injury or the impact it will have on the rest of her life. In preparation for this important conversation with your patient, write about the information you need to share with her about her condition, how you will discuss it, and her possible responses.
5. Think of all the professional members of your team (doctors, nurses, physical therapists, etc.). Identify 2 of them with whom you have had conflicts in the past. Put yourself in their shoes regarding what it's like to do their job. Write about what you discover. Write how you view them and discuss the skills, benefits, and value they bring to the team. Write about what you can do to improve your relationship with them.

SELF-EXAMINATION QUESTIONS
(Answers begin on p. 367)

1. Which of the following is not part of the DESC model?
   A. Explain
   B. Consequence
   C. Satisfy
   D. Describe
   E. State

2. Asking a patient, "Can you please tell me what parts of the home care regimen you're doing and how that's going?" is an example of:
   A. A closed-ended question
   B. An intrusive question
   C. A derogatory question
   D. An open-ended question
   E. An inflammatory question

3. Of the following behaviors, which best describes an important part of conflict resolution?
   A. Focusing on what the other person did wrong
   B. Proving that you're right
   C. Stating the part you played that exacerbated things
   D. Threatening to tell the person's supervisor
   E. Blaming the other person

4. Reflective listening is best characterized by which of the following behaviors of the listener?
   A. Telling the person how he or she can relate by sharing a similar personal story of his or her own
   B. Offering an opinion about the person's situation

C. Paraphrasing back to the person the content of what he or she just heard
D. Telling the person what he or she thinks the person should do
E. Criticizing what the person has said

5. Which of the following best characterizes "I" statements? They:
   A. Promote defensiveness in the listener
   B. Create vulnerability and honesty in the speaker
   C. Are a self-absorbed, narcissistic form of speaking
   D. Keep the speaker focused outward and blaming others
   E. Don't create vulnerability and honesty in the speaker

REFERENCES

1. The Joint Commission, Office of Quality Monitoring. Sentinel event data root causes by event type 2004–2012. The Joint Commission website. http://www.jointcommission.org/assets/1/18/Root_Causes_Event_Type_04_4Q2012.pdf. Accessed February 3, 2014: 5, 8, 19.
2. Lloyd M, Bor R. *Communication Skills for Medicine*. 3rd ed. Edinburgh: Churchill Livingstone Elsevier; 2009:3.
3. Kirby SG. Communication among health care professionals: an essential component of quality care. Newsletter 2010:(No. 4), February 2, 2011 posting: North Carolina Medical Board website. http://www.ncmedboard.org/articles/detail/communication_among_health_care_professionals_an_es sential_component_of_qua. Accessed February 3, 2014.
4. Accreditation Council for Graduate Medical Education (ACGME). Teamwork Section VI.F. Common Program Requirements Effective July 1, 2013. ACGME website. http://www.acgme.org/acgmeweb/Portals/0/PFAssets/ProgramRequirements/CPRs2013.pdf. Accessed February 3, 2014.
5. Gray N, Behm J. Chapter 5: interdisciplinary rehabilitation team. In: Mauk KL, ed. *Rehabilitation Nursing: A Contemporary Approach to Practice*. Burlington, MA: Jones & Bartlett Learning; 2011:54.
6. Patterson K, Grenny J, McMillan R, et al. *Crucial Conversations, Tools for Talking When Stakes Are High*. New York, NY: McGraw Hill; 2002:20.
7. Grenny J. Special report: discouraged doctors, speak up or burn out. *The Physician Executive*. November–December 2006: 26. American College of Physician Executives website. http://net.acpe.org/Resources/Articles/Speak_Up_or_Burn_Out.pdf. Accessed February 3, 2014.
8. Buckley M, Laursen J, Otarola V. Special report: doctor-nurse behavior, strengthening physician–nurse partnerships to improve quality and patient safety. *Physician Exec J*. November–December 2009:26–27. American College of Physician Executives website. http://net.acpe.org/MembersOnly/pejournal/2009/NovDec/Buckley_Michael.pdf. Accessed February 3, 2014.
9. Moore DP. Message from Daniel P. Moore, MD, Professor and Department Chairman. Physical Medicine and Rehabilitation, The Brody School of Medicine. January 19, 2013: East Carolina University website. http://www.ecu.edu/cs-dhs/Rehab/. Accessed February 3, 2014.
10. Maslow AH. A theory of human motivation. *Psychol Rev*. 1943;50(4):370–396.
11. Collins English Dictionary—Complete and Unabridged © HarperCollins Publishers. 2003: The Free Dictionary website. http://www.thefreedictionary.com/empathy. Accessed February 3, 2014.
12. Lloyd M, Bor R. *Communication Skills for Medicine*. 3rd ed. Edinburgh: Churchill Livingstone Elsevier; 2009:18.
13. Patient Safety Authority. Improving the safety of telephone or verbal orders. *PA PSRS Patient Saf Advis*. June 2006:3(2):1, 3–7. Patient Safety Authority, Commonwealth of Pennsylvania website. http://patientsafetyauthority.org/ADVISORIES/AdvisoryLibrary/2006/Jun3(2)/Pages/01b.aspx. Accessed February 3, 2014.
14. Patient Safety Authority. Improving the safety of telephone or verbal orders. *PA PSRS Patient Saf Advis*. June 2006:3(2):1, 3–7. Patient Safety Authority, Commonwealth of Pennsylvania website. http://patientsafetyauthority.org/ADVISORIES/AdvisoryLibrary/2006/Jun3(2)/Pages/01b.aspx. Accessed February 3, 2014.
15. Cohen S, Cox SH, et al. *Core Skills for Nurse Managers: A Training Toolkit*. Danvers, MA: HCPro, Inc.; 2004:(Chapter 5.)
16. Bartholomew K. *Stressed Out: About Communication Skills*. Danvers, MA: HCPro, Inc.; 2007:61–63.
17. Rosenberg MB. *Non-Violent Communication, a Language of Life*. 2nd ed. Encinitas, CA: Puddledancer Press; 2003:6.
18. General Core Competencies, Interpersonal and Communication Skills. *GME-Today Compact Disc Training Program for Residents*. Tamarac, FL: GME-Today; March 2006.
19. Olson DP, Windish DM. Communication discrepancies between physicians and hospitalized patients. *Arch Intern Med*. August 9, 2010;170(15):1302. http://archinte.jamanetwork.com/article.aspx?articleid=775589. Accessed February 3, 2014.
20. O'Leary KJ, Kulkarni N, et al. Hospital patients' understanding of their plan of care. *Mayo Clinic Proc*. 2010:85(1):47. National Center for Biotechnology Information website. http://www.ncbi.nlm.nih.gov/pmc/articles/PMC2800283/#ui-ncbiinpagenav-2. Accessed February 3, 2014.
21. Fallowfield L. Communication with the patient and family in palliative medicine. In: Hanks G, Cherny NI, et al. *Oxford Textbook of Palliative Medicine*. 4th ed. Oxford: Oxford University Press; 2009: Published to Oxford Medicine; 2011: Chapter 6, section 6.1.
22. Peterkin AD. *Staying Human During Residency Training*. 2nd ed. Toronto, ON: University of Toronto Press, Inc., Scholarly Publishing Division; 1998:79–80.
23. Patterson K, Grenny J, McMillan R, et al. *Crucial Conversations, Tools for Talking When Stakes Are High*. New York, NY: McGraw Hill; 2002:143.
24. Patterson K, Grenny J, McMillan R, et al. *Crucial Conversations, Tools for Talking When Stakes Are High*. New York, NY: McGraw Hill; 2002:29.

Sorush Batmangelich

4: Application of Principles of Professional Education for Physicians

GOALS

Demonstrate knowledge and application of principles to the practice of professional education in the physician teaching and learning enterprise.

OBJECTIVES

1. Discuss the principles and practice of adult education in the context of physician professional development.
2. Describe Accreditation Council for Graduate Medical Education (ACGME)'s new accreditation system (NAS), milestones, competencies, clinical competency committee (CCC), clinical learning environment review (CLER), and residency review committee (RRC) roles.
3. Discuss/demonstrate effective techniques for enhancing didactic, clinical, case presentation, psychomotor, and bedside teaching skills.
4. Demonstrate/practice/role-play delivery of constructive feedback.
5. Examine various models of supervision.
6. Review the qualities and characteristics of mentorship.

The continuum of physician education embodies undergraduate medical education (4 years), graduate medical education (another 4 years), and continuing medical education/continuing professional development (up to 40+ years). Although the focus of this chapter and book is on professional development of faculty, residents, and fellows, as well as graduate medical education spanning residency and fellowship training and development, the application and practice of professional education principles applies to the entire spectrum of physician education.

Professional education has evolved into a complex system. Health care is transforming itself and undergoing reengineering of how to best address health care through interprofessional teams. Educating health care professionals should keep up with this transformation. Medical education is about patient-centered care that should exist within the realm of learner-centered education. The objectives for this chapter are to provide tools and strategies for professional development, as well as recommend practical and relevant applications and "how to" guides and tips to complement your clinician educator's portfolio and armamentarium. You should be able to apply many of these skills immediately to enhance and improve your proficiency and techniques as educators. By the end of this chapter, we expect that you will improve your skills as educators and become sensitive to providing, recognizing, sensing, and seizing opportunities for *teachable moments* and *learning moments*. *Teachable* and *learning moments* are brief episodes characterized by intentional and/or unplanned signals and opportunities for bridging resident/fellow education gaps by the clinician educator.

Content areas covered include competencies, milestones, teaching and feedback, evaluation, supervision, and mentorship.

COMPETENCIES

The Oxford dictionary defines the noun *competence* as "the ability to do something successfully or efficiently." The Merriam Webster dictionary defines *competence* as "an ability or skill" with synonyms such as *capability, capableness, capacity, ability*, and *faculty*. Competency is the composite of knowledge, skills, and attitudes/values to allow the individual to effectively perform in one's practice setting and meet the profession's standards. Knowledge, skills, and attitudes/values are the classical three-legged pillars of professional education that shape the judgments essential for interprofessional collaborative practice.

The continuum of physician education is driven by the six core competencies embedded in all residency and fellowship program requirements. These competencies are patient care/procedural skills, medical knowledge, practice-based learning and improvement, interpersonal and communication skills, professionalism, and systems-based practice. Residency and fellowship programs focus on building and demonstrating proficiency in the six core competencies.

The core competencies are core values that constitute the basic foundation for physician development, defined not only by clinical skills but also, equally important, by the skills of the heart, values, and cultivating habits of lifetime practice that is immersed in self-assessment, inquiry, innovation, and discovery. Competence is defined as "the habitual and judicious use of communication, knowledge, technical skills, clinical reasoning, emotions, values and reflection in daily practice for the benefit of the individuals and communities being served"(1).

Physicians are trained to be clinicians and expected to be teachers. The six domains of competencies were articulated and adopted by the ACGME and the American Board of Medical Specialties (ABMS) in the late 1990s and became the essential requirements of organized medicine and physician education across undergraduate, graduate, and continuing medical/professional education development.

Residents must learn and integrate the six competencies into their daily professional conduct. This cannot happen unless faculty members serve as role models for these competencies. You cannot teach competencies and quality care if you are not doing it.

These core competencies inform the culture of continuous improvement and accountability, and have become the common currency and expected standard measures and markers in improvement of quality, safety, and efficiency (triple aim) of the U.S. health care system. In addition to accrediting organizations, insurers, hospitals, and organizations representing quality, credentialing, and the federal government have embodied these core competency values.

The six core competencies, expectations of each competency, and content guide defining each competency is represented by Appendix 1.

ACGME'S NAS AND EDUCATIONAL MILESTONES

Beginning in 2009, the ACGME began to articulate and reorganize its accreditation system to the commonly known NAS, heralded by "milestones" and "levels" as fundamental underpinnings (2). The NAS transitions the ACGME's accreditation system from a "process" orientation to that of "educational outcomes." The NAS has two major objectives: (a) assessment of trainees to determine if the resident/fellow is competent and (b) accreditation of the residency/fellowship program. The milestones support a framework for the assessment of the development of the physician in key dimensions of the elements of physician competency in the given specialty. The milestones for each specialty have been crafted by a working group made up of members of the respective RRC, the ABMS certifying board, program directors, and residents.

The educational milestones are observable developmental steps, organized under the 6 competency areas, that describe a trajectory of progress on the competencies from novice (entering resident) to proficient (graduating resident) and, ultimately, to expert/master.

The new educational milestones are "developmentally based, specialty specific achievements that residents are expected to demonstrate at established intervals as they progress through training. Residency programs in the NAS will submit composite milestone data on their residents every six months synchronized with residents' semiannual evaluations"(2).

Milestones are shared understanding of expectations that map learning experiences to the six core competencies. Milestones serve as metrics across the learning continuum from student to practitioner, providing a rich source of longitudinal tracking and monitoring of important quality indicators that define the educational outcomes of the residency program.

Milestones also match competencies with developmental readiness. In the NAS, programs are expected to document annual evaluation trends and continuing program progress assessment. The six core competencies will remain as anchors for the NAS milestones. The NAS levels comprise five stages of physician professional development, from novice to expert/master, hence Levels 1 to 5, described as follows:

Level 1—Novice: Expected competencies of a graduating medical student
Level 2—Advanced Beginner: Expected competencies of end of physical medicine and rehabilitation (PM&R) postgraduate year (PGY) 1 resident
Level 3—Competent: Expected competencies of end of PM&R PGY 2-year resident
Level 4—Proficient: Expected competencies of end of PM&R PGY 3 graduating resident prepared for unsupervised practice
Level 5—Expert: Expected competencies of advanced resident fellow specialist and practicing physician

The foundation and origins of the five progressive levels of medical education and physician professional development endorsed and adopted by ACGME's NAS were adapted from and first described in the literature by the Dreyfus brothers in 1980 (3), as illustrated below.

Novice—Follows rules (knows right from wrong): *Don't know what they don't know* —Level 1

⇓

Advanced Beginner—Rules + situation: *Know what they don't know*—Level 2

⇓

Competent—Rules + selected contexts + accountable: *Able to perform tasks and roles of the discipline—restricted breadth and depth*—Level 3

⇓

Proficient—Accountable + beginning intuitive; immediately sees what: *Consistent and efficient in performance of task and roles of discipline—know what they know and don't know*—Level 4

⇓

Expert—Immediately sees how; has seen many patterns: *In-depth knowledge of discipline—know what they know*—Level 5

⇓

Master—intuitively integrates with novel patterns (considers different and alternative ways of doing things): *Expert who relishes the unknown, or the situation that breaks the rules—who the experts go to for help—don't know what they know*—Level 5

The process of learning any new skill can be divided into four stages, illustrated as follows, described in 1990 by Neil Whitman (4). These descriptions of learning stages were initially adapted from Noel Burch in the 1970s describing the four stages for learning any new skill. The literature also attributed this model to the founder of humanistic psychology Abraham Maslow's "Hierarchy of Needs" in the 1940s (5).

Unconscious Incompetence (Novice): Don't know that they don't know—Level 1

⇓

Conscious Incompetence: Know that they don't know—Level 2

⇓

Conscious Competence: Know what they know and don't know—Level 3/4

⇓

Unconscious Competence (Expert): Know what they know and don't know that they know—Level 5

MILESTONE EXPECTATIONS AND REPORTING

Milestones consist of knowledge, skills, attitudes, and other attributes for each of the ACGME competencies organized in a developmental framework from less to more advanced. As a resident progresses from entry into residency through graduation, milestones serve as descriptors or markers and targets for performance expectations.

The NAS expects every residency program to establish a CCC whose responsibility is to assess the milestones. The CCC's role is to establish guidelines and thresholds to ascertain whether a resident is competent, and provide supporting information and evidence as to competency. The key characteristic of the CCC is that the member group collectively makes competency decisions through multiple broad consensus, not relying on just the program director or rotation supervisor's judgments. Decisions relating to competency and progressive advancement will be based on dashboards of collective and summative data, and through group conversations and wisdom. Also, if a resident is judged to be deficient in competencies and not achieving the milestones requirements, the remediation strategy is relegated to the CCC. Warnings, probation, repeating rotation, or counseling to consider another specialty or profession's decisions might be options available to the CCC.

Historically, there has been a disconnect between graduate medical education (GME) and chief executive officers of medical centers. ACGME's NAS attempts to address this issue. Academic Institutional Reviews by ACGME of residency sponsoring bodies will now be conducted through the new NAS's CLER, authorized to implement continuous workplace monitoring and assessment. It is estimated that 80% of medical errors are systems based. CLER visits are scheduled every 18 months by a team of visitors, and these engage a different site each visit. CLER will focus on the six domains of (a) quality improvement, (b) patient safety, (c) supervision, (d) transitions of care, (e) duty hours/fatigue management, and (f) professionalism (6,7).

Institutional procedures and outcomes will be reviewed. CLERs will observe and evaluate daily operations by conducting "walk-arounds" of the institution and interview residents, faculty, administrators, quality and safety point persons, nurses and other allied health members, and executives. Significantly, CLERs will engage and interact with and survey chief executive officers, deans, designated institutional officials (DIOs), chief financial officers, chief medical officers, and chief nursing officers, commonly referred to as the "C and D suites."

Milestones are organized into 5 numbered levels. Tracking and monitoring residents from Level 1 to Level 5 coincides with moving from novice (Level 1) to expert (Level 5). These five levels do not correspond with PGY of education, as residents nationally are exposed to clinical experiences during different residency years. Also, milestones are just one source of information for graduation decision making. Ultimately, the program director will have to make a judgment, based on CCC's input, whether the resident "has demonstrated sufficient competency to enter practice without direct supervision."

Residency programs will use milestones as a reporting mechanism for each period. Such a process is designed for programs to use in semiannual review of resident performance and reporting to ACGME. Upon a program's submission of milestones assessments, the ACGME generates a milestones evaluation report for the program. In the initial years of milestones implementation, the RRC will examine milestone performance data for each program's residents as one element in the next accreditation system (NAS) to ascertain whether residents overall are progressing as expected. For a given program, the review committees will compare aggregate program-level data and de-identified milestone data for resident performance against cohorts longitudinally.

Programs will have to review and report for each semiannual period the selection of milestone levels that best describe each resident's current performance and attributes. Selection of a level connotes that the resident substantially demonstrates the milestones in that level, as well as those in lower levels; in other words, a hierarchical structure. For example, a resident demonstrating Level 3 competency is also expected to have demonstrated Levels 1 and 2.

Descriptions of the Milestones Levels (8) are as follows:

Level 1: The resident demonstrates milestones expected of an incoming resident.
Level 2: The resident is advancing and demonstrates additional milestones, but is not yet performing at a mid-residency level.
Level 3: The resident continues to advance and demonstrates additional milestones consistently, including the majority of milestones targeted for residency.
Level 4: The resident has advanced so that he or she now substantially demonstrates the milestones targeted for residency. *This level is designed as the graduation target*, but *does not* represent a graduation *requirement*. Making decisions about

preparedness for graduation is the purview of the residency program director. Over time, study of milestones performance data will be necessary before the ACGME and its partners will be able to determine whether milestones in the first four levels appropriately represent the developmental framework, and whether milestone data are of sufficient quality and rigor to be used for high-stakes decisions.

Level 5: The resident has advanced beyond performance targets set for residency and is demonstrating "Aspirational" goals, which might describe the performance of someone who has been in practice for several years. It is expected that only a few exceptional residents will reach this level.

Progressive implementation of the NAS for ACGME/RRC reviews is being phased in between July 2013 and July 2014 for all 26 ACGME-accredited core specialties. The NAS for PM&R will be phased in beginning July 2014. With respect to the reliability and validity of the milestones—which were developed by working groups of ABMS board members representing major stakeholders—construct, criterion, and predictive validity will be established over time with accumulation of national data (9).

The ACGME/RRC's NAS is characterized by compliance requirements for ongoing annual data collection, tracking and monitoring of evaluation and assessment trends of residents, programs in key performance, and learning outcomes measurement markers. An expected prominent feature of the NAS is to facilitate opportunities for early identification of suboptimal performance. Residency programs will be expected to report aggregated milestone data for their residents every 6 months, synchronized with residents' semiannual evaluations.

The milestones and levels of resident learning outcomes are being defined by each specialty and developed by expert panels. Graduates of all residency programs will have to demonstrate achievement of the required milestones before graduation and entry to unsupervised practice, documented by the programs as the final graduation milestones.

As of this writing, the PM&R RRC has drafted 27 sets of milestones across the 6 domains of core competencies, distributed as follows: patient care (7), medical knowledge (9), professionalism (3), interpersonal and communication skills (2), practice-based learning and improvement (3), and systems-based practice (3).

TEACHING AND FEEDBACK

Multigenerational Workforce

In today's workplace landscape, working effectively together across generations requires sensitivity to, and understanding and appreciation of, the typical attributes of each generation. Generational characteristics such as preferred communication style, leadership styles, rewards, motivators, interaction styles, workplace values, core values, definitions of work, and generational "personalities" have profound implications for learning and teaching outcomes across generations. Unless we are aware and prepared to adapt to these generational differences, we will have missed teaching/learning opportunities and will not do our jobs effectively as educators.

Attendings and residents encompass four age eras: (a) *Traditionalists* (born between 1937 and 1945), (b) *Baby Boomers* (born between 1946 and 1964), (c) *Generation X* (born between 1965 and 1984), and (d) *Millennials or Generation Y* (born between 1985 and 2005). Table 4.1 describes the top 10 multigenerational attributes (10).

What Does It Mean to Teach?

In the age of NAS, teaching and assessing the core competencies is a priority and should be seamlessly integrated with all teaching methods, didactics, journal clubs, mortality and morbidity conferences, seminars, hands-on procedural instruction, and so on.

Think back and remember an exemplary teacher. What qualities and characteristics demonstrated by the teacher influenced your learning? Some of these memorable qualities might be skills in inspiring and "igniting the learning fires," motivating and challenging students, and having the ability to engage and excite the learner and evoke enthusiasm about the content being taught. In fact, these are the same qualities of an effective teacher.

The effective teacher displays skills in creating a "want and need to know" environment. These educators "don't tell" or "don't spoon feed" information, but rather "guide the learner to answers." This is typically known as the Socratic teaching method. Socrates, the Greek philosopher and teacher, was exemplary in pioneering teaching techniques through effective questioning skills, rather than "telling."

The term *doctor* is derived from the Latin word *docer* meaning "to teach." The 4th-century Hippocratic Oath enjoins the physician to teach the craft of healing to younger colleagues. Demonstrating effective teaching skills and the art of teaching draws upon the science of education and is process oriented.

Scholarship is a pillar of professional development. Boyer and Glassick articulated the meaning of scholarship and remind us that physicians must demonstrate competency and commitment to scholarship, including the scholarship of teaching (11–13). The ACGME has adopted Ernest Boyer's definition of the three types of scholarship (11): (a) the scholarship of *discovery* (peer-reviewed funding, peer-reviewed publication of original research), (b) the scholarship of *dissemination* (review articles or chapters in textbooks), and (c) the scholarship of *application* (publication or presentation of case reports, clinical series, lectures, workshops at local, regional, or national meetings; or leadership roles in professional or academic societies). For clarification, *being* scholarly means "improving on others and self," while *doing* scholarship is to advance the field.

Effective teaching components consist of the *content* to be taught, the *learner's* attributes and characteristics, and the *context* within which teaching takes place. The ultimate goal of effective teaching is "delivering the *right learning*, to the *right learner* at the *right time*!" The role of the effective teacher is to take a complex body of knowledge (content) and communicate that at the appropriate learner development stage and level of understanding (learner—Dreyfus Levels 1–5, novice to expert), learner's preferred learning styles (learner), within the particular teaching context, such as didactics, seminars, clinical venue, bedside, journal clubs, or hands-on procedure practicum (context).

Clearly, residency and fellowship programs have an obligation for commitment to education and teaching. Teaching is an

TABLE 4.1 Characteristics of the Four Generations Currently in the Workforce

	ATTRIBUTES	TRADITIONALISTS (1937–1945)	BABY BOOMERS (1946–1964)	GENERATION X (1965–1984)	MILLENNIALS (1985–2005)
1	Age era	Great Depression and World War II	Spiritual awakening, sexual revolution, and women's liberation movement	Oil crisis, economic uncertainty, high divorce rates, and "latchkey care"	Digital media, high-speed communication, abundance in society, doting parents, and high levels of diversity
2	Generational "personality"	Conforming Conservative spenders Oriented to past Hard times in childhood	Competitive driven Soul searchers Willing to "go the extra mile"	Self-reliant Skeptical Risk takers Seek balance and a sense of family	Realistic about the present Optimistic about the future Prefer collective action Tenacious
3	Core values	Dedication/sacrifice Loyalty Honor Patriotism Family	Optimism Personal growth Personal gratification Team player Health and wellness Work	Technoliterate Fun and informality Pragmatism Global thinking Results-oriented Challenge the system	Social consciousness Morality Achievement-oriented Respect for diversity Money
4	Definition of work	Obligation	Adventure	Challenge	Means to an end
5	Workplace values	Respectful of authority Age equals seniority Hardworking Dedicated Reserved Obedient	Avoid conflict Formal Follow protocol Social Idealistic Driven	Fast-paced Independent Confident Value personal time Challenge the status quo Loyal to staff leader	Task oriented Want options Expect feedback Multitask through multimedia Resist rules Value work/life balance
6	Interactive style	Individual	Team player	Entrepreneur	Participative
7	Leadership style	Directive; command and control	Consensus-building	Everyone is equal	Yet to be determined
8	Preferred communication style	Memo	Face-to-face	E-mail	Instant messaging, texting
9	Rewards	Satisfaction in a job well done	Money, recognition, title	Money, freedom	Meaningful work
10	Motivators	"We respect your experience"	"You are valued and needed"	"Forget the rules, do it your way"	"You will work with other bright, creative people"

expectation and a competency in physician education, and monitored by accreditation bodies such as ACGME (responsible for residency, fellowship, and institutional accreditation) and Liaison Committee on Medical Education (LCME; responsible for medical school accreditation). The residents and fellows are student learners first and foremost, and the faculty member's teaching mission must be to create and protect space and environment for teaching and learning. The resident/fellow learner must engage in an iterative cycle throughout the residency, reflecting on the following 3 questions: (a) What am I doing? (b) How am I doing? and (c) How can I improve? In fact, this quality improvement cycle is repetitive throughout the continuing professional development of the physician beyond training well into the Maintenance of Certification (MOC) and Maintenance of Licensure (MOL) phases.

The ACGME is very sensitive to the balance between teaching/learning/education and service rendered by the resident. Despite the importance given to teaching by ACGME and the RRCs, protected teaching time and creating incentives for teaching remain challenges. DaRosa (14) cited major barriers to effective teaching by faculty members, such as lack of faculty development opportunities, attitudes and values faculty might have toward teaching, competition with clinical revenue generation, and limited commitments.

Why learn to teach? The notion that "Teachers are born to teach" and "Teaching is only about knowing the subject matter (content based)" are myths. There is no "gene" for good teaching. Good teaching skills and behaviors are learned and acquired traits and improved with practice and feedback. Physicians improve their individual professional and clinical problem-solving skills through teaching. Teaching is "like learning twice." Learning embodies both education and assessment/evaluation. Faculty serve as role models to resident learners who will spend 20% of their time as residents engaged in teaching peers, medical students, and other team member health professionals. Similarly, medical students receive one-third of their knowledge from attendings and house staff teaching.

Adult Learning Principles and Practice

The foundation of physician learning is embedded in adult education principles and practices, or andragogy (15). The life span of learning is a continuum that moves from pedagogy [how children learn, as articulated by Jean Piaget (16), renowned cognitive child developmental psychologist) to andragogy (how adults learn, as described by Malcolm Knowles (17,18), father of adult education, and Cyril Houle (19)], each with distinct characteristics illustrated in Figure 4.1.

As reflected in Figure 4.1, adults learn best when:

- They are enabled to be actively involved in the teaching/learning activity.
- Their personal *model of reality* is acknowledged and respected, allowing them to pursue their own learning goals, self-reflection, and fostering and supporting self-directed learning.
- Learning that matters is relevant, practical, meaningful, and relates to current tasks, experiences, actual problems, or issues, with immediate direct application.
- Immediate feedback is provided; adults want to know how they are doing.
- Learners' past experience, knowledge, skills, values, and motives are deployed to their existing roles, responsibilities, and resources for learning.

PEDAGOGY to ANDRAGOGY

Pedagogy (Piaget)	Andragogy (Knowles)
• Directed learning • Teacher-centered • Nonreflective learning • Evaluation through external assessment • Competitiveness, grades, tests, quizzes • Learners externally motivated (rewards, competition, grades) • Learners are dependent on others	• Facilitated learning • Active learning • Learner-centered • Learning for immediate application • Self-directed, independent learning • Learners intrinsically/internally motivated, *but* external motivation also plays a role • Self-reflective learning • Evaluation is self-assessment • Immediate feedback • Equality/mutual respect, cooperation/collaboration • Independent study/projects, experimentation

FIGURE 4.1 Learning Continuum Over a Life Span

- Learners treated according to their professional stage identities, developmental readiness, roles/responsibilities, who they are, and their capabilities.
- Learners are clear about *where they are going*, *how they will get there*, and *how they will know when they got there and have succeeded*.

Practice-based learning and improvement (PBLI), one of the six core competencies, is the cornerstone of adult learning and self-directed learning. Lifelong learning (LLL) and self-assessment are hallmarks of adult learning and continuous professional development (CPD). LLL reinforces, expands, and improves core competencies. CPD is the "chronic" habit of looking at your own practice over time longitudinally and comparing it to peers and to acceptable national standards. ABMS's Maintenance of Competency (MOC) and FSMB's (Federation of State Medical Boards) MOL are embedded in a culture of continuous learning, practice improvement, and opportunities for self-directed learning and self-assessment. Competencies for LLL address what you are doing, how you are doing, and how you can improve. Specifically, LLL habits include (a) drawing upon high-quality unbiased evidence-based health care literature and critical thinking; (b) application of clinical and educational information; (c) literature search and retrieval strategies; (d) PBLI methods; (e) self-reflection (developing analogies and new mental models, and improving practice from moving from old to new ways of practicing) and assessment; and (f) skill sets for learning management, drawing upon one's own resource for learning and knowledge management (learning-how-to-learn).

Effective Teaching and Teaching Competencies Strategies

Some common teaching methods and environments during residency include lectures and seminars (didactics); journal clubs; grand rounds; inpatient; outpatient; consultations; bedside teaching; case conferences (case-based learning); hands-on procedures such as electromyography (EMG) and injections (psychomotor); clinics; objective structured clinical examinations (OSCEs); standardized patients (SPs), simulations, actors; and problem-based learning (PBL).

We were brought up in a didactic education world and U.S. medical education is no exception, characterized by predominately being lectured to, referred to as "passive learning." As educators, we know that we should promote a variety of modes of instructional delivery. David Davis's (20) study informs us that high-impact instructional formats that are more likely to result in desired behavior/attitude change when compared to traditional didactic lectures have the following characteristics in common: learner-centered, interactive, meaningful/relevant/personal, reinforcing, successive or repeated, and mixed methods teaching. Foley and Smilansky (21) over 30 years ago informed us that 80% of information delivered by lectures is forgotten within 8 weeks, and that after 20 minutes of lecture, the learner's attention drops dramatically. The lecture is the weakest method for changing behavior.

"Tell me and I'll forget; Show me and I may remember; Involve me and I'll understand." This Chinese proverb reminds us that learning is dramatically improved when the learner

Average Student Retention Rates
National Training Laboratories, Bethel, MD

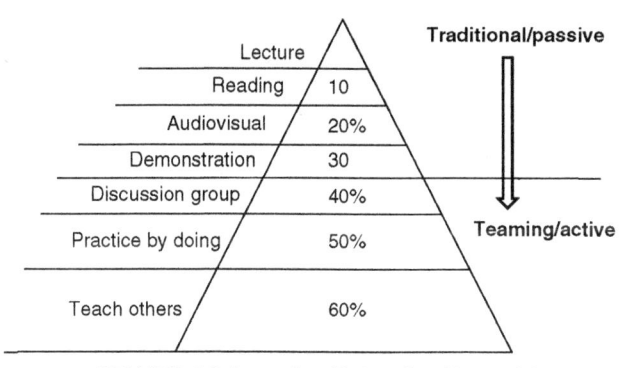

Level	Retention	Type
Lecture		Traditional/passive
Reading	10	
Audiovisual	20%	
Demonstration	30	
Discussion group	40%	
Practice by doing	50%	Teaming/active
Teach others	60%	

FIGURE 4.2 Learning Retention Pyramid

actively does a task, discusses what is taking place, practices, and teaches others, referred to as "active learning." As illustrated in the Learning Retention Pyramid (22), Figure 4.2, retention rate improves progressively as you more actively involve and engage the learner as when you move from passive to active learning. Figure 4.2 demonstrates that we remember only 10% of what we read, 20% of what we hear, 30% of what we see, 50% of what we hear and see (as when we engage in discussion), 70% of what we practice by doing, and 90% of what we teach others.

Teaching is as much an art as it is a science. Artful teachers have the ability to leverage subtle manipulations of emotion, in addition to being content experts. Proficient teachers invariably display the following qualities: (a) establish rapport with learner, be supportive, be accessible, be compassionate, and be organized; (b) create optimal student–teacher dynamics and relationships with frequent exchanges that enlist mutual trust and respect and individual consideration; (c) have passion for teaching; ability to excite, motivate, generate enthusiasm, and emotionally activate learners; (d) early on set up goals, directions, and expectations, and target teaching to learners' level of knowledge and developmental preparedness; (e) give feedback and expect feedback in return; engage in self-evaluation and reflect on one's own teaching; and (f) demonstrate mastery and competence in subject matter being taught.

Learning Styles

As previously stated, the effective teacher considers a learner's preferred learning styles. Educators have known for many years that learning styles affect the way we learn. Highlighted are three well-known assessments used in medical education to identify preferred learning styles and personality indicators: (a) *Myers-Briggs Type Indicator (MBTI)* (23). MBTI is one of the most commonly used psychological personality tests that maps individuals across four sets of coordinates across a continuum: Extroversion (E) ↔ Introversion (I), Sensing (S) ↔ Intuition (I), Thinking (T) ↔ Feeling (F), and Judgment (J) ↔ Perception (P). This excellent instrument can be used to identify and, if desired, intentionally match personalities among residents or faculty, or between faculty supervisor and resident. (b) *Kolb's Learning Style Inventory* (24): This indicator identifies individuals across four dimensions—Convergers, Divergers, Assimilators, and Accommodators. (c) The third inventory tool well validated in the health professions is the *Rezler Learning Preference Inventory (RLPI) (21)*: This is useful in identifying conditions and situations that facilitate individual learning and types of learning situations preferred by the learner. This instrument describes *how* you learn best, but does not evaluate your learning abilities. Scores reflect how you learn across three sets of continuum: Abstract (AB) ↔ Concrete (CO), Teacher-Structured (TS) ↔ Student-Structured (SS), and Interpersonal (IP) ↔ Individual (IN). *AB* learners prefer learning theories, general principles, and concepts, as well as generating hypotheses. *CO* learners prefer learning tangible, specific, practical tasks and skills. *TS* learners prefer well-organized, teacher-directed objectives, with clear expectations, assignments, and goals defined by the teacher. *SS* learners prefer learner-generated tasks, are autonomous, and are self-directed. *IP* learners prefer learning or working with others; emphasis is on harmonious relations between students and teacher and among peer learners. *IN* learners prefer learning or working alone, with emphasis on self-reliance and tasks that are solitary, such as reading or interacting with computers.

Feedback and Educational Contract

The practice of drawing up an "educational contract" between the resident learner and attending supervisor and in providing feedback is extremely useful and important in order to lay out mutual expectations, avoid setting up learners for failure further into the rotation, and ensure a "win–win" situation. "BOGERD" is an acronym for a six-step process described by Bulstrode and Hunt (25) that establishes a teacher–learner education contract that keeps the end in mind from the beginning, as in Day 1 or beginning of the rotation, and is explicit about mutual obligations.

B represents *Background* assessment of a resident's abilities. Invest the time upfront to assess the resident during the first several days or week of the rotation to observe and determine individual strengths and limitations. Begin with a comprehensive assessment of the resident's capabilities and competencies (baseline data) when beginning a rotation, using tools such as knowledge tests, direct observation of skills, Resident Observation and Competency Assessment (RO&CA), Global evaluations, Resident Self-Assessment, and Summative Competency-based evaluation, to name a few. Based on these results, aim teaching to address training needs during the rotation, considering the resident's strengths and weaknesses.

O stands for disclosing and sharing expected *Opportunities* during the rotation, and seeking feedback on opportunities that the resident might be expecting.

G, or *Goals,* is formally articulating on Day 1 or at the beginning of rotation what the rotation covers, such as learning objectives, Dreyfus resident level-specific competencies, and milestones.

E is *Evaluation* informing the resident as to how (e.g., global evaluations, RO&CAs, knowledge tests, multisource

360° evaluations, formative and summative evaluations) and how frequently they will be evaluated, as well as feedback expectations.

R, *Remediation/Rescue*, is to let the resident know what the consequences of not meeting rotation expectations will be and the remediation process, when necessary. And,

D is the contract *Deal*; validate to make sure the resident has fully heard and understands the BOGERD process you articulated and ask him or her to sign off on the learning contract or deal indicating approval by both resident and attending supervisor. This process is illustrated Figure 4.3.

Competency-Based Journal Club

A novel method for teaching core competencies while conducting Journal Clubs in a seamless fashion is described as follows.

1. Residents choose two journal club articles on the topic assigned, of their own choosing, or those designated by their supervisor.
2. The articles must have been from within the past 5 years, unless they are considered classical articles and are still meaningful and relevant.
3. These articles must be chosen at least 4 weeks prior to the journal club and approved by the faculty supervisor.
4. After the attending supervisor approves the articles, residents prepare their presentations.
5. Articles are distributed to all residents and faculty in advance of the journal club date.
6. Presentations may be informal or formal using PowerPoint, although not required.
7. It is expected that all the residents and faculty attending the educational activity will have read the articles.
8. Presentations are expected to be a brief overview of the key elements of the paper, which will then be followed by a discussion.

The following questions should be answered in the journal club (recommend 25–30 min per article, with the suggested time breakdowns as follows):

1. What questions is the article trying to answer (hypotheses)? (1–2 min)
2. Why are the authors trying to answer this question (relevance)? (1–2 min)
3. What is the study design (design)? (2 min)
4. What are their methods (methods)? Include a brief description of the statistical approach (5 min).
5. What did they find (findings)? (5 min)
6. Critique of methods and conclusions (5–10 min)
7. Is this applicable and relevant? Implications for further investigation? Why? (5 min)

To integrate and address ACGME competencies during journal club involves the following:

1. *Patient Care*: Does the article influence patient care practices in PM&R, and, if so, how? **PC**
2. *Medical Knowledge*: What new medical knowledge has been learned as a result of the article? **MK**
3. *Practice-Based Learning and Improvement*: Does the article contribute scholarly evidence to "best practices" in rehabilitation care? Practice-related quality improvement (QI)? Sources for self-study? **PBLI**
4. *Interpersonal and Communication Skills*: Does the article enhance your ability to communicate with patients, families, team members, caregivers, or interprofessional health care colleagues/providers? **IPCS**
5. *Professionalism*: Does the article contribute to learning of humanistic qualities, advocacy, cultural, ethical, diversity, and/or professional issues in rehabilitation care? **PROF**
6. *Systems-Based Practice*: Does the article contribute to understanding of how the health care system works, patient safety, cost-effectiveness, utilization and resource identification, and accessibility, with emphasis on post-acute care strategies? **SBP**

Didactic Lecture Presentations

All residents must be able to acquire skills in conducting didactic presentations. Teaching is an expected competency in all residency training. Having at least one lecture presentation made by resident videotaped, and preferably two to three during the entire residency to track progress and improvement, serves as a powerful resident development instrument. It would be optimal to have a trained observer such as a professional educator or clinician educator assess the presentation using a *skills checklist*, followed by feedback and debriefing for improvement purposes.

Every didactic presentation must have an opening, body, and closing. As indicated previously, optimal lecture presentation length is 15 to 20 minutes, after which, unless you alter the instructional approach (exercises, small group discussions, demonstrations, cases, video triggers, etc.), attention and retention dramatically decline. The two most common errors in didactic presentation are talking too much, and information overload ("stuffing 10 pounds of sugar in a 5-pound bag!"). Focus on two to three key objectives you wish to get across, rather than trying to cover it all in 20 minutes.

The skills checklist for rating a lecture reflects ability in organizing lecture material (clarity and organization), skills

Educational Contract
*"Keep the end in mind from the beginning.
What should happen on Day 1 of rotation"*

Background	→ Assess resident ability
Opportunities	→ Mutual opportunities
Goals	→ Objectives/competencies
Evaluation	→ Assessment/feedback
Rescue	→ Consequences/remedial
Deal	→ Mutual understanding

FIGURE 4.3 BOGERD Process

in use of voice and body movements in delivering a lecture (expressiveness, voice, eye, face, hands coordination), and skills in the use of audiovisual aids. Assessment categories corresponding to the assessor's observations may include "Not Done," "Only Partially or Rarely Done," "Completely or Usually Done," and "Not Applicable or Can't Recall." Perhaps the most important component of the lecture presentation evaluation form is the "comments" section, an open-ended section to capture strengths and weaknesses observed in your videotaped lecture.

At a minimum, have a faculty member observe the presentation and use a checklist to evaluate the presentation skills, followed by constructive feedback. The videotaped presentation can also be used along with the checklist to critique the presentation. It is especially effective to have residents view their videotape independently and use the checklist to self-assess, then compare results of their own self-assessment with those of others who evaluated them. Also, have an evaluation form completed by peers and others in attendance covering presentation skills.

A practical tool to remember when creating PowerPoint slides is the 7 × 7 Rule: No more than 7 words per line, and no more than 7 lines per slide.

Five important rules for learning and teaching are as follows:

1. *Know your audience*: You must take the time to assess what the needs, and level of needs, of your audience are. This will avoid boring the learners because the subject matter is too elementary or fundamental for their level, or conversely, frustrating them because the material is too advanced beyond their level of preparedness. A quick and easy way to assess needs before your presentation is to take some time and directly ask the participants, "Why they are there?" and elicit several topic areas that participants want addressed. This technique is consistent with adult learning practices.
2. *Ordering of content*: Always start with learning objectives for your presentation. For a 1-hour presentation, develop 2 to 3 learning objectives. Start with an opening that draws attention and engages learners; for example, "Why is this topic so important?" or start with an anecdote or a personal story. Your conclusion should summarize the learning objectives you set out to accomplish. Remember this rule: *"Tell them what you are going to say," "Tell them," and "Tell them what you said."* This draws upon the learning power of repetition and reinforcement.
3. *Active participation*: Allow opportunities for the audience to be active participants and engaged in an "active learning" process. This can be accomplished through "mixed method" teaching, which enhances learning efficacy and results in desired behavior/attitude change; or by introducing practical exercises such as case-based breakout sessions, small group discussions, PBL, demonstrations, video triggers, and experiential learning.
4. *Immediate feedback*: An essential rule about adult learners is that they seek immediate feedback and "want to know how they did." We will talk more about feedback later, but for now remember to provide frequent and constructive feedback at the appropriate time.
5. *Draw on learner experiences*: The first rule for learning mentioned earlier is "knowing your audience." Part of this exercise to uncover what the learners want is to also capture their previous knowledge and experiences as a resource for teaching.

CLINICAL TEACHING, CASE PRESENTATIONS, AND FEEDBACK STRATEGIES

Feedback

Feedback is vital, transformational, and enhances relationships. Feedback is important in the learning process because it identifies and reinforces strengths; it also identifies and corrects errors and performance weaknesses. If delivered correctly, feedback can significantly improve the learning process and outcomes. Think back to a time when you received or delivered constructive feedback that was helpful and reflect on why that communication was helpful. Conversely, think back when you delivered or received unhelpful feedback that was challenging and reflect on why the nature of that communication was not helpful. Providing feedback to learners is a key component of adult learning and teaching practices.

Feedback is information that highlights the dissonance between the actual and the intended result. Feedback is information communicated to the learner that is intended to modify the learner's thinking or behavior for the purpose of improved learning (26). Ende states that "Without feedback, mistakes go uncorrected, good performance is not reinforced, and clinical competence is achieved empirically or not at all" (27). Feedback should be both given and solicited. Giving feedback is the communication to a person or group about how their behavior is affecting you. Receiving feedback is the reaction by others about how your behavior is affecting or influencing them.

Listed are some tips, guidelines, and pitfalls for feedback:

1. Feedback requires direct observation, based on objectives and established standards and program requirements. Avoid subjective or arbitrary feedback or comments about personality or attitude that are difficult to change.
2. Plan to limit feedback to three or fewer points during each feedback session.
3. Begin feedback by reminding the resident why the feedback meeting is important, and that the sole purpose of feedback is for continuing professional development in other words, the feedback is improvement oriented.
4. Always begin feedback by first asking for the resident's self-assessment. For example, ask, "How do you think you are doing?" It is more effective when you ask the receiver to give feedback first using his or her own language, which will make your job easier; this also enhances buy-in and receptivity of feedback.
5. Feedback should be well timed to coincide immediately or soon after observed behavior.
6. Feedback should be based on independent, unbiased, firsthand data and personal observations, and not on assumptions, judgments, or what you may have perceived or heard from other second or third parties, such as other attendings or residents.

7. Feedback must be constructive and improvement oriented; it must clearly address specific behaviors a learner can control that are remediable.
8. Constructive feedback behavior fulfills 2 criteria: *descriptive (specific)* and *nonjudgmental*. Describe/articulate specifically what needs to be done to correct the problem. Phrase feedback in descriptive nonjudgmental language that is aimed at specific performance standards or recommendations, not generalizations. Feedback pertains to decisions and actions, and not to personality.
9. Align feedback to developmental readiness of the resident and expected level of task difficulty. Consider expected Dreyfus levels of resident development and milestones trajectory.
10. Express how the observed behavior or task affected you or the patient, and the resulting positive or negative consequences if the mistake is corrected or not corrected. For example, *why* was what you observed great, and conversely, why was what they did incorrectly not a desired behavior?
11. Closure and summarization: Conclude the feedback session by summarizing and ensuring comprehension and agreement, as well as plans for follow-up steps. Reinforce desirable behaviors, repeat corrective actions, and offer encouraging comments.

BEDSIDE TEACHING

One of the weakest and most challenging clinical teaching venues is at the bedside. While resident learners tell us that hands-on bedside teaching is one of the most valuable medical education teaching components, the amount of teaching that takes place at the bedside has been questioned. Typically, during morning rounds, the focus is on administrative aspects of patient care such as patient orders, chart notes, laboratory values, factual information, and whether certain management steps were done or not done. Bedside teaching should be more than administrative management. The bedside must be used for two purposes: patient care and teaching. The patient at the bedside provides an excellent opportunity to teach and integrate the six core competencies. The attending must use the bedside encounter time to (a) demonstrate, observe, or verify technical skills; (b) explain and bridge fundamental principles, concepts, and theory to patient care; (c) demonstrate humanistic and professionalism skills, patient-centered care and empowerment, and team-based care; and (d) provide feedback, evaluation, and reinforcement of directly observed skills, including communication, between patient, resident, and team.

CASE PRESENTATIONS WITH FEEDBACK—SNAPPS AND MICROSKILLS MODELS

Case presentations are one of the most ubiquitous teaching methods used during residency. Clinical case presentations must satisfy 2 purposes: *taking care of the patient* and *teaching the resident*. Case presentations are powerful tools, if executed properly, to integrate the core competencies and teach patient safety and quality, evidence-based PM&R, communication skills, cost-effectiveness, evaluation, and feedback. Case presentations can be effective clinical exercises when attending and resident roleplay. Highlighted further are two effective models for conducting case presentation teaching: Wolpaw's SNAPPS (28), and MICROSKILLS (29), also known as the "One-Minute Preceptor."

The acronym SNAPPS is a six-step case presentation process, described in Figure 4.4:

What makes SNAPPS so effective is that it is *learner-centered*, as the resident presenting the case takes the active lead role driving his or her own learning. This is ideal for a typical 6- to 7-minute case presentation, and ideal even for outpatient settings or clinics. SNAPPS, as described in Figure 4.4, facilitates the transition from a *teachable moment* to a *learning moment*, when both attending preceptor and resident learner contribute and share the educational engagement responsibility. The attending preceptor in SNAPPS assumes the role of "Coach," facilitating the presentation, being a resource, and responding to uncertainties and cues observed from the resident. The preceptor should not provide the answers, but instead ask the resident to independently seek the information and discuss it with the preceptor in a follow-up encounter. Educators have known that the act of looking up information has more learning impact than if the answer were provided on the spot from the attending. SNAPPS is intuitive, easy to learn, and internalized in no time.

Another clinical teaching technique is the five-step MICROSKILLS, also known as the 1-Minute Preceptor model, an effective clinical teaching tool described in Figure 4.5:

Step 1: Solicit a tentative clinical commitment by the resident. This allows the preceptor to gain insight into the learner's skills in medical reasoning and medical judgment by asking for two to three differential diagnoses (hypothesis triggering) and the next plan of action. The preceptor must avoid the

MODEL FOR CASE PRESENTATIONS
■ **S**ummarize briefly the history and findings
■ **N**arrow the differential to two to three: Focus on what's most likely
■ **A**nalyze the differential: Give your rationale
▪ Justify/Compare/Contrast alternatives
■ **P**robe the preceptor by asking questions
▪ Uncertainties? Difficulties? Alternative approaches?
• What else should I include in the differential diagnosis?
• I'm not sure how to examine the knee…?
■ **P**lan management for the patient's medical issues—at least attempt
■ **S**elect a case-related issue for self-directed learning—commit to regular patient-based learning

FIGURE 4.4 SNAPPS Six-Steps (28)

1. Get a Commitment—*What do you think is going on? Differential diagnosis? What do you want to do next in your workshop?*
2. Probe for Supporting Evidence—*What led you to that conclusion? What else might be important?*
3. Provide Feedback—Reinforce. *The history was very clear and... A better way to think about this is...*
4. Teach General Rules—*This sort of problem reminds us that...*
5. Correct mistakes and discuss next steps

FIGURE 4.5 The 1-Minute Preceptor: Five-Step Microskills for Clinical Teaching (29)

temptation for providing cues or prematurely providing the answers (avoid premature closure and pattern recognition), or providing cues for the diagnosis (not fully allowing the resident to entertain alternative hypotheses) and management, so a bad example would be for the attending to say, "Sounds like brachial plexopathy..., don't you think?"

Step 2: Probing for rationale or supporting evidence by asking, "What else did you consider? Why did you rule out that choice? What are the major findings that led to that conclusion?" Encourage the resident to think along evidence-based medicine to justify the strength of the diagnosis, treatment, or management, citing, for example, Cochrane systematic reviews or other meta-analysis review studies. Here the attending preceptor must avoid providing his or her opinion, such as: "I disagree....Do you have any other ideas? This seems to be a classical case of radiculopathy."

Step 3: Repeat and reinforce what the resident learner did right and articulate why by providing effective feedback. For example, the attending might say, "You considered the socioeconomic factors for this patient's medication and discharge to home instructions. That will greatly contribute to patient adherence." On the other hand, a poor example might be to say, "You are right....That was a good decision....Nice presentation," without explaining why.

Step 4: Make a generalizable teaching point such as concepts, general rules, and principles, or find teaching points that can be applied to other clinical situations. For example, the preceptor might say, "The goal of bladder retraining of patients with SCI are....You will have to ensure free flow of urine... empty the bladder generally every 3 hours with consistently <100 ml of residual urine volume...reestablish urinary continence." Similarly, a bad example would be for the attending to say, "The patient has severe cystitis. Don't start bladder retraining."

Step 5: Correct mistakes and discuss next steps with further corrective feedback. A good example would be for the attending to say, "I agree that the patient is probably drug seeking, but we still need to do a careful history and physical exam." Conversely, a poor example would be to reprimand the resident personally or subjectively, rather than being objective, by saying, "You did what?...What were you thinking?"

Avoid making the following common errors when conducting the One-Minute Preceptor (five-step Microskills) clinical teaching: (a) taking over the case; (b) not allowing for sufficient wait time for resident response or being too impatient with interaction; (c) extending the interaction into a mini-lecture; (d) asking leading questions that cue to a particular answer; and (e) pushing the learner too hard.

Questioning Levels

Benjamin Bloom, the father of Bloom's Taxonomy (30), defined 3 major levels of questions:

Taxonomy Level 1: Recall/recognition
Taxonomy Level 2: Simple interpretation of data
Taxonomy Level 3: Problem-solving

In both the Microskills and SNAPPS models of clinical teaching, pay attention to your questioning techniques. Aim questions to uncover a learner's preexisting knowledge and level of understanding. Avoid relying mostly on closed questions that require rote memory-oriented answers, classified as Taxonomy 1, and referred to as "convergent" questions. Instead, focus on higher cognitive-level open-ended questions, Taxonomies II and III, which require data interpretation and problem solving, respectively, also referred to as "divergent" type questions.

Bordage (31) and Connell (32) posited that the hallmark and art of clinical teaching is for the faculty preceptor to get into the resident's mind to articulate his or her thinking during case presentations, and to express and explore uncertainties and difficulties, while allowing the resident the opportunity to learn from mistakes. By doing so, the attending can check and explain the resident's assessment and decision-making competencies.

Procedural Skills Teaching (Psychomotor Skills)

Historically, teaching hands-on technical and procedural skills followed the "See One, Do One, Teach One" model, but this practice is no longer valid. Hands-on technical skills training in the age of core competencies and milestones should follow the "See Some, Practice Many With Feedback, Do One Competently" model. McLeod (33) elucidated the seven principles for proper teaching of procedural skills, listed as follows:

1. *Plan Ahead*: Review competencies and objectives related to instruction of the procedure. Then, assess the learner's previous background and current performance level by direct observation. Use procedural checklists, where entire procedures are broken down into chunks of critical steps, component parts, tasks, procedural steps, segments, or subsets. Such a checklist might include "advance preparation," "instrumentation," "initiation of procedure," "administration of procedure," and "termination of procedure." Good checklists contain five to nine items, and it is best to use several checklists. Checklists must be easy to use, precise, and efficient. Gawande (34) and Nance (35) provided ample convincing evidence in surgery that use of checklists reduces morbidity, mortality, and medical errors; prevents complications; and saves lives.

2. *Demonstrate Procedure*: When you demonstrate the procedure, you are also modeling the skills. We are well into the age of simulations in medicine. Use of simulations is dramatically on the rise in medical and surgical education, and is commonly used when demonstrating, teaching, and evaluating procedures. Simulations are defined as the disaggregation of clinical experience with the real patient in a safe environment that cannot harm the patient. Simulations allow for medical/surgical errors with only "virtual morbidity." The purpose of simulations is both learning and assessment. There are many journals, centers, and membership societies representing medical simulations (*Medical Simulation, The Internet Journal of Medical Simulation, SimLEARN National Center, Simulations in Healthcare, Anesthesiology, Critical Care, Surgery*, Association of Standardized Patient Educators [ASPE], and Society for Simulation in Healthcare [SSH]).

    Some simulations might include SIM MAN (high-fidelity instruction-driven simulator mannequin), OSCEs, virtual patients or SPs (simulated patients, trained actors), and other high-fidelity instruments. When demonstrating procedures, which could be real time or videotaped, make explicit commentary and provide an explanation during the demonstration; for example, what is it that makes what you do work and why? Articulate principles, tricks, and pitfalls. Do allow for questions during the demonstration. Using models and video demonstrations enhances performance and practice.

3. *Allow for Deliberate Practice*: Ericsson (36) submits that deliberate practice is most effective only when it is combined with coaching and feedback during the learning experience. Intentional or effortful practice of a procedure combined with immediate feedback, followed by debriefing used as a Teaching Moment, is most effective in teaching technical skills. Ask a learner to use a checklist when performing a skill. Deliberate practice is when you observe the resident learner in action under progressive supervision, allow for repetitive and iterative practice (doing it over and over again to reach competency), get the resident to describe/verbalize what he or she is doing and why, and what one is seeking to observe, then encourage self-assessment and reflection.

4. *Provide Feedback*: Coaching and proctoring are important components of teaching feedback. As a coach, you are there to make learners perform the procedure well and keep them out of trouble, and not to set them up for failure. Use the checklist items when providing feedback and evaluation. On direct observation, the checklist might reflect "Done Correctly," "Incomplete/Done Incorrectly," and "Not Done." Feedback must be timely, constructive, and frequent. Be specific and descriptive with your feedback. Ensure feedback is nonjudgmental and performance/competency/objective based. Integrate the content of skills exercise to material presented in other parts of the curriculum, such as didactics, in order to bridge what they need to learn and do. Make sure you evaluate their final performance.

5. *Self-Assessment*: Encourage a learner to self-assess perceived level of skill, and to self-assess areas requiring improvement. This might require that the learners be videotaped and have them observe and critique themselves performing. Allow the resident progressive responsibility and begin to fade or progressively decrease supervision (moving along ACGME's defined supervision levels from "direct" to "indirect" to "oversight") when you feel they are ready to assume that role. Allow enough time and opportunity for the resident learner to internalize skills and work out his or her own ways of doing things.

6. *Procedure Complexities*: Allow for practice under complex and less-than-ideal conditions. This can be accomplished by altering and ensuring variability in the complexity of the procedure or technical skills.

7. *Modify Teaching Approach*: Be prepared to modify or alter your teaching approach based on your observation of the learner who might be unprepared or deficient with basic skills expected for his or her level of competency.

EVALUATION AND SUPERVISION

One of the expected major roles of the faculty attending is continuing assessment of the resident's competencies while at the same time providing supervision.

The six core competencies were adopted by ACGME, primarily targeting the resident. However, the ABMS also adopted the core competencies as components of primary certification in core specialties and subspecialties, as well as MOC for physicians in practice. So one assumption for faculty development should be to expect that faculty be held to the same core competency expectations as residents and fellows. Core competency expectations must equally apply to faculty, and include the key skills that make us faculty, such as leadership, teaching, excellence and safety in patient care, support through the learning environment, and supervision and feedback.

Accurate, timely, fair, and honest evaluations are critical to the development of the resident. Effective evaluation identifies gaps between current and expected (desired) competency-based goals, objectives, and individual performance, taking into account Dreyfus levels and milestones.

An unfortunately common problem endemic in U.S. medical education with faculty evaluations of residents is the inconsistency between their verbal assessment communicated to others and what they record and document on the evaluation forms. Roberts and Williams (37) submit that often learners with performance deficiencies are unjustifiably passed on to the next rotation, instead of being asked to remediate, repeat a rotation, or be dismissed. It is important for faculty to recognize that there are hidden costs of not failing residents who deserve to be held back or even failed. Promoting and certifying poorly performing residents is unfair to the public, society, and the profession.

There are typical challenges or pitfalls for reasons why faculty avoid confronting a resident with problems. Some of these, articulated by Franklin Medio (38), include (a) not wanting to upset a resident, or not knowing how a resident will react, or not acting, thinking this would destabilize relationships established with a resident, or even jeopardizing careers. Instead, faculty ought to look at this issue as a "teaching moment" or "learning moment" that confronts and corrects the problem, rather than attacking the person; (b) concerned about legal implications; however, GME-related lawsuits are rare and if you are following the established institutional standards and procedures, this should not be a concern; (c) you as faculty or supervisor might be implicitly or explicitly contributing to the problem and wish to avoid transparency in admitting or recognizing fault; remember, professionalism is a required core competency for both resident and faculty, and being proactive and taking the initiative for acknowledgment of fault in the best interest of the resident is being professional and demonstrates role modeling for professionalism; and (d) reducing the gravity of the problem by perceiving the problem to go away without intervention or feeling that it is "too late" to insist on corrective action; recognize problems early on and immediately address with corrective action and follow-up expectations.

Formative and Summative Evaluation

There are two major categories of evaluation: (a) formative and (b) summative. Features of (a) *formative evaluation* include identifying areas for improvement; early detection of problems during the learning process; identifying developmental needs and developmental readiness; diagnostic and improvement progress-oriented assessment in teaching and learning; helping residents uncover and act upon strengths and limitations or weaknesses; typically not considered part of final evaluation or resident's work performance records; and feedback on degree to which knowledge, skills, and attitudes/values are being mastered.

(b) Qualities of *summative evaluation*, on the other hand, require final judgment and decisions about a resident's performance and competency, and is part of the learner's formal appraisal and becomes a permanent record. Summative evaluation certifies and validates mastery, progress, and competency at the end of the learning experience, such as an end-of-rotation, semiannual evaluation, and final (summative) competency-based evaluation; these require documentation and verification during the final period of education that the resident has demonstrated sufficient competence to enter practice without direct supervision. A common mistake in summative evaluation is when the evaluator is not careful or thoughtful when evaluating; he or she may evaluate everything the same and generalizes an individual's performance, also referred to as the "halo" effect (e.g., all "2s" or all "5s" on a Likert scale). If this occurs, it calls into question the validity and reliability of the assessment instrument.

Through the CCC, Annual Program Evaluation (APE), and the Program Evaluation Committee (PAC), ACGME expects formal documented evaluation of the resident, the faculty, and the program as a whole. There are different evaluation tools for each of the six core competencies commonly used in GME. Some of these are global competency rating evaluation; semiannual evaluations; multisource feedback, also known as 360-degree (attempt for at least 8 people, self, and conduct at least two rounds per year); RO&CA; mini-clinical evaluation exercise (Mini-CEX); chart stimulated recall (record/chart review); OSCE; SP (effective for instruction on dealing with difficult patients, delivering bad news, or dealing with angry patients and families); self-assessment; patient surveys; in-training or in-house quizzes and examinations such as the American Academy of Physical Medicine and Rehabilitation (AAPM&R)'s SAE or American Association of Neuromuscular & Electrodiagnostic Medicine (AANEM). Self-Assessment Examination (SAE) oral examinations; and final summative evaluation submitted to the specialty board. The ACGME recommends aiming to use at least 10 evaluation instruments. NEW INNOVATIONS is a common learning management system to capture, document, summarize, and inform evaluations.

A comprehensive listing and descriptions of assessments are illustrated in Appendix 2.

Under the ACGME's NAS, current evaluation methods illustrated earlier that are being used by programs may continue to be used. Others will be retrofitted to match the milestones, and other tools will be phased in as they are developed. The CCC will utilize assessment data, including faculty attending assessments of residents while on rotation, self-assessments, peer evaluation, and multisource assessments by nurses and other health professionals. The CCC will present each resident for evaluation and will be required to provide evidence as to his or her competence.

Competency-Based Evaluations

Assessment tools must be accurate, useful, practical, and relevant. Listed further are some common evaluation instruments that can be used to evaluate the six core competencies:

Patient Care: global assessment, direct observation, RO&CA, formal oral examination, in-training examination, multisource 360, Mini-CEX, patient surveys, OSCE, simulations, record/chart review, review of drug prescribing, and structured case discussions. Evaluators for these could be faculty members, program director, attendings, supervisors, allied health professional, patients/family members, self, peer residents, and others.

Medical Knowledge: global evaluation, direct observation, in-house or in-training cognitive examination, OSCE, oral examination, record/chart review, review of drug prescribing, structured case discussions, and anatomic models and simulations. Evaluators for these could be faculty members, program director, supervisors, self, peers, and others.

Practice-Based Learning and Improvement: direct observation, global assessment, RO&CA, project assessment such as QI project, multisource 360, record/chart review, in-training examination, models and simulations, and OSCE. Evaluators for these might be faculty members, attending supervisors, program director, allied health professional, families, peer residents, self, and others.

Interpersonal and Communication Skills: multisource 360, direct observation, global assessment, RO&CA, OSCE, patient surveys, simulations, formal oral examination, in-training examination, and project assessment such as QI project. Evaluators for these might be program director, faculty member, patient/family member, self, peer resident, and others.

Professionalism: multisource 360, direct observation, patient survey, global assessment, and project assessment such as

QI project. Evaluators for these might be allied health professionals, program director, faculty attending, supervisors, patient/family member, self, peer resident, patient surveys, and others.

Systems-Based Practice: project assessment such as QI project, global assessment, direct observation, structured case discussions, multisource 360, and RO&CA. Evaluators for these could be program director, allied health professional, faculty member, supervisor, self, peer residents, patient/family member, and others.

SUPERVISION

Quality supervision is the anchor of sound medical education. Clinical supervision is a complex developmental process in the formation of professional identity and competence. Supervision must promote professional development while ensuring patient safety and prevention of adverse events. The major goal of supervision is to meet the resident's needs for increasing responsibility, competence, and autonomy/independence.

Supervision and entrustment are pillars of faculty obligation. Supervision can be defined by the acronyms "MOTIVATED EDUCATORS," represented as follows.

MOTIVATED	EDUCATORS
Manager	**E**ngaged
Open to new ideas	**D**iplomatic
Thoughtful	**U**nderstanding
Innovative	**C**ounselor
Visible	**A**dvocate
Approachable	**T**eacher
Troubleshooter	**O**rganizer
Empathic	**R**esourceful
Disciplined	**S**cholarship

Supervision of residents encompasses two goals: (a) meeting resident's needs for increasing responsibility, competence, and autonomy/independence and (b) engaging in a complex developmental process in the formation of professional identity and competence. "The privilege of progressive authority and responsibility, conditional independence, and a supervisory role in patient care delegated to each resident must be assigned by the program director and faculty members" (ACGME, Common Requirements, VI.D). ACGME expects coordination of resident supervision and graded authority and responsibility to exercise supervision at 3 levels: *direct supervision* (supervising faculty physically present with the resident and patient), *indirect supervision* (direct supervision immediately available or available by phone or electronic modalities), and *oversight* (supervising attending is available to provide review of procedures/encounters with feedback provided after care is delivered).

In a national survey of 36 residency programs, Baldwin (39) studied how residents viewed their clinical supervision and informs us that "what happens during work hours, and what it does to residents matters more than the work hours themselves; and residency experiences are defined by the complex interactions of program characteristics and individual capacities." Some of the problems residents have reported related to supervision include lack of supervision, too little time teaching, excessive workload, amount of scut work, not enough time to think, not enough support personnel, difficulty accessing patient records, underreporting of work hours, lack of computer access, and excessive on call.

Key effective skills in supervision by attendings demonstrate the following 6 characteristics: observation, feedback, coaching, organization/time management, patience, and good bridgers of prerequisite information linked to real-time setting. As with any skill, supervisory skills require intentional deliberate practice and reinforcement, or regression and even extinction may set in.

Current concern about patient safety has heightened adequacy of clinical supervision as a major issue. In the age of NAS, a new understanding of supervision by both faculty and resident is required. The challenge in resident supervision is to balance autonomy with supervisory tasks, and for graduated responsibility in preparing residents for independent practice. Numerous barriers pose a hindrance to effective supervision, including ethical implications, to what is known as the "hidden or informal curriculum," described by Hafferty (40), a medical sociologist. The hidden or informal curriculum is what is not spoken openly, but displayed in the clinical arena that residents observe happening and replicate as "approved behavior." Some examples are not listening carefully to the patient, poor communication and relationship-building skills, and lack of caring and empathy.

ACGME defines the three major levels of supervision (common requirements VI.D.3) and examples illustrated in Figure 4.6: (a) direct, (b) indirect, and (c) oversight.

RIME and Other Models of Supervision

A major challenge with supervising residents is the ability to match the necessary level of supervision to the resident's Dreyfus levels with respect to competence, needs, and abilities at that particular time during their development, PGY 1, 2, 3, or 4.

Faculty attendings can identify the level of supervision a resident or fellow needs, drawing upon several models of supervision available: (a) Pangaro's (41) *RIME model*, (**R**eporter, **I**nterpreter, **M**anager, **E**ducator); (b) *Stages of Learning Model (4,5)* (Unconscious Incompetence, Conscious Incompetence, Conscious Competence, Unconscious Competence); (c) *Dreyfus (3) Model* (Novice, Advanced Beginner, Competent, Proficient, Master); and (d) Hersey-Blanchard's (42) *Situational Leadership Model* (Enthusiastic Beginner, Disillusioned Learner, Reluctant Learner/Cautious Contributor, Expert/Self-Reliant Achiever). The Dreyfus and Stages of Learning Models were addressed earlier in this chapter.

The RIME model is a popular and practical tool that can be applied when determining the level of supervision a resident

Level	Definition	Example
Direct	Attending has direct contact with patient and is physically present with the resident in providing care	EMG
Indirect with direct supervision immediately available	Attending is physically within hospital and is immediately available to provide direct supervision	Attending physiatrist rotating between services
Indirect supervision with direct supervision available	Attending not physically present within hospital but is immediately available by other means of communication (e.g., phone, paper) to provide direct supervision	Discussions with attending physician who is at home while residents are with patient or on call in house
Oversight	Attending reviews care that was delivered by resident after the fact with feedback	Consults

ACGME Standards, 2011

FIGURE 4.6 Types of Supervision

TABLE 4.2 Pangaro's RIME Model

ROLE OF RESIDENT	PGY LEVEL	SUPERVISION LEVEL
Reporter	PGY 1 (Internship)	Resident identifies all or most of the information and relates to them well, but cannot integrate them with basic knowledge to make a diagnosis or interpretation of the problem
Interpreter	PGY 2	Resident identifies all or most of the critical information about the patient and can form a cohesive, integrated vision of the patient and problem, but cannot identify the diagnostic or therapeutic steps or struggles with formulation of this
Manager	PGY 3	Resident identifies the key information, forms a cohesive vision of the patient, and takes the next step of identifying to the team the important diagnostic and therapeutic plan for the patient
Educator	PGY 4	Resident identifies the key information, forms a cohesive vision and plan for the patient, takes the next step in identifying through reading new or unusual diagnostic or therapeutic plans, and shares them with the team

requires based on his or her needs. This model is illustrated in Table 4.2.

Peel (43) illustrated in Figure 4.7 a representation of superimposed similarities of these four models of supervision, and correlated them with the ACGME Supervision Levels (direct, indirect, oversight), with the required amount of support across instruction and feedback. The lower right quadrant is a typical PGY 1 intern; the top right quadrant is the typical PGY 2 resident; the top left quadrant is the PGY 3; and the lower left quadrant represents the graduating PGY 4.

Education of both residents and faculty on supervision is necessary and expected by ACGME. An excellent instructional resource and guiding principle for education of faculty and residents on supervision are the acronym *SAFETY and SUPERB* models developed by Farnan and Arora (44). These two models can be used as rules of thumb for teaching effective supervision.

High ↑ Support ↓ **Low**	Cautious contributor Conscious Competence Manager Competent *Indirect (available)*	Disillusioned beginner Conscious Incompetence Interpreter Advanced beginner *Indirect (immediately available)*
	Self-reliant achiever Unconscious Competence Educator Proficient/expert *Oversight*	Avid beginner Unconscious Incompetence Reporter Novice *Direct*
	Low Instruction & feedback High →	

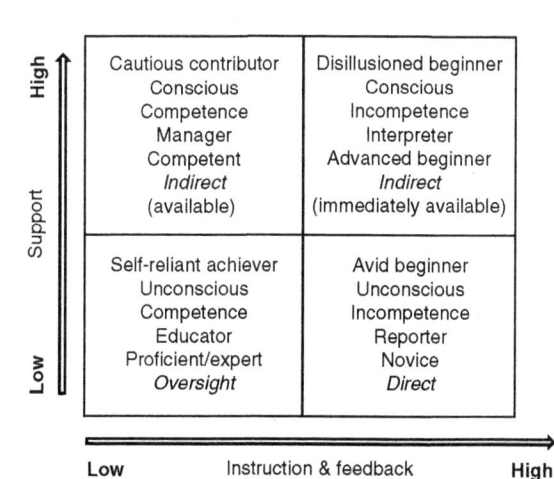

FIGURE 4.7 Representation of Models of Supervision Levels

SAFETY: This is an education model to guide *residents* when to seek attending input.

S*eek attending input early*: To prevent delays in appropriate care, involve your attending early. Attendings are legally responsible for patient care.

A*ctive clinical decisions*: Contact your attending when an active clinical decision must be made such as transfer to surgery, ICU, or another service; invasive procedure; or adverse event.

F*eel uncertain about clinical decisions*: To feel uncertain about clinical decisions is normal. It is expected that a resident should contact his or her attending if one is not sure about a specific decision.

E*nd of life care or family/legal discussion*: Such complex discussions determine the course of patient care. Patients and family should also know that the attending is aware of the discussion.

T*ransitions of care*: Errors often happen during patient transitions. Seek attending input when patient is being discharged or transferred to the ICU, another service, or another hospital.

Y*ou need help with the system/hierarchy*: Despite your best efforts, system complexities and the organization might hinder patient care. Attendings can help expedite care through direct attending involvement with consultants and necessary staff.

SUPERB: This is an education model to guide *attendings* in their supervisory roles.

S*et expectations for when to be notified*: Alert your resident that you expect to be contacted if the patient is being discharged, transferred to the ICU, going to surgery or another service, or expires.

U*ncertainty is a time to contact*: It is normal for a resident to feel uncertain about clinical decisions. Ask your resident to contact you during circumstances of uncertainty about a specific decision.

P*lanned communication*: Set up a specific recurring time to talk before the resident leaves the hospital each day, or during call nights. If a resident gets busy or forgets, the attending will contact the resident.

E*asily available*: Inform the resident how he or she can reach you, by page, phone, and so on.

R*eassure resident not to be afraid to call*: Let your resident know that calling you is not a sign of weakness, or not to feel that you would think this is a stupid question, and that it is OK to wake you up for notification. The attending would rather know what is going on.

B*alance supervision and autonomy for resident*: Tailor supervision for level of resident experience expected. For example: "I want you to be able to make decisions about our patients, but I also know this is your first month as a resident so I will follow closely." Supervision should be tailored to emphasize autonomy for more senior residents.

MENTORSHIP

The term mentor is derived from the character name in Homer's Iliad & Odyssey in Greek mythology, 800 BCE. Mentor was a confidant and trusted advisor to Odysseus, who relegated the responsibility of raising his son, Telemachus, to Mentor while fighting the Trojan wars, 11 to 13th centuries BCE.

Mentorship is a pyramidal relationship that embeds attributes of a guide, coach, preceptor, role model, and ultimately a mentor at the apex, as illustrated in Figure 4.8.

Despite the fact that mentorship is such a fundamental part of medicine, there is limited literature about mentorship in medicine. Most of the studies on mentorship emerge from the fields of education, social sciences, business, and the military. Role modeling behaviors is a central characteristic of effective adult learning practice.

Mentors can support clinical, research, teaching, and administrative missions. In one study by Kirsling (45), among benefits expressed by mentees, 88% indicated that mentors advanced their careers. In another study, Palepu (46) demonstrates that (a) higher career satisfaction scores were indicated for those with mentors, (b) awards for research grants are more likely awarded to faculty with mentors, and (c) research skills and preparation were rated higher for those with mentors.

When asked what mentors do for medical residents, mentees (protégés) say: longitudinal enduring relationships; self-awareness and self-mastery; setting expectations, goals, and priorities; committing to learner and acting as colleagues; opening doors; motivation; approachability and accessibility; support and encouragement; development-oriented feedback; focusing on personal growth and learning leading to change; minimizing hierarchy; and increasing communication, morale, and spirit.

Medical residents have described mentors as sages; docents; those who challenge learners to use their capabilities to be their best; providers of insights and reflections; creators or renewed and expanding ways of thinking; those who impact life pathways and guide explorations. Those who had mentors believe that their mentors were responsible for advancing their careers and resulted in higher career satisfaction. Mentors listened with the heart, served as appropriate role models, self-disclosed, and provided a safe harbor, a place to retreat and regroup when necessary.

Mentorship is a key attribute in medicine that medical students, residents, and fellows expect to learn from and aspire to model. The mentor provides a mirror to the learner protégé.

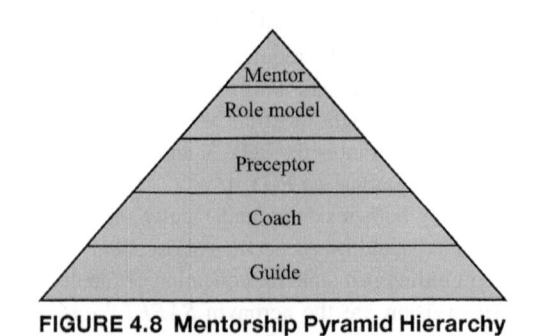

FIGURE 4.8 Mentorship Pyramid Hierarchy

Mentors set high standards. Many professional medical organizations support mentorship programs for their members and colleagues. Education on mentorship and coaching for faculty and resident development activities can be demonstrated and practiced with exercises and case studies conducted around workplace experiences, followed by debriefings.

One of the most rewarding aspects of mentoring is the personal satisfaction of "giving back" and "passing it on." Mentorship is multidirectional in that mentoring never stops—it is both up and down and across all levels of the endeavor. When a mentee asks a mentor how to pay him or her back, the response from the mentor is, "You don't—you just pass it on"! The mentor appears at the start of the journey when the novice mentee is most afraid and uncertain, and in most need of guidance. The mentor's authority and power are considerable at this point. The mentor holds the keys to membership in the world to which the mentee aspires. By the same token, the mentor knows when to retreat and fade away, allowing the protégé center stage as the mentee becomes his or her own teacher when prepared.

Mentors and mentees seek areas of mutual interest, forging symbiotic and synergistic relationships that lead to increased productivity, scholarship, and academic advancement as a result of the relationship (45,46). Mentoring allows seeing the world through professionally younger lenses. Indirectly, academic departments and institutions also benefit from the mentoring relationship through increased visibility and team productivity. Mentees progress to become recruits and magnets for more mentors, again reflecting positively on the institutions where they were trained or worked. Working with mentees also leads to development of future professional and institutional collaborations.

Essential to mentoring habits are reliance on mutual trust and respect, the ability to model and stimulate curiosity, the ability to speak freely and authentically, being flexible, allowing space for uncertainty, humility, and the ability to minimize judgments and promote reflective practice. It is important to stand by and be present for your protégé, and allow him or her to fail. The mentee learns from failing, but knows that the mentor is there to support him or her and celebrate the mentee's successes. Being upfront with your intent and commitment to set up your mentee for success is imperative. Mentors must share their expectations and values, be patient, and be enthusiastic and passionate about their success. Demonstrating the capacity to evaluate and assess a mentee's performance and progress commensurate with effective critique; feedback, both positive and negative; support and encouragement; and sharing insights is fundamental. In return, the mentor must also seek feedback from mentees about themselves.

CONCLUSION

In summary, everything discussed in this chapter is indicative of predisposing or enabling factors that facilitate and enhance learning, called *teachable moments*. Teachable moments are defined as "teaching to learner's learning needs," and are those inadvertent moments the teacher takes to explain a concept that captures the learner's particular interest. Perception and awareness of cues, signals, hints, and questions from the learner that trigger proper timing/setting for teaching and learning may result in powerful and lasting learning outcomes.

Teachable moments, and the corollary, *learning moments*, define the art and skill of an effective teacher who can translate content into meaningful terms for that particular learner in his or her developmental readiness stage, related to his or her immediate needs, work responsibilities, relevance, interests, and concerns, while ensuring it is appropriate for that particular context/setting. Listed further are 16 practical applications to guide you when teaching or learning:

1. Teach to what the learner needs to know.
2. Create a safe learning settings/environment where a learner can freely express his or her learning needs and interests.
3. Recognize moments and opportunities when a learner signals a need to learn. Get to know your learner and what makes him or her "tick."
4. Create a learning culture and environment that emphasizes learner-to-teacher accountability.
5. Develop skills in knowing what the learner is thinking, or the uncertainties and difficulties he or she is expressing, and teach to those needs.
6. Use and gather evidence as an educator while teaching, the same way that you seek data before diagnosing and managing/treating patients.
7. As attending, refrain from spoon-feeding and providing answers, as that prevents signals and cues from the learner to teach to.
8. Learn to seamlessly make the transition from taking care of patients (patient care/management) to tending to/managing the learner's education needs.
9. Use the questions, hints, cues, and signals from the learner to in turn develop questioning techniques to assess learner thinking, quandaries, obstacles, and impediments. This promotes reflection, lifelong learning, and self-assessment—three pillars for continuing professional development.
10. Develop questioning methods that aim at improving critical thinking, problem solving, and judgment skills. For example, during case presentation by resident, for each chief complaint/symptom, ask a learner to develop three differential diagnoses.
11. Allow a learner to make mistakes as long as you use the mistakes as a teaching source to elicit and probe, and to make that a teaching point. Learning from mistakes is a powerful teaching/learning tool.
12. Effective teaching moments are amplified by giving and receiving proper, appropriate, timely, and systematic feedback on an ongoing basis.
13. Effective teaching moments are amplified by proper and systematic role modeling and mentorship.
14. Cultivate a teaching practice to repeat, reinforce, observe, reflect on, and learn from those teaching moments.
15. Teaching moments can be either planned and intentional, or incidental and unplanned. The effect may be the same.
16. As Socrates said, "Effective teaching practice is to seize the opportunity to be a 'midwife to learners pregnant with ideas'."

Parker J. Palmer, a pioneer at ACGME, said "We are who we teach."

SELF-EXAMINATION QUESTIONS
(Answers begin on p. 367)

1. Characteristic of the NAS are tracking and reporting of "milestones" and developmental "levels." Which of the following statements best describes NAS's "Level 4"?
   A. Expected competency at the "Expert" level, typical of an advanced resident or practicing physician
   B. Developmentally based proficiency that the resident is expected to demonstrate with progression from "Advanced Beginner" to "Competent"
   C. Expected competency of a resident who is prepared for unsupervised practice
   D. Developmentally based proficiency of residents who "Know what they know and don't know that they know"
   E. Supervision matched to role of resident as "Manager" in Pangaro's RIME model

2. You are expected to be able to use scientific evidence to investigate, evaluate, and improve patient care practices for your own professional development. Which of the following core competencies does this expectation relate to?
   A. Systems-based practice
   B. Medical knowledge
   C. Professionalism
   D. Practice-based learning and improvement
   E. Patient care

3. Lifelong learning and self-assessment are hallmarks of adult learning (andragogy) and continuous professional development. Pedagogy is the science of how children learn. Which of the following is most characteristic of adult learning?
   A. It is learner-directed and uses reflective learning
   B. Learners' prior experience is not a factor for learning
   C. Learners do not prefer immediate feedback
   D. Learning is relevant and practical with direct application
   E. A and D

4. Bulstrode and Hunt proposed the "BOGERD" model that has valuable applications in GME. Which of the following statements best describes the application of this model?
   A. Learner-centric strategy to conduct case presentations
   B. An educational contract between resident learner and attending supervisor
   C. Implement on Day 1 of rotation
   D. B and C
   E. A and B

5. Which of the following statements describes elements of an effective strategy to conduct case presentations?
   A. SNAPPS six-step model where the resident presenting the case takes the active lead
   B. PDSA cycle where the resident presenting the case takes the active lead
   C. Kern's six-step approach to case presentations where the faculty preceptor presenting the case takes the active lead
   D. Kirkpatrick's four-level model for evaluating case presentation learning outcomes
   E. Moore's conceptual model of faculty preceptor taking the lead in conducting case presentations

6. Which of the following statements most accurately describes ACGME's most desirable suggested best methods for evaluation of competencies?
   A. Professionalism: 360 multisource, patient survey, global rating, OSCE
   B. Systems-based practice: SP, 360 multisource, patient survey, global rating
   C. Interpersonal and communication skills: OSCE, SP, patient survey, procedure/case logs
   D. Patient care: patient survey, OSCE, SP, MCQ examination
   E. Practice-based learning and improvement: record review, chart-stimulated recall, portfolios, MCQ examination

7. As an attending you are responsible for supervising a PGY 2 resident. Using Pangaro's RIME model of supervision and ACGME's definitions of levels of supervision, which of the following best fits expectations of this resident?
   A. Manager, indirect (available) supervision
   B. Reporter, direct supervision
   C. Interpreter, indirect (immediately available) supervision
   D. Educator, oversight supervision
   E. B and D

8. According to the SUPERB/SAFETY model for resident and attending education on supervisory roles, which of the following statements best represents this model?
   A. SAFETY refers to attending supervisory roles, while SUPERB refers to resident asking for attending input
   B. SUPERB refers to attending supervisory roles, while SAFETY refers to resident seeking attending input
   C. Setting expectations for when to be notified is part of the SUPERB guide
   D. Seeking attending input early is part of the SUPERB guide
   E. B and C

9. Identify a QI project that you are interested in exploring. Discuss how you would go about conducting the project using the PDSA (Plan, Do, Study, Act) cycle, and framing each cycle component.

10. Identify a journal club article that you are interested in presenting. Describe how you would present the article directed with questions and discussion to cover content in the 6 core competencies, as applicable.

REFERENCES

1. Epstein RM. Assessment in medical education. *N Engl J Med.* 2007;356:387–396.
2. Nasca TJ, Phillibert I, Brigham T, et al. The next GME accreditation system—rationale and benefits. *N Engl J Med.* March 15, 2012;366:1051–1056.

3. Dreyfus S, Dreyfus H. A five-stage model of the mental activities involved in directed skill acquisition. California University Berkeley Operations Research Center [monograph on the Internet]; 1980. Retrieved from http://www.dtic.mil/dtic/index.html. Downloaded February 11, 2014.
4. Whitman N. *Creative Medical Teaching*. Utah: University of Utah. Department of Family and Preventive Medicine. University of Utah School of Medicine; 1990.
5. Maslow AH. A theory of human motivation. *Psychol Rev.* 1943;50(4):370–396. Retrieved from http://psychclassics.yorku.ca/Maslow/motivation.htm.
6. http://www.acgme.org/CLER/. Accessed February 11, 2014.
7. Weiss KB, Wagner R, Nasca TJ. Development, testing, and implementation of the ACGME Clinical Learning Environment Review (CLER) program. *J Grad Med Educ.* 2012;4(3):396–398.
8. http://www.acgme.org/assets/pdf/NASFAQs.pdf. Accessed November 7, 2013.
9. Swing SR, Clyman SG, Holmboe ES, et al. Advancing resident assessment in graduate medical education. *J Grad Med Educ.* 2009;1(2):278–286.
10. Top 10 Characteristics of the Four Generations Currently in the Workforce. Compiled from the following sources: Ethics Resource Center. Supplemental Research Brief, 2009 National Business Ethics Survey; Hammill G. Mixing and managing four generations of employees. FDU Magazine Online. Winter/Spring 2005. http://www.fdu.edu/newspubs/magazine/05ws/generations.htm; Jones D. Co-existing with Millennials: what we and they need to know to improve the workplace. Presentation at AMWA (American Medical Writers Association) Annual Conference, Jacksonville, October 21, 2011.
11. Boyer E. *Scholarship Reconsidered: Priorities of the Professoriate*. San Francisco, CA: Jossey-Bass; 1990. The Carnegie Foundation for the Advancement of Teaching.
12. Boyer E. Scholarship a personal journey. In: Glassick C, Huber M, Maeroff G, eds. *Scholarship Assessed: Evaluation of the Professoriate*. San Francisco, CA: Jossey-Bass; 1997. An Ernest Boyer Project of the Carnegie Foundation for the Advancement of Teaching.
13. Glassick C, Huber M, Maeroff G. *Scholarship Assessed: Evaluation of the Professoriate*. San Francisco, CA: Jossey-Bass; 1997. An Ernest Boyer Project of the Carnegie Foundation for the Advancement of Teaching.
14. DaRosa DA, Skeff K, Friedland JA, et al. Barriers to effective teaching. *Acad Med.* April 2011;86(4):453–459.
15. Darkenwald GD, Merriam SB. *Adult Education: Foundations of Practice*. New York, NY: Harper & Row, Publishers, Inc.; 1982.
16. McLeod SA. Jean Piaget; 2009. Retrieved from http://www.simplypsychology.org/piaget.html. Accessed February 11, 2012.
17. Knowles M. *The Modern Practice of Adult Education*. rev. ed. Chicago, IL: Association Press/Follett Publishing Co.; 1980.
18. Knowles M. What we know about the field of adult education. *Adult Educ.* 1964;14(2):67.
19. Houle CO. *Patterns of Learning: New Perspectives on Life-Span Education*. San Francisco, CA: Jossey-Bass Inc., Publishers; 1984.
20. Davis D, O'Brien MA, Freemantle N, et al. Impact of formal continuing medical education: do conferences, workshops, rounds, and other traditional continuing education activities change physician behavior or health care outcomes? *JAMA*. Sept 1, 1999;282(9):867–874.
21. Foley RP, Smilansky J. *Teaching Techniques—A Handbook for Health Professionals*. New York, NY: McGraw-Hill, Inc.; 1980.
22. http://www.virtuala.com.au/essays/learningpyramid.html. Accessed February 13, 2014.
23. https://www.cpp.com/products/mbti/index.aspx. Accessed February 13, 2014.
24. http://etec.ctlt.ubc.ca/510wiki/Kolb's_Learning_Styles_Model_and_Experiential_Learning_Theory. Accessed February 13, 2014.
25. Bulstrode C, Hunt V. Assessment at the end of training—a necessity nuisance. *Surgeon.* February 2004;2(1):28–31.
26. Shute VJ. Focus on formative feedback. *Rev Educ Res.* 2008;78(1):153–189.
27. Ende J. Feedback in clinical medical education. *JAMA*. 1983;250:777–781.
28. Wolpaw TM, Wolpaw DR, Papp KK. SNAPPS: a leaner-centered model for outpatient education. *Acad Med.* 2003;78:893–898.
29. Neher JO, Gordon KC, Meyer B, Stevens N. A five-step "microskills" model of clinical teaching. *J Am Board Fam Pract.* July–August 1992;5(4):419–424.
30. Bloom BS. *Taxonomy of Educational Objectives, Handbook I: The Cognitive Domain*. New York, NY: David McKay Co Inc; 1956.
31. Bordage, G. Why did I miss the diagnosis? Some cognitive explanations and educational implications. *Acad Med.* 1999;74:10.
32. Connell KJ, Bordage G, Chang RW, et al. Measuring the promotion of thinking during precepting encounters in outpatient settings. *Acad Med.* October 1999;74(10 Suppl):S10–12.
33. McLeod PJ, Steinert Y, Trudel J, Gottesman R. Seven principles for teaching procedural and technical skills. *Acad Med.* October 2001;76(10):1080.
34. Gawande A. *The Checklist Manifesto: How to Get Things Right*. New York, NY: Metropolitan Books; 2009.
35. Nance JJ. *Why Hospitals Should Fly: The Ultimate Flight Plan to Patient Safety and Quality Care*. Bozeman: Second River Healthcare Press; 2008.
36. Ericsson KA. Deliberate practice and the acquisition and maintenance of expert performance in medicine and related domains. *Acad Med.* 2004;79:S70–S81.
37. Roberts NK, Williams RG. The hidden costs of failing to fail residents. *J Grad Med Educ.* June 2011;127–129.
38. http://www.med.wayne.edu/news_media/streamingmedia/curriculum/gme/download/Remediation%20Handouts.pdf.
39. Baldwin DWC, Daugherty SR, Ryan PM. How residents view their clinical supervision: a reanalysis of classic national survey data. *J Grad Med Educ.* March 2010;2(1):37–45.
40. Hafferty FW, Franks R. The hidden curriculum, ethics teaching, and the structure of medical education. *Acad Med.* November 1994;69(11):861–871.
41. Pangaro L. A new vocabulary and other innovations for improving descriptive in-training evaluations. *Acad Med.* November 1999;74(11):1203–1207.
42. Hersey P, Blanchard, KH. *Management of Organization Behavior: Utilizing Human Resources*. Englewood Cliffs, NJ: Prentice-Hall; 1988.
43. Peel JL, Nolan RJ. UTHSC. Presented at the 2013 ACGME Annual Educational Conference, San Antonio.
44. Farnan JM, Johnson JK, Meltzer DO, et al. *J Grad Med Educ.* March 2010;2(1):46–52. http://www.stritch.luc.edu/cme/sites/default/files/cme/2_8_11_farnan.pdf
45. Kirsling RA, Kochar MS. Mentors in graduate medical education at the Medical College of Wisconsin. *Acad Med.* 1990;65:272–274.
46. Palepu A, Friedman RH, Barnett RC, et al. Junior faculty members' mentoring relationships and their professional development in US medical schools. *Acad Med.* 1998;73:318–323.

Appendix 1

```
                    ACGME/ABMS CORE
                    COMPETENCIES TOPIC
                         GUIDE
```

Patient care/procedural skills

The ability to provide patient care that is compassionate, appropriate, and effective for the treatment of health problems and the promotion of health

- Data gathering
- History taking
- Patient examination
- Diagnosis
- Interpretation/decision making/assessment
- Management/treatment plans
- Preventive care
- Procedures

Medical knowledge

The knowledge about established and evolving biomedical, clinical, and cognate sciences and the application of this knowledge to patient care

- General principles/concepts/theories
- Applied basic sciences
- Applied biomedical sciences
- Applied clinical knowledge
- Epidemiology and psychosocial behavioral sciences
- Population-based medicine/public health

Practice-based learning and improvement

The ability to investigate and evaluate patient care practices, appraise and assimilate scientific evidence, and improve their patient care practices

- Benchmarks/best practices
- Practice-related quality improvement (QI)/practice improvement (PI)
- Evidence-based practice/medicine
- Continuing professional development (CPD)/continuing medical education (CME)
- Practice self-assessment
- Information technology/medical informatics
- Teaching and learning and lifelong learning

Interpersonal and communication skills

The ability to demonstrate interpersonal and communication skills that result in effective information exchange and collaboration with patients, their families, and other health professionals

- Teaming and team leadership skills (interprofessional, multidisciplinary)
- Effective communicator and listener
- Caring, respectful behavior
- Written and verbal communication skills
- Educating/counseling patients and family members
- Teaching skills

Professionalism

Reflects a commitment to carrying out professional responsibilities, adherence to ethical principles, and sensitivity to a diverse patient population

- Physician accountability, initiative
- Humanistic qualities (respect, courtesy, compassion, integrity, trust)
- Professional ethics
- Sociocultural factors (sensitivity to culture, diversity, gender, age, disabilities)
- Lifelong learning
- Advocacy for and responsiveness to patient needs
- Commitment to excellence and quality care, proficient
- Mentorship and role modeling

Systems-based practice

An awareness of and responsiveness to the larger context and system of health care, and the ability to call effectively on other resources in the system to provide optimal health care

- Patient safety
- Cost-effective care/socioeconomics
- Management of resources
- Medical errors
- Continuity of care
- Health care delivery and systems of care models
- Utilization issues
- Risk management
- Electronic medical records and record keeping
- Management and leadership skills

Appendix 2

ACGME Competencies: Suggested Best Methods for Evaluation

COMPETENCY	REQUIRED SKILL	RECORD REVIEW	CHART STIM. RECALL	CHECKLIST	GLOBAL RATING	SP	OSCE	SIMULATIONS & MODELS	360° GLOBAL RATING	PORTFOLIOS	EXAM MCQ	EXAM ORAL	PROCEDURE OR CASE LOGS	PATIENT SURVEY
Patient Care	Caring and respectful behaviors			3		1			2					1
	Interviewing			1		2	1		3					
	Informed decision making		1	2			2					2		
	Develop and carry out patient management plans	2	1	2	3			2	3					
	Counsel and educate patients and families			3		1	1		2					1
	Performance of procedures a) Routine physical examination			2		1	1	1						
	b) Medical procedures			1	3				2				3	
	Preventive health services	1				2	1			3			2	
	Work within a team			3	3				1					

(continued)

Appendix 2
ACGME Competencies: Suggested Best Methods for Evaluation *(continued)*

COMPETENCY	REQUIRED SKILL	RECORD REVIEW	CHART STIM. RECALL	CHECKLIST	GLOBAL RATING	SP	OSCE	SIMULATIONS & MODELS	360° GLOBAL RATING	PORTFOLIOS	EXAM MCQ	EXAM ORAL	PROCEDURE OR CASE LOGS	PATIENT SURVEY
Medical knowledge	Investigatory and analytic thinking		1					2	3			1		
	Knowledge and application of basic sciences							2	3		1	1		
Practice-based learning and improvement	Analyze own practice for needed improvements	2	2			2	2	3	3	1				2
	Use of evidence from scientific studies	1	1			3	2			1	1	1		
	Application of research and statistical methods		2	3	3					1	3			
	Use of information technology					2	2		1	1			2	
	Facilitate learning of others			2	3				1	3				
Interpersonal and communication skills	Creation of therapeutic relationship with patients			3		1	1		2					1
	Listening skills			3		1	1		2					1

Professionalism	Respectful, altruistic		3	1	2		3	1
	Ethically sound practice	2	2		2	1	3	2
	Sensitive to cultural, age, gender, disability issues	2	2	1	3	1	3	2
Systems-based practice	Understand interaction of their practices with the larger system			2		1	3	
	Knowledge of practice and delivery systems	2		3			2	1
	Practice cost-effective care	3	1		2	2		
	Advocate for patients within the health care system		3	2	1	1	2	1

ACGME/ABMS Joint Initiative Attachment/Toolbox of Assessment Methods© Version 1.1 September 2000
Ratings are 1, the most desirable; 2, the next best method; 3, a potentially applicable method.
Toolbox of Assessment Methods© Accreditation Council for Graduate Medical Education (ACGME) and American Board of Medical Specialties (ABMS). Version 1.1.

Sarita Patel
William Donovan
Adrian Cristian

5: Ethical Considerations in the Practice of Rehabilitation Medicine—A Contextual Framework for Addressing Ethical Issues in Rehabilitation Medicine

GOALS

Reflect a professional commitment to carrying out ethical responsibilities and an adherence to ethical principles in the practice of rehabilitation medicine.

OBJECTIVES

1. Demonstrate knowledge of the general principles of ethics and the steps in the methodology of making ethical decisions in the practice of rehabilitation medicine.
2. Demonstrate knowledge of ethical issues in clinical research.

Physiatrists, like other physicians, are taught throughout their training to place the interests and welfare of their patients as their primary responsibility and are familiar with the mantra to "first do no harm." However, all physicians, practicing in this day and age, realize that there are societal factors that continuously insert themselves into the physician's judgment as to what may be the best for one's patient, particularly when treating those with chronic conditions as physiatrists do.

Issues such as quality of life, "futile care," advance directives, funding limits imposed by insurance companies, state and federal governments, and other factors can impact the physician–patient relationship, not only during acute care and acute rehabilitation but also afterward. Such factors can confront the physiatrist and his or her team with the need for decisions far more complex than just how to create an environment and treatment plan geared to maximize and maintain health and quality of life.

It is clear from the examination of different cultures from both a historical and contemporary point of view that doing the right thing by physicians has varied among civilizations and societies depending upon the resources available and prevailing beliefs (1).

The purpose of this chapter, therefore, is not to provide a universal roadmap to guide the physiatrist's judgment for every decision he or she must make, but to provide a vista of general principles to keep in mind and to provide directions to resources when engaged in research and clinical care.

HISTORY

From the dawn of history, humankind has been concerned with doing the "right thing." However, this has been expressed in many forms from primitive societies, including the barbaric, such as allowing human sacrifice, up to civil societies employing the rule of law. In essence, then, it can be said that the "right thing" corresponds to behaviors that the societies in which people live regard as acceptable. Over the years, whether the societies were nomadic, agricultural, peaceful, or hostile, rules of behavior were established and communicated to members by word or script. Those who developed a script that allowed information to be passed through generations and that subsequently allowed archeologists to discover them include civilizations on both hemispheres such as those of ancient Egypt and the Mayas of Mesoamerica (2). These and many other discoveries have confirmed people's desire for order and rules to live by. One of the most famous was the Ten Commandments in Mosaic Law. Others can be found in religious texts such as the Hindu Vedas, Judaic Torah, Christian Bible, and Islamic Quran, or among the edicts of pharaohs and kings who were regarded as gods. Regardless, divine inspiration was deemed by believers to be the source (3).

Since the invention of Gutenberg's printing press in the 15th century and the emergence of philosophers and scientists, especially during the period of the European Enlightenment, authors, particularly John Locke, David Hume, John Stuart Mill, and others, have expanded on rules found in the religious texts, often by exercising reason without claiming divine inspiration (4). Basically, their emphases, particularly those concerned with government and civil society, were on instilling in all people, regardless of their faiths, the virtues of trust, respect, responsibility, and consideration for one another, all of which can be expressed in a single term: ethics (5). Authors who have written on the topic of ethics as it applies to the healing arts are many, the more notable among them being Hippocrates, John Gregory, Francesco Petrarch, and, more recently, Lawrence McCullough (1).

Unlike the holy books mentioned earlier, these authors did not claim divine inspiration but rather were guided by reasoning that people could achieve and live peacefully in a civil society. The idea that the people could do this by governing themselves instead of being governed by a monarch or dictator was a doctrinaire concept until Thomas Jefferson and his 4 colleagues proclaimed it could be done by a nation. Governments, he said, derive "their just powers from the consent of the governed" (6). Since the "governed" rarely speak with one mind, democracies required that all agree to abide by the will of the majority as opposed to the will of a ruler.

Subsequently, as more nations adopted democratic governments with separation of religion and state, it was inevitable that ethics (i.e., doing the right thing in civil societies) became more mutable depending on the choices of the majority. Thus, sometimes disparities can arise between rules created by the majority and rules that certain believers avow were created by God. Abortion is one example. To believers of many faiths, even though it may be legal and ethical to the majority, it is morally wrong and therefore abjured for "how can God be wrong?" Therefore, their views are more refractive to change (1). Some have therefore prescinded those rules of behavior derived from the spiritual from those derived from the secular realms. By placing the former under the rubric of morals and the latter under the rubric of ethics, it is possible to avoid the pejorative of "situational ethics." By designating ethics as derived from man's rules as far as the majority is concerned, it can be realized that ethics can vary within any society, be they primitive or advanced. On the other hand, if we designate morals as derived from God's rules as far as believers are concerned, the era and prevailing opinion do not matter.

When the ethics decided by the majority conflict with the morals held by a minority, avenues are available for resolution through debates, essays, blogs, even litigation and the political process, but not violence since that would be a primitive society's methodology, not a civil one's. It would seem the more diverse a society is, the more Jefferson's ideals could be realized, since as James Madison said, it would be harder for one segment of society to force its will on all the others, thereby fostering compromise—a concept often referred to as "Madisonian democracy" (7).

As health care providers, we have guidelines for ethical behaviors reached by the majority of our representatives in our professional organizations. As will be discussed later, these have evolved over the years and have been influenced by the Hippocratic Oath, the Nuremberg Code, the Helsinki Declarations, the Belmont Report, the Code of Federal Regulations, and the American Medical Association's Code of Medical Ethics, which was compiled by its Council on Ethical Affairs (1). The latter provides guidance for hospital ethics committees and all health care providers. It contains judicial rulings and expert opinions garnered by the committee and is an extremely valuable resource that provides precedence for difficult decisions one may be called upon to make, helping the reader to balance patient autonomy with professional beneficence in the society in which we live.

RESEARCH

All practicing physiatrists, whether contributing to the advancement of knowledge in physical medicine and rehabilitation (PM&R) through research activities or keeping pace with that advancement through educational activities, have an interest in the quality of research, whether it might be anticipated as a breakthrough, simply an explanation of an existing phenomenon, or an improvement upon a prevailing treatment.

Durable, credible research must be planned, executed, and analyzed honestly, without bias. The Nuremberg Code, crafted in 1947 following the atrocities committed by Nazi researchers, provided the first path for medical investigators to follow.

Its essential ingredients include: (a) The voluntary consent of the human subject is essential. There must be no coercion, no deceit, and a full explanation of risks and benefits by the investigator(s). (b) There must be an expectation of gaining useful knowledge. (c) Thorough preliminary studies must be conducted before human studies. (d) Avoidance of unnecessary suffering or injury is mandatory. (e) There must be no expectation of death or injury as an outcome. (f) Risks must not exceed benefits. (g) Proper facilities are required. (h) Only qualified investigators should be allowed. (i) Subject(s) can withdraw at any time. (j) Investigator must terminate the study if harm seems likely (8,9).

Subsequently, the Helsinki Declarations, the Belmont Report, and 45CFR46, as noted earlier, expanded on the Nuremberg Code's initial guidelines. 45CFR46 is now law in the United States, which all investigators in the health care realm must abide by. Academic researchers also have on-site guidance from their Institutional Review Board (IRB). Manufacturers of pharmaceuticals and medical devices have the Food and Drug Administration (FDA) to advise them and approve their discoveries before they can be marketed (1).

While these entities provide guidance to researchers for the conduct of credible, scientific research, other regulatory and advisory bodies exist to protect the subjects and the public. The Office of Research Integrity (ORI) in the U.S. Department of Health and Human Services (HHS) has published "points for discussion," which addresses many pitfalls that should be avoided in order to conduct research that is honest and unbiased. These include research misconduct (lying during any phase of the research), conflicts of interest (receiving payment from a commercial entity whose product one is investigating), data mismanagement ("bending" the data to fit a preconceived expectation), pressures to speed discovery and bring products to market, inadequate mentoring and supervision (by the principal investigator and the institution), and inadequate peer review by the institution and/or the scientific journals (being alert for "repetitive publications, supernumerary authorship, lack of disclosure, among others") when publication of a manuscript is sought (10,11).

Readers of published work and society in general expect that researchers will truthfully report what works, what just seems to work, what seems not to work, and what doesn't work at all. Patients in turn trust that practitioners will truthfully convey that information to them. The National Academy of Sciences (NAS) has warned that trust in all these areas must never become eroded or the results would be calamitous; they have even expressed the fear that such breaches of ethics could be an expression of a broader pattern of deviation from traditional norms. Hopefully, this fear will never materialize (12). Nevertheless, realizing that scientists are only human and subject to the same temptations and distractions as anyone else, the ORI has pointed out that the responsibilities to safeguard adherence to honesty and ethical principles lie with several entities along the research process. The scientists, their scientific societies, and their institutions must create an environment where carelessness, apathy, and fraud will not be tolerated. This applies not only to the conduct of the research but also to other aspects such as honest time–effort reporting, full disclosure of funding sources, priorities of coauthorship, conflicts of interest, pressures to ascend the academic or business ladder, and/or overstatement of conclusions, which must not be allowed to stain the process of discovery (13). By adherence to such ethics in research, a proper example is shown to young investigators as they in turn strive to seek funding, secure space and recognition, and pass on their respect for honesty in their investigations to their protégés.

ETHICAL FRAMEWORKS

Medical ethics has been described as a system of moral principles that apply values and judgments to the practice of medicine. As a scholarly discipline, medical ethics encompasses its main practical application in clinical settings (14).

The art and science of medical ethics on one level is fundamental and timeless and on the other level is constantly changing and evolving. A physician must be prepared to reaffirm what is fundamental, like the physician–patient relationship, and learn new emerging issues ranging from confidentiality and electronic medical records to human biological material and research.

From genetic testing before conception to dilemmas at the end of life, physicians, patients, and their families are called upon to make difficult decisions. This section is intended to facilitate the process of making ethical decisions in clinical practice. The goal is to teach and explain underlying ethics principles, as well as the physician's role in society and with colleagues, with specific issues and cases relevant to the field of physical medicine and rehabilitation.

In the medical profession, practitioners put the welfare of the client or patients above their own welfare. Professionals have a duty that might be thought of as a contract with society. As modern medicine brings a plethora of diagnostic and therapeutic options, the interaction of the physician with the patient and society becomes more complex, potentially raising the ethical dilemmas. The American Board of Internal Medicine and the European Federation of Internal Medicine have jointly proposed that medical professionalism should emphasize 3 fundamental principles (15).

1. Primacy of patient welfare
2. Patient autonomy
3. Social justice

The professional responsibility of *primacy of patient welfare* emphasizes the fundamental principle of the medical profession and helps provide a moral compass that is not only grounded in tradition but also adaptable to the current practice of medicine. The physician's altruism must not be affected by economic, bureaucratic, and political challenges that are faced by the physician and the patient.

Altruism is a central trust factor in the physician–patient relationship. Market forces, societal pressures, and administrative exigencies must not compromise this principle. There is concern, however, that, in today's health care environment, the physician's commitment to the patient is being challenged by the conditions of medical practice and external sources (16).

The principle of *patient autonomy* asserts that physicians make the recommendations, but patients make the final decisions. The physician is an expert advisor who must inform and empower the patients to base a decision on scientific data and how this information can and should be integrated with the patient's preferences. The patient's decision about his or her care must be paramount, as long as those decisions are in keeping with ethical practice and do not lead to demands for inappropriate care. Only in the latter part of the 20th century did the public begin to view the physician as an advisor.

The importance of *social justice* symbolizes that a patient–physician interaction exists in a community or society. The physician has a responsibility to the individual patient and a broader society to promote access and to eliminate the disparities in health and the health care system. This calls upon the profession to promote a fair distribution of health care resources (17).

Physicians should work actively to eliminate discrimination in health care, whether based on race, gender, socioeconomic status, religion, or any other social category. Physicians who use these and other attributes to improve their patent's satisfaction with care are not only promoting professionalism but also reducing their own risk for liability and malpractice (18).

METHODOLOGY—ETHICAL DECISION MAKING

The Decision-Making Process

The conjoint decisions made by patients with physical impairments and disabilities and their physicians can profoundly affect the quality of a patient's life. When physicians and patients face ethical decisions about emotionally charged issues such as withholding or withdrawing life-sustaining treatment, the *model of shared decision making* can ensure communication and respect for the multiple and sometimes conflicting needs of physicians, patients, and family members.

When making decisions about ethical issues, all parties should be involved in an identified decision-making process. One example of such a decision-making process was developed by the Hastings Center and has been modified for use in this book (19).

Steps in the Process for Making Ethical Decisions
1. Professional commitment
2. Systematic evaluation of the case
3. Communication among all involved
4. Consider ethical principles
5. Make the decision
6. Document the decision
7. Implement the decision and change it when necessary
8. Respond to objections and challenges

Step 1. Professional Commitment
Every physician has an obligation to uphold ethical and professional behavior and redouble his or her commitment to professionalism, especially when dealing with ethical dilemmas. The American Board of Internal Medicine, ACP-ASIM Foundation, and the European Federation of Internal Medicine have jointly proposed "the charter on Medical Professionalism" (15) that comprises three principles and ten commitments:

A. *Three fundamental principles*: (a) primacy of patient welfare, (b) patient autonomy, and (c) social justice.
B. *Ten professional commitments*: (a) professional competence, (b) honesty with patients, (c) patient confidentiality, (d) maintaining appropriate relations with patients, (e) improving the quality of care, (f) improving access to care, (g) just distribution of finite resources, (h) scientific knowledge, (i) maintaining trust by managing conflicts of interest, and (j) professional responsibilities.

Step 2. Systematic Evaluation of the Case
When complicated issues require a formal decision-making process, a thorough evaluation of the patient's situation is the necessary first step. Often what appears to be a complex moral dilemma may be nothing more than a disagreement based on inaccurate or inadequate knowledge of clinical facts, biographical facts, or cultural facts. It is the responsibility of the care provider to gather all relevant information about the decision to be made. Potentially important questions to be answered are related to the aspects of clinical status, preferences of the patient, surrogate and others involved, life history, risks and benefits of proposed treatments, and decision making. Every clinical case, when seen as an ethical problem, should be analyzed by means of four topics (20).

1. Medical indications
2. Patient preferences
3. Quality of life
4. Contextual features

Adapting to this method, a practical approach in the form of a "four-box model" is organized and presented by the American Academy of Hospice and Palliative Medicine.

CLINICAL FACTS	BIOGRAPHICAL FACTS
QUALITY OF LIFE	CULTURAL FACTS

1. *Clinical Facts:*
   - What is the patient's diagnosis and prognosis?
   - How has the patient's condition changed? Are symptoms adequately controlled?
   - What is the proposed intervention?
   - What is the intention of the proposed intervention?
   - What are the potential benefits and burdens of each proposed intervention?

2. *Biographical Facts:*
   - What is known about the patient's wishes and values?
   - How does the patient describe his or her quality of life?
   - What is known about the wishes of surrogates, family members, and other involved parties?
   - Does the patient have the capacity to make decisions about medical treatments?
   - Who is involved in making the decision and what is his or her involvement?
   - What is the recommendation of the interdisciplinary team?

3. *Quality of Life:*
   - How does this patient describe his or her quality of life?
   - What brings meaning to or sustains the patient?
   - How has the patient made treatment decisions in the past?
   - What types of treatments would provide a satisfactory outcome for the patient's life?
   - What is achievable with regard to the patient's preferences?

4. *Cultural Facts:*
   - Who is this patient?
   - What are the patient's life story and primary values?
   - What is the patient's relationship with family members and significant others?
   - What are the patient's cultural, religious, and spiritual values?
   - What are the potential benefits and burdens of each alternative for the patient and family, including financial and emotional costs?
   - What are possible alternatives?
   - What are the legal considerations?
   - How will the decision affect the patient and family physically, emotionally, spiritually, socially, and economically?

This four-box model can help evaluate the vast majority of ethical dilemmas in clinical practice.

This model also provides a hierarchy to keep in mind: Clinical and biographical facts focus on what makes sense medically, respects the patient's wishes, and are given more weight than quality of life or cultural facts. The quality of life and cultural facts are not insignificant and attuned to the avoidance of unnecessary conflicts or dilemmas. The sample case analysis demonstrates how this model can be practically used.

Step 3. Communication Among All Involved
Effective communication is honest, compassionate, open, and unhurried, and it is essential to understanding and alleviating a patient's suffering. Sharing of adequate and accurate knowledge

of the patient's condition, the patient's wishes, and the potential benefits and burdens of proposed treatments, as well as consequences of nonintervention, are cornerstones of effective communication. The wishes of a competent, well-informed patient take priority over other opinions. On occasion, patients may wish to withhold information from family members or members of the interdisciplinary team. Balancing a patient's right to privacy with the family and team's need for information can present ethical dilemmas. In most cases, patients are willing to negotiate the sharing of information, a process that protects the patient's right to privacy and helps ensure the families and team's ability to intervene effectively when needed. In any case, the patient's right to confidentiality should be given great weight.

Step 4. Consider Ethical Principles

There are some main beliefs that can be invoked to address bioethical dilemmas encountered in clinical activities. These can be broadly categorized into four groups—principle based, virtue based, caring based, and respect for personhood.

A. PRINCIPLE BASED. The four generally accepted values that make up the foundation of modern medical ethics are beneficence, autonomy, nonmaleficence, and justice (21,22).

Beneficence: Promote the patient's well-being. The principle of beneficence, which is synonymous with the Hippocratic obligation to always act in the best interests of the patient, is grounded in the concept of promoting the patient's well-being. In physical and rehabilitating settings, the principle of beneficence implies positive acts, including effective treatments for physical and cognitive impairments and pain and the provision of psychosocial and emotional support.

Limitations: Although the obligation to promote a patient's well-being is basic to the physician–patient relationship, its implementation can be problematic. For example, the development of medical technologies such as ventilators and total parenteral nutrition has resulted in confusion about when and for how long such treatments should be provided to ensure a patient's well-being and the provision of ethical patient care. Their existence makes it difficult to remember that they are ethically neutral; when considered alone, medical treatments offer neither benefit nor burden. It is only within the context of applying a particular medical intervention to a specific patient that the treatment's contribution to a patient's well-being can be determined.

Autonomy: Respect the patient's self-determination. The principle of autonomy, or patient's self-determination, recognizes the right of a patient with decision-making capacity to make decisions about treatments according to his or her own beliefs, cultural and personal values, and life plan, even when these decisions differ from what has been advised or recommended by a physician.

Patient autonomy means any patient with decision-making capacity is free to reject, without coercion or fear of retribution, any form of medical therapy, including life-prolonging or life-sustaining therapy. A patient's right to refuse unwanted treatment, including nutrition and hydration, is absolute. In physical and rehabilitation settings, the principle of autonomy includes the patient's right not only to refuse a particular course of treatment but also to ask that the treatment be modified to meet other needs, such as the need for privacy, mental alertness, or care in a particular setting at a specific time.

Limitations: Although the emphasis on patient autonomy may challenge health care professionals, they are obligated to respect a patient's considered choices about treatment. Autonomy is not served when a physician makes unilateral decisions or recognizes a patient's right to make health care decisions only when those decisions concur with the physician's opinion. Furthermore, a patient's disagreement is not grounds for a determination of diminished capacity to make decisions (19).

The principle of autonomy upholds the patient's right to reject any form of medical therapy, but it does *not* extend to the patient a right to demand any and all treatment regardless of its likely benefit or cost. The principle does not require the provision of treatments that, in the judgment of the physician and the interdisciplinary team, are likely to be harmful or futile or that counter the ethical principle of justice, nor does autonomy always outweigh other ethical principles.

Nonmaleficence: Do no harm. The principle of nonmaleficence is synonymous with the Hippocratic obligation to avoid doing harm to a patient. Nonmaleficence obligates respect for the inherent worth and dignity of every patient and the avoidance of treatments and interventions that may harm them. The principle of avoiding harm is particularly applicable to patients in the physical and rehabilitation setting, many of who are frail, frightened, and vulnerable when receiving care.

The following are examples of possible violations of the principle of nonmaleficence:

- Failure to minimize the risk of iatrogenic hypoglycemia or hypotension in patients undergoing inpatient rehabilitation
- Prescribing medications that can lead to cognitive and balance impairments and subsequent falls in an inpatient rehabilitation setting
- Prolonged or inappropriate use of indwelling urinary catheters that can predispose the patient to urinary tract infections
- Failure to follow aspiration precautions in high-risk patients that can subsequently lead to aspiration-related complications
- Failure to prescribe adequate prophylaxis for prevention of venous thromboembolic events in high-risk patients
- Aggressive range of motion of limbs in spinal cord-injured patients that can lead to fractures
- Aggressive pulmonary physical therapy interventions over ribs that have metastatic lesions
- Failure to observe limited weight-bearing status precautions (e.g., patients with metastatic lesions in limbs; hip fracture repair)
- Promoting polypharmacy
- Failing to provide adequate pain relief with appropriate medications
- Failure to provide immunization in patients with spinal cord injuries and at risk for pneumonia
- Insisting that patients confront the reality of their disability
- Destroying or creating false hope
- Providing unnecessary devices.

- Failing to stop treatments when their burdens begin to exceed their benefits (e.g., continuing the provision of artificial nutrition when patients are actively dying or continuing IV fluids for dyspneic patients with congestive heart failure).

Lack of knowledge and clinical misinformation can generate apparent ethical quandaries. For example, some physicians fail to prescribe adequate amounts of pain medication because they fear that the required dosages may inadvertently affect the patient's ability to participate in physical therapy, shorten his or her life, or lead to addiction. They tend to grossly overestimate the toxicity of carefully titrated dosages of opioids and erroneously invoke the principle of nonmaleficence. Carefully titrated opioid dosages are unlikely to shorten the patient's life and may actually lengthen it when effective pain control improves appetite, eases movement, and enhances the will to live.

Justice: Provide fair allocation of resources. Justice is the principle that has come under the most scrutiny and reinterpretation since the development of traditional medical ethics. The rising costs of health care and concerns about the equitable distribution of health care resources have contributed to the development of the principle of justice as a means of addressing not only the protection of vulnerable patients but also the well-being of society (23,24). When applying the principle of justice, a physician's first obligation is to the patient, not to a committee concerned with cost cutting and economic pressures (25).

Limitations: Nonetheless, in some cases, distributive justice may appropriately limit personal autonomy when the needs of others intrude on the patient's desires (26). As the costs of health care rise, society cannot be expected to pay for futile treatments, even when these treatments are desired by the patient and family and are funded by private insurance.

It is also the obligation of the physician to use medical technology and resources judiciously. In an era of increased financial pressures, resources to offer the full complement of rehabilitation interventions (physical, emotional, psychological, and social) may become threatened. Health care professionals involved in all aspects of PM&R care must use interdisciplinary care in the most efficient and effective ways to improve a patient's quality of life and conserve resources. Neither society nor physicians are obligated to, nor should they, provide treatments that offer no reasonable expectation of benefit (27,28).

B. VIRTUE BASED. The following virtues define the character of a good physician:

- *Fidelity to trust and promise*—honoring the ineradicable trust of the patient–physician relationship
- *Effacement of self-interest*—protecting the patient from exploitation and refraining from using the patient as a means of advancing power, prestige, profit, or pleasure
- *Compassion and caring*—exhibiting concern, empathy, and consideration for the patient's plight
- *Intellectual honesty*—knowing when to say "I do not know"
- *Prudence*—deliberating and discerning alternatives in situations of uncertainty and stress.

C. CARING BASED. The ethics of caring assume that connections to others are central to what it means to be human. Caring requires receptiveness to the patient with empathy and compassion, responsibility toward the patient with actions that meet the patient's needs, and creation of an educational environment that fosters caring.

D. RESPECT FOR PERSONHOOD. Respect for personhood proposes the following:

- Treatment of patients must reflect the inherent dignity of every person regardless of age, debility, dependence, race, color, or creed.
- Actions must reflect the patient's current needs.
- Decisions must value the person and accept human mortality.

Step 5. Make the Decision

Because ethical decision making often requires consideration of complicated, emotionally charged issues, the views of all parties in this process must be respected. This includes the views of the patient or surrogate, patient's family members, attending physician, specialists, and other interdisciplinary team care providers. All parties in the decision-making process depend on effective, honest communication to recommend a course of action and achieve the goal of improving the patient's quality of life.

A. Identify the Key Decision Maker(s): The patient is the key decision maker, with authority to give binding consent or refusal of treatment regardless of family wishes as long as the patient retains decision-making capacity. The previously stated wishes of a patient with decision-making capacity do not become void when capacity diminishes; instead, they should be honored.

- If a patient with diminished decision-making capacity has completed a durable power of attorney for health care, the designated surrogate becomes the decision maker and should follow the patient's wishes.
- When a patient lacks decision-making capacity and has no identified surrogate, state statutes may identify specific family members as surrogates. If the identified person is unable or unwilling to act as a surrogate, family members should work with the physician when making decisions. If consensus cannot be reached, a single surrogate should be identified.
- When no family member is available or willing to act as a surrogate or when family members cannot agree on a single surrogate, the court can designate one. However, court proceedings rarely are necessary when all parties use effective, open communication.

B. Evaluate the Patient's Decision-Making Capacity

Competence. Physicians often misunderstand the term *competence* because it has acquired a somewhat technical but imprecise legal meaning (20). Competence refers to a person's ability to understand the nature and consequences of decisions; however, the term is restricted to describing a person's legal status. A person may be declared incompetent in business or financial matters but retain decision-making capacity to consent to or refuse medical care. A proper legal authority, usually a judge, determines competence.

Decision-Making Capacity. A patient is presumed to have decision-making capacity unless proved otherwise. In medical settings, it is the physician's responsibility to determine decision-making capacity. Capacity may change depending on the patient's condition and the complexity of the decision. To have capacity to make a specific decision, a patient needs to be able to:

- Understand relevant information and the implications, including benefits, risks, and alternatives of various treatment choices (Communication)
- Reflect on information in accordance with personal values and draw conclusions (Comprehension)
- Voluntarily make and communicate a choice to health care professionals (no Coercion)
- These can be thought of as the "three Cs" of informed consent—Communication, Comprehension, and no Coercion (29).

In clinical settings, physicians should first assess the patient's mental status and then, if necessary, look for treatable physical conditions that may be interfering with the patient's ability to process information and draw conclusions. Decision-making capacity can be temporarily compromised by conditions such as delirium, dementia, metabolic imbalances, severe pain, and life-threatening infections. Decision-making capacity may also fluctuate hour by hour because of high dosages of drugs sometimes needed to control symptoms, shifts in levels of consciousness caused by advancing disease, and psychological factors such as the patient's denial of serious illness (30).

Despite continued emphasis on a patient's right to make health care decisions, recent studies verify difficulties with assessing decision-making capacity in terminally ill patients. The method used to determine capacity may affect the outcome of the assessment. Although some professionals base their decisions about capacity on cognitive and psychological examination data, such as a patient's responses to the Mini-Mental State Examination, decision-making capacity may be unrelated to performance on mental status examinations. Other professionals base their decisions primarily on daily observations and impressions (30). Asking patients specific questions about their condition, including diagnosis and prognosis, or using hypothetical case vignettes may be a more valid approach (31). In any case, family members and other health care professionals, particularly those with day-to-day contact with the patient, should be included in the assessment process. When determining decision-making capacity, physicians should avoid excessive reliance on test scores or a single assessment of decision-making capacity.

When a patient's capacity fluctuates or is uncertain, further clarification of decision-making capacity is necessary if the physician, the patient or surrogate, and the family disagree on treatment decisions. When disagreements about treatment occur, the best course of action is to wait until the patient regains decision-making capacity. If the patient's lack of decision-making capacity is likely to continue indefinitely, the designated surrogate has the authority to make decisions as long as the patient's advance directive is followed. If an advance directive is not available, apply the patient's previously stated preferences and values (32). If these are unknown, consider the decisions a reasonable person would make under the patient's circumstances (the best interests standard) (19,33).

Step 6. Document the Decision

Documentation is critical. Whenever complex decisions are made, documentation in the patient's medical record should include information about how, why, and with whom decisions were made. It is critical that this documentation is available when needed and follows the patient across care settings. Documentation protects the interests of all involved by ensuring adherence to a decision and orderly reviews when needed (34).

For example, a decision to withhold cardiopulmonary resuscitation (CPR) must be documented to prevent resuscitation efforts during a terminal event. It can be documented in institution-specific forms such as a MOLST form—Medical Orders for Life-Sustaining Treatment or POLST form—Physician Orders for Life-Sustaining Treatment (35).

Videotaping is another way to document a patient's explanation of changes in a will. Signing the new will helps avoid legal difficulties after the patient's death.

Step 7. Implement the Decision and Change It When Necessary

When implementing decisions, it is important to recognize and acknowledge that most medical illnesses, including the dying process, are dynamic processes. The concept of time-limited trials can be helpful for patients and physicians as they work together to improve the patient's quality of life during a terminal illness (36). A time-limited trial reinforces patient participation in the treatment process and helps support the hope that an effective combination of drugs and other treatments including rehabilitation will be found.

Time-limited trials may also show that certain treatments do not achieve the goals hoped for and present an opportunity to reinforce the concept that treatment options can be altered. Because clinical facts often change, the patient's treatment plan should be revised as needed to avoid doing harm. When a decision is changed, documentation in the patient's medical record should reflect who participated in the decision and how and why the change was made. A patient or surrogate can change any decision at any time, including a decision to continue with an aggressive curative treatment, limited medical intervention, and exclusive comfort approach to care.

Step 8. Respond to Objections and Challenges

Effective, honest, and compassionate communication reduces the number of requests for bioethics consultations. However, the procedures for resolving objections and challenges should include full discussion with concerned parties and, if necessary, referral to an identified ethics committee.

A. Challenges to Determining a Lack of Capacity

Ultimately, a court determines legal competency and the capacity to make health care decisions. However, because the decision-making capacity of terminally ill patients tends to deteriorate rapidly, lengthy court proceedings rarely are practical or helpful for making clinical decisions. Ethics committees may serve as more practical intermediaries.

A patient, family member, or surrogate can challenge a determination of decision-making capacity. When a challenge arises, the importance of continued open communication and reevaluation cannot be overemphasized. If the challenge cannot be resolved, it should be referred to a psychiatrist skilled in assessing decision-making capacity.

B. **Challenging a Surrogate**
When a surrogate's designation or decision is challenged, and the matter cannot be resolved, it should be discussed at length to clarify the biographical, cultural, and clinical facts behind the challenge. Most problems can be resolved in this manner. Occasionally, a challenge must be referred to an ethics committee, but a court is rarely needed.

C. **Disagreement Among Members of the Interdisciplinary Team**
Because rehabilitative programs try to meet the patient's physical, emotional, spiritual, and social needs, the skills and resources of an entire interdisciplinary team are needed. As with any group, differences of opinion are bound to occur among members of the team. In fact, they are an expected part of the creative process of working together. When skillfully managed by a group facilitator or team leader, differences can usually be resolved in a manner that results in better patient care and professional growth for all concerned. On occasion, differences cannot be resolved by discussion. If consultation with an ethics committee or counseling by a supervisor does not resolve the problem, specific staff members may need to be reassigned.

Neither physicians nor other health care professionals are required to participate in treatments in opposition to their ethical or religious principles. However, physicians are responsible for communicating their concerns to patients and arranging for the patient's transfer (with the patient's consent) to another physician or institution if necessary.

D. **Withdrawal of a Health Care Professional or Institution**
Physicians with ethical or religious objections to providing or withdrawing treatments demanded by a patient or surrogate must communicate these concerns to the patient or surrogate and arrange for the patient's transfer of care to another physician, if necessary. If another member of the team has ethical or religious objections to a decision, the institution should honor a request for removal from the case, if necessary (37).

When a patient or surrogate is adamant about obtaining treatments that the program cannot ethically provide, as a last resort, the patient can be discharged or transferred to another institution. If a case requires transfer to another provider or institution, a referral to the institution's ethics committee and legal department should be considered.

Principle of Double Effect: Double effect is an important ethical principle designed to ensure safe and adequate patient care and to protect health care providers who treat these patients. It validates the use of treatments that are aimed at relieving suffering even in the event that these interventions may inadvertently shorten a patient's life. The intent of treatment must be to relieve symptoms, not to end life.

The four elements of the doctrine are:

1. The good effect has to be intended (pain or dyspnea relief with opioids).
2. The bad effect can be foreseen but not intended (awareness of shortening of life).
3. The bad effect cannot be the means to good effect (cannot end life to relieve dyspnea).
4. The symptoms must be severe enough to warrant taking risks. (This is proportionality.)

How Do Principles "Apply" to a Certain Case?

Principles in current usage in health care ethics seem to be of self-evident value. For example, the notion that the physician "ought not to harm" any patient appears to be convincing to rational persons. One might argue that we are required to take all of the previous principles into account when they are applicable to the clinical case under consideration. Yet, when 2 or more principles apply, we may find that they are in conflict.

For example, consider a patient who has sustained a cerebrovascular accident with resulting expressive and receptive aphasia and impaired swallowing, which makes it very difficult for him to obtain adequate hydration and nutrition. The medical goal should be to provide adequate nutrition and hydration to the patient, through the use of a feeding tube. On the other hand, surgery and general anesthesia to insert the feeding tube carries a degree of risk, and the physician is under the obligation "not to harm" the patient. The rational calculus holds that the patient is in far greater danger from harm from inadequate hydration and nutrition if we do not act, than from the surgical procedure and anesthesia associated with inserting the tube.

In other words, we have a *prima facie* duty to both benefit the patient and "avoid harming" the patient. However, in the actual situation, we must balance the demands of these principles by determining which carries more weight in the particular case. Moral philosopher W. D. Ross claims that *prima facie* duties are always binding unless they are in conflict with stronger or more stringent duties. Weighing and balancing all competing *prima facie* duties in any particular case determine a moral person's actual duty.

Although ethical principles provide a framework for discussing ethical issues, they cannot be used as straightforward guides for making clinical decisions, nor can they be ranked in any definitive manner when they appear to conflict with one another. Application of the principles and how they are balanced when they appear to conflict with one another depend on the clinical, biographical, and cultural facts of each particular case.

Two of the principles—beneficence and nonmaleficence—were based on the Hippocratic ethic, but autonomy and justice are new and appear to contradict more traditional principles in some situations. Although the principle-based approach to medical ethics is being challenged, universally accepted alternatives have not emerged. Many health care professionals believe that the principles should be respected unless a strong reason exists to overrule them. Nevertheless, difficulties may arise when the principles are applied to clinical situations.

Questions about the limitations of principle-based medical ethics have contributed to renewed interest in alternative frameworks such as virtue-based ethics, the ethics of caring, and a system of ethics based on respect for personhood described earlier. Thus, other frameworks may be required to augment the four basic principles previously outlined. Regardless, at the core of clinical fidelity lies faithfulness to persons, not adherence to disembodied principles.

ADDRESSING AND RESOLVING ETHICAL CONFLICTS

There is no formula or small set of ethical principles that mechanically or magically gives answers to bioethical dilemmas. Instead, medical practitioners should follow an orderly analytic process.

1. Practitioners need to obtain the *facts* relevant to the situation.
2. They must delineate the *basic bioethical issue.*
3. It is important to *identify all the crucial principles and values* that relate to the case and how they might conflict.
4. Because many ethical dilemmas have been analyzed previously and subjected frequently to empirical study, practitioners should *examine the relevant literature*, whether it is commentaries or studies in medical journals, legal cases, or books. With these analyses, the particular dilemma should be reexamined; this process might lead to reformulation of the issue and identification of new values or new understandings of existing values.
5. With this information, it is important to *distinguish clearly unethical practices* from a range of ethically permissible actions.
6. It is important not only to come to some *resolution of the case but also to state clearly the reasons behind the decisions,* that is, the interpretation of the principles used and how values were balanced.

Selected Ethical Issues in the Practice of Physical Medicine and Rehabilitation

Ethical issues are very common in the care of individuals living with impairments, activity limitations, and participation restrictions and they can be encountered in acute in-patient, subacute, and outpatient settings. Physiatrists are encouraged to be alert for their presence and apply the methodology described in this chapter to address ethical conflicts as they arise. Some examples are listed in Table 5.1 along with ethical principles that apply.

Sample Case Analysis

CASE. A 61-year-old man, an electrician by occupation, who was recently told of a suspected diagnosis of amyotrophic lateral sclerosis (ALS), was admitted for worsening of his right hand weakness. He says his symptoms have made it difficult to manipulate wires and grip tools when working.

Physical examination revealed right upper extremity muscle weakness, fasciculations, atrophy and hyperreflexia, and normal sensation. After further workup for ALS and excluding the treatable mimics, two experienced neurologists independently confirmed a diagnosis of ALS.

Upon learning from an "Internet search" that this is an incurable progressive disease, he felt extremely anxious. He explained his situation to his physiatrist and requested help committing suicide. When the physiatrist refused, the patient reassured him that he did not plan to attempt suicide any time soon. But when he went home, he ingested all his antidepressant medicine after pinning a note to his shirt to explain his actions and to refuse any medical assistance that might be offered. His wife and children, who did not yet know about his diagnosis, found him unconscious and rushed him to the emergency room without removing the note.

What should the care team at the emergency room do?

Clinical Data. There are two diagnoses/prognoses that merit consideration. The underlying complex neurodegenerative disease of ALS has no available treatment and a bleak long-term prognosis. However, there are effective treatments available for the acute diagnosis of drug overdose. How does the chronic diagnosis affect our response to the acute condition?

Biographical Data. We know from the patient's suicide note that he is refusing all medical treatment. However, what do we know about these statements of preference? Were they informed? Was the patient competent to make that decision? The answers to these questions remain unclear, but we do know that the patient does not have decision-making capacity for the present decision of whether to proceed with the gastric emptying. Is there a surrogate decision maker available?

Quality of Life. Life with ALS can be difficult with the onset of spasticity and cognitive abnormality. The patient was somewhat familiar with the quality of life associated with living with ALS as he researched extensively about this disease on the Internet. On the other hand, he does have a supportive family and continues to be able to work for the time being. How should the diminished quality of life that is anticipated in the future affect the current decision?

Cultural Data. Several factors in the context of this case are significant. While the patient has a legal right to refuse treatment, he is currently unconscious and his surrogate (his wife) is requesting treatment. There are also certain emergency room obligations to treat emergent conditions. How should the emergency staff weigh the various competing legal and regulatory duties?

Analysis

This is a case of treatment refusal of potentially life-sustaining treatment when the competency of the patient to decide is questionable. Also at issue is the distinction between the acute and chronic conditions of the patient.

The precedent for cases such as this one is fairly clear. When the patient's preferences are unclear, and the acute condition is easily treatable, and the harm of not treating is very great, medical teams can feel comfortable about providing the treatment for the immediate life-threatening condition, creating an opportunity to talk with the patient about his preferences regarding his chronic condition at a later time.

TABLE 5.1 Clinical Applications of Ethical Principles

ETHICAL ISSUE	PRIMARY ETHICAL PRINCIPLES INVOLVED
End-of-life care and advance directives	Principle based: autonomy, beneficence Virtue based: compassion and caring; fidelity to trust and promise; prudence Caring based: empathy and compassion Respect for personhood
Use of opioid medications in the treatment of nonmalignant musculoskeletal pain—patient wishes vs. physician recommendations and concerns	Principle based: autonomy, beneficence, nonmaleficence Virtue based: compassion and caring; fidelity to trust and promise; prudence Caring based: empathy and compassion Respect for personhood
Informed consent for treatments and research in individuals with cognitive impairments	Principle based: autonomy, nonmaleficence, justice Virtue based: compassion and caring; fidelity to trust and promise Caring based: empathy and compassion Respect for personhood
Refusal of rehabilitative treatment plan by patient against the recommendations of the physiatrist	Principle based: autonomy, beneficence Virtue based: compassion and caring
Limitations on health insurance coverage for rehabilitation resources recommended by the rehabilitation team (e.g., treatments, durable medical equipment, limits on length of stay on in-patient acute rehabilitation facility dictated by health insurance company)	Principle based: justice, beneficence, nonmaleficence Virtue based: compassion and caring Caring based: empathy and compassion Respect for personhood
Admitting a frail medically complex patient to an in-patient rehabilitation facility that cannot tolerate 3 hours of therapy per day to maintain high occupancy percentage on the in-patient rehabilitation facility	Principle based: justice, nonmaleficence Virtue based: fidelity to trust and promise; effacement of self-interest; compassion and caring; prudence Caring based: empathy and compassion Respect for personhood
Dual role of physiatrist—providing clinical care to a patient with neurologic disease as well as acting as a primary investigator in a research protocol in which that patient is a research participant	Principle based: beneficence, nonmaleficence, justice Virtue based: fidelity to trust and promise; effacement of self-interest; compassion and caring; intellectual honesty Respect for personhood
Providing unnecessary tests to a patient to increase reimbursement revenue	Principle based: beneficence, nonmaleficence, justice Virtue based: fidelity to trust and promise; effacement of self-interest

Notice that the facts of this particular case determine whether the precedent case is applicable. If the medical team was very familiar with this patient's expressed preference to refuse any medical treatment or if the available treatment for the acute condition was considerably less certain to be effective, the case could be decided differently. The patient was managed for the drug overdose and discharged home.

Two years later:

Over the course of 2 years, the patient received treatment from a team of clinicians including a psychiatrist, neurologist, and physiatrist as well as a speech pathologist, physical therapist, and occupational therapist. The management was largely supportive and directed toward relieving symptoms, prolonging independence, and improving quality of life. This time the patient gets admitted with dysphagia, weight loss, dehydration, and dyspnea associated with depressed mood and apathy. The patient was noted to have head ptosis and speech difficulties. He refuses any life-sustaining interventions for fear of further suffering, but expressed that he may want to live for his daughter's wedding, which is a few months later, if he can preserve his functions to some extent. The wife and children support the decision and are prepared to do whatever is needed.

Looking at the case in light of the aforementioned four topics at this time in the patient's life, we must consider the patient's current clinical condition, preferences, and quality-of-life indicators as well as the current contextual data.

Clinical Data (Medical Information)

Questions to consider: Consider each medical condition and its proposed treatment. Ask the following questions: Does it fulfill any of the goals of medicine? With what likelihood? If not, is the proposed treatment futile?

Data: For poor nutritional status, options include percutaneous gastrostomy (PEG) tube placement and diet counseling. For respiratory difficulty, options include initiating noninvasive positive pressure ventilation. For speech difficulty, options include recommending an augmentative communication device by speech pathologist. A physical therapist can offer exercises, braces, and adaptive devices. This admission is also an opportunity to clarify the goals of care regarding the long-term plan.

Biographical Data (Patient Preferences)

Questions to consider: What does the patient want? Does the patient have the capacity to decide? If not, who will decide for the patient? Do the patient's wishes reflect a process that is informed? Understood? Voluntary?

Reported data to consider: The patient wants to live longer but doesn't want suffering and added burden.

He has insight into his medical condition and is fully informed about different options of care.

Quality of Life

Questions to consider: What is the patient's subjective acceptance of likely quality of life? What are the views of the care providers about the quality of life? Is quality of life "less than minimal?" (i.e., qualitative futility).

Reported data to consider: The patient is OK with his current quality of life, and can go on for a few months if his clinical condition remains same. The care providers approve of his decision.

Both patient and family would like to preserve his current level of functioning and are likely to accept interventions that support their goal.

Cultural Data (Contextual Features)

Social, legal, economic, and institutional circumstances in the case can influence the decision or be influenced by the decision (e.g., inability to pay for treatment and inadequate social support).

The aspect of family/social obligation is also defining the goals of care.

These topics help clinicians understand where the moral principles meet the circumstances of the clinical case. It is advisable to review the four topics in order to see how the principles and the circumstances together define the ethical problem in the case and suggest a resolution.

It is rare that an ethical problem involves only one ethical principle. Every actual ethical problem is a complex collection of many circumstances. Good ethical judgment consists in appreciating how several ethical principles should be evaluated in the actual situation under consideration.

SELF-EXAMINATION QUESTIONS
(Answers begin on p. 367)

1. Which of the following best describes essential understanding of the Nuremberg Code?
   A. Voluntary consent of the human subject is not essential
   B. Coercion, deceit, and not explaining the risks and benefits are acceptable on the part of investigators under the right circumstances
   C. Avoidance of unnecessary suffering or injury is mandatory
   D. Risks can exceed benefits
   E. Once the subject has started participating in a study, he or she cannot withdraw from the study

2. The three fundamental principles of medical professionalism proposed by the American Board of Internal Medicine and the European Federation of Internal Medicine are
   A. Primacy of patient welfare, patient autonomy, and social justice
   B. Patient autonomy, social justice, and beneficence
   C. Physician paternalism, social welfare, and patient dependence
   D. Physician welfare, social welfare, and social injustice
   E. Physician autonomy, patient dependence, and social justice

3. Which description best characterizes the principle of social justice?
   A. Physician's primary responsibility is to ensure that patient's family has access to health care if they can afford it
   B. Physician has a responsibility to promote a distribution of health care resources only to the patients who can afford to pay for health care
   C. The physician has a responsibility to the individual patient and a broader society to promote access and to eliminate the disparities in health and the health care system
   D. Physicians don't have to promote access to health care and eliminate disparities in health care systems since this is the job of hospital administrators
   E. Physicians don't have to promote access to health care and eliminate disparities in health care systems since none exist

4. The principle of patient autonomy is best characterized by
   A. Physician determines what is in the best interest of the patient and the patient must follow recommendations
   B. Physician makes the recommendations, but patient makes the final decision
   C. The patient's wishes must be honored by the physician, regardless of whether they go against ethical practice or not
   D. Patient's family determines what is in the best interest for the patient, and physician must comply with the wishes of the family
   E. Physician makes the recommendations, and patient's family makes the decision for the patient

5. Which of the following is one of the ten professional commitments included in the Charter of Medical Professionalism?
   A. Professional incompetence
   B. Dishonesty with patients
   C. Maintaining inappropriate relations with patients
   D. Maintaining trust by managing conflicts of interest
   E. Distributing finite health care resources to those who can pay for them

6. Which of the following best describes the elements of the principle of double effect?
   A. Bad effect can be a means to a good effect
   B. Good effect does not need to be intended
   C. Bad effect cannot be the means to good effect
   D. Symptoms don't need to be severe to warrant taking risks
   E. The intent of treatment is to end life

REFERENCES

1. Donovan WH. Ethics, health care and spinal cord injury: research, practice and finance. *Spinal Cord.* 2011;49:162–174.
2. Mann CC. *1491.* New York, NY: Vintage Books (division of Random House); 2011: 242–247.
3. Bowker J. *God a Brief History.* London: Dorling Kindersley; 2002;56–373.
4. Macintyre AC. *A Short History of Ethics.* London: Routledge; 1998:11–14.
5. McCullough LB. John Gregory and the invention of professional relationships in medicine. *J Clin Ethics.* 1997;8:11–24.
6. Bernstein RB. *Thomas Jefferson.* New York, NY: Oxford University Press; 2003:15–35.
7. Labrunski R. *James Madison and the Struggle for the Bill of Rights.* New York, NY: Oxford University Press; 2006:3–23.
8. Katz J. The Nuremberg code and the Nuremberg trial-A reappraisal. *JAMA.* 1996;276:1662–1666.
9. Barondess JA. Medicine against society—lessons from the Third Reich. *JAMA.* 1996;276:1657–1661.
10. Office of Research Integrity. RCR—Points for Discussion. [Online] 2008 [cited February 22, 2010]. Retrieved from http://ori.hhs.gov/education/point_all.shtml.
11. Sigma Xi, The Scientific Research Society. *Honor in Science.* New Haven, CT: Sigma Xi; 1997:18.
12. National Academy of Sciences, National Academy of Engineering, Institute of Medicine. Responsible Science. *Ensuring the Integrity of the Research Process.* Vol. 1. Washington, DC: National Academy Press; 1992: 1–35.
13. Weber LJ, Wayland MT, Holton B. Health care professionals and industry: reducing conflicts of interest and established best practices. *Arch Phys Med Rehabil.* 2001;82:S20–S24.
14. Baker RB, Caplan AL, Emanuel LL, et al., eds. *The American Medical Ethics Revolution: How the AMA's Code of Ethics Has Transformed Physicians' Relationships to Patients, Professionals, and Society.* Baltimore, MD: Johns Hopkins University Press; 1999.
15. Project of the ABIM Foundation, ACP–ASIM Foundation, and European Federation of Internal Medicine*
16. Hafferty FW. Professionalism—the next wave. *N Engl J Med.* 2006;355:2151–2152.
17. Owens DK, Qaseem A, Chou R, et al. Clinical Guidelines Committee of American College of Physicians. High-value, cost-conscious health care: concepts for clinicians to evaluate the benefits, harm, and cost of medical interventions. *Ann Intern Med.* 2011;154(3): 174–180 (PMID:21282697).
18. Stelfox HT, Gandhi TK, Orav EJ, et al. The relation of patient satisfaction with complaints against physicians and malpractice lawsuits. *Am J Med.* 2005;118:1126–1133.
19. Hastings Center. *Guidelines on the Termination of Life-Sustaining Treatment and the Care of the Dying.* Bloomington, IN: Indiana University Press; 1987.
20. Jonsen AR, Siegler M, Winslade WJ. *Clinical Ethics: A Practical Approach to Ethical Decisions in Clinical Medicine.* 4th ed. New York, NY: McGraw-Hill, Inc.; 2010.
21. Nash RR, Nelson LJ. *UNIPAC 6—Ethical and Legal Issues—a Resource for Hospice and Palliative Care Professional.* 4th ed.; Glenview, IL: American Academy of Hospice and Palliative Medicine, 2013.
22. Gordon JS. Global ethics and principlism. *Kennedy Inst Ethics J.* 2011;21(3):251–276.
23. Beauchamp TL. Principlism and its alleged competitors. *Kennedy Inst Ethics J.* 1995;5(3):181–198.
24. Halvorsen K, Forde R, Nortvedt P. The principle of justice in patient priorities in the intensive care unit: the role of significant others. *J Med Ethics.* 2009;35(8):483–487.
25. Smith C. Between the Scylla and Charybdis; physicians and the clash of liability standards and cost cutting goals within accountable care organization. *Ann Health Law.* 2011;20(2):165–203.
26. Petrini C. Triage in public health emergencies; ethical issues. *Intern Emerg Med.* 2010;5(2):137–144.
27. Niederman MS, Berger JT. The delivery of futile care is harmful to other patients. *Crit Care Med.* October 2010:38(suppl 10):S518–S522.
28. Snyder L. American College of Physicians. Ethics Manual: 6th ed. *Ann Intern Med.* 2012;156(1, pt 2):73–104 (PMID:22213573).
29. Terry PB. Informed consent in clinical medicine. *Chest.* 2007;131(2):563–568 (PMID:17296662).
30. Scott JF, Lynch J. Bedside assessment of competency in palliative care. *J Palliat Care.* 1994;10(3):101–105.
31. Fazel S, Hope T, Jacoby R. Assessment of competence to complete advance directives: validation of a patient centered approach. *BMJ.* 1999;318(7183):493–497.
32. Luce JM. End-of-life decision making in the intensive care unit. *Am J Respire Crit Care Med.* 2010;183(1):6–11.
33. Pope TM. The best interest standard: both guide and limit to medical decision on behalf of incapacitated patients. *J Clin Ethics.* 2011;22(2):134–138.
34. Hickman SE, Hammes BJ, Moss AH, et al. Hope for the future: achieving the original intent of advance directives. *Hastings Center Rep.* 2005;(Special Repo. S26: 28–31).
35. New York State Department of Health MOLST web page http://www.health.ny.gov/professionals/patients/patient_rights/molst/. Published in June 2010. Revised May 2013.
36. Quill TE, Holloway R. Time-limited trials near the end of life. *JAMA.* 2011;306(13):1483–1484.
37. Kinzbrunner BM. Jewish medical ethics and end-of-life care. *J Palliat Med.* 2004;7(4):558–573.

---

*This charter was written by the members of the Medical Professionalism Project: ABIM Foundation: Troy Brennan, MD, JD (*Project Chair*), Brigham and Women's Hospital, Boston, Massachusetts; Linda Blank (*Project Staff*), ABIM Foundation, Philadelphia, Pennsylvania; Jordan Cohen, MD, Association of American Medical Colleges, Washington, DC; Harry Kimball, MD, American Board of Internal Medicine, Philadelphia, Pennsylvania; and Neil Smelser, PhD, University of California, Berkeley, California. ACP–ASIM Foundation: Robert Copeland, MD, Southern Cardiopulmonary Associates, LaGrange, Georgia; Risa Lavizzo-Mourey, MD, MBA, Robert Wood Johnson Foundation, Princeton, New Jersey; and Walter McDonald, MD, American College of Physicians–American Society of Internal Medicine, Philadelphia, Pennsylvania. European Federation of Internal Medicine: Gunilla Brenning, MD, University Hospital, Uppsala, Sweden; Christopher Davidson, MD, FRCP, FESC, Royal Sussex County Hospital, Brighton, United Kingdom; Philippe Jaeger, MB, MD, Centre Hospitalier Universitaire Vaudois, Lausanne, Switzerland; Alberto Malliani, MD, Università di Milano, Milan, Italy; Hein Muller, MD, PhD, Ziekenhuis Gooi-Noord, Rijksstraatweg, the Netherlands; Daniel Sereni, MD, Hospital Saint-Louis, Paris, France; and Eugene Sutorius, JD, Faculteit der Rechts Geleerdheid, Amsterdam, the Netherlands. Special Consultants: Richard Cruess, MD, and Sylvia Cruess, MD, McGill University, Montreal, Canada; and Jaime Merino, MD, Universidad Miguel Hernández, San Juan de Alicante, Spain.

Frantz Duffoo
Adrian Cristian

6: Professionalism

GOALS

Demonstrate a commitment to carrying out professional responsibilities, adherence to ethical principles, and sensitivity to a diverse patient population applicable to rehabilitation medicine.

OBJECTIVES

1. Demonstrate compassion, integrity, and respect for others, as well as sensitivity and responsiveness to diverse patient populations, including but not limited to diversity in gender, age, culture, race, religion, disabilities, and sexual orientation.
2. Role model respect for, beneficence, least harm, respect for autonomy, and justice as applicable and relevant to the practice of medicine.
3. Exhibit qualities of accountability to self, patients, society, and the profession.
4. Demonstrate how to conduct patient-centered care and patient-centered decision making.
5. Identify and discuss the 10 professional responsibilities from the Physician Charter.
6. Describe the key components of the American Academy of Physical Medicine and Rehabilitation (AAPM&R) Code of Conduct.
7. Define the terms *financial conflict of interest*, *impaired physician*, and *disruptive physician*.

Picture this scenario. A physician comes to work late and proceeds to walk into his office, sloppy in appearance. He lounges at his desk, which is cluttered with patients' files he has not reviewed yet. Then, the physician proceeds to make his morning rounds while showing a lack of interest and caring toward his patients. The physician ignores his mistakes, does not accept the advice of his colleagues, and basically does just enough to get by until he goes home. If this physician were a machine, he would meet the criteria to be recalled by his manufacturer, the way cars and other machines are recalled when they are found to be defective. Unfortunately, poorly trained physicians cannot be removed from circulation that easily.

The *Merriam-Webster Dictionary* defines *professionalism* as the skill, good judgment, and polite behavior that is expected from a person who is trained to do a job well. It also defines professionalism as the conduct, aims, or qualities that characterize or mark a profession or a professional person. The ACGME/ABMS's expectation of professionalism as a core competency is "reflecting a commitment to carrying out professional responsibilities, adherence to ethical principles, and sensitivity to a diverse patient population." The ACGME requires that program directors attest to a trainee's competence in those qualities and mode of conduct that are important to medical professionalism. The attestation can be done by documenting the abilities the trainee possesses at a given stage of his or her training (milestones) and/or by documenting what tasks the resident can be trusted to perform (entrustable professional activities). In order for program directors to attest to a trainee's competence in the medical profession (1), the trainee must first be taught how to provide compassionate care; how to show respect for patients and their relatives; and how to communicate with integrity, trust, and honesty.

Compassionate care is patient centered. Patient-centered care ensures patient safety and addresses the needs of patients rather than the self-interest of the treating physician. This model of care also takes advantage of the latest information technology to prescribe, communicate, track results, monitor performance, and facilitate performance improvement projects. Effective communication and interpersonal skills are cornerstones of physicians' professional identities, and constitute an expected ACGME/ABMS core competency (Interpersonal and Communication Skills). The successful physician must be able to establish therapeutic doctor–patient relationships.

Residents must learn to advocate for their patients, superseding self-interests and motivations, and maintain excellent patient relationships; work as a team with other providers; integrate and coordinate patient care across multiple settings; manage population health; enhance access by meeting patient needs in a timely manner; use data to improve patient care; and lead practice change and improvement. This must be done with empathy and concern for a diverse patient population without bias toward a patient's race, culture, religion, gender, or sexual orientation. In addition, residents at any institution must act as teachers of other residents and students, a role facilitated by the same skill set. They must learn how to form therapeutic physician–patient relationships via patient interviewing and physical examination. As they learn, they will show an increasing ability to communicate with other members of their health care team, including nurses, care managers, respiratory therapists, physical therapists, pharmacists, and social workers. Focused care coordination contributes to developing the ACGME/ABMS core competencies of professionalism, patient care, systems-based practice, and interpersonal and communication skills. The medical residents will learn that the patient-centered model of care strengthens the clinician–patient relationship, leading to a safer, higher quality of care; more empowered patients; and a renewal of the patient–provider relationship.

Respect comes from *respectare*, a Latin word meaning to "look again" or to "look with new eyes." Respect, along with courtesy, compassion, integrity, and trust, is part of the constellation of professionalism traits. To look with new eyes means asking clinical questions designed to elicit information from patients about their ideas regarding what they think might be wrong with them; their feelings and fears about their illness, rather than the standard questions used in everyday practice.

Kleinman and colleagues (2) published more than 30 years ago the key questions that must be asked; they are as follows:

1. What do you think caused the problem?
2. Why do you think it happened when it did?
3. What do you think your sickness does to you?
4. How severe is your sickness?
5. What kind of treatment do you think you should receive?
6. What are the most important results you hope to receive from this treatment?
7. What are the chief problems your sickness has caused for you?
8. What do you fear most about your sickness?

These types of questions will convey to the patient that the resident is able to see the nature of the problem from the patient's point of view. The residents must also be taught effective listening skills; how to understand silent body language (nonverbal communication); and how to show transparency, receptivity, and openness during communication. They must be taught to be tolerant and to be nonjudgmental about patient preferences; to learn to listen with sympathy and understanding to the patients' perception of their illness; to avoid confrontation; and to respond to each patient's unique characteristics and needs.

The 10 professional responsibilities from the Physician Charter published by the American Board of Internal Medicine Foundation and the American College of Physicians Foundation in 2002 (3,4) must be used to guide the education of residents about professionalism. They are subsequently listed in italics and each one is followed by the respective plan of action for the trainees.

1. *Commitment to professional competence. Physicians must be committed to lifelong learning and be responsible for maintaining the medical knowledge and clinical and team skills necessary for provision of quality care.* The residents must be taught how to identify areas for self-improvement and how to implement strategies to enhance their knowledge, skills, attitudes, and behaviors.

2. *Commitment to honesty with patients. Physicians must ensure that patients are completely and honestly informed before the patient has consented to treatment and after treatment has occurred. Physicians should also acknowledge that in health care, medical errors that injure patients do sometimes occur.* An entrustable professional activity based on the process of obtaining informed consent must be documented for all residents after they have been taught the knowledge, skills, attitudes, and behaviors needed to obtain informed consent.

3. *Commitment to patient confidentiality. Earning the trust and confidence of patients requires that appropriate confidentiality safeguards be applied to disclosure of patient information.* Residents must be taught the key elements of the Privacy Rule including who is covered, what information is protected, and how protected health information can be used and disclosed.

4. *Commitment to maintaining appropriate relations with patients. Given the inherent vulnerability and dependency of patients, certain relationships between physicians and patients must be avoided. In particular, physicians should never exploit patients for any sexual advantage, personal financial gain, or other private purpose.* Residents must learn how to advocate for their patients and how to maintain excellent patient relationships with empathy and compassion.

5. *Commitment to improving quality of care. Physicians must be dedicated to continuous improvement in the quality of health care. This commitment entails not only maintaining clinical competence but also working collaboratively with other professionals to reduce medical error, increase patient safety, minimize overuse of health care resources, and optimize the outcomes of care. Physicians must actively participate in the development of better measures of quality of care and the application of quality measures to assess routinely the performance of all individuals, institutions, and systems responsible for health care delivery. Physicians, both individually and through their professional associations, must take responsibility for assisting in the creation and implementation of mechanisms designed to encourage continuous improvement in the quality of care.* Residents must learn the key principles of quality improvement that include W. Edwards Deming's Plan, Do, Study, and Act (PDSA) cycle. The PDSA cycle was originally developed by Walter A. Shewhart as the Plan-Do-Check-Act (PDCA) cycle. W. Edwards Deming modified Shewhart's cycle to PDSA, replacing "Check" with "Study" (5).

6. *Commitment to improving access to care. Medical professionalism demands that the objective of all health care systems be the availability of a uniform and adequate standard of care. Physicians must individually and collectively strive to reduce barriers to equitable health care.* Residents must learn the concept of Patient-Centered Medical Home (PCMH). They must learn about National Committee for Quality Assurance (NCQA) standards for PCMH.

7. *Commitment to a just distribution of finite resources. While meeting the needs of individual patients, physicians are required to provide health care that is based on the wise*

and cost-effective management of limited clinical resources. They should be committed to working with other physicians, hospitals, and payers to develop guidelines for cost-effective care. The physician's professional responsibility for appropriate allocation of resources requires scrupulous avoidance of superfluous tests and procedures. The provision of unnecessary services not only exposes one's patients to avoidable harm and expense but also diminishes the resources available for others. Residents must learn about issues of cost–benefit analysis in medical care, fostering the ability to practice in a cost-effective manner. They must learn about the concepts of high-value care.

8. *Commitment to scientific knowledge.* Much of medicine's contract with society is based on the integrity and appropriate use of scientific knowledge and technology. Physicians have a duty to uphold scientific standards, to promote research, and to create new knowledge and ensure its appropriate use. The profession is responsible for the integrity of this knowledge, which is based on scientific evidence and physician experience. Residents must learn to cultivate a spirit of inquiry and improvement; this spirit supports both innovations in daily practice that translate into better service to patients, system improvements, and improved patient outcomes.

9. *Commitment to maintaining trust by managing conflicts of interest.* Medical professionals and their organizations have many opportunities to compromise their professional responsibilities by pursuing private gain or personal advantage. Physicians have an obligation to recognize, disclose to the general public, and deal with conflicts of interest that arise in the course of their professional duties and activities. Relationships between industry and opinion leaders should be disclosed, especially when the latter determine the criteria for conducting and reporting clinical trials, writing editorials or therapeutic guidelines, or serving as editors of scientific journals. Residents must learn how to maintain ethical relationships with industry and how to interact with pharmaceutical representatives and other members of industry.

10. *Commitment to professional responsibilities.* As members of a profession, physicians are expected to work collaboratively to maximize patient care, be respectful of one another, and participate in the processes of self-regulation, including remediation and discipline of members who have failed to meet professional standards. The profession should also define and organize the educational and standard-setting process for current and future members. Physicians have both individual and collective obligations to participate in these processes. These obligations include engaging in internal assessment and accepting external scrutiny of all aspects of their professional performance. Residents must be taught how to transition the care of their patients both within and outside of their institution. That entrustable professional activity will help to prepare them to interface with their colleagues in various disciplines of health care.

The education of residents about these 10 professional responsibilities will make professional formation an explicit area of focus in residency training and help to cultivate in the residents a spirit of collaborative practice that is patient-centered, compassionate, caring, altruistic, and trustworthy. The physician discussed at the beginning of this chapter should not only learn about the 10 professional responsibilities but must also read Francis Peabody's article "The Care of the Patient" that was published in JAMA in 1927 (6).

PROFESSIONALISM IN REHABILITATION MEDICINE

The Ethical Issues Subcommittee of the Medical Practice Committee of the American Academy of Physical Medicine and Rehabilitation (AAPM&R) developed a Code of Conduct for the practice of rehabilitation medicine. This code is meant to "serve as a guideline for professional and personal behavior and to promote the highest quality of physiatric care. It is a statement of ideals, commitments and responsibilities of the physiatrist to patients, their families, other health professionals, society and to themselves" (7). The code is meant to outline ethical practice for physiatrists.

The code addresses relationships between physiatrists and their patients and families, members of the rehabilitation team, other physicians, the community, and government. It also addresses research and scholarly activities. A brief summary of this Code of Conduct is provided next.

Ethics Relating to Patients and Patients' Families

The physiatrist will provide the best possible care for his patient. This implies that the physiatrist will strive to maintain excellence in the practice of rehabilitation medicine through continuing medical education activities. He should be aware of the limits of his education and competence and seek out consultations from other clinicians with more experience when it is in the best interest of the patient. The patient's privacy and confidentiality must be preserved at all times.

Impaired physicians can have a significant negative impact on patient care as well as on the effectiveness of the team providing care to the patient. According to the Federation of State Medical Boards, the definition of an impairment is "the inability of a physician to practice medicine with reasonable skill and safety as a result of a mental disorder or physical illness or condition, including but not limited to those illnesses or conditions that would adversely affect cognitive, motor or perceptive skills or substance-related disorders including abuse and dependency of drugs and alcohol" (8).

The Code of Conduct addresses the issue of physician impairment by stating that physiatrists will not provide patient care while under the influence of alcohol, drugs, or illness that can place the patient's well-being at risk. Additional information on this topic is available from resources of the American Medical Association and American College of Physicians (9,10).

The issue of patient abuse is also addressed in the Code of Conduct. Physiatrists must not abuse patients physically, sexually, or psychologically.

Transfer of care from one physiatrist to another is also addressed in the Code of Conduct. If a patient requests that the care be transferred to another provider or if the physiatrist believes that it is in the best interest of the patient to transfer the patient's care to another provider, the current treating physiatrist has an obligation to transfer care to another physician in a safe manner.

The Code addresses conflicts of interest that can impact patient care by stating: "Conflicts of interest must be resolved in the best interest of the patient" (7). Financial conflicts of interest have been described in the 6th edition of the *American College of Physicians Ethics Manual*. According to this manual, some examples of potential conflicts of interest that can involve physicians include (a) incentives to overutilize (fee for service arrangements) or underutilize (capitation arrangements) resources, (b) business relationships or gifts from medical device or pharmaceutical companies, and (c) referring patients to medical facilities in which they have financial investment or ownership. Physicians must identify potential conflicts of interest and disclose them to their patients (10).

In the practice of rehabilitation medicine, some examples of potential conflicts of interest include (a) referring patients to a physical therapy facility in which the physiatrist has financial interest or ownership and (b) physiatrist writing prescriptions for prosthetic limbs while owning stock or financial investment in a company that manufactures prosthetic limbs.

The Code of Conduct also addresses the issue of access to physiatric care by stating that the physiatrist must not refuse to provide care to a patient "on the basis of their race, religion, nationality, disability or gender" (7). The Code also addresses the role of the physiatrist with respect to the patient's family, surrogates, or proxy decision makers.

Relationships With Members of the Rehabilitation Team

Physiatrists are members of a team that often includes physical therapists, occupational therapists, nurses, psychologists, vocational counselors, recreational therapists, and social workers. It is therefore important that physiatrists respect and honor the rights and privileges of other team members and encourage them to work for the betterment of the patients and within the scope of practice of their professions. Physicians can adversely affect the functioning of the rehabilitation team and the care of the patient when their behavior is disruptive.

The Federation of State Medical Boards has defined disruptive behavior as "behavior exhibited as a pattern of being unable, or unwilling, to function well with others to such an extent that his or her behavior, by words, attitude, or action has the potential to interfere with quality health care. The physician's behavior (attitudes, words or actions) intimidate and demean others potentially resulting in a negative impact on patient care" (8). The issue of disruptive physicians is an important one and a full discussion of this issue is beyond the scope of this chapter. The reader is referred to resources from the American College of Physicians and Joint Commission of Accreditation of Healthcare Organizations for additional information (10,11).

Physician-to-Physician Relationships

The Code of Conduct addresses how physiatrists should behave with respect to other physicians. This includes a responsibility to teach other physicians, students, and health care providers and the importance of not slandering other physicians.

According to the Code, physiatrists "should assist in the identification and rehabilitation of an impaired colleague." If they themselves are identified as being impaired, they should seek care and rehabilitation prior to resuming patient care.

Relationship With Community and Government

This section of the Code describes the relationship between physiatrists, the community they serve, and government. Physiatrists shall obey the pertinent laws of the land as well as the rules and regulations of the facilities in which they practice and refrain from unlawful activity. However, they should support changes to laws that they believe work against the best interest of patients. This section also describes how a physiatrist shall provide expert testimony. It is important to note that, according to the code, physiatrists "have an obligation to be involved in community and world activities, especially those matters affecting health."

Research and Scholarly Activity

The physiatrist is encouraged to participate in research that can advance the field of Physical Medicine and Rehabilitation. However, when he or she participates, the physiatrist is expected to obtain informed consent from participants and follow the rules governing research activities in the institution in which he or she works. The Code also addresses the issue of research data being accurately presented and subject to peer review prior to being publicized. Plagiarism is considered unethical (7).

It is important for physiatrists conducting research to be aware of potential conflicts of interest associated with research activity. One example is a physiatrist receiving research grants for treatment of spasticity from a company that sell products to treat spasticity while also providing clinical treatment of patients with spasticity and recruiting patients from the clinical practice for the research protocols. It is important for physiatrists to disclose this information to prospective research participants and the research department in the institution in which the research is being carried out.

SELF-EXAMINATION QUESTIONS
(Answers begin on p. 367)

1. Which of the following statements best defines an impaired physician according to the Federation of State Medical Boards?
   A. An inability of a physician to practice medicine with reasonable skill and safety as a result of a mental disorder, physical illness, or a substance-related disorder
   B. An inability of a physician to practice medicine with reasonable skill and safety as a result of both lack of financial compensation and substance-related disorder
   C. An inability of a physician to practice medicine with reasonable skill and safety as a result of both lack of adequate training and physical illness
   D. An inability of a physician to practice medicine with reasonable skill and safety as a result of both number of years practicing as a physician and substance-related disorder
   E. An inability of a physician to practice medicine with reasonable skill and safety as a result of both a language barrier and mental disorder

2. Which of the following statements best describes the AAPM&R Code of Conduct?
   A. It addresses relationships between physiatrists and their patients
   B. It addresses relationships between physiatrists and the state licensing boards
   C. It addresses relationships between physiatrists and American Board of Physical Medicine and Rehabilitation
   D. It addresses relationships between physiatrists and the American Medical Association
   E. It addresses relationships between physiatrists and the media

3. Which of the following best describes the AAPM&R Code of Conduct related to conflicts of interest for physiatrists?
   A. Conflicts of interest must be resolved in the best interest of the hospital
   B. Conflicts of interest must be resolved in the best interest of the physiatrist
   C. Conflicts of interest must be resolved in the best interest of the patient
   D. Conflicts of interest must be resolved in the best interest of the health insurance company
   E. Conflicts of interest must be resolved in the best interest of the referring physician

4. Which of the following best reflects the type of question that will convey to the patient that the resident is able to see the nature of the problem from the patient's point of view?
   A. What is the impact of your illness on your doctor?
   B. What type of health insurance do you have and why did you pick this one?
   C. What does your doctor fear most about your illness?
   D. What are the chief problems your sickness has caused for you?
   E. What do your friends think about the treatment you should receive?

5. According to the Physician Charter, which of the following is one of the 10 professional responsibilities?
   A. Commitment to professional incompetence
   B. Commitment to dishonesty with patients
   C. Commitment to professional responsibilities
   D. Commitment to promoting conflicts of interest
   E. Commitment to an unjust distribution of finite resources

REFERENCES

1. Snyder L. American College of Physicians Ethics Manual. *Ann Intern Med*. 2012;156:73–104.
2. Kleinman A, Eisenberg L, Good B. Culture, illness, and care: clinical lessons from anthropologic and cross-cultural research. *Ann Intern Med*. 1978;88(2):251–258.
3. ABIM. Medical professionalism in the new millennium: a physician charter. *Ann Intern Med*. 2002;136(3):243–246.
4. Blank L, Kimball H, McDonald W, et al. Medical professionalism in the new millennium: a physician charter 15 months later. *Ann Intern Med*. 2003;138(10):839–841.
5. Deming WE. *The New Economics for Industry, Government, and Education*. Cambridge, MA: The MIT Press; 2000.
6. Peabody FW. The care of the patient. *JAMA*. 1927;88:877–882.
7. http://www.aapmr.org/about/who-we-are/Pages/aapmr-code-of-conduct.aspx. Accessed January 26, 2014.
8. http://www.fsmb.org/pdf/grpol_policy-on-physician-impairment.pdf. Accessed January 26, 2014.
9. http://www.ama-assn.org/resources/doc/physician-health/policies-physicain-health.pdf. Accessed January 26, 2014.
10. http://www.acponline.org/running_practice/ethics/manual/manual6th.htm. Accessed January 26, 2014.
11. http://www.jointcommission.org/assets/1/18/SEA_40.pdf. Accessed January 26, 2014.

Adrian Cristian

7: Systems-Based Practice in Rehabilitation Medicine

The Accreditation Council of Graduate Medical Education (ACGME) defines systems-based practice as "an awareness of and responsiveness to the larger context and system of health care and the ability to effectively call on system resources to provide care that is of optimal value" (1).

Based on this definition, Graham et al. identified six expectations that resident physicians must fulfill relevant to their clinical specialty: (a) work effectively in various health care delivery systems, (b) coordinate patient care in the health care delivery system, (c) incorporate cost-awareness and risk–benefit analysis in patient care, (d) advocate for quality and optimal patient care, (e) work in professional teams to enhance patient safety and improve patient care quality, and (f) participate in identifying system errors and implementing potential solutions (2).

Graham et al. also enumerated classifications for assessing resident physician competency in the key domains of systems-based practice. In this taxonomy, they defined five roles: (a) system consultant, (b) care coordinator, (c) resource manager, (d) patient advocate, and (e) team collaborator. They defined appropriate behavior and context for each of these roles as well as provided examples for supervising physicians to consider (2).

These expectations can be applied to the practice of physical medicine and rehabilitation. Physiatrists should:

A. Have a working knowledge of the delivery of rehabilitation services in a variety of health care delivery systems;
B. Understand the role of rehabilitation medicine within the context of larger health care delivery systems;
C. Be able to coordinate effective patient care across the health care delivery system;
D. Have a working knowledge of rehabilitative service payers and their expectations as well as costs associated with the delivery of rehabilitation services and strategies to minimize costs while maintaining high-quality care;
E. Possess the skill set necessary to identify medical errors and patient safety issues across health care delivery systems;
F. Use said skill set to improve the safety of rehabilitative services; and
G. Work effectively as a team member and leader in maximizing patient safety and improving the quality of rehabilitative care.

GRADUATE MEDICAL EDUCATION AND SYSTEMS-BASED PRACTICE

Medical education focuses on obtaining medical knowledge about the diagnosis and treatment of diseases at the individual physician–patient level and tends to put less emphasis on the system as a whole, as well as its impact on patient care, safety, and quality (3). Training in systems-based practice during residency is not much developed (3).

Ziegelstein differentiated between the two ACGME competency protocols, namely Practice-Based Learning and Improvement (PBLI) and Systems-Based Practice (SBP), by using the metaphors of a mirror and a village. PBLI is the "mirror" that a resident looks in to assess himself as a basis for self-improvement, whereas SBP refers to the "village" within which the physician practices (the health care system). In this village, he collaborates with other clinicians to provide patient care (4).

In a recent survey of residents in three PMR training programs in New York, New Jersey, and Pennsylvania, residents noted that there is a lack of training with regard to PMR policy issues, documentation, rehabilitative care delivery models, and knowledge about insurance companies at the system level (5).

Health Care Systems

A health care system has been defined as "a complete network of agencies, facilities, and all providers of health care in a specified geographic area" (6). The delivery of health care is very complex and generally known to be made up of a number of interdependent components and microsystems. These microsystems are usually comprised of small groups of individuals working together on very specific tasks (e.g., neurosurgical team, cardiovascular surgical team, and rehabilitation team specializing in spinal cord injury medicine). These microsystems can have multiple connections with other microsystems in the same organization. Clinical staff can simultaneously be part of several microsystems within an organization, which only complicates matters further. The actions of individuals are not always predictable; however, given their connected and interdependent nature, actions of one can affect others within that microsystem and organization (3). Health care systems are also subject to external forces from payers, regulators, competitors, changing demographics, and market forces.

Systems Thinking

According to Peter Senge, systems thinking is the practice of seeing wholes. It is a framework for identifying significant relationships *between* the influences of macrocosmic forces and structures rather than within them. It is seeing patterns of change, rather than static snapshots. It is a focus on "circles of causality" and interrelationships rather than linear cause-and-effect chains and underscores the maxim that "every influence is both cause and effect. Nothing is ever influenced in just one direction" (7).

As mentioned earlier, health care organizations are made up of small and large microsystems, with an interdependence defined by relationships between policies, procedures, regulations, and staff. Each of these microsystems affects others around it and in turn is affected by other microsystems. They are individual parts of a larger whole. As a systems thinker, the physiatrist needs to understand the role of rehabilitation medicine in his or her own health care system, his or her own role within that system, and look for patterns of interdependencies. This is important, because in application of systems thinking, all individuals and their microsystems share in the responsibility for the success and failures generated by their interdependent health care system. Senge also writes that mastering systems thinking "lies in seeing patterns where others only see events and forces to react to" (7). Systems thinkers realize that health care systems have a dual complexity—detail and dynamic complexity.

Detail complexity refers to the various variables that need to be considered, whereas dynamic complexity refers to the subtle causes and effects that are not linear, yet connected in time and space in such a way that their impact is not necessarily obvious.

Dynamic complexity is at work when an action has both local consequences in the health care system and also distant consequences somewhere else in that system. Situations wherein an action with ostensibly localized consequences can grow and have more significant consequences are also illustrative of dynamic complexity. For example, a bedbound diabetic patient whose disease is aggressively treated on an acute medical service in one part of the health care organization may experience hypoglycemia once the patient starts his or her rehabilitation program on an acute inpatient rehabilitation unit in another part of the organization.

Systems thinkers also recognize that they cannot always see the long-term consequences of their actions because of the limited time frame from which the provider must form an analysis. For example, a physiatrist administering a trigger point injection to a patient with myofascial pain may inadvertently cause a pneumothorax; however, the physiatrist may not know this if the patient is not readily available for follow-up and receives treatment for this complication at a hospital in a distant setting.

A systems thinker might, in addition to temporal constraints, meet with organizational limitations on their analyses. They cannot always see the impact of their actions on more removed parts of the institution. For example, a policy decision to address increased length of stay on a medical ward by earlier discharges to an inpatient rehabilitation ward in the same institution may lead to more acute discharges, higher costs of care, and decreased functional outcomes from provision of rehabilitation services due to increased medical acuity of the admitted patients earlier than they might otherwise be considered fit to undergo 3 hours of therapy per day.

Still, systems thinkers become experts at looking for delays and bottlenecks in the health care system as well as workarounds. These can be indicators of system-wide issues.

To be an effective systems thinker, a physiatrist needs to:

- Identify the system, key stakeholders in that system—including themselves—and the connections between all involved;
- Describe the detail and dynamic complexity in that system;
- Identify any changes in that system (lack of funds, key personnel, change in policy, or priorities for the organization);
- Identify the delays, bottlenecks, and work-arounds in that system and their impact;
- Identify symptoms as well as root causes for the problems (e.g., decreased quality of services provided; underinvestment) (7).

To become a systems thinker, one must learn to practice effective reflection, inquiry, and dialogue. Senge commented that "reflective openness leads to looking inward, allowing our conversations to make us more aware of the biases and limitations in our own thinking, and how our thinking and actions contribute to problems" (7). This should be done at the individual level as well as collectively at the group level.

Through thorough and consistent inquiry, we can challenge our mental models for how things work and should work in a health care organization. Senge asserts that mental models are often flawed because they focus on only readily visible variables, miss critical feedback relationships, misjudge time delays, see the system in overly simplistic terms, and are dominated by linear thinking.

Through effective inquiry, the systems thinker develops a collective understanding of the health care system—warts and all—from different perspectives and thus creates a collective mental model.

Dialogue refers to the collective review of the system among the key stakeholders in that system, especially after an unexpected event or outcome has occurred. Some points to consider include (39):

- What happened?
- What should have happened?
- Why did it happen?
- What can be learned from this event?
- How can it be prevented or encouraged (depending on whether the outcome was not favorable or favorable)?

These models and the discussion presented here underscore the reality that health care is not delivered in a vacuum.

Proficient systems thinking in health care requires that the physician develop an understanding of how individual patient care relates to the health care system as a whole and how to improve the delivery of individual patient care by improving the health care system (3).

THE PHYSIATRIST AS SYSTEMS CONSULTANT IN REHABILITATION HEALTH CARE DELIVERY SYSTEMS

Following acute hospitalizations for illness or injury, individuals are often referred for postacute care (PAC). This care is usually provided in inpatient rehabilitation facilities (IRFs), skilled nursing facilities (SNFs), and home-based care. The goal of PAC is to improve the level of function to the highest level possible and to assist with the transition from hospital to the community (8).

Inpatient Rehabilitation Services

It has been reported that Medicare is the payer in approximately 70% of patients admitted to IRFs. In 2006, there were 404,000 Medicare discharges from IRFs (9).

Section 1886(j) of the Social Security Act authorized the prospective payment system (PPS) for the payment of inpatient rehabilitation services. The Centers for Medicare and Medicaid Services has described IRFs as "free standing rehabilitation hospitals and rehabilitation units in acute care hospitals. They provide an intensive rehabilitation program and patients who are admitted must be able to tolerate 3 hours of intense rehabilitation services per day" (10).

In this system, payment is based on information collected from patient assessment instruments (PAIs). This information includes data about the patient's clinical diagnosis, comorbidities, impairment group, swallowing status, level of function (based on the Function of Independence Measure) at admission and discharge, interruptions to their rehabilitation program, discharge destination, complications encountered during the course of a rehabilitation program, and quality indicators about pressure ulcers and catheter-associated urinary tract infections (11).

Patients are grouped into rehabilitation impairment categories and mixed-case groups, then subsequently into four tiers within each mixed-case group where the costs associated with the patient's comorbidities are factored in to determine a higher or lower level of payment. The payment level is also adjusted if the patient had a length of stay less than 3 days or one that was shortened due to a transfer. Other factors that are considered in the payment include (a) geographic differences in labor costs, (b) whether the facility is located in a rural area, (c) whether the facility treats a high proportion of low-income patients, and (d) whether the facility has a residency training program.

In order for an IRF to be paid under the PPS instead of the acute care hospital inpatient PPS, the facility must treat patients with one of 13 medical conditions for a minimum of 60% of its total inpatient population. This compliance threshold is known as the "60 percent rule." These medical conditions are stroke, spinal cord injury, congenital deformity, amputation, major multiple trauma, hip fracture, brain injury, and neurological disorders (multiple sclerosis, motor neuron disease, polyneuropathy, muscular dystrophy, Parkinson's disease, and burns).

To substantiate the need for admission to an IRF, complexity of the condition can be taken into consideration in some clinical scenarios such as (a) severe arthritic conditions in which less intensive rehabilitation programs were not successful, (b) the patient underwent bilateral knee or hip joint replacement surgery just before the admission to the IRF and was obese (body mass index of at least 50 at the time of admission to IRF) or is 85 years or older at the time of admission to the IRF. The patient must be medically stable to participate in the rehabilitation program and have a need to be medically supervised during the rehabilitation stay (12). Quality indicators must be reported for catheter-associated urinary tract infections and pressure ulcers by the IRF facility. Failure to report leads to a two-percentage point penalty in payment effective in 2014 (13).

Conditions for payment under PPS also stipulate that patients directly admitted from the community to the IRF following a first illness are responsible for a deductible, whereas those admitted from an acute care hospital to the IRF are not. The patients would also be responsible for copay for the 61st to 90th day according to Medpac (14).

Outpatient Rehabilitation Services

A course of outpatient rehabilitation commonly includes services provided by physical therapists, occupational therapists, speech pathologists, and physiatrists. Medicare pays for services provided by "skilled professionals that is appropriate, effective for a patient's condition and are reasonable in terms of frequency and duration. The beneficiary must be under the care of a physician, have a treatable condition, and be improving." "Medicare does not cover maintenance-level outpatient therapy services." Speech pathologists may bill Medicare directly. Certain services provided by physical and occupational therapy assistants are also covered if performed under the supervision of a qualified therapist who bills for these services. For most services, Medicare pays the provider 80% of the fee schedule amount and the patient pays a 20% copayment. Medicare has therapy caps for outpatient rehabilitative therapy services provided by physical therapists, occupational therapists, and speech and language pathologists, unless they are provided in a hospital outpatient therapy department (15).

Skilled Nursing Facilities

Medicare covers costs of an admission in a skilled nursing facility for patients following a hospital stay of at least 3 days that requires specialized nursing and/or rehabilitative care. Medicare pays the SNF on a predetermined per diem rate for up to 100 days through a PPS. The base payment rate takes into account geographic differences in labor costs and case mix. Case mixes enable the Resource Utilization Groups (RUGs), which have nursing and rehabilitative therapy weights that are applied to the base payment rate (16). Patients are assigned to an RUG based on the following: (a) number of minutes of therapy that the patient will need (e.g., need more or less than 45 minutes of therapy per week), (b) need for specialized services such as respiratory therapy, (c) presence of certain conditions, and (d) patient's level of function for eating, toileting, bed mobility, and ability to transfer (16).

The daily rate is based on the following: (a) skilled nursing needs; (b) therapy needs; and (c) SNF costs for room, board, and administrative costs (16). For the fiscal year 2009, Medicare daily base rates for an urban SNF were as follows: (a) $151.74 for nursing, (b) $114.30 for therapy, and (c) $77.44 for other costs (16).

Home Services

Home health agency (HHA) personnel provide care in the patient's home. This typically includes skilled nursing, physical therapy, occupational therapy, speech pathology, social work, and home health attendants. The Center for Medicare and Medicaid Services (CMS) pays HHAs for these services for 60-day episodes based on a PPS. Patients are assigned to 1 of 153 home health resource groups (HHRGs) based on their level of function and required need of services using the Outcome and Assessment Information Set (OASIS). The HHRGs range from those comprised of uncomplicated cases to very complicated patients in need of extensive rehabilitative resources. The base rate for the HHRGs takes into account geographic differences in labor and administrative costs, and whether the patient needs more or less than five visits, and whether the payment is subject to a high cost or short stay outlier, respectively. The PPS also pays for nonroutine medical supplies (17).

PATIENT CARE COORDINATION IN THE PRACTICE OF REHABILITATION MEDICINE

Patient care is often delivered in multiple settings and is provided by multiple different providers. It is not uncommon for patients to be admitted to a medical or surgical ward of a medical center for an acute illness or injury and be cared for by a team of physicians, nurses, and therapists, and then, once stabilized, be transferred to another ward, only to be cared for by another team. Subsequently, admissions to a medical rehabilitation facility and/or a skilled nursing facility and care by other teams often ensue.

Coordination of the patient care across this health care continuum requires a working knowledge of the following: (a) the health care system and its rules, regulations, and policies; (b) health insurance companies—their policies, rules, and regulations as they apply to the patient and his or her diagnosis; (c) community resources; and (d) effective communication and interpersonal skills and an ability to work with a team that consists of different clinicians and administrative staff.

The physiatrist is well suited for this role by virtue of his or her training in the team approach to patient care. The patient's best interests should remain paramount in the mind of the physiatrist at all times and serve as the primary driver of care and decision making—a concept known as patient-centered care.

In the inpatient setting, interdisciplinary team meetings and interactions are ideal opportunities to coordinate the care of the patient with a coalition that might at any point include therapists, nursing staff, social worker, psychologist, and recreational therapists. In these settings, the team can set goals, discuss medical complications that are affecting the patient's ability to reach functional goals, and determine length of stay and postdischarge plan of care. The physiatrist can also coordinate clinical care among medical and surgical consultants and communicate information to treating therapists.

Coordination of care is especially important at transition points when attention to detail is paramount. The information passed from one treating team to another should be complete and include key information about the following:

- The patient's hospital course and complications
- Past medical and surgical history
- Laboratory and imaging results
- Operative and procedure reports
- Medications
- Allergies
- Advance directives (e.g., do not resuscitate/do not intubate)
- Contact information for key clinical staff that is knowledgeable about the patient's condition and medical history

If this information is not complete, the physiatrist should obtain it from the most credible source and subsequently ensure that it is passed along to the next team caring for the patient in the inpatient or outpatient setting.

The time of discharge from an inpatient rehabilitation facility to another facility or to a home setting is another opportunity for ensuring that care coordination is effectively handled. This includes contacting the physicians at the receiving institution or the patient's primary care physician in the community, and verbally discussing the key aspects of the patient's care and any concerns or pending test results that need follow-up.

If the patient is to receive home health services, discussing the patient's care with the nurse or therapist in the home setting can also ensure that the patient's care is not interrupted and that an appropriate treatment plan is carried out. Telemedicine technology can play a significant role in patient care coordination with monitoring of the patient's condition in the home setting using monitors for vital signs and periodic phone calls from nurses or physicians.

One should take care to remember that the patient and family members are integral partners to the physiatrist in care coordination. The physiatrist should take the time to educate his or her patient about key aspects of the patient's diagnosis, potential problems, and how to best manage them as well as how to self-advocate for their needs.

THE PHYSIATRIST AS RESOURCE MANAGER

There is evidence that patients discharged from comprehensive medical rehabilitation facilities gain functional improvement relative to their condition at the time of admission in the context of a variety of conditions, such as hip fractures, stroke, brain injury, medical debility, and lower limb joint replacement. In addition, the vast majority of patients with these conditions are discharged back to the community.

However, according to several reports by the Uniform Data System for Medical Rehabilitation, which reviewed data for an 8- to 10-year period beginning in 2000, there has been a general trend in admitting patients with a lower level of function to medical rehabilitation facilities and then discharging them at a similarly unsatisfactory level of functioning at the end of the reporting period. In addition, length of stay and discharge rates back to the community also decreased; however, efficiency of care remained stable for stroke, traumatic brain injury, and traumatic spinal cord injury. The efficiency of care improved for patients admitted with lower limb joint replacements and medical debility. The authors raised the possibility that policy changes affecting factors such as classification, reimbursement, and/or documentation processes may have had a role in these findings (18–23).

Ottenbacher and Graham described four types of barriers to access for rehabilitation services: financial, personal, structural, and attitudinal.

Financial barriers include insurance coverage and out-of-pocket expenses for treatments. Personal barriers include lack of understanding of rehabilitative resources available, lack of knowledge about how to access these services by patients, and socioeconomic factors. Examples of structural barriers include referral patterns restricted to specific providers and institutions, and the 3-hour rule, which limits access to certain types of rehabilitation facilities. Attitudinal barriers are based on individual beliefs and preferences about rehabilitation services and their outcomes (24).

Chan discusses the impact that changes in the payment systems for PAC have on quality, outcomes, and access to rehabilitation services. He raises concerns that while the changes in the payment systems carry financial incentives for different providers of rehabilitative services, there is conspicuous lack of information about where the incentives should be placed to ensure the most effective and efficacious treatments for different types of patients to achieve the best outcomes. There is also a lack of knowledge about the future impact of these payment system changes on the care of individuals with conditions such as traumatic brain injury and spinal cord injury, as well as the potential for racial, ethnic, or sociodemographic barriers to receiving adequate PAC (25).

Financial factors can be powerful motivators for facilities and HHAs providing PAC. Different payment structures can lead to different utilization patterns and differences in PAC sites that provide care. These in turn can affect patient outcomes. Buntin provides an example in which SNFs are incentivized to keep daily costs down since they are payed a per diem rate, even as incentives for decreasing length of stay are considerably less robust. Buntin also raised concerns with respect to access to PAC rehabilitation, specifically for severely ill patients who are at higher risk for the following:

- Reduced access to care
- Receiving rehabilitation services with lower-than-optimal intensity
- Premature discharge from a PAC facility or program
- Receiving less medical care
- Receiving unnecessary care

This concern was compounded by lack of "clear evidence about which sites of care and treatment intensities are appropriate for many types of patients" (26).

Accountable care organizations (ACOs) have been described as part of the Patient Protection and Affordable Care Act of 2010. Their goal is to provide high-quality care at a low cost through incentives that focus on improving quality and efficiency, as opposed to volume-based care (27). The idea is that by improving care coordination among health care providers and hospitals and linking them through quality metrics, health care costs would also be reduced. Pay for performance metrics would also be used to incentivize high-quality care. As of 2011, PMR-specific performance metrics were limited (27).

Patient-centered medical homes have been proposed as an integral aspect of ACOs. These are primary care practices in which care is coordinated among clinical teams for specific diagnoses. An opportunity may exist, through their close alignment with primary care practices, for the physiatrist to play a role in the coordination of team management efforts as they apply to TBI, SCI, and osteoarthritis patient populations, among others. Electronic health records are an important part of this care coordination.

However, in spite of overall interest in ACO demonstration projects, significant obstacles were reported relating to cost of these projects, operational challenges to implementation, and lack of evidence-based treatment protocols (27).

Risk–Benefit Analysis in the Practice of Rehabilitation Medicine

Medical decision making often requires an analysis of the risks and the benefits for a particular medical test or treatment plan. In a risk–benefit analysis, the following steps may be of help:

- Identify the relevant patient and situational characteristics that are pertinent to the risk–benefit analysis.
- Identify the risks associated with a treatment or medical test.
- Assign a risk value to the risk (e.g., low risk or high risk).
- Identify the benefits of the test or treatment.
- Assign a benefit value to the test or treatment (e.g., low benefit or high benefit).
- Review the pertinent scientific literature, consult with a local expert, and review applicable medical center rules, policies, procedures, or local laws for additional relevant information.
- Discuss with the patient the risks and benefits and note his or her wishes.
- Compare risks vs. benefits.

If the benefits significantly outweigh the risks and the patient is motivated, the test or treatment plan should be carried out. If the risks significantly outweigh the benefits, then the decision is made against carrying out the test or treatment plan. The challenge arises when the risks and benefits are closely matched such that both the risks and benefits are significant. In the practice of rehabilitation medicine, there are additional considerations since tests and/or treatment plans also have a cost associated with them and one must also consider how to effectively make use of available resources.

For example, in deciding whether or not to order a head CT scan for a patient who fell on an inpatient rehabilitation unit and hit his or her head against a sink in the room, one must first analyze the patient's condition in the context of his or her illness. Key factors to consider include: Is this a patient with a history of anticoagulant therapy? Is this a patient with a recent neurosurgical procedure? Is there a change in mental status or neurologic findings on physical examination? Next, one must consider the risks of performing a CT of the head. Will the information obtained be important to change management of the patient's condition? Is there potential harm to the patient from the CT of the head (e.g., exposure to radiation) or added costs, and if so, is the risk from harm mild or severe. Next, one should review the scientific literature on the risk–benefit analysis of CT of the head in such a scenario or consult with a local expert. Next, one should discuss the pros and cons with the patient or health care proxy to obtain his or her wishes.

Once all of this has been completed, the risks and benefits of performing the CT are compared. In this example, if there is a neurological change in the context of trauma to the head and anticoagulant use, a CT of the head could potentially change management if an acute hemorrhage is identified and neurosurgical intervention is needed. This benefit would outweigh the risks associated with performing a CT of the head.

In contrast, if the patient was not on anticoagulant therapy and the trauma to the head was minimal with no neurologic findings on examination, the benefit of performing the CT of the head may not significantly outweigh the associated risks and costs of the procedure.

Medical Necessity: IRF vs. SNF

The American Academy of Physical Medicine Medical Inpatient Rehabilitation Criteria Task Force Report titled "Standards for Assessing Medical Appropriateness Criteria for Admitting Patients to Rehabilitation Hospitals or Units" described the various factors that need to be considered when a physiatrist needs to make a decision on whether a patient is better served by undergoing rehabilitation in an IRF as opposed to a skilled nursing facility (SNF). These factors consider both patient characteristics and organizational characteristics (28). Patient characteristics include the following:

- Patient's physical and/or cognitive impairment as well as their severity
- Patient's motivation to participate in a rehabilitation program
- Patient's medical stability to undergo 3 hours of rehabilitation therapies per day
- Patient's perceived ability to return to the community setting
- Patient having clear functional goals that can be achieved in a realistic time frame

Organizational characteristics of IRF and SNF were described with some clear distinctions drawn between them. Some of these are given in Table 7.1.

The task force characterized the patient admitted to the IRF as one having had a recent serious illness or exacerbation of a serious illness that decreased that individual's ability to perform activities of daily living or ambulate safely. They are considered in need of close medical monitoring of their illness or comorbidities, need rehabilitation nursing services 24 hours per day and 7 days per week, can actively participate in a rehabilitation program of 3 hours per day for 5 days per week, can achieve realistic goals in a reasonable period of time, and can safely be discharged to home or a community setting.

The decision to admit to an IRF should be made by a physician with the necessary experience and training to make such a decision and should be based on medical data and sound judgment. The facility should only accept patients who are medically stable for whom it can provide adequate resources and staff for optimal medical rehabilitation.

According to the task force, the cost–benefit analysis on whether or not to admit to an IRF or a SNF should be made by considering various questions:

- Will intense therapy (e.g., 3 hours per day) change the discharge plan and level of independence?
- Can the patient tolerate 3 hours of therapy per day? If so, will the patient need close medical monitoring?
- Does the patient need 3 hours per therapy per day to achieve his or her goals or will less than 3 hours suffice? (28)

Patient Advocacy for Quality and Optimal Care

The physiatrist can have a significant impact on the quality of care rendered to individuals with disabilities through their clinical care, surveillance for system issues having an impact on

TABLE 7.1 Comparison of Organizational Characteristics of Inpatient Rehabilitation Facilities and Skilled Nursing Facilities

IRF (INPATIENT REHABILITATION FACILITIES)	SNF
Availability of physicians and nurses with specialized training in medical rehabilitation 24 hours per day and 7 days per week.	Physicians provide "general medical supervision" and are required to visit patient every 30 days (every 60 days after the first 3 months). Physicians are not required to manage therapy services. Twenty-four-hour nursing is not required. Rehabilitation nursing is not required.
Patient receives 3 hours of therapy per day.	Whereas physical therapy, occupational therapy, and speech and language pathology services must be available, 3 hours of therapy per day is not required.
Registered or licensed physical therapy, occupational therapy, recreational therapy, and respiratory therapy are provided.	Laboratory, radiological, or emergency visits are not required to be available on site.
Psychologists, social workers, vocational counselors, prosthetist, orthotist, and dieticians or nutritional counselors must be available.	No requirement that SNF needs to provide prosthetic or orthotic services.
Medical, surgical, and behavioral medicine specialists are available.	Social work services must be available.
Weekly team meetings held to discuss goals and discharge planning.	Interdisciplinary team meetings are not required.

patient safety, and advocating for their patients' needs in a variety of forums. The Center for Disease Control has some suggestions and resources for clinicians (29,30).

Some examples include:

1. Ensuring that clinical care is provided in medical offices that are wheelchair accessible, have low examining tables to facilitate patient transfers, and have equipment that can be used to thoroughly examine individuals with disabilities.
2. Minimize delays for the patient while in the health care system through effective care coordination (e.g., expediting appointments with consultants and expediting transfers from one setting to another setting along the health care continuum of care).
3. Allow ample time to examine and talk to someone with a disability. Utilize a holistic approach to the patient's needs.
4. Provide appropriate preventative care through cancer screenings, immunizations, smoking cessation therapies, and weight control.
5. Optimize medical management of diseases such as diabetes mellitus, coronary artery disease, and hypertension to minimize the impact of their associated complications such as stroke and myocardial infarctions.
6. Maximize patient safety by incorporating into the treatment plan measures that minimize the risk of pressure ulcers, contractures, urinary tract infections, aspiration-related complications from impaired swallowing, falls, medication-related side effects, deep vein thrombosis, and burns associated with use of heat modalities.
7. Learn and subsequently apply quality improvement methodology tools to analyze health care systems for barriers to care for individuals with disabilities and then implement interventions that could improve health care and remove barriers.
8. Advocate with payers of the patient's health care costs for the right rehabilitation services, right intensity, at the right time, in the right place, and by the right providers, that will maximize the patient's level of function in the health care system and improve his or her overall health.
9. Educate the patient and his or her family about the illness and its associated impairments, activity limitations, and participation restrictions. The education should also include strategies to best navigate the health care system and advocate for the patient's health care needs to ensure optimal health.
10. Advocate at the community level for access to transportation for people with disabilities.
11. Optimize transfer of care at transition points through appropriate hand-offs.
12. Effective utilization of clinicians and administrative personnel in the health care, community, workplace, and school settings to optimize level of function and overall health for the patient.
13. Be involved in emergency preparedness training for individuals with disabilities.

Team Collaborator: Systems-Based Practice and Teams

In their book titled *Educating Physicians: A Call for Reform of Medical School and Residency*, the authors described the challenges facing modern medical education and the importance of motivating physicians for continuous learning and improvement. They stated that there is a need for "fundamental change in medical education that will require new curricula, new pedagogies and new forms of assessment." The authors recommended that physicians should learn to work collaboratively with other health professionals such as medical assistants, nurses, pharmacists, physical therapists, and social workers and to be responsible for quality of care and their team performance (31).

Whereas it is important for the physiatrist to understand the health care systems in which he or she works, it is equally important for the physiatrist to understand the roles and responsibilities of the various team members involved in the rehabilitation of the patient. Ideally, the physiatrist should spend time learning about the systems involved in the delivery of rehabilitative care from the different perspectives of disciplines such as physical therapy, occupational therapy, speech pathology, vocational rehabilitation, social work, psychologists, and rehabilitation nursing.

This knowledge is invaluable in truly understanding the complexity of delivery of rehabilitative service. It can be obtained through discussions with clinicians in these disciplines as well as activities in which the physiatrist can observe the clinician at work. Discharge planning and interdisciplinary team meetings are other opportunities to work closely with team members and to learn from them. The physiatrist can use this information as well as the expertise of his or her colleagues to improve the quality of delivery of rehabilitative services both within the institution and outside the institution using quality improvement methodology.

The Physiatrist as Leader in Improving Health Care Quality and Patient Safety in Rehabilitation Medicine

To ensure quality and safety in the practice of rehabilitation medicine, leadership and management skills are essential for the physiatrist. Leadership has been defined as "working with people and systems to produce needed change" (32). Management has been defined as "working with people and systems to produce predictable results" (32).

According to Reinertsen, leadership is important because change is essential for quality improvement. The effective physiatrist leader often has to function in both of these roles to improve patient safety and quality in rehabilitative care. These are briefly described as follows:

The physiatrist as leader should embody personal integrity, honesty, humility, passion, trustworthiness, and a commitment to providing the highest quality of patient care and safety. As an addendum, Goleman describes the importance of emotional intelligence in the leader. This includes self-awareness, self-regulation, empathy, and social skills (33).

The effective leader also possesses competency in three areas, according to the National Center for Healthcare Leadership: people skills, transformational skills, and execution skills (34).

People skills: Effective leaders are highly professional. They are confident in their own abilities, value the people with whom they work, and are genuinely interested in their own others' professional development. They are enthusiastic coaches and mentors, skilled at building and maintaining relationships and adept at resolving conflicts in a mutually satisfactory manner to all parties involved. Effective leaders recognize the importance of rewards, incentives, and praise as tools to use to obtain the best performance from the people with whom they work.

Transformational skills: Effective leaders are capable of facilitating transformation and can develop a shared vision, setting direction for quality and safe rehabilitative care both among members of their team and the larger health care organization of which they are a part. They are analytical systems thinkers who look for patterns, relationships, and linkages in systems (7). They understand the "big picture" perspective, are able to break it down into its fundamental components, and can articulate the nature of these to the people around them in order to effect change and develop a shared vision (35). Effective leaders possess sound financial skills and have a deep understanding of quality improvement methodology as it applies to systems. Effective leaders are able to successfully establish meaningful links between patient safety, quality, and markers important to the organizations (e.g., quality, financial links, and business goals) (32). Effective leaders are innovative strategic thinkers who apply their skill set to improve the quality and safety of health care delivery.

Execution is the "ability to translate a vision and strategy into optimal organizational performance" (34). The effective leader has an awareness and understanding of his or her health care organization, is a collaborator, and has excellent interpersonal and communication skills, as well as abilities to manage projects. These skills can be used toward exerting influence to bring about change.

A leader looks for ways to align people within departments of rehabilitation medicine as well as in other parts of the health care system with the overarching goal of providing high-quality and safe patient care through improved policies, procedures, and processes.

The leader uses four "reference frames" to better understand the organization's strengths, weaknesses, opportunities, and threats. They are oriented around structural, human resources, symbolic, and political frames.

According to Bolman, the structural frame refers to the rules and policies within the organization. The human resources frame refers to the skills, wants, needs, and fit of the people working in the health care organization. The political frame refers to the power structure within the organization. The symbolic frame refers to the organizational culture, rituals, symbols, and ceremonies (36).

Once the physiatrist understands the organization through these four frames of reference, they need to understand the environment in which their health care system has to survive, in order to improve the quality and safety of rehabilitative care delivered in that system. To accomplish this, Porter described a "five-force" strategy analysis with respect to the payers, suppliers, competitors, potential new providers, and substitutes for products (37). It is important to familiarize oneself with these since the forces acting on the delivery of rehabilitative services both from within and from outside the health care system can have a direct impact on the quality and safety of the rehabilitative services delivered.

The effective physiatrist leader is good at managing teams such that they are able to provide optimal and safe rehabilitative care. This involves selecting the right team members; setting ground rules, goals and deadlines; managing conflicts; mentoring; providing feedback; and dealing with marginal performers.

The effective physiatrist leader excels in the practice of both ground-up *and* top-down leadership. One realizes that he or she cannot effectively improve quality and safety just from sitting behind a desk in one's office, but rather by walking around the institution, effectively listening to people, and empowering, mentoring, and inspiring others about the importance of safety and quality in rehabilitation medicine. The physiatrist leader is effective at breaking down silos and rebuilding multidisciplinary connections between key stakeholders involved in the delivery of rehabilitation services in the health care organization and encourages processes that—and people who—engage in shared decision making for the greater good.

Reinertsen offers some examples for leaders in health care to help in their efforts to transform themselves into quality improvement leaders. They are listed as follows:

- Personally interview a patient and his or her family who sustained serious harm in the health care organization and the impact that it had on them.
- Personally interview a staff member who was involved in an error that caused serious harm.
- Listen to a patient daily.
- Learn and use quality improvement methodology.
- Perform regular safety rounds with a team.
- Use purposeful reflection on a regular basis on their roles as leaders (32).

He also described the "seven deadly sins of leadership":

1. Embracing the role of victim
2. Not matching the words with the deeds (talk more about quality improvement without providing the resources)
3. A love for the trappings of the leader role more than the work itself
4. A focus on popularity as opposed to leadership
5. Maladaptively seeking peace and avoiding conflict
6. Lack of sustained focus on one idea
7. Not admit to making mistakes (32)

PATIENT SAFETY, SYSTEMS ERRORS, AND QUALITY IN REHABILITATION MEDICINE

In its landmark report titled "Crossing the Quality Chasm," the Institute of Medicine (IOM) identified six aims to improve health care. Health care should be safe, effective, and patient centered, timely, efficient, and equitable.

The IOM defined safe health care as care in which patients are not harmed by the health care provided. Effective health care is based on sound scientific knowledge and avoids underuse or overuse of health care services. In patient-centered care, the patient's values, wishes, and preferences are paramount in guiding clinical care. Timely care aims to reduce delays and waits accrued during the delivery of health care. Efficient care avoids waste and equitable care is defined as care "that does not vary in quality because of personal characteristics such as gender, ethnicity, geographic location, and socioeconomic status." Their recommendation was that "all health care organizations, professional groups, and private and public purchasers should adopt as their explicit purpose to continually reduce the burden of illness, injury, and disability, and to improve the health and functioning of the people of the United States" (38).

These aims are especially important in the care provided to individuals with impairments, activity limitations, and participation restrictions who are particularly vulnerable with respect to the six aims outlined by the IOM.

SYSTEM EVALUATOR: IDENTIFYING ERRORS AND IMPLEMENTING POTENTIAL SYSTEMS SOLUTIONS

In order to identify system errors, the physiatrist should become familiar with the basics of quality improvement methodology and how to perform a root cause analysis (RCA). The Institute for Healthcare Improvement has an online curriculum that provides training on patient safety, communication with patients after adverse events, culture of safety, leadership in health care, quality improvement methodology, and performing RCA (39).

According to the IHI, the purpose for performing an RCA is to understand the systems failures that led to the adverse event in order to prevent it from happening again in the future. An RCA seeks to learn what happened, why, and what can be done that both prevents reoccurrence and maintains confidence in patient safety measures in the future.

To perform an RCA, a team of those involved in the system is assembled to answer the aforementioned questions. There are six steps in performing an RCA: (a) determine what happened, (b) review what should have happened, (c) determine the causes for the event, (d) write the causal statement, (e) identify a list of recommendations to prevent a similar event from happening again in the future, and (f) communicate findings with key stakeholders. It is important that the RCA team uses a blame-free approach to the RCA. In determining causes, the IHI recommends that the question *why* is asked five times to get to the underlying root cause. Causes can then be grouped into categories using tools such as fishbone diagrams. The causal statement links the cause with the effect and the event. It should be written in a neutral, nonpunitive, nonjudgmental, blame-free manner (39).

Once an issue in the quality of health care has been raised, it is important to use quality improvement methodology to identify systems issues and implement interventions that would improve the quality. It is important to note that as part of the American Board of Physical Medicine and Rehabilitation Maintenance of Certificate, physiatrists are currently required to complete and report a clinical care practice improvement project (40).

A quality improvement project typically involves the following steps: (a) identifying the team members, (b) defining the problem to be addressed, (c) identifying appropriate data to be collected as well as appropriate benchmarks, (d) defining the steps in the process in need of improvement—both as it currently is and as it should be, (e) identifying the barriers to the process, (f) identifying interventions, (g) implementing interventions, (h) collecting and analyzing data and comparing with benchmarks, (i) reflecting on the findings, (j) adopting interventions that worked, and (k) communicating the findings with the appropriate stakeholders (41).

Another commonly used quality improvement methodology is the PDSA cycle. There are four components to this methodology: plan, do, study, and act.

In the "**P**lan" phase, a plan is developed that will be carried out during the cycle. In the "**D**o" phase, the plan is carried out and data are collected and analyzed. In the "**S**tudy" phase, the effect of the change is compared against the goals and benchmarks and lessons learned are summarized. In the "**A**ct" phase, the interventions and changes found to be successful are implemented. In this phase, the decision to carry out a future plan is considered.

There are several tools and utilities that a physiatrist can use to improve the quality of rehabilitative care systems. These include control charts, histograms, cause-and-effect fishbone diagrams, Pareto charts, affinity diagrams, matrix diagrams, and priorities matrices. The reader is referred to an easy-to-use reference that describes these tools in greater detail (42).

In Failure Mode and Effects Analysis (FMEA), the focus is on prevention of failure in a system. Griffin and Haraden describe key components of FMEA:

- Identifying the steps in the process
- Describing what could go wrong
- Describing why failure would happen
- Describing the consequences of failure
- What is the likelihood that the failure will not be detected?
- What is the likelihood of harm from this failure?

In improving health care systems, these authors also cautioned against automation of faulty processes and overuse of technology. They advised to automate processes that are working well, as well as minimize and standardize steps in a process so that users of different skill levels can easily follow (43).

Some areas of particular concern when assessing safety during the delivery of rehabilitation medicine within inpatient facilities that should be considered include the risks for/of:

- Hypotension
- Hypoglycemia
- Falls
- Contractures
- Aspiration-related complications
- Catheter-associated urinary tract infections
- Medication-related side effects
- Contractures
- Venous thromboembolism

Some areas of safety concerns in the outpatient setting are related to the use of injections—trigger point injections, spinal injections, peripheral joint injections, to name a few—as well as the use of modalities (e.g., application over insensate areas).

SELF-EXAMINATION QUESTIONS
(Answers begin on p. 367)

1. Which of the following best describes the root cause analysis?
   A. Following an event in which a patient was harmed, it seeks the answer what happened, why did it happen, and how can this be prevented from happening again
   B. The purpose of performing a root cause analysis is to assign blame for an adverse clinical event
   C. Its main purpose is to understand failures of doctors and less to understand system failures in health care

D. Root cause analysis is best performed by one individual—usually the chairman of the department
E. Root cause analysis is best performed by one individual to assign blame and to decide the punishment

2. According to the American Academy of Physical Medicine Medical Inpatient Rehabilitation Criteria Task Force Report titled "Standards for Assessing Medical Appropriateness Criteria for Admitting Patients to Rehabilitation Hospitals or Units," which of the following best describes the differences between rehabilitation services provided in inpatient rehabilitation facilities vs. skilled nursing facilities?
    A. In skilled nursing facilities, patients are required to receive 3 hours of therapy per day
    B. In skilled nursing facilities, weekly interdisciplinary team meetings to discuss goals and discharge planning are required
    C. In inpatient rehabilitation facilities, patients must be medically stable to participate in rehabilitation programs, are required to receive 3 hours of therapy per day, and physicians and nurses with specialized training in medical rehabilitation need to be available 24 hours per day, 7 days per week
    D. Rehabilitation nursing is mandatory in skilled nursing facilities
    E. In skilled nursing facilities, patients are required to receive 5 hours of therapy per day

3. Which of the following is a barrier to access to rehabilitation services?
    A. Financial barriers such as insurance coverage and out-of-pocket expenses
    B. Attitudinal barriers such as the beliefs of the friends of the patient regarding the patient's medical care
    C. Personality and attitudinal barriers on the part of the patient
    D. Oversupply of rehabilitative services referral options for patients
    E. Personality and attitudinal barriers on the part of the physicians

4. The minimum compliance threshold for inpatient rehabilitation facilities under the prospective payment system to treat patients is
    A. 6% of its total inpatient population
    B. 16% of its total inpatient population
    C. 45% of its total inpatient population
    D. 60% of its total inpatient population
    E. 90% of its total inpatient population

5. Which of the following is true with respect to Medicare payment for outpatient rehabilitation services?
    A. The beneficiary must be under the care of a physician, have a treatable condition, and be improving
    B. Medicare pays for maintenance-level outpatient therapy services
    C. Medicare pays the provided 50% of the fee schedule and the beneficiary pays a 50% copayment
    D. Outpatient rehabilitation services are rarely necessary and therefore not covered by Medicare
    E. Medicare pays the provided 40% of the fee schedule and the beneficiary pays a 60% copayment

6. Which of the following is true with respect to Medicare coverage of costs for an admission to a skilled nursing facility (SNF)?
    A. Medicare pays the SNF on a predetermined annual rate for up to 30 days through a prospective payment system
    B. Medicare pays the SNF on a predetermined per diem rate for up to 100 days through a prospective payment system
    C. The base payment rate does not take into account geographic differences in labor costs and case mix
    D. Medicare does not cover costs to a skilled nursing facility for rehabilitation
    E. Medicare pays the SNF on a predetermined per diem rate for up to 50 days through a retrospective payment system

7. Which of the following is the best choice about systems thinking?
    A. Focuses on the role of the individual in a system and less about interrelationships between structures
    B. Focuses on the interrelationships between health care systems
    C. Systems thinking is a framework for seeing interrelationships between structures, circles of causality where every influence is both cause and effect
    D. Focuses on linear cause-and-effect thinking
    E. Systems thinkers are taught to focus on short-term consequences of their actions and their impact in their immediate part of the system

REFERENCES

1. http://www.acgme.org/outcome/comp/GeneralCompetencies Standards21307.pdf.
2. Graham MJ, Naqvi Z, Encandela J, Harding KJ, Chatterji M. Systems-based practice defined: taxonomy development and role identification for competency assessment of residents. *J Grad Med Educ.* September 2009;1(1):49–60.
3. Johnson JK, Miller SH, Horowitz SD. Systems-based practice: improving the safety and quality of patient care by recognizing and improving the systems in which we work. In: Henriksen K, Battles JB, Keyes MA, et al., eds. *Advances in Patient Safety: New Directions and Alternative Approaches* (Vol. 2: Culture and Redesign). Rockville, MD: Agency for Healthcare Research and Quality (US); August 2008. http://www.ncbi.nlm.nih.gov/books/NBK43731/.
4. Ziegelstein RC, Fiebach NH. "The mirror" and "the village": a new method for teaching practice-based learning and improvement and systems-based practice. *Acad Med.* January 2004;79(1):83–88.
5. Elwood D, Kirschner JS, Moroz A, et al. Exploring systems-based practice in a sample of physical medicine and rehabilitation residency programs. *PMR.* March 2009;1(3):223–228. doi:10.1016/j.pmrj.2008.10.009. Epub 2009 February 6.
6. Mosby, Inc. *Mosby Medical Dictionary*, 8th ed. St. Louis, MO: Elsevier/Mosby; 2009.

7. Senge PM. *The Fifth Discipline: The Art and Practice of the Learning Organization.* New York, NY: Doubleday; 2006.
8. Beeuwkes Buntin M. Access to postacute rehabilitation. *Arch Phys Med Rehabil.* 2007;88:1488–1493.
9. http://www.medpac.gov/documents/MedPAC_Payment_Basics_08_IRF.pdf. Accessed December 2, 2013.
10. http://www.cms.gov/Medicare/Provider-Enrollment-and-Certification/GuidanceforLawsAndRegulations/InpatientRehab.html.
11. http://www.cms.gov/Medicare/Medicare-Fee-for-Service Payment/InpatientRehabFacPPS/Downloads/IRF-PAI-FINAL-for-Use-Oct2014-updated-v4.pdf.
12. http://www.cms.gov/Outreach-and-Education/Medicare-Learning-Network-MLN/MLNProducts/downloads/InpatRehabPaymtfctsht09-508.pdf.
13. http://www.cms.gov/Medicare/Quality-Initiatives-Patient-Assessment-Instruments/IRF-Quality-Reporting/.
14. http://www.medpac.gov/documents/MedPAC_Payment_Basics_08_IRF.pdf.
15. http://www.medpac.gov/documents/MedPAC_Payment_Basics_08_OPT.pdf. Accessed December 2, 2013.
16. http://www.medpac.gov/documents/MedPAC_Payment_Basics_08_SNF.pdf. Accessed December 2, 2013.
17. http://www.medpac.gov/documents/MedPAC_Payment_Basics_08_HHA.pdf. Accessed December 2, 2013.
18. Granger CV, Karmarkar AM, Graham JE, et al. The uniform data system for medical rehabilitation: report of patients with traumatic spinal cord injury discharged from rehabilitation programs in 2002–2010. *Am J Phys Med Rehabil.* April 2012;91(4):289–299.
19. Granger CV, Markello SJ, Graham JE, et al. The uniform data system for medical rehabilitation: report of patients with traumatic brain injury discharged from rehabilitation programs in 2000-2007. *Am J Phys Med Rehabil.* April 2010;89(4):265–278.
20. Granger CV, Reistetter TA, Graham JE, et al. The uniform data system for medical rehabilitation: report of patients with hip fracture discharged from comprehensive medical programs in 2000-2007. *Am J Phys Med Rehabil.* March 2011;90(3):177–189.
21. Granger CV, Markello SJ, Graham JE, et al. The uniform data system for medical rehabilitation: report of patients with lower limb joint replacement discharged from rehabilitation programs in 2000–2007. *Am J Phys Med Rehabil.* October 2010;89(10):781–794.
22. Granger CV, Markello SJ, Graham JE, et al. The uniform data system for medical rehabilitation: report of patients with stroke discharged from comprehensive medical programs in 2000–2007. *Am J Phys Med Rehabil.* December 2009;88(12):961–972.
23. Granger CV, Markello SJ, Graham JE, et al. The uniform data system for medical rehabilitation: report of patients with stroke discharged from comprehensive medical programs in 2000–2007. *Am J Phys Med Rehabil.* December 2009;88(12):961–972.
24. Ottenbacher K, Graham JE. The state of the science: access to postacute care rehabilitation services. *Arch Phys Med Rehabil.* 2007;88:1513–1521.
25. Chan L. The state of the science: challenges in designing postacute care payment policy. *Arch Phys Med Rehabil.* 2007;88:1522–1525.
26. Buntin M. Access to postacute rehabilitation. *Arch Phys Med Rehabil.* 2007;88:1488–1493.
27. Melvin JL, Worsowicz G. What are the implications of accountable care organizations for physical medicine and rehabilitation practices? *PMR.* 2011;3(11):1068–1071.
28. http://www.aapmr.org/advocacy/health-policy/medical-necessity/Documents/MIRC0211.pdf. Accessed December 2, 2013.
29. http://www.cdc.gov/Features/DisabilitiesDay/index.html. Accessed December 4, 2013.
30. http://blogs.cdc.gov/publichealthmatters/2013/01/4994/. Accessed December 4, 2013.
31. http://www.carnegiefoundation.org/elibrary/summary-educating-physicians. Accessed February 1, 2014.
32. Reinertsen JL. Physicians as leaders in the improvement of health care systems. *Ann Intern Med.* 1998;128:833–838.
33. Goleman D. What makes a leader? *Harvard Business Review.* January 2004.
34. www.nchl.org
35. Kotter JP. Leading change: why transformation efforts fail? *Harvard Business Review.* March–April 1995.
36. Bolman LG, Deal TE. *Reframing Organizations: Artistry, Choice, and Leadership.* 3rd ed. Hoboken, NJ: John Wiley and Sons; Hoboken, NJ: 2008.
37. Porter ME. The five competitive forces that shape strategy. *Harvard Business Review.* January 2008.
38. National Research Council. *Crossing the Quality Chasm: A New Health System for the 21st Century.* Washington, DC: The National Academies Press; 2001.
39. www.ihi.org. Accessed December 7, 2013.
40. www.abpmr.org. Accessed December 7, 2013.
41. Harvard School of Public Health-HCM 711. *Quality Improvement and Quantitative Methods* Dr. Mark Bloomberg, Dr. Josko Silobrcic.
42. Brassard M, Ritter, D. *Memory Jogger 2—Healthcare Edition.* Salem, TN: GoalQPC Inc.; 2008.
43. Griffin FA, Haraden C. Patient safety and medical errors. In: Ransom ER, ed. *The Healthcare Quality Book.* 2nd edition. Chicago, IL: Health Administration Press; 2008.

Kristjan T. Ragnarsson

8: Essentials of Leadership in the Field of Physical Medicine and Rehabilitation— A Personal Perspective

OBJECTIVES

1. Discuss characteristics of leadership based upon personal observations and experience.
2. Describe qualities of effective leaders.

Several years ago, I was asked to discuss the essentials of leadership in the field of Physical Medicine and Rehabilitation (PM&R) with a group of young academic physiatrists. In this regard, I was asked by the group's leader to describe my own leadership style and how it has changed over time, name the qualities that I believe are important for a leader to possess, and describe skills that are essential to acquire to be an effective leader.

To describe one's own leadership style is difficult, since your own views are likely to be very different from the opinions of those you are supposed to lead. Frankly, your own views of your leadership style matter less than what others think. To capture what others think of one's leadership style, one should ask others about the characteristics of excellent leaders with whom they have directly worked and whose leadership they have directly observed, followed by the same for your colleagues' perceptions of your leadership style. Therefore, I asked a couple of my faculty members' opinion of my leadership style. I was pleasantly surprised, although I realized that they would carefully avoid describing the negative aspects of my style! Nonetheless, I will humbly include some of their observations below, which I can only hope are correct!

One of my associates described my leadership style in the following ways: You bring in the people you trust, you give them authority, and you stay out of their way while their performance is good. You keep an open-door policy, so you are easy to approach to listen to my concerns and give me advice. You don't rush to make a decision, but rather try first to get all essential information in order to eliminate bias and then you make a sound decision.

Another one, in less than 5 minutes, wrote up the following: You have a spotless international reputation; you command respect and have multiple levels of involvement in the field of PM&R and within our own academic institution. You do not put people in a position they don't want to be in, which plays to the satisfaction of those working for you. For example, you allowed me to develop my interest in medical education, which has kept my job interesting for me and helped me in my career. You work as hard as or harder than those around you. You give credit to those working for you and you share your success with your associates, even your personal success, such as when you receive awards. You are willing to make changes in your own performance based on feedback of coworkers; for example, you increased the time you spend with our residents when they complained that they did not interact enough with you. You provide mentorship and make relevant suggestions to your faculty and staff in order to enhance their performance.

My third associate wrote the following: You listen to all staff and appropriately act on their concerns. You lead by example. You are a visionary thinker. You believe in the mission of rehabilitation medicine and you have created one of the best rehabilitation centers in the country (world) in an academic center where rehabilitation medicine was barely known before. You continue to make the center even better, despite the excellent reputation that it enjoys, which is a major reason why key staff members stay. You are an analytical thinker who also thinks "outside the box." You develop novel solutions to difficult problems. You carefully select your staff, guide their development, and help maximize their potential. You are a highly skilled physician, which is essential for a successful physician leader. You are always willing to share or even give up the spotlight to others. You set the highest ethical standards and you adhere to them yourself. You are reliable, easy to respect and trust, which is fundamental.

Has my leadership style changed over time? I don't think so, but it is hard for me to judge. I would have to evaluate by using reliable leadership style assessment tools over time in order to track and monitor changes in my leadership style. What happens over time is that your credibility and influence increases if your performance has been consistent and significant. People listen to you more carefully, which also means that you must be more careful in what you say and do. Your words may have a surprising influence, for better or for worse!

These observations of many of the leadership traits identified by my associates parallel the literature on leadership characteristics from distinguished thinkers and contributors such as Peter Senge, Warren Bennis, Tom Peters, Jack Welch, and Steve Covey.

QUALITIES THAT LEADERS MUST HAVE

The broadest definitions of leadership are "roles played by key individuals to facilitate change." Leadership competencies include (a) vision, (b) focus, (c) direction, (d) communication, and (e) mentorship. Some core traits of a good leader include drive, motivation, honesty/integrity, self-confidence, intelligence, and knowing the business. Being considerate of others as individuals is also a key characteristic of effective leaders. True to the mission of your organization, good leaders are proficient in clarifying, defining or framing issues, setting goals, and coordinating action steps. Leadership is all about being mentored and mentoring others.

Integrity, Which Will Inspire Trust

I believe reliance on mutual trust and respect is fundamental and most important of all qualities. A person without integrity cannot be trusted and should never be selected to a leadership position at any level.

A leader must be honest, truthful, and consistent. Your word should be as good as your signature. My mentor, Howard A. Rusk, MD, used to say, "Always tell the truth, then you will never have to remember what you said!" However, this is only one reason of many why you should always tell the truth if you say anything at all.

There should be no surprises in your behavior. Your constituents must always be able to figure you out. Inconsistent reactions and behavior will make it difficult for your faculty and staff to tolerate you.

A leader must never exploit one's people or one's constituents. An example of such exploitation occurred a decade ago when the president of Enron told his staff to buy the company's stock, when he himself was selling his own stock in anticipation of the company's implosion. The leader must never manipulate his constituents by not giving them the full story. A leader must be trusted as the best advocate for his or her constituents. The leader must try to protect his constituents from difficult and threatening situations in order to allow them to do their job in peace and without fear.

As a leader, you must know yourself, be candid about yourself, and have the capacity to self-disclose, at least to an extent. You must admit to your own mistakes, at least when they are obvious to others. You don't always have to try to have the last word in order to make your opinion prevail, especially when others on your staff are unconvinced.

If you are able to inspire trust in your constituents, there is a wonderful payback (i.e., you will also be able to trust the people who report to you). This is fundamental for a strong leadership (i.e., mutual trust).

Unfortunately, I do not believe that integrity can be learned, although it can and must be practiced by what we think and do in our daily lives. Integrity is a quality a leader must have. Integrity cannot be acquired on the job.

Competency

Of course, a leader must be competent. Expertise is an essential component of leadership. You have to know what you are doing. In selecting leaders, competency can usually be judged quite easily by examining the track record of the applicant and speaking directly with those listed as references.

If you are to lead an interdisciplinary rehabilitation team, a PM&R practice, or an academic department, you have to know and thoroughly understand what each member of your faculty and staff does and is capable of doing. You also need to know what you as the leader need to do in order to succeed.

Competency is something you cannot acquire after you obtain a leadership position. You must have it before.

Energy and Endurance

A leader must be able to work hard and not just in spurts, but consistently over long periods of time, even for years or decades. As a leader, you must be ready to come in early, leave late, work on weekends, and delay or cancel vacations and trips, when your effort is needed within your organization.

You have to be able to adhere to deadlines and consistently deliver on time. Answer e-mail, telephone calls, and so on, at once or as soon as possible. If there will be a delay, let the sender know. Those who develop a reputation for being unresponsive or slow to respond are often rejected as candidates for leadership positions. Being too busy is not a good excuse, because we all are. Similarly, it is important to be punctual and not keep your constituents waiting. Their time is valuable, just like yours. By consistently being punctual as a leader, you send a strong message for others to act likewise.

By being the hardest worker, you will serve as a role model for your constituents. This should be fairly natural for most leaders, because it is by hard work that most got to the top (i.e., it is more by perspiration than by inspiration). Paradoxically, you don't have to be driven all the time. You must be able to relax in between. More than a century ago, John Ruskin (1819–1900) wrote: "In order that people may be happy in their work, these three things are needed: they must be fit for it, they must not do too much of it and they must have a sense of success in it." You must be able to handle stress well, be able to smile and laugh, even when things are tough.

Energy and endurance can hardly be acquired on the job once you are in a leadership position. On the other hand, there are certain things that can be practiced.

- Establish good work habits. Come to work early and tackle first those things that you least want to do.
- Try to thrive on pressure (i.e., if nobody demands top performance of you, demand it of yourself).
- Try never to let up. If it appears that you have succeeded, you should be aware that there is no status quo. The environment changes and failure may lurk just around the corner. Therefore, try to retain a sense of urgency.

Passion and Compassion

Most leaders feel passionate about their work and are champions for inspiring others toward a desired mission. We know that one of the most evident qualities of an effective leader is the charisma and ability to inspire. Leaders must enjoy or even love what they are doing. They must passionately believe in the mission, be eager to get involved, and look at their work as an opportunity to do even more. In this regard, I passionately believe that our department and institution must provide the best services possible for people with physical disability and those suffering from painful musculoskeletal disorders. Failing to achieve that goal terrifies me and keeps me awake at night.

Passion without compassion is not good. You have to be compassionate and sensitive to the needs of your colleagues, staff, and patients, be supportive and helpful to them, and indeed serve them in every way. You do not do this for power or money, but for the cause you believe in.

Passion and compassion cannot be learned on the job, you must have it before. I find that your passion for your work may increase, but if you lose it, it is time to quit or do something else.

SKILLS THAT A LEADER SHOULD ACQUIRE AND PRACTICE

Vision and Foresight

Leaders are proactive in shaping the future. It is always a good idea to think before you act. A leader must know where the program, practice, department, organization, or even the entire health care enterprise is going and what the conditions in the future will be. As somebody once said, if you don't know where you are going, you can go very fast in the wrong direction! Another wise person said that not having a vision is like flying a plane on a dark night without radar. You will most likely crash.

In order to be a visionary leader, you must be knowledgeable about what is going on around you and you must be able to anticipate the changes that are coming. Therefore, you must go to meetings, serve on committees, and get involved, and then you have to be able to dream a little. Without dreaming about the good things you want to see happen, they will never materialize. Yes, dreaming of better things to come is important for every good team and supports their sense of meaning. As a leader, you must use your imagination in a positive and in a constructive way. Do not think primarily about the bad things that may happen, think about how you can make things better.

I believe it is important to develop a mission statement, which is your program's reason for being, and your entire constituency should be able to buy into the mission statement with excitement and enthusiasm. Often, it is also important to develop a vision statement with setting of goals, objectives, and priorities, listing the strategies to achieve these. If you want early success, you will have to identify the "low lying fruits" (i.e., objectives that are relatively easy to achieve). In general, your mission, your vision, your goals, and objectives need to fit the goals of the entire organization (e.g., the medical school or the hospital, not only your practice or the department). Building on your mission statement, you need to be able to turn it into a document describing ways to achieve improved quality, healthy finance, logical planning, and good management. A vision statement may and often should challenge the current way of thinking and status quo. Preferably, it should define a new and better way of doing things.

My personal style is such that outside of a small circle of my closest colleagues, I generally do not talk much about my dreams, desires, and goals, until there is a realistic way to make them happen, often through a great deal of preparatory work. Talking too much about all the things you want to happen—and then not having them happen—will just undermine your credibility.

Vision and foresight can be acquired. You must sit down, study the facts, feel the trends, know the plans, think, speculate, discuss, and dream in a constructive way!

Interpersonal and Communication Skills

We lead by example, and everything we do sends a message, sets a tone, and indicates to your people what to do, or not to do. Creative communication of vision, purpose, sense of urgency, and clear boundaries is key.

Clearly, good interpersonal and communication skills are highly desirable for a leader. Fortunately, I believe that these can be acquired and be improved with practice. A few things are worth bearing in mind:

1. Clarify your ideas before communicating. The more you think about an idea and discuss it with your closest confidants, the easier it will be to communicate to your entire constituency.
2. Know the true purpose of each communication. Are you trying to boost your constituents' spirit, start a new project, win support, change the current way of thinking or what? You must try to make each message of communication of real value to the receiver.
3. Let your constituents know what you stand for, but try to keep it simple. If you can, use simple words that will stir the emotions. Everybody must understand what you want and where you are going.
4. Never underestimate the power of a speech. No matter what the size of the audience or the setting. Remember that your faculty and staff are a very influential audience.
5. Consider the importance of nonverbal communication (e.g., your body language, your tone of voice, your passion, and your sincerity). We all know that meaning and intent are expressed in other ways than by words. Often, it is helpful to be able to smile and look confident when you present new ideas. This is not always easy.
6. You also have to demonstrate that you are receptive to the audience's reactions. Your own actions are also a means of nonverbal communication. Don't say one thing and do another. You cannot let your words contradict what you actually do, or nobody will listen seriously to you.
7. Follow-up on your communication. Find out as soon as possible how your message was received. Were you just wasting your time and effort, or did you indeed succeed in expressing what you meant and what you want of your constituents?
8. Be a good negotiator and be skilled in conflict resolution to ideally attain a win–win situation.

9. Be a good listener. Leaders are effective listeners. They don't just hear, but they listen, read body language, and internalize messages that have a deeper meaning. Listen much more than you speak and be attentive. Be able to state exactly what the other party means and wants. Show people that you truly understand what they were saying. After you have done that, you can express your own view without being argumentative, even if your view is very different from theirs. As you listen, you have to learn when to keep your mouth shut and just look wise and attentive. Don't gossip with your constituents. I strive never to quote anybody directly, who has not expressed a view or knowledge publicly. Your communication with your constituents is usually not in the form of memos and speeches, but rather it is in your everyday interaction with them. How do you greet your constituents? Do you do it by name, by eye contact, and so on? What do you know about them personally? Do you take personal interest in their well-being? Do you help them when they have a professional or even personal problem? Most people agree that it is important for a leader to be able to smile, even when things are tough, and show that he or she can have fun, both in and out of the office.
10. Pour on the praise, but only on those who deserve it. Empty praise is not good. Send a note, pick up the telephone, and mention their accomplishments at staff conferences. (I must admit that I could be much better in this regard.) When you are recognized for things well done, give them credit and allow them to share the spotlight with you. Most of the time, you could not have done it without them. Being able to encourage and motivate facilitates the change you are aiming for or helps to maintain a high standard.
11. Similarly, you must know how and when to criticize. This can be both uncomfortable and difficult for you, but necessary from time to time as a leader. However, it is important to be constructive in your criticism, which should make it clear that you are trying to help. Continuous or regular feedback based on direct observation of behaviors and performance is critical and facilitates improvement.
12. Always try to be positive and reject negativity. Don't be pessimistic before you tackle a problem or at the beginning of a task. However, you must be able to accept and adjust to change. But try to develop a "can do" attitude. In the final analysis, it is important for you as a leader and as a communicator to:
    - Know who you are, and what your values and priorities are. It will help you to be confident in your communications.
    - Keep an open mind and be flexible and adaptable to new ideas.
    - Keep a professional attitude. Try to behave as is expected of you, but still be yourself. There is no need to be perfect. It may even be better not to be perfect so that you can come across as a real human being, not a robot. If you are successful in what you do, you should try to be more of yourself, not less.
13. Be a coach and a mentor. As a coach, the leader must be able to help staff members to perform their jobs effectively, while they serve under his or her employment. Mentoring is different. Mentoring is a very personal and often long-term relationship, which is built on mutual respect and desire. The mentor is the more experienced person who wants to help the mentee to develop and succeed, not just in the current position, but also in building a satisfying and successful career wherever they may be. The mentee must be genuinely interested in seeking the guidance and help of the mentor, and be able to show appreciation and ability to follow the mentor's advice.

Mentoring relationships can be either informal or formal, or both. Until a few years ago, my own mentoring of faculty members was mostly informal, a relationship that developed naturally during daily interactions. A formal mentoring program was established at my medical school a few years ago, which required at least an annual face-to-face meeting and a review of the faculty member's accomplishments or lack thereof. This meeting is followed by a letter from me, summarizing our discussions and goals agreed on, to which the mentee responds with a letter. Whether mentoring is formal or informal, the mentor needs to be nonjudgmental, responsive, focused on the mentee's needs, supportive, and respectful, but still inviting a degree of informality, which eliminates barriers and strengthens personal bonds. Being a good mentor does not come naturally to all. Most leaders would benefit from learning mentoring techniques and by gaining understanding of the pitfalls to avoid. Communication skills may not always come naturally, but can be learned and must be practiced.

Ability to Delegate and Build a Team

Leaders are proficient in empowering others. Empowerment of your staff helps you to achieve your mission and vision. You cannot do it all by yourself, so you must ask others to do certain tasks. Select the people well and ask them to do things that they really want to do. Recruitment and retention of good people may take much time and effort, but is essential and will make your job easier and your program more successful. Give them responsibility and authority. Find out what they like to do and can do well. Then help them to do more of it. Help them to become better at doing the job—even better at it than you. Now that takes considerable ego strength. Don't ever delegate tasks so you can sit back, waste time, or be absent. You must always work harder than your staff.

Leaders build consensus, outline an agenda, and expect positive outcomes. Building a team is in large part a delegation of tasks, but it is also much more. A workgroup with a single leader is not a team if it only serves the leader's goals. A real team is motivated by common mission, vision, and goals. Members on a true team should be considered equal and accountable to each other. No single individual should stand to gain more than another by the team's success or lose by its failure. It is only the group that is affected. A collection of superstars does not guarantee a good team!

On a true team, each member understands the roles of all team members and is able and willing to fill each role when needed. It is worth remembering that your goal is not to make yourself or any of your team members indispensable, your goal as a leader is to make sure that the show will go on without you.

Fortunately, most people can learn to delegate and even build a team, although the success of the team may vary.

Decisiveness and Ability to Implement

It only helps to be decisive if you consistently make the right decisions. Decisions are preceded by gathering of lots of facts and by extensive discussions with your most trusted coworkers. Decisions should not be made impulsively and without knowing all the facts, risks, opportunities, and so on.

However, when making important decisions you should not let your closest associates block your view. You should also listen to outsiders, the people who may be critical of you and your decisions. You should make them your partners if feasible.

Ultimately, you as a leader must move the agenda item from discussion to a decision. Once a decision is made, you must see to it that it is implemented, but you should try to leave the actual implementation to your management and staff. As a leader, you are responsible for the vision, strategy, and decision, but usually not for implementation and day-to-day management.

The real measure of success as a leader is whether you are able to manifest your talents through others. Have you inspired others to learn and do more and given them the will to carry the mission on to make the world better? That is the question. Nobody can consistently do all these things or have all the leadership qualities described in this chapter; such a person would hardly be of the human race. But you can practice the qualities and actions each day and in turn you will be able to do better.

In summary, effective leaders exhibit the following characteristics:

- Lend purpose to mission, vision, meaning, direction, and focus: Who are we? What business are we about? What business are we not in? What target and priorities are we aiming for, short term and long term? What values and principles should define our relationships and what we do? How does each individual's job expectation fit into the organization, and what is expected of him or her? How should feedback, learning, and self-improvement be expected?
- Be able to make decisions (sometimes shared and sometimes alone as the circumstance requires), identify problems, and problem-solve.
- Be a systems thinker. Systems-Based Practice is one of the ACGME/ABMS core competencies.
- Understand and be sensitive to the interdependence and interaction between individuals and human behavior psychology.

We each have the obligation as PM&R leaders to approach leadership with renewed vigor.

II: Core Clinical Competencies

Nicole Sasson

9: Upper Extremity Limb Loss

PATIENT CARE

GOALS

Provide patient care that is compassionate, appropriate, and effective for the treatment of the adult with an upper extremity amputation.

OBJECTIVES

1. Describe the key components of the assessment of the adult with an upper extremity (UE) amputation.
2. Describe potential injuries associated with UE amputation.
3. Formulate the key components of a rehabilitation treatment plan for the adult with UE amputation.

The evaluation and assessment of the patient with an upper extremity (UE) amputation drives the rehabilitation process. UE amputations can be divided into two categories: congenital and acquired. Most acquired UE amputations are traumatic in nature (1). It is essential to obtain a detailed medical and surgical history including the cause and nature of the amputation and surgical interventions as well as any complications encountered. A patient with an upper limb amputation is unique and no two amputations are the same. A person with an UE amputation is initially devastated and more so if the amputation is bilateral, as we as humans are dependent on the use of our arms and hands. Patients are usually unable to perform a simple task initially.

Patients with UE amputations may have suffered concomitant traumatic brain injury and brachial plexus injury, which might impact their rehabilitation program.

In cases where resection of a malignancy was the cause of the amputation, it is important to obtain information about the type and stage of the cancer as well as treatments used. The treatments may have included prior surgical resections, chemotherapy, or radiation therapy.

The past medical history should document previous hand dominance. There should be a detailed history concerning the existence of comorbid vascular, endocrine, rheumatologic, orthopedic-musculoskeletal, and neurologic diseases. Renal impairment and fluctuations in fluid retention are important issues when prescribing a prosthesis.

A complete *review of symptoms* of overall health and comorbidities, is necessary for the team to consider before pursuing prosthetic options on an individual basis. The presence of phantom limb sensation, phantom limb pain, and presence of neuromas and the need to treat (and with what classes of medications) should be documented. It is also important to ask the patient about musculoskeletal pain in the residual part of the amputated extremity, visual symptoms, and the presence of depression or anxiety—all of which can potentially have an adverse effect on the successful rehabilitation of the patient.

The *past surgical history* should document all interventions including bony fixations, myodesis, myoplasty, cineplasty, and angulation-osteotomy (see Table 9.3). Fracture interventions; revascularization attempts; placement of skin grafts and type, including presence of surgical scars and associated adherence to the underlying residual structures; and presence of neuromas are all very important to record and consider.

A *functional history* should be taken, documenting the performance of activities of daily living including personal hygiene, dressing, feeding, and vocational activities. Vocational and leisure needs provide important information for the team to consider in prescribing an appropriate prosthetic limb and engagement into the rehabilitation process.

Physical examination of the UE amputee should document pertinent points in the past medical history and past surgical history already mentioned. Residual limb length and shape should be recorded and assessed with the following points in mind.

Ideal Residual Limb Length and Shape

1. *Transradial*—Ideally, the residual limb retains the configuration of an intact UE limb. The longer, the better for the lever arm, with more physiologic pronation and supination. This is ideal for a body-powered UE prosthesis. This can be used to perform manual labor. Presence of the brachioradialis muscle results in improved elbow movement. Residual limbs shorter than the medium length (<55% transradial length) are ideal

89

candidates for externally powered prostheses such as a myoelectric or a hybrid prosthesis.
2. *Transhumeral*—Ideally, the residual limb should be cylindrical in nature with retention of the tuberosity of the deltoid. The longer the better for the lever arm, where retention of the affected humerus compared with the sound limb is 50% to 90%.

Range of motion and presence of contractures of the residual limb should be recorded. Skin integrity is also an important concern since it is needed to suspend the prosthesis and control the terminal device of an UE prosthesis.

On inspection, it is important to look for scars, bony or soft-tissue deformities, and burns.

On palpation, it is important to feel for skin adhesions and tender areas as well as ascertain for the presence of neuromas, which can be a source of pain for the patient.

In UE amputations secondary to trauma, key neurologic or vascular structures in the limb may have been injured; therefore, an assessment is warranted. This should include an evaluation of the muscles and key sensory areas supplied by the brachial plexus and its terminal branches, as well as performing an evaluation of the vascular supply to the limb. Motor strength of key muscle groups in the affected UE as well as in the sound extremity is important to record. Sensory testing should include light touch, pinprick, and proprioception.

A brief cognitive evaluation can also be helpful in cases where significant trauma was associated with the limb amputation since the presence of a brain injury can signal challenges in learning how to use the prosthesis safely and may require additional testing. Level of alertness, orientation, attention span, immediate and delayed recall, and judgment are some key areas to focus on.

Visual acuity plays an important role while using UE devices and deficits should be recorded.

Imaging and Other Diagnostic Studies
Imaging studies such as x-rays and MRIs of the residual limb can provide significant information regarding the osseous and soft-tissue integrity of that limb. Electrodiagnostic studies can provide information regarding injury to the brachial plexus and its terminal branches.

Rehabilitation of the Upper Extremity Amputee
Successful outcomes in rehabilitation for the UE amputee, whether unilateral or bilateral, are dependent on multiple factors including early posttraumatic intervention, an experienced team approach, patient-directed prosthetic training, patient education, and on-going patient evaluation and follow-up (2).

The use of rigid dressings and early fitting in patients with transhumeral or more distal amputations encourages the resumption of bimanual activities, promotes wound healing, and decreases edema. This can lead to a greater acceptance and use of the prosthesis. There is a known direct relationship with time of fitting of prosthetic device and long-term prosthetic use. Which usually should happen in the first month following the amputation (3). Earlier application of the UE prostheses also helps to decrease the incidence of phantom limb pain that can disrupt prosthetic training and use.

There are multiple steps in the rehabilitation of the UE amputee (Table 9.1). Ideally, the physiatrist should be involved early and in all of the steps. Preamputation counseling involves education on the specific surgical intervention, the subsequent rehabilitation, and basic prosthetic design options as well as peer visitation and psychological counseling. Pain control is tantamount to successful rehabilitation. Once stable surgically, range of motion, strengthening, massage and desensitization, and wound care of the residual limb must be stressed to prepare for successful prosthetic fitting and use. Avoiding contracture development is important in postfracture priority. The transhumeral residual limb's preferable shape is cylindrical with retention of the deltoid tuberosity.

Unilateral UE amputees usually perform all tasks and activities of daily living (ADLs) with their intact side. Commonly, they will experience overuse syndromes and must be educated to avoid this. Overuse injuries are more common, the more proximal the amputation. They can present with decreasing frequency in the elbow, shoulder, and least commonly in the wrist joint.

Pain syndromes are common in UE amputees. Phantom sensation is felt by nearly all "acquired amputees," but is not always troublesome (1). Aggressive preamputation pain management leads to better postsurgical pain states. Use of a patient-controlled analgesia (PCA) system is the standard pre- and postoperatively followed by scheduled parental/oral analgesia. Therapeutic desensitization modalities to assist in pain management are introduced first with edema control, light touch and

TABLE 9.1 Steps in UE Amputee Rehabilitation

STAGES OF AMPUTATION REHABILITATION
Preamputation counseling
Amputation surgery
Acute postamputation period
Preprosthetic training
Preparatory prosthesis fitting
Prosthetic fitting and training
Reintegration into the community/advanced functional skills training
Long-term follow-up

STAGES OF REHABILITATION
Acute care
Support
Pain management
Wound care
Preprosthetic training
Comprehensive evaluation
Edema control and limb shaping
Pain control
Adaptation to body image
Soft-tissue desensitization/ROM/strength training
Maximize left/right dominance retraining hand dominance
Myo-site testing

tapping, and transcutaneous nerve stimulation. Virtual imaging techniques, mirror therapy, and acupuncture (4) have also been found to be quite helpful. Severe cases might necessitate nerve blocks: ganglion, epidural nerve blocks with steroids. Surgical intervention is deemed as a last resort as it is not as successful.

It is important to be fit with the first prosthesis as soon as possible. The first UE prosthesis is intended to promote residual limb maturation and desensitization, increase wearing tolerance, and allow the patient to become a functional UE prosthetic user (1). This is usually accomplished with a body-powered prosthesis. A period of several months of wearing and use is usually needed before fitting with a more permanent prosthesis. This is usually followed with serial circumferential measurements of the limb.

Bilateral UE amputees perform ADLs with their feet—especially when congenital in nature; however, as the child ages, he or she should be fit with prostheses. The rule when prescribing prostheses for pediatric patients is "fit to sit (5)." This occurs by 6 months of age with an initial prosthesis that has a passive terminal device. When no "normal limbs" remain for comparative measurement, the normal upper arm length is estimated by multiplying the patient's height by 0.19 and normal forearm length is estimated by multiplying the patient's height by 0.21 (6).

The health care certifying organization, Joint Commission (JCAHO), has standards for spiritual care that state that each patient's "spiritual care be assessed, accommodated, and attended to in ways that are important to them" (7). These standards are typically followed upon admission to the hospital. The admissions personnel ask patients to state their religion and whether or not they would like to see a chaplain. But the chaplain can also serve as a member of the interdisciplinary rehabilitation team and assist the patient in his or her rehabilitation program. JCAHO stresses that the cultural and spiritual beliefs of our patients are met (7), whereas the Commission on Accreditation of Rehabilitation Facilities (CARF) advocates a more holistic approach to the care of the amputee, treating the mind and the body of the patient. CARF emphasizes delivery of exceptional medical care as well as meeting the cultural, spiritual, and educational needs of this population (8).

MEDICAL KNOWLEDGE

GOALS

Demonstrate knowledge of established and evolving biomedical, clinical, and epidemiological sciences pertaining to UE amputees, as well as the application of this knowledge to guide holistic patient care.

OBJECTIVES

1. Describe the epidemiology of upper limb loss.
2. Describe the common anatomical levels of upper limb amputations and their relevance to prosthetic prescription.
3. Review the prosthetic prescription for the individual with upper limb loss.

Each year approximately 185,000 persons undergo an amputation of their limbs (1). There are more than 1.9 million persons living in the United States with limb loss (9). Lower extremity (LE) amputations are most commonly due to dysvascular disease, whereas upper limb amputation is relatively rare and mainly traumatic in origin, affecting 41,000 persons or 3% of the U.S. amputee population (1,9). Major amputations of the upper extremity (UE) (other than digital amputations) account for 3% to 15% and are approximately 20 times less common than LE amputations. UE amputations can be broken down into two groups: congenital and acquired. Reasons for congenital malformations are largely unknown but are thought to be due to exposure to teratogenic agents and/or environmental radiation. Approximately 60% of limb deficiencies in children are congenital and involve the UE compared with the LE in a 2:1 ratio. The most common deletion of the UE is the absence of the left transverse radius (10). Most amputees (68.6%) who have lost limbs to traumatic injuries have lost an upper limb (9,11). Traumatic amputation is the major reason for UE limb loss in the military. This population has grown in particular with the last two military conflicts, Operation Iraqi Freedom and Operation Enduring Freedom in Afghanistan. UE amputations are more common in men than in women: 4 to 6/1 ratio. The majority of these amputations occur in the 20- to 40-year-old age group. Most of the service men and women who undergo amputation will have polytraumatic injuries, including traumatic brain injuries and multiple amputations. OSHA regulations over the past decades have decreased the incidence of occupational workplace incidents. Malignant tumors are the primary reasons for shoulder disarticulation and forequarter amputations (12) (Table 9.2).

Length of the residual limb should be preserved using microvascular anastomosis, distal free flaps, and spare part flaps from the amputated limb, if possible (12), as the level of amputation is the single most important determination of function. However, transcarpal amputation and wrist amputation are seen less frequently because of limited functional outcome (1) with an UE prosthesis (Tables 9.3 and 9.4).

Prosthetic Prescription

Prostheses prescription for the UE amputee has become quite intricate with new technology and componentry being developed since the 1980s. High technology is not required of all users and should be determined by the interdisciplinary team. UE amputees have chore-specific arms fabricated, with body powered being the staple one.

TABLE 9.2 Etiology of Upper Limb Amputations (Decreasing Frequency)

Trauma (80%–90%)
Congenital (9%)
Cancer (8%)
Vascular complications of disease (6%)

TABLE 9.3 Levels of Amputation (Distal to Proximal) and Lengths of Residual Limbs

Transcarpal
Below-Elbow Amputation
Wrist disarticulation
Transradial
Long 55%–100%
Short 35%–55%
Very short <35%
Elbow disarticulation
Above-Elbow Amputation
Transhumeral
Standard 50%–90%
Short 30%–50% or less
Shoulder disarticulation
Interscapulothoracic disarticulation "forequarter"

TABLE 9.4 Surgical Techniques

Myodesis: Direct suturing of residual limb musculature or tendon to the bone/periosteum.
Myoplasty: Suturing of agonist–antagonist muscle pairs to each other.
Cineplasty: Surgical isolation of a loop of muscle (biceps/pectoralis most common) covering it with skin.
Angulation–Osteotomy: Skeletal alteration of the humerus aiding in suspension of a prosthesis, facilitating rotation.
Osseointegration (12)
Targeted muscle reinnervation: Rerouting of nerves to existing unused residual limb musculature.
Hand transplants (13)

Terminal Device

The functional activities of the hand are intricate but can be separated into two groups: nonprehensile and prehensile. Voluntary opening terminal devices are normally held closed by a spring or a rubber band and open when the control cable is pulled. It takes the shape of a "c" configuration. Each rubber band produces approximately 0.45 kg (1 lb of prehensile force) between the hook fingers. A version of this type of terminal device is the most commonly prescribed type of terminal device in our country because of its versatility and reliability. The type of metal used depends on the length of the residual limb. A transradial amputee would probably receive a stainless steel hook, whereas a transhumeral amputee would probably receive an aluminum alloy hook to ease the weight and effort needed with elbow flexion.

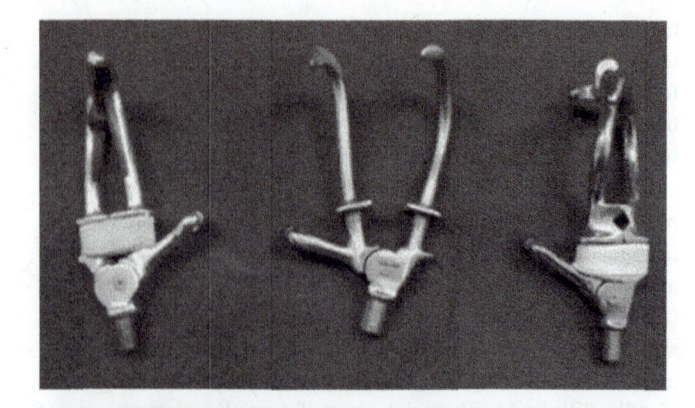

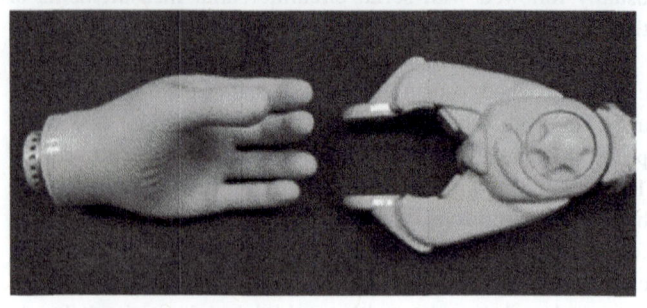

FIGURE 9.1 Prehensile and Nonprehensile Devices

- *Transradial amputation* (TR) may allow lifting of 20 to 30 lbs
- Terminal device (TD) is the most important functional part of the upper extremity prosthesis
  - Passive–cosmetic
    - Flexible passive mitts–sports/task specific
    - Voluntary–opening (VO) split hook type; usually made of aluminum, more lightweight; most common and practical
    - Specialized work hook-type (i.e., farmer's hook); made of stainless steel, heavier in nature
    - CAPP (Child Amputee Prosthetics Project) alligator or helper
    - Prehensile forces are determined by the number of rubber bands. Can use up to 10 bands
    - Nonamputee male pinch force is 15 to 20 lbs
  - Voluntary–closing (VC) hook type is not limited by rubber band strength or springs
    - Gradient of pinch is dependent on the force exerted
    - Provides better control of closing pressures, but active effort is required to maintain closure or items may be dropped
    - Myoelectric hands—offer spherical/palmar grasp with grip forces greater than VO/VC TDs. More cosmetically appearing but more fragile
    - One-site two-function controllers use weak versus strong contractions of the same muscles to operate the TD
    - Two-site two-function controllers use different muscles to open and close the TD
- Wrist unit
  - Friction wrist units
    - Constant—friction wrist units
    - Allows passive pronation/supination, but rotates when holding heavy objects
  - Active pronation/supination

- Passive pronation/supination
- Quick-disconnect wrist unit
- Wrist flexion units—spring assisted, useful for midline activities: eating, hygiene, toileting, and dressing not usually seen in unilateral but **bilateral** amputees because of increased weight at the end of the prosthesis
- Rotational wrists—lock in place
- Elbow unit
  - Attaches to the triceps pad and to the prosthetic forearm
  - Flexible hinges—Dacron webbing; leather or metal cable allowing approximately 50% of residual rotation for amputations through the distal one-third of the forearm
  - Rigid hinges—for amputations at or above the mid-forearm level; eliminates rotation
  - Single axis hinges—for shorter residual limb set in pre-flexion to prevent hyperextension of the elbow.
  - Polycentric hinges—for short transradial amputees; provides room in the cubital fossa increasing range of motion (ROM)
  - Step-up hinges—split socket configuration; enhances flexion
    - For a short TR amputation used to provide a 2:1 ratio of flexion to socket motion
  - This requires the amputee to use approximately twice as much force to flex the prosthesis
    - Sliding action joint
    - Geared joint
- Socket double walled for optimal fit
  - Outer wall is rigid and serves to connect to other components
  - Inner wall is fit precisely to the shaped residual limb
  - Suction socket can provide self-suspension without straps
    - Munster supracondylar socket can provide suspension to a very short transradial amputee but precludes full elbow extension; can be used for externally powered TD
- Harness
  - Figure of 9—for a long transradial amputation or a wrist disarticulation; requires a self-suspending socket, is generally more comfortable than a "figure of 8."
  - Figure of 8—short transradial or more proximal amputation
  - Axilla loop—Primary Anchor from which two other straps originate; encircles the shoulder girdle on the non-amputated side.
  - Anterior support strap or the "inverted Y suspensor."
  - Connects to the triceps pad or half arm cuff, usually with an elbow hinge one cable or single control system that attaches proximally to one of the nonelastic straps of the harness and distally at a prehension device or TD
  - Bilateral Transradial Harness—omits the axilla loops
- **Transhumeral (TH) amputation may be able to lift 10 to 15 lb**
- Terminal device—as above
- Wrist unit—as above
- Elbow unit has an alternator lock that alternately locks and unlocks with the same movement
  - With the elbow unlocked, body movements will flex or extend the elbow with the cable
  - With the elbow locked, the cable will operate the TD
- Outside locking hinges—Elbow disarticulation/transcondylar amputation
- Inside Locking Hinges—Transhumeral amputations, if 5 cm proximal to the elbow joint
- Flail—arm hinges—postbrachial plexus lesions
- Ratchet hinge—postbrachial plexus injury works like a beach chair positioning
- Friction units—lightweight, passive positioning
- Flexion assist—counterbalances the weight of the prosthetic forearm
- Nudge control unit—originally designed to lock and unlock the elbow
  - Can also be adapted to operate other components, including flexion and rotation wrist units
- Shoulder unit
  - Bulkhead-humeral segment is connected directly to the socket; makes the prosthesis lightweight
  - Friction loaded-passively moveable; provides assistance with dressing and tabletop activities
  - Single axis—permits abduction
  - Double axis—permits abduction and flexion
  - Triple axis—permits passive motion
  - Ball and socket—permits passive motion
  - Locking shoulder—can stabilize the shoulder in 36 different flexion positions; can be used with an externally powered terminal device (TD); a second friction-controlled hinge provides abduction and adduction stabilization
- Socket—double walled for optimal fit
  - Suction socket can provide self-suspension without straps
  - Munster supracondylar socket can provide suspension to an elbow disarticulation by encasing the humeral condyles; can be used for externally powered TDs.
- Harness
  - Figure of 8—short transradial or more proximal amputation (see previous)
  - Shoulder Saddle with chest straps frees the opposite shoulder
  - Relieves the pressure caused by the axillary loop of the "8"
  - Heavy loads are tolerated better
  - Poor cosmesis
  - Donning requires assistance and is more difficult
- Endoskeletal upper limb prostheses vs. exoskeletal upper limb prostheses
  - Systems with tubular humeral and forearm elements
    - Encasement in a cosmetic foam cover and components above
    - Lightweight compared to exoskeletal UE prostheses
- Necessary movements for body-powered prosthesis control
- *Transradial (TR) Amputations*
- Glenohumeral forward flexion
  - Natural movement
  - Generates good force to reach and activate TD or flex an elbow
  - Biscapular abduction
  - Generates weak force that may activate TD while it remains still to perform midline activities
- *Transhumeral (TH) Amputations*
- Glenohumeral forward flexion

- Biscapular abduction
- Glenohumeral depression, extension, and abduction
  - Unnatural and difficult
  - Unlocks or locks elbow
- Scapular adduction/chest expansion
  - Unnatural
  - Unlocks or locks elbow
  - Allows TD functions
- Scapular elevation
  - Requires another strap-waist belt
  - Unlocks or locks elbow

The Krukenberg procedure is classically indicated for a person with bilateral transradial amputations who was also blinded in the same incident/accident. This is usually from an exploded hand grenade or improvised explosive device. This procedure restores a functional and sensitive grip; however, it is not natural in appearance. It is mainly performed in places where prosthetic fabrication and costs are prohibitive (i.e., developing nations). The operation is the conversion of a transradial residual limb into sensate, muscle-powered radial and ulnar pincers creating a unique form of prehension. Postoperative distraction of the radial and ulnar pincers is key to the success as well as initiating postoperative exercises within 12 to 14 days to open and close the bifid forearm and to take advantage of the somatosensory plasticity of the brain. The procedure is contraindicated in transradial amputees younger than 2 years old and in the elderly who are dependent on others for their ADLs. It is also contraindicated with severe elbow contractures or when the residual limb is too short for effective pincer function (<10 cm in adults). Patients who undergo a Krukenberg procedure can also be fit for a prosthesis. As with all prosthetic prescriptions, type chosen/prescribed is dependent on the intended use.

Comorbidities may interfere with the rehabilitation of an individual with an UE amputation. Many persons may have suffered concomitant multiple trauma, which may even include a brain injury, a spinal cord injury, and multiple amputations, which need to be addressed by the interdisciplinary rehabilitation team. These comorbidities may preclude training and use of certain prosthetic components. Patients with pain syndromes not stabilized on a pharmacological regimen might have fluctuations in cognitive functions, which may interfere with progress. The best way to deal with these patients is to provide good patient and support system education. Peer visits from the Amputation Coalition of America or Wounded Warriors provides additional emotional support and guidance in recovery and reintegration.

UE amputee care involves a holistic approach to the care of the patient while using the latest highly technical prostheses when appropriate. Significant advances have been made in the componentry and fabrication of the UE prosthesis. These have been assisted by the military and the government embarking on several research ventures since the Gulf War and continued military efforts. Two advanced upper limb prosthetic solutions are being developed. One uses neural control, the other uses a "strap and go system," that can be controlled by noninvasive methods. The Department of Veteran Affairs (VA) has partnered with the Defense Advanced Research Projects Agency (DARPA) and DEKA Integrated Solutions since 2008 to optimize the function of an advanced prosthetic arm system (the later system) that will enable greater independence and function (14) to meet the needs of military amputations. These projects have also fueled the Department of Veteran Affairs to develop an amputation system of care with centers of excellence. Since all teams are not versed in the varying types of technology, care can be shared with these centers of excellence through telemedicine venues, which will eventually be duplicated in the civilian health care system based on need.

PRACTICE-BASED LEARNING AND IMPROVEMENT

GOALS

Develop an understanding and exhibit the importance of continuing professional development; lifelong learning; continuous self-assessment; goal setting; teaching skills for team, patient, family, and colleagues; and systematic analysis and improvement of the clinical practice of the physiatrist as it applies to quality care of the upper limb amputee, with support of evidence-based practice.

OBJECTIVES

- Describe the importance of "clinical reflection" in the professional growth and improvement of the physiatrist taking care of the upper limb amputee.
- Identify key references and resources, including evidence-based reviews, important to the care of the upper limb amputee.
- Demonstrate ongoing lifelong professional development and self-assessment with linkage to quality, safety, and efficiency in patient care.
- Describe the key elements of effective patient education methodology as it applies to the care of the upper limb amputee.

As mentioned earlier, UE amputations are not as common as lower limb amputations; therefore, physiatrists may not have significant opportunities to care for these patients. Therefore, it is important for physiatrists to perform a self-assessment of their medical knowledge about the care of these patients as well as the various types of prosthetic components currently available on a periodic basis as well as when asked to be involved in the clinical care of an amputee. Gaps that are identified in that self-assessment can be used to identify areas in need of further education, which can then be used to direct educational activities. Some areas that are important in that self-assessment include (a) ability to evaluate and treat musculoskeletal and neuropathic pain syndromes, (b) ability to prescribe a UE prosthesis, and (c) ability to prescribe a rehabilitation program for the UE amputee that would address the various impairments, activity limitations, and participation restrictions commonly affecting these patients.

Alternatively, physiatrists can "reflect back" on the care they provided to a UE amputee and use that opportunity to assess their knowledge base about the various issues involved in the care of that patient.

Once the gaps are identified, there are several resources and strategies that one can use to address them. One useful approach is "reading around your patient." In this approach, one updates clinical and treatment skills as they apply to their specific patient. This may include reading on relevant topics in various textbooks and pertinent journal articles as well as seeking out clinical expertise from physiatrists, prosthetists, and physical and occupational therapists who have significant experience in the care of these patients. Various institutions also offer courses on prosthetics and orthotics for clinicians as part of continuing medical education activities for those interested in pursuing this option. Online resources include Knowledge NOW sponsored by the American Academy of Physical Medicine and Rehabilitation.

Patient educational materials are aimed individually at the style that the patient is known to best learn. This can be with written materials at a fourth-grade to sixth-grade reading level in their native language, videos, Internet access, demonstration, and through appropriate individual or support groups. Models and prosthetic samples are quite effective mediums used in teaching sessions. Patients and their families are educated on proper skin care and inspection of their residual limbs, maintaining maximal range of motion, and techniques to achieve pain relief. There is also an emphasis on maintaining sexuality with the patient's new impairment.

INTERPERSONAL AND COMMUNICATION SKILLS

GOALS

Develop an understanding and appreciation for the importance of effective verbal, nonverbal, and written communication with patients, their families, and professional colleagues in building effective relationships and resolving conflicts.

OBJECTIVES

- Describe effective verbal, nonverbal, and written communication skills in the care of the upper limb amputee.
- Identify the key elements of effective and timely medical record documentation as a communication tool among and between colleagues.
- Propose strategies to resolve conflicts between the upper limb amputee patient and the clinical staff providing care for him or her.

Effective communication requires multiple attributes from all team members. Remember that the patient is an essential team member in patient-centered care. Family members and significant others are used to enlist support. Progress toward goals should be presented in a manner that is nonjudgmental and unemotional. An effective communicator is able to function independently; accepts differences in the perspectives of others; is able to negotiate with other team members; is able to form new values, attitudes, and perceptions; tolerates ongoing review and challenge of ideas; takes risks; possesses personal integrity; and mostly accepts the team philosophy. Conflict resolution is an important part of the communication process of the interdisciplinary rehabilitation team who has the UE amputee patients' best interests and good care at heart.

A comprehensive medical record is an essential communication tool between colleagues caring for the UE amputee. The record must be accurate, stating goals and barriers in regard to medical, rehabilitation, psychosocial, vocational, and prosthetic issues and needs to be completed in a timely manner. The use of electronic medical records comes with new challenges of unnecessary duplication in the medical record, which needs to be addressed.

PROFESSIONALISM

GOALS

Develop an understanding and appreciation for the importance of commitment, excellence, responsibility, adherence, ethics, and sensitivity to diversity as they apply to quality care of the upper limb amputee.

OBJECTIVES

- Discuss and exemplify the importance of accountability, respect, courtesy, altruism, integrity, trust, honesty, compassion, and empathy in the care of the upper limb amputee.
- Describe and demonstrate the importance of being proactive in team-based patient-centered care, advocacy and responsiveness to patient needs, confidentiality, respect for privacy and autonomy, shared decision making, and informed consent as they apply to the care of the upper limb amputee.
- Explain and model the importance and impact that the patient's sociocultural factors such as cultural beliefs, age, gender, and disability have on the care of the upper limb amputee.
- Describe and reflect adherence to the ethical principles for issues that can come up in the care of upper limb amputees.

The physiatrist providing care for the UE amputee is accountable for the overall rehabilitation, prosthetic prescription, and management of specific impairments and issues that pertain to the individual with UE limb loss. The care should be patient centered and delivered with the respect for the patient and his or her cultural and religious beliefs, age, and gender. The physiatrist should deliver care in an ethical manner that is based on trust, compassion, and empathy for the patient.

A prosthetic limb cannot adequately replace the sensibility of the hand, and the function of a prosthetic limb decreases with higher levels of amputation (11). A UE amputation is initially devastating, even with today's most advanced prostheses. It is very important to provide the best care while being honest, empathetic, and respectful of the patient and his or her family.

The patient and his or her ongoing needs and wants are the center of the interdisciplinary care team's efforts from step one of the process—the preoperative phase of the rehabilitation process.

Patients need to be addressed on an individual basis. Their needs, hobbies and activities, and functional status all play a role in the specific prostheses prescribed. UE prosthetic needs are task specific; therefore, patients receive several to perform necessary tasks, from a cosmetic prosthesis for formal events to task-specific body-powered prostheses with dynamic and fixed terminal devices.

Physiatrists should employ a proactive approach to the needs of the UE amputee at every stage of the rehabilitative process and serve as an advocate for the patient while respecting the privacy and wishes. Shared decision making is an important component of the effective physician–patient collaboration. Some examples of advocacy for the patient include (a) advocating for appropriate rehabilitative services and adequate pain management with other clinicians involved in the care of the patient as well as the patient's health insurance carrier and (b) advocating for the patient to receive the most appropriate prosthesis that will enable him or her to meet one's life goals (e.g., work, school, family, and community roles).

The ethical principle of autonomy is of paramount importance in medical and rehabilitative care. It implies that the patient's wishes are to be respected and honored. Whereas the physiatrist should provide the appropriate counseling and education about various treatment options, the competent patient with intact medical decision-making capacity makes the final decision regarding his or her care. This can sometimes pose an ethical conflict if there is a disagreement between the physiatrist and patient regarding issues related to prosthetic components and rehabilitation. Another ethical conflict can occur when a patient who could benefit from a particular type of prosthesis cannot receive it due to limited health insurance coverage or lack of expertise in fabricating it in that part of the country.

It is important for the rehabilitation team to be educated in local laws and have policies and guidelines for navigation in challenging situations. Further ethical challenges are seen with the advances in medicine in regard to limb transplants and use of technology like telemedicine and virtual care with specialized amputation care teams, as have been developed throughout the Veteran's Administration Healthcare System with the Amputation System of Care. It may not be unusual that patients with severe pain syndrome seek consideration for elective limb amputation when all modes of conventional intervention have been exhausted. All outcomes of this definitive intervention must be explored. It is possible that there in fact might be no improvement in the current pain level with this drastic measure.

SYSTEMS-BASED PRACTICE

GOALS

Develop an awareness, responsiveness, and understanding of the strengths, challenges, and cost considerations of different settings in which rehabilitation services are provided for amputees, with specific reference to the importance of interprofessional teamwork and patient advocacy, and the impact of system-related errors as they apply to the safe care of the upper limb amputee.

OBJECTIVES

- Describe the different inpatient and outpatient settings that provide rehabilitation services to amputees and effective resource management and coordination of care between these settings.
- Examine patient safety concerns and systems-related errors in the care of upper limb amputees and identify strategies to prevent them.

The rehabilitation of the UE amputee usually occurs in the outpatient setting; however, regrettably, multidisciplinary resources are often scarce. Ideally, a physiatrist-led team consisting of a prosthetist, occupational therapist, or physical therapist is well suited to provide care for this patient. At times, the patient may require additional clinical expertise depending on any associated impairments. This may include a neuropsychologist if the patient has a traumatic brain injury, orthopedic surgeon, or oncologist if the patient has an underlying malignancy. The physiatrist is well suited to coordinate and lead the team's efforts to optimize the patient's level of function and reintegration into his or her life roles.

The VA Amputation System of Care is a model system of care of all amputees. It uses resources most efficiently with the greatest benefit to U.S. veterans. There are four key levels of care. Regional Amputee Centers have the most comprehensive levels of care for amputees with care coordinators, followed by Polytrauma Amputation Network Sites, and then by Amputation Care Teams, followed by Amputation Points of Contact. This system allows for the efficient and complete continuum of care and allocates appropriate resources to each level of care.

There are several patient safety concerns that physiatrists should be aware of in the rehabilitation of the UE amputee. Rehabilitative interventions can potentially cause harm to the residual limb of the patient through aggressive range of motion, strengthening or weight-bearing exercises in individuals with risk for fracture in the residual limb due to prior injury (e.g., traumatic amputation), or malignancy as reason for amputation (e.g., risk of pathological fracture). Use of heat modalities for pain management over insensate areas or in patients with cognitive impairments can potentially cause burns. Use of medications to treat pain can be associated with excessive sedation and impaired cognitive function, which in turn can lead to harm when operating heavy machinery or driving. A poorly fitting or functioning prosthesis can be a source of injury as well when using a device for performing various functions in the course of work or performing activities of daily living.

Hand-off of patients from one level of care to another provides an opportunity for these patients to fall between the cracks in our health care system. This is where the rehabilitation team, and the physiatrist in particular, serves to be the patient advocate and play the most crucial role of team coordinator of services across the continuum of care. Education about proper residual UE care—range of motion, skin care, and pain management—is essential to having any future success when fit with a prosthesis.

Poor communication between physicians, prosthetist, physical, occupational, and nursing therapy at various transition points in care along the health care continuum can predispose to injury. Information that is important to transmit between health care providers as it pertains to the UE amputee includes (a) reason for amputation, surgery performed, and complications following surgery; (b) weight-bearing precautions and range of motion restrictions; (c) comorbid medical conditions; and (d) current medications, their indication, dose, and adverse effects.

CASE STUDY

A 25-year-old African American married male apache helicopter mechanic with two children is admitted to an inpatient rehabilitation unit 2 weeks posttraumatic amputation of his bilateral upper extremities when there was a tire explosion, rendering him a left transhumeral as well as a right transradial amputee. He also sustained loss of consciousness and visual and auditory injuries from the blast. He complains of pain in the residual limbs that is temporarily relieved by pain medications. He has a tendency to keep his upper extremities internally rotated and adducted. His wife is busy caring for their 2 children younger than 5 years and he lives with them in an apartment with stairs to enter. Prior to surgery he was an active young man, whose hobbies were graphic design and building custom furniture.

CASE STUDY DISCUSSION QUESTIONS

PATIENT CARE. Formulate the postoperative clinical management, rehabilitative care, and prosthetic recommendations for this patient in the acute hospital, acute inpatient rehabilitation unit, and outpatient settings. Write a prosthetic prescription for this patient.

MEDICAL KNOWLEDGE. What are the different types and levels of upper limb amputations and their incidence and prevalence? What are the common causes of pain in the upper limb amputee? What are the clinical guidelines for the care of a patient with bilateral UE amputations, long transradial (dominant side), and long transhumeral (nondominant side) amputations?

PRACTICE-BASED LEARNING AND IMPROVEMENT. What are some possible quality-of-care issues, including benchmarks and best practices, in the rehabilitation of UE amputee patients? Describe a quality improvement project for the provision of care in upper limb amputees—include a description of the methodology and outcome measures, as well as evidence-based practices. What are the key points of a patient education program that emphasizes minimizing the risk of complications after a UE amputation? What are some key resources and references that the patient should know about?

INTERPERSONAL AND COMMUNICATION SKILLS. Describe some strategies to be used in communicating with the patient and his or her family members about his or her care.

PROFESSIONALISM. Describe the "patient-centered care" approach and "shared decision making" as they apply to this patient. Are there any cultural issues that affect the patient's adherence to the treatment or to an understanding of the disease? Any privacy concerns? Any ethical issues raised in the diagnosis and care of the patient?

SYSTEMS-BASED PRACTICE. Are there any access-to-care issues? Are there any issues with affordability of medications or insurance coverage? Are there any patient safety concerns? Describe the advantages and disadvantages of caring for this patient in different inpatient and outpatient settings. What are the cost considerations in prescribing the prosthetic components?

SELF-EXAMINATION QUESTIONS
(Answers begin on p. 367)

1. Which of the following is the ideal shape of a transhumeral residual limb for optimal prosthetic fitting?
    A. Conical
    B. Cylindrical
    C. Dog-eared
    D. Pointy
    E. Choked

2. Which of the following is the best first step to avoid phantom limb pain in a new amputee?
    A. Leave wound open without compression dressing
    B. Place residual limb in a rigid compressive dressing
    C. Provide a prosthesis 8 months after the amputation
    D. Encourage lack of movement of involved limb
    E. Leave residual limb in anatomically comfortable position

3. Which of the following care paradigms has JCAHO and CARF stressed in recent years for amputee care?
    A. Patient responsibility for long-term care
    B. Physician-centered care proposals
    C. A holistic and spiritual approach
    D. Focus on amputation-related issues only
    E. Dependence on family for activities of daily living

4. Of the following, who is the most important team member in the interdisciplinary rehabilitation team?
    A. The physiatrist
    B. The prosthetist
    C. The surgeon
    D. The patient
    E. The social worker

5. When a patient who has a history of wrist disarticulation and other LE amputations comes to clinic asking for an elective hand transplant, which of the following is the most appropriate recommendation?
    A. Further amputation resulting in a long transradial amputation to facilitate prosthetic fabrication
    B. Psychological evaluation for candidacy
    C. Commencing dominance retraining
    D. Ethical consultation
    E. Candidacy for a Krukenberg procedure

6. Of the following, which step in the system continuum of care process is communication between team members the most important for avoiding medical errors?
   A. Transition points in care
   B. During long-term follow-up in a stable patient
   C. During the interview process with the patient
   D. In the immediate postsurgical period
   E. After receipt of appropriate prosthesis

REFERENCES

1. Braddom RL. *Physical Medicine and Rehabilitation*. 4th ed. Philadelphia, PA: Saunders Elsevier; 2010.
2. Smith, D. *Atlas of Amputations and Limb Deficiencies: Surgical, Prosthetic, and Rehabilitation Principles*. 3rd ed. American Academy of Orthopedic Surgeons; 2004.
3. Malone JM, et al. Immediate, early and late postsurgical management of upper limb amputation. *J Rehabil Res Dev*. 1984;21:33.
4. Pinzur M. Functional outcomes following traumatic upper limb amputation and prosthetic limb fitting. *Jnl of Hand Surg*. 1994;19a(5).
5. Nelson VS. Limb deficiency and prosthetic management. *Arch Phys Med Rehabil*. March 2006;87(supp 1).
6. *Krusen's Handbook of Physical Medicine and Rehabilitation*. 4th ed. Philadelphia, PA: Saunders, 1990.
7. Joint Commission on Accreditation of Healthcare Organizations. *Joint Commission Guide to Allied Health Professionals*. Oakbrook Terrace, IL: Joint Commission on Accreditation of Healthcare Organizations; 2010.
8. Commission on Accreditation of Rehabilitation Facilities, www.carf.org 6951 East Southpoint Road, Tucson, Arizona 85756. 2013 Medical Rehabilitation Standards Manual.
9. National Limb Loss Information Center. Amputation statistics by cause. Limb loss in the United States. NLLIC fact sheet 2008. http://www.amputee-coalition.org/fact_sheets/amp_stats_cause.pdf. Accessed January 2013.
10. Nelson et al. Limb deficiency and prosthetic management. *Arch Phys Med Rehabil*. March 2006; 87(suppl 1).
11. Ziegler-Graham K, et al. Estimating the prevalence of limb loss in the United States: 2005 to 2050. *Arch Phys Med Rehabil*. 2008:89:422–429.
12. Canale ST, Beaty JH. *Campbell's Operative Orthopaedics*. 12th ed. Mosby Elsevier; 2012.
13. Branemark R, et al. Osseointegration in skeletal reconstruction and rehabilitation. *J Rehabil Res Dev*. April 2001;38(2).
14. Resnik L, et al. Advanced upper limb prosthetic devices: implications for upper limb prosthetic rehabilitation. *Arch Phys Med Rehabil*. April 2012;93.
15. Kelly, BM. Orthotic and prosthetic prescriptions for today and tomorrow. *Phys Med Rehabil Clin N Am*. 2007;18:785–858.
16. Monga TN, et al. Acupuncture in phantom limb pain. *Arch Phys Med Rehabil*. May 1981;62(5): 229–231.

Gail Latlief
Christine Elnitsky
Robert Kent

10: Lower Extremity Amputation

PATIENT CARE

GOALS

Provide competent patient care that is compassionate, appropriate, and effective for the evaluation, treatment, education, and advocacy for lower extremity amputee (LEA) patients across the entire spectrum of care, from the acute injury until death, and the promotion of good health.

OBJECTIVES

1. Perform a comprehensive interdisciplinary assessment of the adult with a lower limb amputation.
2. Describe the key components of a rehabilitation program for the lower limb amputee, including long-term follow-up.
3. Identify the main components of an effective patient education strategy for this population to prevent further limb loss as well as potential complications associated with lower limb loss.

Assessment of a person with a new amputation is a vastly important undertaking. This overall assessment will help define the rehabilitation process, identify key areas of possible success or failure, and allow for the highest quality of care for that patient. The first step in the assessment of a person with a lower limb amputation should be developing a clear medical history, including the cause of the amputation and a comprehensive understanding of comorbidities. Description of the amputation surgery, date of surgery, and postoperative complications are all important factors to document.

The *past medical history* should include direct questioning regarding coronary artery disease, peripheral vascular disease, diabetes mellitus, peripheral neuropathy, stroke, chronic obstructive pulmonary disease, contralateral limb history of ischemia, foot ulcers, trauma, fractures, depression, glaucoma, cataracts, osteoarthritic and rheumatological disorders, end-stage renal disease, and dialysis (including dialysis schedule).

The *past surgical history* review should include documentation of prior revascularization attempts and their dates, limb salvage surgeries, and prior amputations. Prior amputations should be outlined to demonstrate the progression of the disease. For example, if a person has peripheral vascular disease and has multiple amputations starting with a toe amputation progressing to a transfemoral amputation, the timeline should be identified to help understand the disease process and the patient's experience. This will aid in further development of a care plan.

Review of systems should include a basic overall review of symptoms with some issues highlighted due to common comorbidities as well as rehabilitation planning. The presence of chest pain, shortness of breath, or other signs of cardiac or respiratory deficiency should be documented. Impaired vision, pain secondary to musculoskeletal conditions (e.g., low back pain) or nerve injury, hand dexterity difficulties, impaired memory and concentration, anxiety, depression, skin issues, and contralateral limb issues should all be documented. Included in the review of systems for specific patient subsets, especially in traumatic amputations, is a clear history of burns or skin grafts. Assessment of burns and skin grafts is necessary for appropriate rehabilitation planning as well as prosthetic design.

Allergies and medications should be reviewed as in any patient. Certain key points in medication review should include pain medications for appropriate pain control and identification of medications that may lead to balance or cognitive deficits.

Social and functional history is an important part of the physiatric assessment and is especially important in amputees. Level of independence with ambulation and activities of daily living prior to and post amputation, employment and hobby history, home environment, presence of stairs and level of support from family, as well as smoking, alcohol, and drug abuse history, should be documented. The physical examination should be thorough and comprehensive (Table 10.1).

Patient and family education is of utmost importance in dealing with amputee patients due to the possibility of negative sequelae that can develop chronically by poor mechanics or skin

TABLE 10.1 Physical Examination Components

- Cognitive evaluation (alertness and orientation, attention, working memory, speed of mental processing, executive functioning, visual–spatial skills)
- A depression screen
- Cardiopulmonary evaluation
- Describe how patient arrives to clinic such as power wheelchair, walking with AD
- Neurological evaluation—motor, sensory, reflexes, proprioception, balance
- Musculoskeletal evaluation—range of motion of the limbs and spine; evaluation for flexion contractures, especially in the hips and knees; posture; habitus; and gait
- Residual limb examination: shape, length, circumferential measurements, incision line integrity, tenderness, sensation, pulses proximal to the amputation
- Contralateral limb examination: ischemic changes, pulses, foot deformities, sensory loss, calluses
- Skin examination of the residual limb, contralateral limb, pressure points of a prosthesis, and pressure wound sensitive areas in specific patients at risk
- Functional level of independence and ability to perform bed mobility, transfers from bed to chair; hopping with assistive device and ambulation with a prosthesis if applicable, 2-min walk, "get up and go" test
- Diagnostic studies: laboratory tests, imaging reports, vascular study results as needed for each individual patient

care, progression of disease and disability, and the need for continued patient-driven rehabilitation. Patients and their families should be educated on proper foot and skin care of the contralateral limb to minimize the risk of limb loss, strategies to minimize the risk of knee and hip flexion contractures, appropriate biomechanics, diabetic education if the patient is diabetic, medication management, pain management techniques including patient-performed physical modalities (e.g., desensitization techniques), fall prevention strategies, safe ambulation and transfers with appropriate assistive devices, and smoking cessation. These educational strategies should take into account the patient's age, level of education, language preference, preferred method of learning, and ethnicity. Educational content should be presented in multiple formats and repeated to maximize comprehension.

The assessment of the patient will continue and change as the plan is developed and the patient progresses through the rehabilitation process. There are some key things to identify and discuss concerning each individual at this point. Identifying a K level is important to quickly describe an amputee's overall functional level. This rating was developed by Medicare (Table 10.2).

MEDICAL KNOWLEDGE

GOALS

Demonstrate knowledge of established evidence based on evolving biomedical, clinical, epidemiological, and sociobehavioral sciences pertaining to LEA, as well as the application of this knowledge to guide holistic patient care.

OBJECTIVES

1. Describe the epidemiology, etiology, anatomy, physiology, and pathophysiology of LEA.
2. Identify the major medical problems faced by amputees and their management.
3. Describe the five phases in the rehabilitation of the LEA.
4. Describe the components of a comprehensive rehabilitation program in the adult with a major limb amputation.
5. Describe the different levels of amputations of the lower limb and the choices of prosthetic limb components in the LEA.
6. Describe postamputation complications in the LEA.
7. Identify causes of gait abnormalities in the LEA ambulating with a prosthesis.
8. Describe management considerations in unique populations with an amputation such as brain injury, spinal cord injury, coronary artery disease, and renal disease.

TABLE 10.2 K-Level Rating With Brief Description

- K0—Patient does not have the ability to ambulate or transfer safely, and a prosthesis would not enhance his or her quality of life
- K1—Patient has the functional ability to use a prosthesis on a level surface at a fixed cadence (household ambulator)
- K2—Patient has the functional capacity for ambulation and ability to traverse low-level environmental barriers or uneven surfaces (limited community ambulatory)
- K3—Patient has functional capacity to ambulate with variable cadence and navigate uneven surfaces, and prosthetic utilization may include vocational, therapeutic, or exercise demands beyond simple locomotion
- K4—Patient has functional capacity beyond ambulation and may participate in high-impact activities with exceptional energy expenditures (1)

In the United States, there are approximately 1.6 million people living with limb loss. It has been estimated that 1 of every 200 people in the United States has had an amputation, with dysvascular amputations accounting for 82% of all causes of limb loss. Lower limb amputations are the most common types of amputations. In patients with dysvascular amputations, 15% to 28% will undergo contralateral amputation within the next 3 years after their initial amputation. In elderly patients, only 50% survive longer than 3 years after their initial limb amputation. Greater than half of all diabetic amputees will face a second amputation within 5 years. Traumatic amputations account for 6% to 25% of all amputations. Malignancy-related causes are responsible for roughly 5% of all amputations, most commonly occurring in children and adolescents between 10 and 20 years of age. It is estimated that by 2050 there will be 3.6 million people living with amputations (2). Trauma is seen as a cause of amputation in higher instances in specific populations, including military patient subsets (2–5). Congenital abnormalities are the most common cause for amputation in young pediatric populations. Recent wars have resulted in an increase in traumatic amputations. The Department of Defense–Department of Veterans Affairs Extremity Trauma and Amputation Center of Excellence reports a total of 1,577 Operations Enduring Freedom, Iraqi Freedom, and New Dawn patients with amputations in all military facilities; of these 273 have upper extremity involvement (personal communication, December 20, 2012).

Important elements in the care of the individual with a lower limb amputation include optimizing the management of medical, surgical, and psychiatric comorbidities; optimal treatment of painful conditions; minimizing the risk of future amputations in both the ipsilateral and contralateral limbs; preventing the development of additional impairments; optimal use of a well-fitted prosthesis; and maximizing functionality. These elements of care are important throughout the continuum of care of the amputee, beginning before the amputation surgery and continuing in the preprosthetic and prosthetic phases of rehabilitation and throughout the lifetime of the amputee. The rehabilitation of the lower limb amputee can be divided into five distinct phases: (a) preoperative, (b) acute postoperative, (c) preprosthetic, (d) prosthetic, and (e) long-term follow-up.

In the preoperative phase, the patient is educated on the amputation surgery, the rehabilitative process, basic prosthetic design, and strategies to minimize the risk of contralateral limb loss. Additional education on smoking cessation and nutrition is also important. Rehabilitative efforts during this phase include general strengthening programs for key muscle groups in the upper and lower extremities as well as endurance training to optimize the patient's physical condition. Psychological counseling and peer counseling can be very helpful in this phase to optimize the patient's mental state prior to the surgery. In the acute postoperative period, limb shaping should be initiated and strict pain control should be attempted. Prior to transfer to an acute rehabilitation floor or a skilled nursing facility, a person's medical condition must be optimized so it does not interfere with the rehabilitation process and the person's safety once transferred.

In the preprosthetic phase, the following are important: (a) pain management of residual limb and phantom pain using pharmacological and nonpharmacological interventions; (b) optimization of wound healing of the residual limb; (c) minimization of risk of contractures of the residual limb; (d) management of medical comorbidities such as hypertension, coronary artery disease, diabetes, and chronic obstructive pulmonary disease; (e) optimization of nutrition and hydration; and (f) evaluation and treatment of adjustment disorder, depression, anxiety, and substance abuse as needed. Rehabilitation interventions during this phase include (a) range of motion exercises to the noninvolved extremities and the residual limb; (b) strengthening exercises to key muscle groups in the upper and lower extremities as well as core trunk muscles; (c) bed mobility, transfer training, wheelchair mobility, and gait training with appropriate assistive devices; and (d) training in activities of daily living such as bathing, grooming, dressing, and hygiene. A common question asked by clinical staff and persons with an amputation has to deal with the issue of an appropriate timeline for preprosthetic training during this period. While every patient is different and this should only be seen as a basic reference, the acute postoperative period usually lasts from postoperative day (POD) 1 to day 4; POD 4 to 3 weeks out, continue wound healing with preprosthetic rehabilitation; 3 to 4 weeks after amputation, suture or staple removal and temporary prosthesis fitting and continued physical therapy. Throughout preprosthetic training, crutches are avoided due to possible development of poor gait mechanics with crutch use. Ambulation with a walker is an adequate gauge of the patient's functionality and relative energy expenditure with the eventual prosthesis (1). During the preprosthetic rehabilitation phase, it is important to identify the patient's ability and capacity beyond K level and understand the increased energy demands by differing levels. This will allow the clinician to tailor appropriate rehabilitation planning to each individual patient (Table 10.3).

Volume management and protection of the residual limb are an integral part of residual limb management and need to progress during the preprosthetic period. Rigid limb dressings and wrapping of the residual limb are often used to accomplish these goals. Ace wrapping with the figure eight method of wrapping is often the most effective for volume management in the initial postoperative period, but this must be done several times a day and is dependent on proper technique. It is also important to monitor the surgical incision line for evidence of infection and to treat the infection when present. Contractures can occur in the residual limb with the most common sites: (a) knee flexion and (b) hip flexion and hip abduction. Interventions during this phase to minimize the risk of contractures include prone lying and active range of motion. Strategies and techniques for residual

TABLE 10.3 Energy Demands by Level of Limb Amputation

AMPUTATION LEVEL (6)	ENERGY ABOVE BASELINE (%)	SPEED (m/min)	OXYGEN COST (mL/kg/m)
Long transtibial	10	70	0.17
Average transtibial	25	60	0.20
Short transtibial	40	50	0.20
Bilateral transtibial	41	50	0.20
Transfemoral	65	40	0.28
Wheelchair	0–8	70	0.16

limb pain management include desensitization techniques, medications, and strategies for volume control and shaping of the residual limb. The preferred shape for the transfemoral residual limb is conical and for a transtibial residual limb it is cylindrical. Improved outcomes for a shorter transfemoral residual limb are noted with preservation of the greater trochanter and hip adductors attachment. In a transtibial amputation, the tibial tuberosity with patellar attachment is a key structure to save. Other important interventions in this phase include fall prevention strategies and strategies to minimize the risk of additional amputations.

In the prosthetic phase, there is continuation of the interventions started in the earlier phases with the addition of fitting and training in the use of the lower limb prosthesis. Rehabilitation interventions focus on preservation of range of motion in all the limbs with added focus on strategies to reduce and/or treat contractures, strengthening protocols of key muscle groups in the limbs and trunk, balance training—static and dynamic with the prosthesis—as well as gait training. Gait training often begins in the parallel bars and is progressed to other flat surfaces indoors with an appropriate assistive device. As the person becomes more confident, ambulation up and down stairs is added to the training program, as is ambulation on different types of terrain outdoors (i.e., gravel, grass, up/down inclines). Car transfers and driver training are also often offered to amputees as well as opportunities to return to work and sports with modifications. For transtibial amputees, 4 to 6 weeks of physical therapy is usually appropriate, whereas transfemoral amputees often need 6 to 12 weeks. Patient education includes pain control strategies, residual limb care, prosthetic education, care of prosthesis, donning/doffing of the prosthesis, sock management, monitoring of skin for evidence of skin breakdown, coping strategies, patient safety, and weight management.

Long-term follow-up of the patient with a lower limb amputation is recommended for proper fit of the prosthesis, counseling on weight control, smoking cessation, and strategies to preserve the contralateral limb and to ensure appropriate community reintegration. Continued long-term follow-up should be at least annually if not more often, and the condition of components of the prosthesis should continue to be monitored in conjunction with prosthetist in the community or facility.

Prosthetic Fit and Design

Understanding the different types of amputation and the prosthetic options will always help a clinician develop a more effective rehabilitation program with the appropriate prosthetic device. Different levels of amputations of the lower limb will lead to different choices of prosthesic components. While transfemoral and transtibial are the most common lower limb amputations, other amputations, such as knee and hip disarticulations or the Symes procedures, may be seen in the rehabilitation setting as well. A Symes procedure is an ankle disarticulation with the heel pad attached to the distal tibia and accounts for about 3% of lower limb amputations. Transtibial amputations account for 59% of lower limb amputations, transfemoral amputations account for 35% of lower limb amputations, hip disarticulations account for 2% of lower limb amputations, and knee disarticulations account for 1% of lower limb amputations (7). There are also a number of partial foot amputations that should be reviewed by clinicians as well. Another factor to consider in deciding on an appropriate prosthesis is the length of the residual limb length (Tables 10.4 and 10.5).

TABLE 10.4 Transtibial Residual Limb Length

Short: <20% of limb below the knee remains
Standard: 20%–50% of limb below the knee remains
Long: 50%–90% of limb below the knee remains

When choosing a transtibial prosthetic socket design (Table 10.6), the most commonly used is the total contact socket. This type of socket has a medial tibial flare, with relief areas built in for the hamstring tendon and femoral head and a patellar bar for contact at the patellar tendon. Pressure-tolerant areas include the patellar tendon, popliteal fossa and gastroc-soleus complex, pretibial musculature, medial tibial flare, and lateral fibular surface. Pressure-sensitive areas include fibular head, tibial condyles, distal fibula, and hamstring tendons. The development of heterotopic ossification, anatomic variability, and type of surgical amputation performed can all lead to differences in prosthetic fit. A close working relationship with the prosthetic team is integral to rehabilitation success. Transfemoral amputation prosthetic fitting is more complicated for a number of reasons, including use of a prosthetic knee joint, difference in biomechanics, and increased energy expenditure (Table 10.7). Transfemoral amputations are fitted in slight flexion and adduction for improved mechanical advantage to hip extensors and abductors.

The current concepts in amputee care revolve around two major themes: technology and holistic approach to the amputee. In recent years, significant advances have been made in both the fabrication and quality of prosthetic components. Lower limb prostheses are more dynamic and lighter and often incorporate microprocessor technology to improve patient safety, gait, and comfort of use. However, it is important to identify the appropriate candidate for use of this technology since a significant cause of limited use or abandonment of technology is lack of clinician assessment of appropriateness of technology for a patient (1). While patients may wish for the latest technology, it may not always be available to every patient nor indicated, and this should be openly discussed with each individual patient.

Select Postamputation Complications

Phantom pain can start soon after the amputation or years later. It is extremely important to differentiate between phantom sensation and phantom pain. Up to 79% experience phantom sensation and 72% experience phantom pain (8). Physical modalities should be considered prior to initiation of medication, and it is important to remember that use of a prosthesis and weight bearing tends to decrease phantom pain. Physical modalities may include massage

TABLE 10.5 Transfemoral Residual Limb Length

Short: 0%–35% of the femur remains
Standard: 35%–60%
Long: >60%

TABLE 10.6 Transtibial Prosthetic Sockets and Suspension

Differential pressure

Silicone suction with shuttle lock
- Consider for patient with stable limb volumes, good hand dexterity

Anatomic

Brim suspension
- Uses extension of socket over femoral epicondyles
- Easy to don/doff
- Useful for short limb, knee instability

Supracondylar cuff
- Not for short residual limbs or knee instability
- Add fork strap and waist belt for physically active

Sleeve
- Good for short limbs and also for hyperextension control if necessary

COMMON FOOT–ANKLE ASSEMBLIES

Solid ankle-cushioned heel (SACH foot)—most common one used
- Light, durable, stable, inexpensive
- Soft heel simulates plantar flexion
- Well suited for flat, level surfaces

Single-axis foot
- Heavier, less durable than SACH
- Better for transfemoral amputees, better knee stability, quicker foot flat
- Only sagittal axis movement

Multiaxis foot
- Plantar, dorsiflexion, inversion, eversion, rotation
- Improved balance and coordination
- Good shock absorption, better on unlevel ground
- Heavy, expensive, frequent adjustments

Dynamic elastic response
- "Energy storing feet"
- No actual change in energy expenditure when compared to SACH foot (19)
- Very light, rare adjustments

Microprocessor and power foot/ankles

TABLE 10.7 Transfemoral Prosthetic Sockets and Suspension*

Quadrilateral design
- Narrow anterior and posterior, posterolateral reliefs for gluteal maximus, anterolateral relief for rectus femoris, posteriomedial relief for hamstring tendons, anteriomedial relief for adductor longus, bulges for scarpas triangle anteriorly, ischial seat posteriorly
- Not as effective for short residual limbs

Ischial containment design
- Better for short residual limbs
- Bony lock incorporates ischial tuberosity, pubic ramus, greater trochanter
- Narrow mediolateral design for more efficient energy cost

SUSPENSION OPTIONS

Suction
- Good for active patient with good limb length, stable limb volume

Silesian belt
- Belt attaches at greater trochanter and wraps around opposite iliac crest

Total elastic suspension belt
- Elastic belt wraps around proximal prosthesis and waist

Pelvic band and belt suspension
- Rigid belt connected to metal joint overlying lateral hip
- Improves mediolateral and rotational stability especially
- Heavy, bulky, interferes with sitting

KNEE COMPONENTS

Single axis
- Durable, cheap
- Cadence is fixed, stability is poor, more appropriate for level surfaces

Stance control or safety knee
- Will not flex during weight bearing, stability during stance phase
- Common with geriatrics, poor hip control
- Some uneven surface ambulation
- Delayed swing phase due to need to unload knee to flex

Polycentric
- 4-bar linkage
- Increased stability
- Heavy, expensive, increased maintenance

Fluid controlled
- Automatic swing phase control at variable cadence, smoother, natural gait
- Expensive, heavy, maintenance
- Manual or fixed locking
- Best stability, poor gait, and increased energy consumption

*Foot components will be the same as listed in Table 10.6.

and desensitization techniques, ultrasound, wrapping, mirror therapy, short-wave diathermy, and transcutaneous electrical nerve stimulation (TENS). Medications that may have a positive effect on phantom pain include beta-blockers, neuromodulators such as gabapentin, tricyclic antidepressants, calcitonin, and topical analgesics. One topical analgesic that is being used more commonly in peripheral neuropathy is topical ketamine. The mechanism of action is unknown peripherally, as NMDA receptors have only been found centrally; however, research and the efficacy of use have led to the hypothesis that peripheral NMDA receptors are targeted by topical ketamine, thereby providing peripheral pain relief.

Gabapentin is often the first-line medication and can be a successful treatment; however, renal function and cognitive impairment need to be identified in this patient group. Increasingly, interventional procedures are being used. Some of the techniques that may be used in refractory cases include trigger point, ultrasound-guided neurolysis, and peripheral nerve stimulation. Narcotics are often used but are not recommended for neuropathic pain.

Choke syndrome can lead to distal limb edema with verrucous hyperplasia. This commonly occurs when there is proximal limb pressure and lack of total contact with prosthesis leading to pistoning in the socket. This is more common in dysvascular patients (1). The choking effect of the residual limb can be treated effectively by adding a pad to the distal end of the socket, correcting the faulty prosthetic suspension and relieving the pressure from the proximal portion of the socket. However, sometimes this may require a new socket.

Other complications and issues to continually monitor in amputee patients include skin care and biomechanics. Skin care of the residual limb and the contralateral limb is important to avoid downtime from prosthetic use, further amputations, and life-threatening infections.

Biomechanics, specifically in gait related to prosthetic use, can be difficult to correct; however, this needs to be addressed as early as possible. Tables 10.8 and 10.9 outline some common stance and swing phase problems.

Special Populations

Multitrauma, Traumatic Brain Injury, and Amputations

The diversity in pathologies that lead to amputations or exist as comorbidities can complicate the rehabilitation process. Multitrauma patients, such as patients who sustain blast injuries, motor vehicle accidents, or gunshot wounds with concomitant

TABLE 10.8 Stance Phase Problems

Excessive trunk extension/lumbar lordosis during stance phase
■ Pelvic rotation, hip flexion contracture, weak hip extensors
Foot slap
■ Foot too far posterior or excessive socket flexion
Knee instability
■ Knee axis—too anterior, insufficient plantar flexion, failure to limit dorsiflexion, large hip flexor contractures, posterior foot placement, weak hip extensors
Lateral bending
■ Prosthesis is too short, abduction contracture
■ Insufficient lateral wall, abducted socket
Vaulting
■ Prosthesis is too long, too much knee friction, poor suspension
Whip
■ Abrupt rotation of heel at end of stance phase—whip
■ If heel moves medial, medial whip; if heel moves lateral, lateral whip
■ Caused by poor knee axis alignment, free-moving socket

TABLE 10.9 Swing Phase Problems

Abducted gait
■ Prosthesis is too long
■ Abduction contracture
■ Medial wall of socket encroaching on groin
Circumducted gait
■ Prosthesis is too long, difficulty with knee flexion, abduction contracture
Foot drag
■ Inadequate suspension
■ Prosthesis is too long, insufficient knee or hip flexion of contralateral limb
Excessive heel rise
■ Insufficient knee friction or excessive knee flexion
Terminal swing impact
■ Insufficient knee friction

traumatic brain injuries, pose particular safety concerns. As for patients who suffer traumatic brain injuries along with amputation of one or multiple limbs, understanding and identifying key safety features in the rehabilitation process are integral to patient safety. These patients are prone to falls for having cognitive impairment that is compounded by an amputation, along with further issues such as spasticity, visual impairment, impulsivity, or vestibulo-cochlear deficits.

Another important consideration is patients who undergo craniectomy after the initial event, which leads to increased possibility of severe injury if a fall were to occur. While wearing a helmet is not usually a consideration for a noncomplicated amputee, in this patient population it is our practice to always have a helmet in place during gait training in any patient with a craniectomy.

Along with fall issues, understanding the etiology and ramifications of the patients' other injuries is important to map out a safe rehabilitation process. Patients with multiple injuries may have an amputation along with weight-bearing restrictions on other joints that complicate safety issues. When progressing weight bearing, the use of a tilt table or overhead tracts and harness systems allows for offloading weight in order to continue to work on balance, mobility, and upright tolerance.

Polypharmacy is a major concern when it comes to patients with traumatic brain injuries, and this again is compounded when a patient has an amputation. The sedating side effects of pain medications, neuromodulators, and antispasticity medications can impact cognitive therapies and ability to participate as well as decrease safety in cognitively impaired patients.

Heterotopic ossification of joints and soft tissue can cause pain, skin integrity, and mobility issues. The treatment of heterotopic ossification can also be limited by the presence of other healing fractures. This is an extremely important area for prosthetists to work closely with therapists and providers to make socket modifications, such as windows, as well as identify pain with increased weight bearing or any skin breakdown that may be due to the underlying heterotopic ossification. An interdisciplinary team approach to manage these patients is of utmost importance to identify safety concerns as early as possible. Working within these teams, educating family members of patients with amputations with concomitant cognitive deficits needs to be a focus to ensure safety and help prevent complications. Patient families need to be educated on issues such as skin monitoring, stump sock management, donning and doffing prosthesis, residual limb hygiene, componentry inspection, and maintenance.

Spinal Cord Injuries and Amputations

Another complex subset of amputee patients are those with spinal cord injuries. These injuries can be cervical, thoracic or lumbar, complete or incomplete, with varying degrees of ability to tolerate a prosthesis, ambulation, skin complications, and level of independence or expected independence. Working closely with the patient's primary spinal cord injury team is integral to optimize safety. Identifying team and patient goals—often dictated by their level of injury—is important to be able to choose the most appropriate prosthesis. While some persons may only wish to have a prosthesis for cosmesis, others may be able to progress on to future ambulation, and the most appropriate prosthetic limb for their individual situation will help them safely attain these goals. Working within an interdisciplinary team here again is in the patient's best interest. Identification of pain issues, early skin issues, progress of limb shaping, or changes in independence will need to be monitored to assure the highest level of safety for these patients while they progress through rehabilitation.

Renal Disease and Amputation

Renal patients are of special concern and offer their own specific complexities. While the list of comorbidities can be extensive, patients with amputations secondary to dysvascular issues are more likely to have renal impairment as well. With changes in limb size due to fluctuating edema, prosthetic fit needs to be monitored closely to identify early skin breakdown or further complications such as pistoning, which could also lead to falls. Dosing of medications that are cleared by the kidneys and creatinine clearance should be monitored, and close co-management with the patient's nephrologist is recommended. Gabapentin is often used in phantom limb pain and requires especially close monitoring as it can cause further renal damage, and the dosing will change depending on clearance issues. It is also important to keep an updated dialysis schedule if the patient's renal issues have progressed to that point. Comorbidities such as visual impairment, diabetes mellitus, cardiovascular issues, and increased metabolic demand should all be closely monitored in patients with severe renal disease to optimize safety. Patients with poorly controlled diabetes mellitus should have their blood glucose levels regularly checked to identify and correct for extreme changes in blood sugar that could compromise safety.

Coronary Artery Disease

Coronary artery disease is prevalent in patients with lower extremity peripheral vascular disease, especially among those who go on to amputation. The use of dipyridamole-thallium imaging in these patients may improve the ability to diagnose asymptomatic coronary artery disease before initiating an exercise program, thereby allowing adequate treatment and preventing complications during rehabilitation.

Exercise testing using lower extremity exercise has been the "gold standard" for screening for coronary artery disease, but many patients with peripheral vascular disease and those with amputations have difficulty performing this type of exercise. Arm ergometry is a safe and effective exercise alternative for detecting asymptomatic coronary disease in those unable to exercise their lower extremities and can be used to determine safe upper extremity exercise levels in poorly conditioned patients and those with known coronary disease. Arm ergometry testing is also useful for providing prognostic information concerning functional outcome after a rehabilitation program. Exercise testing is therefore indicated in all vascular amputee patients before beginning an exercise training and prosthetic rehabilitation program. Exercise training can safely and inexpensively enhance the functional capacity of amputee patients with peripheral vascular disease (PVD) (9).

PRACTICE-BASED LEARNING AND IMPROVEMENT

GOALS

Demonstrate competence in continuously investigating and evaluating your own LEA patient care practices, appraising and assimilating scientific evidence, and continuously improving your patient care practices based on progressive self-evaluation and lifelong learning.

OBJECTIVES

1. Describe learning opportunities for providers, patients, and caregivers with experience in LEA.
2. Use methods for ongoing competency training in LEA for physiatrists, including formative evaluation feedback in daily practice, evaluating current practice, and developing a quality improvement and clinical practice improvement activity strategy.
3. Locate resources including available websites and professional organizations for continuing medical education and continuing professional development in LEA.
4. Describe some areas paramount to self-assessment and lifelong learning such as "clinical reflection"; review of quality care markers: current guidelines, including evidence-based, in treatment and management of patients with LEA; and the role of the physiatrist as the educator of patients, families, residents, students, colleagues, and other health professionals.

Self-assessment is a central component of practice-based learning and improvement. In providing rehabilitative care for the patient with LEA, the physiatrist should self-assess for the following: (a) his or her ability to obtain a medical history and perform a physical examination that specifically targets this population; (b) knowledge base regarding the different levels of amputation, lower limb amputation surgical techniques, and current prosthetic components; (c) gait abnormalities in the lower limb amputee ambulating with a prosthesis; (d) common medical and rehabilitative issues in the care of the LEA and their management; and

(e) interpersonal and communication skills with his or her patient and the multidisciplinary team providing care for this patient. This self-assessment can be completed through reflection on one's clinical practice, seeking feedback from colleagues as well as patients, and through self-assessment examinations.

Once gaps have been identified during the self-assessment, there are several resources available to physiatrists to increase their skills and knowledge base. Some of them are available through the American Academy of Physical Medicine and Rehabilitation (AAPMR) such as articles through Knowledge NOW and online prosthetics and orthotics courses in the Maintenance of Certificate series (www.aapmr.org). Others include prosthetics and orthotics courses sponsored by academic institutions and even advanced fellowship training.

The VA/DoD clinical guidelines released in January 2008 (10) identify 5 distinct phases of rehabilitation: (a) preoperative, (b) acute postoperative, (c) preprosthetic, (d) prosthetic training, and (e) long-term follow-up. Within each of these phases, the guidelines identify 11 key interventions that should be examined and acted upon to allow for the most effective rehabilitation process. Interventions are:

1. Pain management
2. Medical comorbidity management
3. Behavioral health, psychological, and cognitive function
4. Residual limb management
5. Patient education
6. Prosthetic
7. Discharge planning
8. Rehabilitation interventions—range of motion, strengthening, cardiovascular, balance, mobility, and designing of a home exercise program
9. Functional activities and activities of daily living
10. Community
11. Equipment

These guidelines provide an excellent checklist for each period or rehabilitation and each intervention that needs to be addressed. This also supplies a strong framework for a quality analysis and improvement project.

For continued practice-based learning and quality improvement, effective measurement tools are instrumental in clinical assessment and improvement. One of these tools, the Orthotics and Prosthetics User's Survey (OPUS), has been an effective tool in initial and follow-up assessment of patients' satisfaction with their prosthetics and continues to gain popularity as an invaluable clinical tool (11). Use of other standardized tools such as the Groningen Activity Restriction Scale (GARS) and clinical tests such as the 2-min walk and the "get up and go" test can develop a clearer clinical picture and monitor patient functional improvement or decline (12).

Quality assurance is an important tool in monitoring overall amputee patient care and identifying care issues. It is important to have objective outcome measures that can track the effectiveness of an amputee rehabilitation program based on the above core components. Some examples include (a) next available appointment with a physiatrist, physical therapist, occupational therapist, and prosthetist with significant experience in the care of amputees; (b) quality of life measure instrument; (c) incidence of wounds in residual limb; (d) incidence of contralateral amputations; and (e) prosthetic fit questionnaire. Data collected can be analyzed and compared to external or internal benchmarks, and performance improvement projects can be initiated if a deviation from benchmarks is identified. Both qualitative and quantitative factors should be identified with actions and recommendations that are measurable and manageable.

INTERPERSONAL AND COMMUNICATION SKILLS

GOALS

Demonstrate interpersonal and communication skills that result in the effective exchange of information and collaboration with LEA patients, their families, and the rest of the rehabilitation team.

OBJECTIVES

1. Demonstrate skills used in effective verbal and nonverbal communication, listening skills, conflict resolution, and collaboration with LEA patients and their caregivers across socioeconomic and cultural backgrounds.
2. Delineate the importance of the role of the physiatrist as the interdisciplinary team leader and consultant pertinent to LEA.
3. Demonstrate proper and timely medical record documentation and effective communication between health care professional team members in patient care as it applies to LEA.
4. Identify key areas for physicians to counsel patients and families specific to LEA.

Effective interprofessional and multidisciplinary communication between and among the physiatrist, the patient, his or her family, and health professional colleagues is one of the cornerstones of good patient care. The key components of effective communication and conflict resolution are (a) relationship building; (b) listen, reflect, redirect, and validate; (c) shared understanding and common ground; (d) frame and reframe the issues; (e) collaborative brainstorming and shared decision making; and (f) aligned expectations. Relationship building with the patient is an important way of establishing good rapport and needs to be initiated at the first meeting. It is important to get to know the patients and find out what is truly important to them, what their values are, their preferred style of communication, their role in their family and community, hobbies, and interests.

It is equally important to recognize the emotional impact of the amputation on the patient and review and summarize the situation often using the patient's own words to describe his or her challenges. Show respect for the patient's efforts to address the problem. Be humble and don't be afraid to show vulnerability. Be a coach and advisor to the patient and not be judgmental.

To be an effective communicator requires active listening on the part of the physiatrist. Ask open-ended questions initially, followed by more focused questions. Reflect back on what the patient says, using his or her own words whenever possible. If the patient goes off on tangent, redirect him or her.

A shared understanding of the issues involved in the care of the LEA requires an understanding of the problem from several different perspectives—the physiatrist, the patient, her family, and at times the institution or setting where the patient is receiving rehabilitative care. Once these have been defined, a "shared understanding" of the problem that combines the perspectives of all the stakeholders can be developed. Based on this shared understanding, the issues can be framed in a mutually acceptable way and common ground achieved. A productive perspective is the cooperative efforts of the physiatrist and the patient, working for the maximum benefit of the patient while confronting the challenges faced in lower limb amputation. The patient with an amputation must build confidence and assume the role of active participation in the treatment process, becoming committed and taking responsibility for self-management as he or she transitions to outpatient status (13).

Communication highlights the importance of the role of the other partner in the consultation, the patient. Patients may vary in what they want to discuss in the consultation as well as the role they want to take in decision making (14). A key role of communication is the exchange of ideas and preferences from the patients' perspective. Patient-centered care calls for providers to consider the person, not just the disease, and support the patients' individual preferences and lifestyle considerations (15). Providers must often support the patients' preferences even if they disagree with clinical recommendations (15).

Once a common understanding has been developed, shared goals can be developed that are based on the goals of the physiatrist, patient, family, and often the interdisciplinary team caring for the patient. Based on these shared goals, collective brainstorming occurs in which all the treatment options and potential consequences of options are discussed, and the patient is assisted in his or her risk–benefit analysis and decision making.

In providing feedback, the physiatrist should use objective markers of success that are mutually agreed upon with the patient, use positive statements as often as possible, and emphasize the positive things that the patient is doing in his or her care plan. The progress and issues should be presented in specific, nonjudgmental, and nonemotional approaches. The clinician should check for understanding. In giving negative feedback, it is important to be tough on the expected behavior and easy on the person. Ask for reasons why the behavior is occurring (the why, how, what, who, when of the problem) and focus on key discrepancies. Describe the expected behavior and the discrepancy and don't play "Gotcha"! Tell the patient in advance the topic of discussion so that he or she can formulate a response. Create opportunities and encouragement for the patient to be honest. It can be very helpful to enlist support from family members whenever possible.

The clinician should speak at a moderate pace, varying the tone of speech for emphasis and pausing effectively when making a point. It is also important to take frequent turns while speaking and avoiding dual monologues. Do not interrupt the patient while he or she is talking. Nonverbal communication is equally important. Some useful strategies include the following: (a) maintain good eye contact; (b) sit at eye level with the patient; (c) remove barriers between the physiatrist and the patient (i.e., furniture, telephone, etc.); (d) keep an open posture; (e) face the patient; (f) sit next to the patient, rather than across from him or her; and (g) don't fold arms across chest or cross legs.

A good medical record is an essential tool of communication between clinicians caring for the lower limb amputee. The documentation should be provided on a timely basis; reflect the patient's medical, rehabilitative, psychosocial, and prosthetic barriers, and offer a treatment plan to address the barriers. In an age of electronic medical records, it is essential that the physiatrist refrain from "cut, copy, paste" of medical record material from one note to another.

Patients should be taught at an appropriate reading level. Educational strategies should take into account the patient's special population needs, educational level, language and cultural beliefs, as well as preferred learning style. Important educational components for the patient, family, caregivers are listed in Table 10.10.

Models and sample prosthetics have been effective tools used to demonstrate possible prosthetic components and outline individual benefits and disadvantages. To illustrate this process for patients and practitioners, in conjunction with the University of South Florida PMR and James Haley VA prosthetics departments, we have created "The Mannequin project." Through a team effort we transformed an everyday mannequin into an indispensable teaching tool. The team created a quad "amputee" from a mannequin and, through the processes we use in everyday amputee care, we fitted the mannequin's residual limbs with several different prosthetic devices, creating a showpiece that we are able to use in all facets of our patient's care. One of the most difficult things for a new amputee is to visualize the device that he or she will be eventually utilizing as well as grasping the importance of comprehensive amputee care. We have found by having a concrete visual figure we are better able to address

TABLE 10.10 Important Educational Components for Patient, Family, and Caregivers

- Strategies to minimize the risk of future amputations
    - Check the bottom of foot for skin breakdown; don't walk barefoot; seek appropriate footwear and foot care, use a long-handled mirror
- Smoking cessation techniques
    - Relationship to pain and increased risk for further PVD-related amputations as well as pulmonary and cardiac decline make this an extremely important and understressed topic
- Proper donning/doffing of prosthesis and care of the residual limb and prosthesis
- Continued physical modalities for pain relief
- Constant reminders on appropriate biomechanics
    - Proper gait
    - Positional corrections—limb and axial
    - Lifting techniques
- Fall avoidance strategies
    - Medication reviews

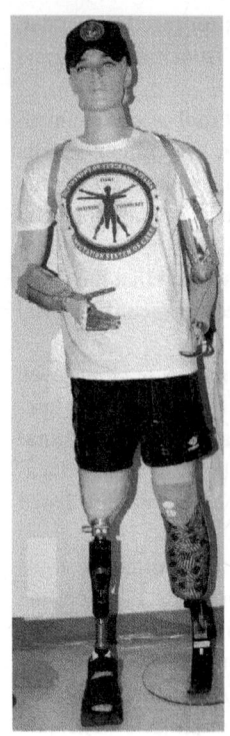

FIGURE 10.1 Educational mannequin fitted with prosthetic limbs.

patient questions and alleviate fears and reservations that they have regarding their future as an amputee (Figure 10.1).

To further delineate the process of amputee care we created a hub-and-spoke model showing the integrated team approach that will take place in the patient's ongoing care. Through the involvement of both PM&R and prosthetic residents in this project, an innovative teaching approach to core competency development was created, and all ACGME core competencies were integrated and instructed in a patient-centered setting (16).

PROFESSIONALISM

GOALS

Reflect a commitment to carrying out professional responsibilities and an adherence to ethical principles in caring for patients with LEA.

OBJECTIVES

1. Exemplify the humanistic qualities as a provider of care for patients with LEA such as respect, altruism, integrity, honesty, compassion, and empathy.
2. Demonstrate ethical principles and responsiveness to patient needs superseding self and other interests.
3. Demonstrate sensitivity to patient population diversity, including culture, gender, age, race, religion, disabilities, and sexual orientation.
4. Demonstrate and respect patient-centered care, confidentiality, patient privacy, autonomy, shared decision making, and informed consent as applicable to LEA.

A major limb amputation of the lower extremity is a life-altering event for an individual. It can have a profound impact on the person's self-image; ability to work, care for him- or herself and his or her provide self-care and care for the family; and engage in activities that were once meaningful prior to the amputation. It is very important to show respect, compassion, and empathy for the patient at this time in his or her life when he or she is most vulnerable and to provide the best possible care in an honest and respectful manner.

It is important that all attempts be made to have the patient and his or her needs at the center of the care plan of the interdisciplinary team. Systems and processes should support this fundamental tenet of patient care. The physiatrist and interdisciplinary team members should work together with the patient in a collaborative manner in making clinical care decisions that are consistent with the patient's wishes and values, and this should be initiated at first visit, preferably preoperatively if possible. An example of shared decision making is in determining the right prosthetic prescription for the patient. The physiatrist and the prosthetist have the clinical expertise to guide the patient on the most appropriate prosthesis; however, the patient provides input on the types of activities that will require the use of a prosthesis. Together they share in the decision-making process, and this leads to a team approach that will lead to improved function and patient satisfaction.

The patient's age and cultural beliefs can also have an impact on the care of the lower limb amputee. For example, an individual's advanced age should not be an automatic disqualifier in the decision to prescribe a prosthesis. The person may have the necessary motivation, patience, and medical stability to learn to ambulate safely with a prosthesis, despite an advanced age. This is also true of comorbid disabilities. While some comorbidities such as impaired vision may be a contraindication in some clinician's opinion, it is in no way an absolute contraindication. Each patient should be examined on an individual basis.

There are also times when a person's cultural and religious beliefs and pursuits may become a factor in his or her care. For example, there may be instances when a lower limb amputee may not be able to ambulate with a prosthesis for long distances, but it may be important for that person not to be perceived as having a disability. She may require a more limited use of the prosthesis for activities that are meaningful to her or important to her culturally or psychosocially, and these should be respected.

Ethical issues can come up in care of the lower limb amputee. One example is whether or not to prescribe a prosthesis to a person who is unsafe to ambulate yet still demands to have it. Alternatively, a lower limb amputee may ambulate with a prosthesis in an unsafe manner, placing himself or herself at risk for falls and injury that would require a discussion concerning ongoing use of the prosthesis. There are times when a patient's health care insurance dictates the types of rehabilitation services provided, the location of where they will be provided, and even the type of prosthesis that will be prescribed. In all these instances it is important to (a) define and understand the ethical issues in question from the perspectives of all of the stakeholders, (b) compare and contrast the importance of the various ethical factors in question (i.e., is there one that takes a higher priority), and (c) review existing laws, policies, and guidelines for guidance.

Other ethical considerations that lay on the forefront of medicine include telemedicine, limb transplant, and elective limb amputation. An example of elective limb amputation that has been brought to clinicians often before involves patients with complex regional pain syndrome (CRPS). At this time, there is no research to support amputation as a cure for CRPS, and with the unknown true pathology of CRPS, the extent of peripheral versus central neuropathic pain, amputation may be of no benefit and may lead to more pain and decreased functional outcomes.

SYSTEMS-BASED PRACTICE

GOALS

Awareness and responsiveness to systems of interdisciplinary care delivery, and the ability to access, evaluate, recruit, and coordinate effectively resources in the system to provide optimal continuum of care and outcomes as it relates to LEA.

OBJECTIVES

1. Identify the key components, interprofessional team providers, systems of care delivery, services, referral patterns, coordination of care, and resources in the rehabilitation continuum of care, including inpatient and outpatient settings, for the LEA patient.
2. Identify patient safety issues as they apply to LEA.
3. Describe optimal follow-up care for the LEA patient.
4. Describe markers of quality in the care of LEA patient.
5. Describe cost/risk–benefit analysis, utilization, and management of resources as they apply to LEA.

The Commission on Accreditation of Rehabilitation Facilities (CARF) has advocated a holistic approach to the care of the lower limb amputee (17). In this model of care, the individual living with lower limb loss is evaluated and treated by a team of professionals across a continuum of lifelong care to ensure optimal medical, surgical, psychiatric, and functional well-being. For a person who has undergone the psychosocial trauma of limb loss and its functional sequelae and related comorbidities, a team approach using a holistic model of patient care is integral to the achievement of short-term and lifelong rehabilitation goals.

The rehabilitation of the lower limb amputee often occurs in a variety of settings. These include the medical/surgical unit of an acute care medical center, an acute inpatient rehabilitation unit, a subacute rehabilitation unit in a skilled nursing facility, and visiting therapy services in a patient's home and in outpatient rehabilitation centers. It should be a goal of an amputee rehabilitation team to meet with the patient preoperatively if possible for patient–clinician relationship building, education, and prognostic expectations. On the medical/surgical unit of an acute medical center, the lower limb amputee typically receives physical therapy and occupational therapy at the bedside or in the facility's rehabilitation gym. Physiatry consultation and prosthetic services may or may not be available. Following his or her stay on the medical/surgical unit, the patient is typically transferred to either an acute rehabilitation ward in the medical center or a hospital or skilled nursing facility that specializes in rehabilitation medicine. The decision whether to transfer the patient to a skilled nursing facility vs acute rehabilitation setting is often dependent on the patient's medical stability and comorbidities, the patient's current level of function, and the number of hours per day that the patient can participate in a rehabilitation program. Additional factors include level of support at home and health care insurance program. If the patient's residual limb has not fully healed following the surgery, he or she may be sent home with visiting nursing and therapy services or to a skilled nursing facility until the wound has healed. The physiatrist has a critical role in the coordination of services across this continuum of care to ensure that the patient receives the right care at the right place and at the right time and to minimize the potential for fragmented care. This is an area where physiatrists need to be even stronger advocates for their patients.

Cost considerations and risk–benefit analysis are an important part of the decision-making process in the care of the lower limb amputee. This is especially evident in the selection of prosthetic components. There is a wide selection of prosthetic components, and it is important to match the patient's level of function, lifestyle, and hobbies with the right prosthetic components. For example, a predominantly sedentary patient residing in a skilled nursing facility may not require a high-tech and expensive prosthetic foot meant for runners.

The interdisciplinary team that is involved in the care of the lower limb amputee typically includes physiatry, physical therapy, occupational therapy, prosthetics, rehabilitation nursing, social work and psychology, vocational specialists, driver training, and recreation therapists. This team is usually seen in rehabilitation wards/hospitals and skilled nursing facilities but may be present in a different composition on the medical/surgical wards, outpatient settings, and in the provision of home services. It meets on a regular basis to discuss the patient's progress and barriers to discharge. Based on the team's evaluation, appropriate services are identified, and a treatment plan is developed and carried out within an agreed-upon time frame. In private institutions, it is important to consider rehabilitation time and the stability of a patient. Most third-party payers will initiate rehabilitation as soon as the patient is transferred from the acute surgical/recovery unit. Once transferred, the allotted time allocated by each payer starts, and once it starts, any transfers back to acute care beds will still be counted as rehabilitation days. This is one of the reasons why it is so important to consider the patient's stability and comorbidities before transferring to inpatient rehabilitation.

The lower limb amputee encounters several potential safety risks during his or her rehabilitation across the continuum of care described earlier. These can include (a) falls, (b) medication errors, and (c) trauma to the residual limb. The increased risk of falls is often multifactorial in the lower limb amputee and can be due to a combination of acuity of medical condition, limited insight, medications, advanced age of the patient, poor vision, impaired balance, improper wheelchair use, poorly fitting prosthesis, and environmental factors (9). Leadership in ensuring good communication between rehabilitation team members, patient, and family is an essential factor in minimizing these risks. This communication is especially important at transition points as the patient moves through the continuum of care. At these points, clinicians should (a) review medications, (b) educate the patient about the risk of falls and strategies to minimize them, and (c) minimize disorientation as the patient gets acclimated to his or her new environment. Strategies and equipment to protect the residual limb from trauma and minimize contractures are also important.

Veterans Affairs Amputee System of Care

The Veterans Affairs Amputee System of Care has been designed specifically for amputees. It provides the most efficient use of resources and with the greatest benefit to these patients. It was first initiated in 2008, and 2009 was the first funded year for integration. This design is a complex hub-and-spoke system with four key components: Regional Amputee Center (RAC), Polytrauma Amputation Network Sites (PANS), Amputation Care Team (ACT), and Amputation Points of Contact (APOC). The RAC of a region has the most comprehensive level of care for an amputee with an APOC having simply a point of contact to enter the VA system of care. The RAC is the hub of a region and has the most specialized treatment options and expertise. These centers are used for the most complex amputee cases and medically complicated patients. The RAC care teams are comprised of comprehensive groups of providers including physicians; physical, occupational, and vocational therapists; social workers; prosthetists; and a designated care coordinator (18). The development of this system of care allows for ease of transition between levels of care, appropriate access to care, and efficient allocation of resources to serve the amputee population within the VA system.

CASE STUDY

A 65-year-old Hispanic-American man is admitted to an inpatient rehabilitation unit 2 weeks post transtibial amputation. He has coronary artery disease, peripheral vascular disease, diabetes mellitus, and peripheral neuropathy. He complains of pain in the residual limb that is temporarily relieved by pain medications. He has a tendency to keep his knee bent. He lives alone in an apartment with stairs to enter. He has an involved daughter that lives nearby. Prior to surgery, he was a limited, household ambulator.

CASE STUDY DISCUSSION QUESTIONS

MEDICAL KNOWLEDGE: What are the different types and levels of lower limb amputations and their incidence and prevalence (MK)? What are the common causes of pain in the lower limb amputee? Write a prosthetic prescription for this patient. What are the clinical guidelines for the care of a patient with a transtibial amputation?

PATIENT CARE: Formulate the postop clinical management, rehabilitative care, and prosthetic recommendations for this patient in the acute hospital, acute inpatient rehabilitation unit, and outpatient settings.

PRACTICE-BASED LEARNING AND IMPROVEMENT: What are some possible quality of care issues, including benchmarks and best practices, in the rehabilitation of amputee patients? Describe a quality improvement project for the provision of care in lower limb amputees—include a description of the methodology and outcome measures, and evidence-based practices. What are the key points of a patient education program that emphasizes minimizing the risk of future limb loss? What are some key resources and references that the patient should know about?

SYSTEMS-BASED PRACTICE: Are there any access-to-care issues? Are there any issues with affordability of medications or insurance coverage? Are there any patient safety concerns? Describe the advantages and disadvantages of caring for this patient in different inpatient and outpatient settings. What are the cost considerations in prescribing the prosthetic components?

PROFESSIONALISM: Describe the "patient-centered care" approach and "shared decision making" as they apply to this patient. Are there any cultural issues that affect the patient's adherence to the treatment or to an understanding of his disease? Any privacy concerns? Any ethical issues raised in the diagnosis and care of the patient?

INTERPERSONAL AND COMMUNICATION SKILLS: Describe some strategies to be used in communicating with the patient and his family members about his care.

SELF-EXAMINATION QUESTIONS
(Answers begin on p. 367)

1. Which of the following best describes the reason for assessing hand dexterity and function in the patient with a lower limb amputation?
   A. It aids in the decision regarding prosthesis and socket as donning/doffing issues may arise
   B. It is the most helpful factor in deciding the type of prosthetic foot to prescribe for the patient
   C. It is the most important factor in determining whether or not to prescribe a prosthesis
   D. It is the most important factor in determining if a patient is a good candidate for inpatient rehabilitation
   E. It aids in the decision on the best location in which to provide rehabilitative services

2. Which of the following is the best first step to avoid choke syndrome in an amputee who is having difficulty with his or her new prosthesis?
   A. Remake the patient's prosthesis
   B. Initiate further gait training
   C. Place a distal socket pad
   D. Change angulation of the foot component
   E. Place a lateral heel wedge in the shoe of the nonamputated limb

3. Which of the following care paradigms has the Commission on Accreditation of Rehabilitation Facilities stressed in recent years for amputee care?
   A. Focus on patient responsibility for long-term care
   B. Focus on a physician-centered care approach to patient care
   C. Focus on a holistic approach to patient care

D. Focus on amputation-related issues only
E. Focus on a therapist-centered care approach to amputee care

4. Which of the following best describes physician communication with a patient with a lower limb amputation?
   A. Speak at a fast pace using technical jargon
   B. Speak in a low volume and monotone manner
   C. Don't allow much time for the patient to ask questions
   D. Limit eye contact with the patient
   E. Use nontechnical jargon in discussions with the patient

5. In order to avoid medical errors, where in the following system process is communication between team members the most important?
   A. Transition points in care
   B. During long-term follow-up in a medically stable patient
   C. During the interview process with the patient
   D. In the immediate postsurgical period for a medically stable patient
   E. During therapy sessions for a medically stable patient

REFERENCES

1. Braddom RL. *Physical Medicine & Rehabilitation*. 3rd ed. Philadelphia, PA: Saunders Elsevier; 2010.
2. Ziegler-Graham K, et al. Estimating the prevalence of limb loss in the United States—2005 to 2050. *Arch Phys Med Rehabil.* 2008;89:422–429.
3. Adams PF, et al. Current estimates from the National Health Interview Survey, 1996. *Vital Health Stat.* 1999;10:200.
4. AmpFact Sheet: Amputation Statistics by Cause. (n.d.). *Amputee Coalition ... Saving Limbs. Building Lives.* Retrieved from http://www.amputee-coalition.org/fact_sheets/amp_stats_cause.html
5. Centers for Disease Control and Prevention. (n.d.). *Centers for Disease Control and Prevention.* Retrieved from http://www.cdc.gov
6. Waters R. The energy expenditure of normal and pathologic gait. *Gait Posture.* 1999; 9.3:207–231.
7. Amputee Resource Foundation of America, Inc. (n.d.). *Amputee Resource Foundation of America, Inc.* Retrieved from http://www.amputeeresource.org
8. Ehde DM, Czerniecki JM, Smith DG, et al. Chronic phantom sensations, phantom pain, residual limb pain, and other regional pain after lower limb amputation. *Arch Phys Med Rehabil.* 2000;81:1039–1044.
9. Latlief G, Kent R, Elnitsky C, et al. Patient safety in the rehabilitation of the adult with an amputation. *Phys Med Rehabil Clin N Am.* 2012;23.2:377–392.
10. National Guideline Clearinghouse. VA/DoD clinical practice guideline for rehabilitation of lower limb amputation, Version 1.0 2007 (n.d.). *National Guideline Clearinghouse | Home.* Retrieved from http://www.ngc.gov/content.aspx?id=11758
11. Heinemann AW, Bode RK, Oreilly C. Development and measurement properties of the Orthotics and Prosthetics Users' Survey (OPUS): a comprehensive set of clinical outcome instruments. *Prosthet Orthot Int.* 2003;27:191–206.
12. Kempen GI, Miedema I, Ormel J, et al. The assessment of disability with the Groningen Activity Restriction Scale. Conceptual framework and psychometric properties. *Soc Sci Med.* 1982;43.11: 1601–1610.
13. Speedling EJ, Rose DN. Building an effective doctor-patient relationship: from patient satisfaction to patient participation. *Soc Sci Med.* 1985;21(2):115–120.
14. Bensing J. Bridging the gap. The separate worlds of evidence-based medicine and patient-centered medicine. *Patient Educ Couns.* 2000;39:17–25.
15. Lupinacci M. Developing physician leaders of patient-centered care. *PM&R.* 2010;2:983–986.
16. Kent R, Standley J, Latlief G, et al. The Manny project. *Arch Phys Med Rehabil.* Pre-print (2013).
17. CCAC. NP. (n.d.). *CARF International. Commission on the Accreditation of Rehabilitation Facilities.* Retrieved from http://www.carf.org/Resources/
18. Sigford B. Paradigm shift for VA amputation care. *J Rehabil Res Dev.* 2010;47:15–19.
19. Torburn L, Powers CM, Guiterrez R, Perry J (1995). Energy expenditure during ambulation in dysvascular and traumatic below-knee amputees: A comparison of five prosthetic feet. JRR&D 32(2) 111–119.

Matthew Bartels

11: Cardiopulmonary Rehabilitation

The goal of achieving competency in cardiopulmonary rehabilitation is to be able to provide rehabilitation for two groups of patients. There are patients with primary cardiac and pulmonary disease who need cardiac/pulmonary rehabilitation and then there are patients with other disabilities who have a cardiac or pulmonary secondary disability. This includes patients with respiratory failure and patients who have need for ventilatory support. The incidence of dual-disability patients is now rising as more rehabilitation patients are elderly and have multiple comorbidities. Applying the principles of cardiac rehabilitation to the programs of these patients broadens the number of patients with stroke, vascular disease, or other conditions who can be included in active cardiac and pulmonary rehabilitation programs.

In order to apply cardiac and pulmonary rehabilitation for patients with cardiopulmonary disease, it is necessary to understand the basic principles of cardiac and pulmonary physiology and apply these principles to improve the exercise capacity of these patients. The principles of normal exercise physiology also need to be understood in order to apply the correct adaptations for patients with abnormal cardiopulmonary physiology.

A basic understanding of the historical and present models of cardiopulmonary rehabilitation along with an assessment of several systems in which these are currently delivered will be reviewed and will include inpatient and outpatient settings as well as the need for developing methods of allowing for maintenance programs and potential use of telemedicine.

Cardiac and pulmonary rehabilitation are among the most underutilized yet most effective treatments for patients with cardiopulmonary disease. It is essential for rehabilitation specialists to know how to provide cardiopulmonary rehabilitation and to have an important role in the delivery of cardiopulmonary rehabilitation services to patients with primary and secondary cardiopulmonary disability.

PATIENT CARE

GOALS

Provide competent patient care that is compassionate, appropriate, and effective for the evaluation, treatment, education, and advocacy for patients diagnosed with cardiopulmonary disorders all along the health care continuum.

OBJECTIVES

1. Describe the key components of the assessment of the patient with cardiac and pulmonary diseases.
2. Formulate comprehensive interdisciplinary rehabilitation treatment plans for the patient with cardiac and pulmonary diseases.
3. Evaluate individuals diagnosed with cardiac and pulmonary diseases for physical impairments, activity limitations, and participation restrictions.

ASSESSMENT OF CARDIOPULMONARY FUNCTION

History and Physical Examination

It is essential to have a complete cardiopulmonary history and physical examination as part of the evaluation for patients with cardiac or pulmonary disease who are to undergo rehabilitation. The history may reveal issues to be addressed and help to develop the rehabilitation program. Important parts of the history are from both verbal and nonverbal cues and will allow the patient and physician to establish mutual goals and improve compliance with the treatment program.

History

Historical information should include the patient's emotional state, concurrent illnesses, other disabilities, functional history, occupational history, social history, personal habits, family dynamics, and the effect of disability and cardiopulmonary illness on the patient's performance in the community. It is essential that symptoms at rest and with activity are reviewed. Some specific aspects of the history are discussed in the following text (1).

Dyspnea. Shortness of breath (SOB) is often the chief presenting complaint for patients with cardiopulmonary disease. The description of dyspnea needs to be complete in order to differentiate the contribution of cardiac or pulmonary disease to the underlying dyspnea. Pulmonary causes of dyspnea include pulmonary vascular disease, restrictive lung disease, and obstructive lung disease. Primary cardiac issues include ischemic heart disease, congestive heart failure (CHF), valvular heart disease, and arrhythmias. Often, both cardiac

TABLE 11.1 Causes of Dyspnea

DISORDER	SITE OF PATHOLOGY	PATHOPHYSIOLOGY
Airflow limitation	Lung	Mechanical limitation to ventilation
Restriction (intrinsic)	Lung	Poor lung compliance
Restriction (extrinsic)	Chest wall	Poor chest wall compliance
Valvular disease	Heart	Limited cardiac output
Coronary disease	Heart	Coronary insufficiency
Heart failure	Heart	Limited cardiac output
Anemia	Blood	Limited oxygen-carrying capacity
Peripheral circulation	Peripheral vessels	Inadequate oxygen supply to metabolically active tissues
Obesity	Adipose tissue	Increased work of movement Respiratory restriction if severe
Psychogenic	Emotional	Hyperventilation
Deconditioning	Multiple organ systems	Loss of ability to effectively distribute systemic blood flow
Malingering	Emotional	Inconsistent results
Acute pulmonary disease	Lungs	Increased V/Q mismatch

and pulmonary problems may be present simultaneously. In both conditions, physical conditioning should be ascertained. Patients should also have assessment of their psychological state as they may also have anxiety, which heightens dyspnea. Dyspnea may or may not be associated with hypoxemia and this should be assessed as well with pulse oximetry. See Table 11.1 for an outline of common causes of dyspnea.

Chest Pain. Chest pain, tightness, and burning are the classic symptoms of coronary insufficiency, but they may also be present in patients with valvular heart disease or arrhythmia. The history may help differentiate the causes of chest pain and the duration, quality, provocation, and location of the pain; in addition, any ameliorating factors should be noted. Precipitating factors for chest pain are of particular interest as they may affect the design of the therapy program and may be a cause of functional limitations experienced by the patient. There may also be chest pain associated with certain lung conditions, including pressure and tension with both obstructive and restrictive lung disease. Chest pressure is also commonly experienced with exertion in patients with pulmonary vascular disease.

Palpitation. Palpitations are a sensation of an irregular or forceful heartbeat and can be indicative of serious arrhythmias.

Syncope. Cardiac syncope is usually abrupt with no warning or only a brief warning (with the patient feeling as if he or she were about to pass out). Pulmonary syncope is often slower in onset and may be due to hypercarbia, hypoxemia, or pulmonary vascular disease. Syncope may indicate the presence of aortic stenosis, idiopathic hypertrophic subaortic stenosis (IHSS), primary pulmonary hypertension (PH), hypercarbia, hypoxemia, ventricular arrhythmias, reentrant arrhythmias, high-degree atrioventricular (AV) block, or sick sinus syndrome. Postural syncope can be due to autonomic dysfunction, neurological disease, vagal stimuli, or psychological stimuli.

Edema. Peripheral edema may be an indication of CHF, and in pulmonary disease may indicate right heart failure and PH.

Fatigue. Fatigue is common in cardiopulmonary disease, and there may be other causes that may coexist that contribute to fatigue. A good history can help to identify depression, physical exhaustion, medication side effects, and deconditioning.

Cough. Cough is common in restrictive and interstitial lung disease (ILD) and is often a component of obstructive lung disease, with or without sputum production. Cough may also be caused by cardiac congestion. "Cardiac" cough is characterized by postural changes, with little or no sputum production, and is often relieved by assuming an upright position. Cardiac cough is often nocturnal and episodic.

Limitations of the History. Often patients may not be able to give a complete or accurate history, and even though history does not allow for risk assessment or exercise prescription, it is still an essential part of cardiopulmonary rehabilitation evaluation.

PHYSICAL EXAMINATION

The physical examination of the cardiopulmonary patient is complex, and a full review is beyond the scope of this chapter. Still, we will review some of the important unique elements. The general survey of the patient can reveal exophthalmos (which might be a clue to thyrotoxicosis) or xanthelasma (indicating hypercholesterolemia). Extremities can reveal acrocyanosis (chronic hypoxemia) or clubbing (chronic hypoxemia). Ankylosis is associated with aortic valve disease and conduction defects, and Down syndrome may have associated cardiac abnormalities. Myasthenia or neuromuscular disease may be related to both cardiomyopathy or conduction disease and ventilatory failure.

The details of the cardiopulmonary examination are well described in basic physical examination textbooks, so only a few key points are highlighted here.

Cardiac auscultation can show a fixed splitting of the second heart sound, which can indicate an atrial septal defect. A murmur may indicate valvular heart disease. PH typically produces a heightened second heart sound, and a mid-systolic click may indicate mitral valve prolapse. A noncompliant ventricle can be detected via an atrial gallop at the cardiac apex, and a left ventricular gallop may reveal heart failure. Aortic valve sclerosis, which is common in older patients, may cause an aortic systolic murmur. The combination of pulse contour, the nature of the splitting of the heart sounds, and the quality of the murmur can help differentiate aortic sclerosis from aortic stenosis. Younger patients should be evaluated for pulmonary stenosis and valvular heart disease and may be hard to differentiate from IHSS. Diastolic murmurs can hint at mitral stenosis or PH with pulmonary valve regurgitation. Continuous murmurs may indicate ventricular septal or atrial septal defect. The physical examination can then lead to further evaluation, which may then avoid complications in cardiac rehabilitation.

Pulmonary examination may reveal decreased breath sounds (obstructive disease) or a barrel chest with increased anteroposterior (AP) diameter. Patients may have diffuse crackles or basilar crackles that indicate ILD. There may be inspiratory stridor indicating upper airway obstruction or expiratory wheezing or rhonchi that indicate obstruction or secretions. Patients with suspected respiratory compromise should also have assessment of their symmetry of breathing, looking for accessory muscle use and for possible compromise to diaphragmatic function.

Cardiopulmonary examination and history are important in the detection of patients at risk for complications in a cardiac rehabilitation program, which can often be started in the physiatrist's office with the basic history and physical examination.

The rehabilitation of the patient with cardiac disorders commonly includes the following: (a) education about risk factor modification, lifestyle modification, stress management, and medications; and (b) conditioning and strengthening programs. The rehabilitation of the patient with a pulmonary disease includes the following: (a) strengthening and conditioning exercise programs; (b) smoking cessation; and (c) education about nutrition, stress and anxiety management, medications, supplemental oxygen use, and breathing techniques.

Most of the activity limitation and participation restriction that arises from cardiopulmonary disease stems from the exercise limitation that goes along with impaired cardiopulmonary function. Fatigue is a very common issue, with most patients with heart failure and chronic obstructive pulmonary disease (COPD) reporting chronic fatigue. A major symptom limiting activity in both cardiac and pulmonary patients is dyspnea, with chest pain more common in cardiac patients. Hypoxemia is the major physical limitation, leading to activity limitation and participation restriction in pulmonary patients, while decreased cardiac output (CO) is the most common physical limitation, leading to activity limitation and participation restriction in patients with cardiac diseases. These limitations (fatigue, hypoxemia, dyspnea, chest pain, and low CO) can be deceptive to detect and many observers will not appreciate the degree of disability that they can cause, in their worst forms limiting patients to their homes or bedrooms and causing major limitations in their lives.

MEDICAL KNOWLEDGE

GOALS

Demonstrate knowledge of established evidence-based and evolving biomedical, clinical, epidemiological, and sociobehavioral sciences pertaining to cardiac and pulmonary diseases, as well as the application of this knowledge to lessen impact of physical and functional impairments and guide treatment.

OBJECTIVES

1. Review important principles of cardiac and pulmonary anatomy, as well as normal and abnormal cardiac and pulmonary physiology.
2. Review general principles of cardiac and pulmonary rehabilitation.
3. Review principles of cardiac rehabilitation following myocardial infarction (MI), revascularization procedures, post-cardiac transplantation, and in patients with cardiomyopathy, valve disease and cardiac arrhythmias.
4. Review principles of pulmonary rehabilitation in diseases such as emphysema, intrinsic lung disease, ventilatory failure, and PH.
5. Review principles of cardiac and pulmonary rehabilitation as they apply to physically disabled populations.

REVIEW OF CORONARY ANATOMY AND PHYSIOLOGY

Cardiac Anatomy

All physicians involved in cardiac rehabilitation need to be familiar with the normal distribution of the major arteries of the heart, cardiac valvular anatomy, and the structures at risk from ischemia or infarction in these distributions.

Overall, the heart consists of paired atria and ventricles, with deoxygenated venous blood entering the right atrium, traversing the right ventricle via the tricuspid valve, entering the pulmonary artery through the pulmonic valve. Oxygenated blood reenters the heart via the left atrium, entering the left ventricle through the mitral valve, where it is then ejected into the aorta through the aortic valve. Proper heart valve function ensures unidirectional unobstructed flow of blood, and proper atrial function can help to augment cardiac function, adding up to 15% to 20% to the total CO. Atrial contribution is greater with increased heart rate (HR) and in conditions with decreased ventricular compliance

(2). The loss of the contribution of atrial "kick" is especially important to consider in disease conditions where atrial dysfunction is seen, such as atrial fibrillation.

The cardiac conduction system is a specialized system of muscle cells (myocytes), which allow coordinated contraction of the atria and ventricles at a controlled rate. The SA node is the usual cardiac pacemaker located in the right atrium. The electrical pulse travels through three atrial internodal pathways to the AV node where conduction is delayed to cause sequential atrial and ventricular contraction. Below the AV node, the signal passes into the bundle of His and divides into left and right bundles. The left bundle has anterior and posterior fascicles, and all bundles then end in terminal branches to excite the myocytes and cause contraction. MI, aging, and other conditions can alter the conduction system and create heart block and sick sinus syndrome. Congenital defects and accessory pathways can be seen in Wolff-Parkinson-White (WPW) syndrome.

Variation of Arteries

Normally, there can be several different variations of coronary circulation. The left main coronary artery usually divides into the left anterior descending and the circumflex arteries, while the right coronary artery continues on as a single vessel. The most common anatomy (60%) is right dominant circulation, while left dominant circulation (10%–15%) is seen when the posterior descending artery arises from the left circumflex. The remaining 30% of individuals have balanced circulation where the posterior descending arises from the left circumflex and right coronary arteries (2) (Table 11.2).

Cardiac Physiology

Cardiac myocytes are highly metabolically active with nearly 65% oxygen extraction at all levels of activity (compared with 36% for the brain and 26% for the rest of the body). Carbohydrates are the preferred energy source (40%), with fatty acids making up most of the remaining 60%. This high oxygen extraction and coronary blood flow only during diastole predisposes the heart to ischemic injury, especially in the endocardium. Normally, coronary vasodilation increases blood flow with exertion, via nitric oxide pathways. It is the goal of most medical and surgical therapies for ischemia to restore or preserve myocardial perfusion, through vasodilation or bypass or endovascular procedures. Exercise is also a very effective therapy, as regular exercise can increase cardiac collateral circulation and improve arteriolar vasodilation (2).

Appropriate fluid balance is also important in cardiac care, as adequate venous return can maintain appropriate cardiac "preload," while fluid overload with excessive venous return can exacerbate heart failure. For mechanical cardiac constriction, surgery can allow greater dilation of the ventricle to restore CO, and in dilated heart failure, medical treatment may decrease the size of the ventricles in order to increase CO. Left ventricular assist devices (LVADs) and cardiac transplantation can be used for the most refractory cases.

REVIEW OF PULMONARY ANATOMY AND PHYSIOLOGY

Pulmonary Anatomy

Basic pulmonary anatomy includes the upper and lower airways (the oropharynx, larynx, trachea, mainstem bronchi, and smaller bronchi), the lung parenchyma itself, and the chest walls and musculature (diaphragm, accessory muscles of breathing, rib cage, pleura). Abnormalities in any of these structures can cause pulmonary limitations and may lead to decreased exercise capacity. The pulmonary vasculature includes pulmonary arteries and veins, which deliver deoxygenated blood to the lungs and deliver oxygenated blood to the left atrium, as well as intrinsic pulmonary artery circulation, which delivers oxygenated blood to the respiratory tree.

Upper airway obstruction from vocal cord paralysis or tumor may cause stridor. Reactive airway disease may cause asthma and be associated with dyspnea. Patients with parenchymal lung disease may have a loss of alveoli with loss of intrinsic recoil of the lung and subsequent hyperinflation and dyspnea (emphysema, COPD) or may have interstitial scarring with increased recoil and decreased ability to diffuse oxygen through the lung tissues (ILD, pulmonary fibrosis). In some conditions

TABLE 11.2 Coronary Artery Anatomy

ARTERIES	MAIN BRANCHES	DISTRIBUTIONS	VARIATIONS
Right coronary artery	Nodal branch	Right atrium and SA node	
	Right marginal branch	Right ventricle to apex	
	Posterior intraventricular (descending) branch	AV node, posterior third of septum, right bundle of His	AV node in 85%–95% of individuals, distal anastomosis to the left circumflex artery
Left coronary artery	Anterior intraventricular (descending) branch	Anterior left and right ventricles, anterior two-thirds of septum, left bundle of His, AV node	AV node in 5%–15% of individuals, 40% with some contribution
	Circumflex artery	Left atrium, superior portions of left ventricle	

there may be an interplay of both restrictive and obstructive diseases, although usually one is predominant over another (cystic fibrosis, sarcoidosis). Assessment of the lung parenchyma can be made with imaging or physiological testing such as pulmonary function tests (1).

Pulmonary Physiology

Normal breathing is governed by the respiratory center in the medulla oblongata of the brain. Injury to that part of the brain can cause respiratory failure and need for ventilatory support. Signals for inspiration are carried via the phrenic and other somatic nerves to the diaphragm and secondary inspiratory muscles (intercostals, sternocleidomastoids, pectorals) and cause rhythmic breathing via negative pressure in the chest wall. Normal exhalation is a passive process dependent on elastic recoil of the chest wall and the lung parenchyma. In pulmonary disease such as COPD and emphysema, exhalation can become active with the need for abdominal muscles to cause exhalation and markedly increasing the work of breathing. Any disease affecting the brain, spine, or phrenic nerves; the muscles; or the mechanical properties of the chest wall or diaphragm will affect normal respiration. In ILD, the compliance of the lung tissue can become so severe that the lung volumes decrease and hypoventilation can result (1).

Pulmonary vascular disease can lead to PH, and this can be either primary or secondary. Primary pulmonary vascular disease can be idiopathic or can result from vasculitis, thromboembolic disease, or as a part of the progression of intrinsic parenchymal disease. Secondary hypertension is usually a result of left heart failure and may eventually develop a component of intrinsic vascular compromise. Chronic exposure to hypoxemia may also create pulmonary vascular compromise and can be seen with obesity, obstructive sleep apnea, and high-altitude exposure. Hypoxemia leads to pulmonary vascular constriction and in a chronic state will lead to vascular intimal hypertrophy and the development of fixed pulmonary vascular resistance and PH.

Basic Terminology

AEROBIC CAPACITY Aerobic capacity (VO_2max) is the measure of the work capacity of an individual. Aerobic capacity is expressed as the oxygen consumed by the individual (liters of oxygen per minute or in milliliters of oxygen per kilogram per minute). Oxygen consumption (VO_2) increases linearly with workload, increasing up to a plateau, which occurs at the VO_2max. Knowing a person's maximal exercise capacity can help with assessing disability and planning exercise and recovery programs (1).

HEART RATE HR is used to guide exercise as it has a linear relationship to VO_2. Maximum HR is determined by age and can be estimated as: peak HR = 220 − age or by the Karvonen equation. The slope of the relationship of HR and VO_2 is determined by physical conditioning, with a lower slope representing improved conditioning. HR is mediated by the interaction of vagal and sympathetic tone and circulating catecholamines and can be altered by medications (1).

STROKE VOLUME Stroke volume (SV) is the quantity of blood ejected with each left ventricular contraction. Normally, maximal SV can be increased with exercise. SV increases the most during early exercise and is sensitive to postural changes, changing little when one is supine but increasing in a curvilinear fashion until it reaches maximum at approximately 40% of VO_2max. SV declines with advancing age, in cardiac conditions that result in decreased compliance, after MI, and in heart failure (1).

CARDIAC OUTPUT This is the product of the HR and SV and increases linearly with work. Peak CO is the primary determinant of VO_2 max and is maximized in upright work compared with supine work (1).

MYOCARDIAL OXYGEN CONSUMPTION Myocardial oxygen consumption (MVO_2) is the oxygen consumption of the heart and rises in a linear fashion with workload. Angina occurs when the MVO_2 exceeds the maximum coronary artery oxygen delivery. MVO_2 can be estimated with the rate pressure product (RPP), calculated as the product of the HR and the systolic blood pressure (SBP) divided by 100. Upper extremity and isometric exercises have a higher MVO_2 for a given VO_2. Supine exercises demonstrate a higher MVO_2 at low intensity and a lower MVO_2 at high intensity compared with erect exercises. MVO_2 is also increased in the cold, extreme heat, after smoking, or after eating (1).

For pulmonary exercise assessment, basic static lung volumes and dynamic responses to exercise need to be assessed. A full discussion of pulmonary function testing is beyond the scope of this chapter, but important values include the following:

Total Lung Capacity (TLC). The volume of air in the lungs at full inspiration.
Vital Capacity (VC). Volume change of air through the mouth between full inspiration and full expiration.
Forced Expired Vital Capacity (FVC). Maximum volume that can be expired from the lungs after a maximal forced expiration.
Forced Expiratory Volume in 1 Second (FEV_1). The FEV over 1 second is the most commonly reported value and is severely limited in airway obstruction.
Maximal Voluntary Ventilation (MVV). Measurement of the maximum minute ventilation over 15 seconds.
Residual Volume (RV). Volume of air in the lungs after a full expiration.
Tidal Volume (TV). The volume of a regular nonforced breath at rest.
Diffusion of the Lung for Carbon Monoxide (DLCO). This measures the ability of gases to diffuse across the alveolar membrane.

The capacity to exercise in cardiac and pulmonary conditions is best assessed with cardiopulmonary exercise testing and is useful for diagnostic, prognostic, and exercise prescription in both populations. The effects of various physiological conditions on the interpretation of pulmonary exercise testing are shown in Table 11.3.

TABLE 11.3 Effects of Physiological Conditions on the Interpretation of Pulmonary Testing

ABNORMALITY	PHYSIOLOGIC ABNORMALITY	GAS EXCHANGE
Obesity	Increased work with activity	Rapid alveolar–arterial pA–PaO$_2$ fall with exercise
Peripheral vascular disease	Claudication limits exercise	Low VO$_2$max Low anaerobic threshold
Pulmonary vascular disease	Impaired pulmonary blood flow	Decreased O$_2$ uptake at maximum work Low anaerobic threshold Rapid pulse at low exercise
Anemia	Low oxygen-carrying capacity	Low VO$_2$max Low anaerobic threshold Rapid pulse at low exercise
Chronic obstructive pulmonary disease	Restricted expiratory phase of breathing Decreased alveolar ventilation	Low VO$_2$max Low anaerobic threshold Rapid pulse at low exercise Submaximal heart rate achieved
Restrictive lung disease (intrinsic)	Poor diffusion capacity Poor pulmonary compliance	Low VO$_2$max Low anaerobic threshold Tachypnea Low pulmonary reserve High alveolar–arterial pA–PaO$_2$ difference
Restrictive lung disease (extrinsic)	Poor pulmonary compliance	Low VO$_2$max Low anaerobic threshold Tachypnea Low pulmonary reserve Submaximal heart rate achieved
Asthma	Restricted expiratory phase of breathing Decreased alveolar ventilation In exercise-induced asthma, peak flows drop 5–10 min into exercise	Most findings normal when not symptomatic, resemble obstructive with acute attack
Ventricular failure	Compromised pulmonary blood flow	Low VO$_2$max Low anaerobic threshold Tachypnea Exaggerated heart rate response to exercise
Ischemic heart disease	Chest pain/cardiac ischemia Can precipitate ventricular failure	Often normal Can appear like mild ventricular failure Can have inability to raise BP
Metabolic acidosis	Metabolic acidosis, low HCO$_3$	Normal diffusion Exaggerated response of ventilation to exercise

AEROBIC TRAINING

Aerobic training is a physical exercise that increases the cardiopulmonary capacity (VO$_2$max). The basic prescription for aerobic training requires four components: intensity, duration, frequency, and specificity.

Intensity is how hard an exercise is and can be indicated by a target HR, metabolic level (MET level), or intensity (wattage). For cardiac training in primary prevention, the target HR can be set at 80% to 85% of the predicted maximum HR or peak HR on an exercise tolerance test (ETT). Exercises above 60% of the maximal HR will have training effect. This is also true in pulmonary disease.

Duration is how long a bout of exercise will be. Cardiopulmonary conditioning exercise should be 20 to 30 minutes, with a 5- to 10-minute warm-up and cool-down period. Exercise at lower intensity will require a longer duration to achieve a similar training effect.

Frequency is how often exercise is performed over a fixed time period, usually expressed in sessions per week. At a minimum, training programs should be done three times per week, increased to five times per week for low-intensity programs.

Specificity describes the activity to be done in exercise. Training benefits are most specific to the activities that are performed; for example, cycle ergometry is not as beneficial for improving walking as a treadmill training program. Specificity of a training program should take into account the needs of a particular patient. For example, upper arm ergometry for a spinal cord patient or cycle ergometry over treadmill for patients with lower limb arthritis. This is the law of specificity of conditioning and is commonly referred to in cardiopulmonary conditioning programs (1).

The benefits of aerobic training are as follows:

Aerobic Capacity. Increased with training. The resting VO_2 does not change, and the VO_2 at a given workload does not change. The changes are also specific to the muscle groups that are trained.

Cardiac Output. The maximum CO increases. Resting CO does not change, but resting HR will decrease, with increased SV. This leads to lower MVO_2 at rest and submaximal exercise.

Heart Rate. The HR is lower at rest and at any given workload. Maximum HR is not changed.

Stroke Volume. SV is increased at rest and at all levels of exercise and allows for maintenance of CO at a given workload with a lower HR and RPP at a given level of exertion.

Myocardial Oxygen Capacity. The maximum MVO_2 does not usually change but is lower at a given workload after training. This can allow individuals to perform more activities below the anginal threshold with fewer symptoms and increased safety. Pharmacological interventions or revascularization procedures can also improve maximum MVO_2.

Peripheral Resistance. The peripheral vascular resistance (PR) decreases in response to exercise training. This is often referred to as "afterload." The decrease in PR is due to the increased vasodilatation in peripheral vascular beds. This causes a lower RPP and a lower MVO_2 at a given workload and at rest.

Minute Ventilation. As a person has improved conditioning, he or she will require a lower VO_2, and thus a lower VE for a given activity. This can decrease dyspnea in patients who have pulmonary and cardiac diseases.

Tidal Volume. As patients improve with exercise, they can sustain a higher TV, meaning a decrease in respiratory rate and a decrease in subjective dyspnea.

Respiratory Rate. This will decrease as TV is able to improve and will be lower for a given minute ventilation, helping to lower dyspnea.

By remembering the basic physiology described earlier, cardiopulmonary rehabilitation specialists can improve function, decrease symptoms, and have a positive effect on outcomes in their patients. The main benefits of cardiac conditioning are reduced cardiac risk and improved cardiac conditioning. The reduction of cardiac risk is established historically in numerous studies. As long ago as 1989, pooled data from 22 randomized studies of exercise in 4,554 patients following acute MI demonstrated a 20% to 25% reduction in all-cause mortality, fatal MI, and cardiac mortality in a 3-year follow-up (3). The benefits of cardiac rehabilitation apply to the elderly, women, and in postbypass patients (3).

Pulmonary rehabilitation is also effective in COPD; it helps to decrease hospitalizations and improve function and quality of life (4–7). An overview of the pulmonary rehabilitation program is in Table 11.4.

TABLE 11.4 Goals and Methods of Pulmonary Rehabilitation

GOALS	METHODS
Prevention	
Smoking cessation	Enroll in a cessation program, emotional support, monitor abstinence
Immunization compliance	Assure proper immunizations, communicate with primary physician
Prevent exacerbations	Self-assessment skills taught Self-intervention taught Instruct on accessing private physician
Appropriate medication use	Review medications and dosing schedules Review interactions and side effects Review appropriate use of inhalers and nebulizers
Pulmonary toilet	Review bronchial hygiene Teach proper cough techniques Use of chest physiotherapy as needed Teach chest physiotherapy techniques to family as appropriate
Appropriate use of oxygen therapy	Teach use with exertion Review self-monitoring Review use of equipment Encourage acceptance of the need for O_2 Review importance of use and consequences of failure to use oxygen
Nutritional counseling	Counseling to achieve ideal body weight Counseling to avoid high carbohydrate diet Instruction in avoidance of high sodium diets Encourage balanced nutrition, avoidance of fad diets

(continued)

TABLE 11.4 Goals and Methods of Pulmonary Rehabilitation (continued)

GOALS	METHODS
Family training	Teaching regarding: COPD Pulmonary toilet Medication use Oxygen use Family support group Counseling as needed
Dyspnea Relief—Exercise Training	
Exercise	Multifaceted program individualized to each patient's needs
Strengthening	Emphasis on gradual increase in strength Focus on proximal muscle groups Avoid injury to weakened musculotendinous structures Focus more on high-repetition, low-intensity training
Conditioning	Work to gradually increase exercise tolerance Cross-training program Emphasis on the development of an independent training program Increase ambulation endurance with gait training Appropriate oxygen titration during exercise
Respiratory muscle training	Inspiratory and expiratory muscle training Isocapnic hyperpnea Inspiratory resistance training Inspiratory threshold training
Upper extremity training	Increase strength Increase capacity for sustained work Improve shoulder girdle strength
ADL training	Energy conservation techniques Adaptive techniques Relieve anxiety and stress Encourage pacing in activities
Breathing retraining	Pursed lip breathing Diaphragmatic breathing
Anxiety reduction	Stress relaxation techniques Paced breathing Autohypnosis Visualization Medications as needed Treat anxiety Treat depression

(continued)

TABLE 11.4 Goals and Methods of Pulmonary Rehabilitation (continued)

GOALS	METHODS
Improve confidence	Build compensatory techniques Build confidence in ability to exercise
Disease Management	
Disease acceptance	Education regarding disease process Reassurance about aggressive treatment
Coping skills	Support group Psychology and social work intervention as needed Treat depression as needed
Quality of life improvement	Improve ADL tolerance Improve coping skills Improve disease management
Advance directives review	Counseling regarding: Health care proxy Resuscitation orders Help in preparing paperwork
Encouragement	Support group Social work support Psychological support
Continuing compliance	Team encouragement Physician counseling Involve primary care physician in plan Family education

Abnormal Physiology

Heart

Physiatrists should be familiar with the alterations of normal cardiac physiology in disease in order to order effective cardiac rehabilitation. Cardiac disease is due to either decreased CO or ischemic disease, with a degree of overlap. During ischemic episodes, the myocardium becomes less compliant with less contractility and a subsequent decrease in SV, while valvular heart disease decreases maximum CO through either stenotic valves (e.g., aortic or mitral stenosis) or valvular regurgitation (e.g., aortic or mitral insufficiency). Finally, CHF has decreased CO with low SV, associated with a lower VO_2max, higher resting HRs, and often a greater MVO_2 at a given VO_2.

Arrhythmias usually decrease the CO through decreased SV and increased HRs. This may be due to a loss of atrial contribution (atrial "kick") with supraventricular arrhythmias (e.g., atrial fibrillation of supraventricular tachycardias), or from high HRs without atrial coordination (e.g., ventricular tachycardias and ventricular bigeminy).

Surgical treatments of cardiac disease either aim to restore coronary circulation (e.g., bypass and intravascular procedures) or aim to restore normal anatomy (e.g., valve replacement). Medical therapy for ischemic disease aims to improve coronary circulation, and treatment for heart failure aims to decrease afterload, reduce fluid overload, and increase inotropy with surgical treatment including LVADs. Medical treatment of arrhythmias with medications has been difficult, but implantable defibrillators and pacemakers have been very efficacious treatment for these conditions. For intractable heart disease, cardiac transplantation or LVAD are final possible treatments. All of these conditions, including transplant and LVAD patients, benefit from cardiac rehabilitation. An understanding of the underlying physiology of all of these conditions is essential to successful rehabilitation. Pretransplant patients have abnormalities, including CHF, intractable ischemia, or arrhythmia, while posttransplant patients have persistently high resting HR and a limited ability to increase SV and peak exercise HRs that can limit exercise response. The outline for programs of rehabilitation of all of these syndromes is discussed subsequently (1).

Lung

Patients with pulmonary disease have essentially three types of impairment: obstructive or restrictive lung disease, or pulmonary vascular disease. Two of these may often be present in one patient and may increase the morbidity of the individual. A basic understanding of the underlying physiology will help in the design of the exercise program for the patients.

A basic way to think of pulmonary impairments is to divide intrinsic lung limitations into either obstructive or restrictive conditions. In obstructive lung disease, there is an inability to exhale, either due to upper airway or large airway disease (sleep apnea, tracheomalacia, vocal cord disease, asthma, bronchitis) or due to secretions or lung parenchymal disease (emphysema, bronchiectasis), and there may also be an acute condition (asthma) versus chronic condition (chronic obstructive lung disease [COPD]). The hallmark of COPD is carbon dioxide retention and active exhalation. Medical treatments in obstructive disease are aimed at relieving the obstruction via bronchodilation for reactive airways, use of steroids and antibiotics for inflamed or infected airways, or surgery for emphysema (lung volume reduction surgery [LVRS]). In end-stage disease, lung transplantation may be the only option.

For patients with restrictive lung disease, there is a limitation to tidal volumes from inability to expand the chest wall (extrinsic restriction) or from very noncompliant lung tissue (intrinsic restriction). Forms of extrinsic restriction include neuromuscular disease, paralysis, and kyphoscoliosis. These conditions often respond to mechanical ventilation and respiratory muscle training, if possible. The intrinsic restrictive lung diseases include pulmonary fibrosis and sarcoidosis and may have profound associated hypoxemia due to decreased diffusion capacity of scarred lung tissue. These patients classically have severe hypoxemia and may need high-flow supplemental oxygen. In the end stage of intrinsic restrictive disease, patients can suffer severe ventilatory failure with hypercarbia and hypoxemia. Since many of these conditions may be progressive, lung transplantation is often a treatment option in selected candidates with end-stage disease. Table 11.5 shows some of the lung pathologies and effects on inspiratory reserve and RV (obstructive diseases), and Table 11.6 shows the effects of various conditions on lung compliance (restrictive diseases) (8).

TABLE 11.5 Lung Pathology

LOSS OF INSPIRATORY RESERVE	INCREASE IN THE RESIDUAL VOLUME
Intrinsic	**Intrinsic**
- Lung fibrosis	- Bronchial obstruction
- Obliteration of alveoli	- Airways collapse
- Pulmonary edema	
Extrinsic	**Extrinsic**
- Chest wall rigidity	- Respiratory muscle weakness
- Respiratory muscle weakness	- Chest wall rigidity
- Chest wall restriction from bracing	

TABLE 11.6 Causes of Alterations in Lung Compliance

INCREASED COMPLIANCE	DECREASED COMPLIANCE
Intrinsic	**Intrinsic**
- Decreased elastic recoil	- Alveolar obliteration
- Loss of alveolar walls	- Increased alveolar stiffness
	- Increased alveolar wall thickness
	- Decreased surfactant
Extrinsic	**Extrinsic**
- Flail chest	- Chest wall stiffness
- Multiple rib fractures	- Chest wall deformity
	- Chest wall bracing

Cardiac Rehabilitation

Cardiac rehabilitation programs come in 2 forms: primary prevention, which includes risk factor modification and education before a cardiac event; and secondary prevention, which is cardiac rehabilitation after the establishment of cardiac disease and includes exercise and risk factor modification.

Primary prevention programs are not usually performed in a rehabilitation setting but are in primary care settings. Primary prevention includes a focus on the reduction of cardiac risk factors with education for at-risk patients and includes community-based cardiac disease prevention. Primary prevention can have a profound effect on the rate of cardiac disease with a decrease in obesity, blood pressure, and lipid profiles. Behavior modification should ideally begin in childhood in order to establish healthy behavior patterns to be maintained throughout life. This is also important in disabled populations who are generally sedentary and may have other risk factors. Primary prevention can include the use of medications to treat hypertension, lipid abnormalities, and antiplatelet agents. These are all cost-effective approaches and can decrease mortality and morbidity on a population-based scale, in addition to the individual benefits (9–11).

Secondary risk factor modification programs are an essential part of cardiac rehabilitation programs for individuals after onset of cardiac disease. Secondary risk factor modification programs include all of the features of primary prevention programs with the addition of disease-specific education and formal exercise. Smoking cessation is an essential part of both primary and secondary prevention programs (12–14).

Pulmonary Rehabilitation

Patients with pulmonary disease follow a similar pattern to cardiac patients with regard to their programs of rehabilitation. Since most pulmonary diseases are chronic and progressive, there is not a model of acute inpatient rehabilitation, but early mobilization programs are now working to limit debility in patients who undergo exacerbations. The essential components of outpatient rehabilitation for pulmonary disease are the same as for cardiac patients. Primary prevention for pulmonary disease includes smoking prevention and cessation, occupational safety, and prevention of exposure to environmental and infectious agents. Secondary prevention is in the form of medication adherence and education, smoking cessation, oxygen supplementation, and environmental modification to prevent recurrent exposure to environmental triggers (5,7).

For patients with ventilatory failure, lung transplant may be a treatment, and these patients can benefit from rehabilitation both before and after transplantation. Pretransplant rehabilitation is focused on the underlying condition and posttransplant rehabilitation is focused on education and restoration of muscle strength, which is impaired from the medical regimen for posttransplant patients.

Cardiac Rehabilitation of the Post-MI Patient

Standard cardiac rehabilitation following MI usually follows the classical model of cardiac rehabilitation, as first described by Wenger et al. in 1971 (1). Since revascularization is now common and infarcts are smaller than in the past, cardiac rehabilitation usually has three stages or phases, eliminating the classical stage 2 recovery phase. The comparison of the old and new programs of mobilization is seen in Table 11.6.

The exception to this paradigm is postsurgical patients who may need an intermediate recovery phase from their surgery before launching into the training phase of rehabilitation. To recount, the first phase is the acute phase in hospital period immediately following the cardiac event that ends at discharge. The second phase is the rehabilitation training phase, with intense education and aerobic conditioning to achieve the desired results of exercise. The third phase is the maintenance phase, which is devoted to the continued aerobic exercise and maintenance of lifestyle modifications. Risk factor modifications are taught and reemphasized throughout all phases. A similar model exists for pulmonary disease patients. All patients who are identified to have cardiopulmonary disease can start directly into the second phase without a hospitalization.

TABLE 11.7 Wenger Protocol—Then and Now

ORIGINAL PROGRAM	MODERN PROGRAM	ACTIVITY
Day 1	Day 1	Passive range of motion (ROM), ankle pumps, introduction to the program, self-feeding
Day 2	Day 1	As above, also dangle at side of bed
Day 3	Day 1	Active assisted ROM, sitting upright in a chair, light recreation, and use of bedside commode
Day 4	Day 1	Increased sitting time, light activities with minimal resistance, patient education
Day 5	Day 1	Light activities with moderate resistance, unlimited sitting, seated ADL
Day 6	Day 2	Increased resistance, walking to bathroom, standing ADL, up to 1-hr-long group meetings
Day 7	Day 2	Walking up to 100 feet, standing warm-up exercises
Day 8	Day 2	Increased walking, walk down stairs (not up), continued education
Day 9	Day 2	Increased exercise program, review energy conservation and pacing techniques
Day 10	Day 3	Increase exercises with light weights and ambulation, begin education on home exercise program
Day 11	Day 3	Increased duration of activities
Day 12	Day 3	Walk down two flights of stairs, continue to increase resistance in exercises
Day 13	Day 3	Continue activities, education, and home exercise program teaching
Day 14	Day 3	Walk up and down two flights of stairs, complete instruction in home exercise program and in energy conservation and pacing techniques

Acute Phase (Phase 1)

The basics of the early mobilization program are outlined in Table 11.7. The educational program relating to risk factor modification should be introduced during phase 1 as many patients are ready to listen to advice in their acute hospitalization. With or without revascularization, the acute mobilization should be done with cardiac monitoring and under the supervision of a trained physical or occupational therapist or nurse. The post-MI HR rise with activity should be kept to within 20 beats per minute (bpm) of baseline and the SBP rise within 20 mmHg of baseline. Any decrease of SBP of 10 mmHg or more should be considered worrisome and exercise halted. The major goal of the phase 1 program is to condition the patient to perform activities up to four METs, which is within the range of most daily activities at home postdischarge.

For patients with pulmonary disease, similar goals exist with new emphasis now being placed on early mobilization in the intensive care unit (ICU), even while still on the ventilator. Treatments such as extracorporeal membrane oxygenation (ECMO) are also now coming to the fore and will allow for mobilization of patients since they will be alert and not sedated on a ventilator, thereby allowing the ability to walk with assistance in the ICU setting. After discharge, patients should be enrolled in pulmonary outpatient programs to allow for consolidation of early gains and a full program of education and exercise.

Inpatient Rehabilitation Phase (Phase 1B)

In order to distinguish between patients who have a rapid recovery after their cardiopulmonary event (pure phase 1) and those patients who require either acute or subacute rehabilitation treatment prior to discharge home, the designation of phase 1B rehabilitation has been established. With advanced age or significant comorbidities or other disabilities that make mobilization more difficult, many rehabilitation specialists will care for these phase 1B patients. The guidelines for exercise are the same as they are for the phase 1 patients, but with a longer recovery period extending their hospitalized care to an acute or subacute rehabilitation setting prior to discharge.

Training Phase (Phase 2)

The training phase of the cardiopulmonary rehabilitation is classically started after a symptom-limited full-level ETT for cardiac patients, or a Cardiopulmonary exercise test (CPET) for complex pulmonary patients. Target HR or intensities can be taken from the exercise test and used as guidelines during aerobic training. For low-risk patients, 85% of the maximum HR is generally regarded as safe. For individuals who are at greater risk, exercise programs at lower target HRs can be tailored to individual patients based on the results of the exercise test and the reason for cessation of exercise. Generally, for patients with life-threatening arrhythmias or chest pain, lower target HRs are chosen. Pulmonary patients with hypoxemia are given oxygen as needed up to high flow (15 L/min or more) in order to maintain saturation for safe exercise. In patients with higher risk, a target HR of 65% to 75% of maximum can be safe and effective in a regular exercise program (50), and target rates as low as 60% can still yield a training benefit. For the patients at higher risk, it is appropriate to monitor individuals at each increase in activity.

A classic cardiopulmonary training program is three sessions per week for approximately 8 to 12 weeks. The major limitation of cardiopulmonary rehabilitation is a lack of referral and a lack of facilities for rehabilitation in many areas. In order to assist in increasing access to cardiopulmonary rehabilitation, creative programs have been developed, including at-home programs for low-risk patients, telemedicine programs, and community- and home-based programs. A key to success in home-based programs is assuring that patients are able to perform self-monitoring during their exercise program. Guidelines for self-monitoring are outlined in the standard references (15,16). Just as in the supervised programs, all exercise sessions should begin with a stretching session, followed by a warm-up session, the training exercise, and end with a cool-down period. It is important to remember that conditioning benefit is related to the specificity of training, and that the conditioning applies to the specific muscles exercised.

Maintenance Phase (Phase 3)

Despite usually receiving the least attention, the maintenance phase of a cardiopulmonary rehabilitation is the most important part of the program. If the patient stops exercising, the benefits gained from phase 2 can be lost in a few weeks. From the beginning of the rehabilitation program, the importance of an ongoing exercise program needs to be emphasized and efforts need to be made to integrate exercise and lifestyle modifications into the patient's life. For moderate-level exercises, patients should perform exercise at the target intensity learned in their rehabilitation program for at least 30 minutes 3 times a week. For low-level exercise, exercise should be done 5 times a week. For pulmonary patients, home pulse oximetry monitoring can be helpful and is cost-effective and easily learned (8).

Cardiac Rehabilitation Programs in Specific Conditions

Angina Pectoris

The goal of cardiac rehabilitation for angina is to decrease angina and improve fitness. The exercise benefit in angina is derived from improving efficiency and improved collateralization.

Cardiac Rehabilitation After Revascularization Procedures

Postcoronary Artery Bypass Grafting

Cardiac rehabilitation can consolidate the benefits after revascularization by emphasizing secondary prevention and adding the benefits of regular exercise to prevent recurrence of the coronary disease. Close monitoring needs to be considered for patients with low ejection fractions and CHF. Full programs of rehabilitation often need to be delayed for up to 6 weeks in patients with sternotomy to allow for sternal healing, but for patients without sternotomy, it can begin as soon as the patient has recovered from the procedure. The rehabilitation of patients after percutaneous interventions (PCIs) is essentially the same as after surgical bypass.

Cardiac Rehabilitation After Cardiac Transplant Surgery

Typically, cardiac transplant patients suffer from months of preoperative invalidism and general muscle weakness and have depression and anxiety. The transplant itself usually resolves the cardiac disability, but a comprehensive approach to the patient is necessary. Due to the complexity of the procedure and the occurrence of vascular and neurological complications, some of these patients also require phase 1B programs and may come to acute or subacute rehabilitation settings.

Because of cardiac deinnervation and immunosuppressive medications, the physiology of the posttransplant patient is altered from the normal cardiac patient. Transplantation causes cardiac denervation, with loss of both sympathetic and vagal connections to central regulation. Loss of vagal inhibition to the SA node creates a mild baseline tachycardia of 100 to 110 bpm. With exercise, there is no direct sympathetic stimulation to the heart and chronotopic response is mediated by circulating catecholamines, causing a blunted and delayed HR response to exercise. Peak HR is usually 20% to 25% lower than in matched controls. There is also resting hypertension, due to the renal effects of calcineurin inhibitors (e.g., cyclosporine and tacrolimus) and prednisone, and diastolic dysfunction may also be seen. Finally, maximum work output and maximum oxygen uptake are reduced to about two-thirds of the age-matched population, similar to lung transplant recipients. Transplant patients thus have higher than normal perceived exertion, minute ventilation, and ventilatory equivalent for oxygen at submaximal exercise levels. At maximum effort, transplant patients demonstrate lower work capacity, CO, HR, SBP, and oxygen uptake, while resting HR and SBP are higher than in normal individuals. Finally, both resting and exertional diastolic blood pressure are higher after cardiac transplantation than in normal individuals (1).

The training regimen in transplant patients must address overall conditioning and education. Aerobic exercises should be done at 60% to 70% of peak effort for 30 to 60 minutes 3 to 5 times weekly with rating of perceived exertion (RPE) targets, using the Borg scale, at 13 to 14, with the level of activity increasing incrementally to stay at this level. Education for posttransplant patients includes the complicated medical regimen, vocational, and psychological needs. The outcomes of rehabilitation in the cardiac transplant population have been generally favorable. Patients usually achieve increased work output and improved exercise tolerance, even resuming competitive athletics (1).

Cardiomyopathy

Despite not being covered by many insurance plans, CHF patients are a growing subset of the cardiac rehabilitation population. New Medicare regulations now will cover rehabilitation for CHF starting in March 2014, and it is hoped that many other insurance plans will follow suit. CHF patients have increased complications compared to coronary artery bypass graft (CABG) or post-MI population, with a higher risk of sudden death, depression, and chronic cardiac disability. They may also have inconsistent responses to exercise with increased fatigue and with possible exertional hypotension, as well as syncope. Low endurance and chronic fatigue are common, but may be improved with appropriate exercise. Since many CHF patients have very low exercise capacity, even a small improvement in VO_2 can mean improved quality of life and even living independently for a patient with heart failure with ongoing rehabilitation (3).

Since CHF patients have higher risk than most cardiac rehabilitation patients, a graded ETT is essential before starting. Due to poor adaptation to exercise in CHF, long warm-up and cool-down periods are required with exercise at a limited workload. Dynamic exercise is preferable with a target HR at 10 bpm below any significant endpoint found with cardiopulmonary exercise testing. Isometric exercises need to be avoided since they increase diastolic pressure and cardiac afterload. Cardiac exercise should be started under supervision with cardiac monitoring initially. Patients with severe left ventricular dysfunction will need telemetry during warm-up, exercise, and cool-down. Once the patient can self-monitor, he or she can start a self-monitored program. CHF patients also need to closely follow body weight (to observe for fluid accumulation), and blood pressure and HR responses to exercise (3).

For more end-stage heart failure, management may include pharmacologic inotropic support or left ventricular mechanical support. Exercise can be done on intravenous inotropes with the same precautions as in other CHF patients (3). LVAD patients will usually follow the usual past surgical course, with phase 1 and 1B rehabilitation followed by phase 2 and 3 programs. Rehabilitation of LVAD in rehabilitation acute and subacute units requires a trained staff, close cooperation with the LVAD team, and familiarity with the devices that are used locally. Since CO is typically well sustained with the device, patients can have good exercise tolerance with the limit to peak exercise capacity limited by the peak flow of the device. Family and patient education are also essential parts of rehabilitation post LVAD (1).

Valvular Heart Disease

Cardiac rehabilitation for valvular heart disease is similar to rehabilitation for CHF. Postsurgical management is also similar to other postsurgical cardiac patients with the one issue of anticoagulation postoperatively for patients with mechanical valves. With anticoagulation, exercises need to avoid high-impact exercises to prevent hemarthroses and bruising and includes education regarding injury avoidance (3). The overall training program is similar to that discussed for the post-CABG patient (3).

Cardiac Arrhythmias

Patients with cardiac arrhythmias need closer telemetry monitoring for any change in intensity levels of exercise and new exercises. Patients identified as high risk of cardiac arrhythmias will need a monitored setting rather than a self-directed home program. For those patients with life-threatening arrhythmias, automatic implantable cardiac defibrillator (AICD) is commonly used. With AICD, exercise programs need to avoid the HR at which the device is set to fire. A pre-rehabilitation exercise stress test and cardiac precautions with target HR set well below the trigger threshold is a sufficient modification for the exercise program. As with other treatments, education and emotional support are an important part of the program (1).

Pulmonary Rehabilitation Programs in Specific Conditions

Emphysema

COPD rehabilitation is essentially standard pulmonary rehabilitation. The goals of the program are disease management and improvement of exercise capacity. Since the rehabilitation program cannot improve the function of the lungs, the goal is to allow for more work with the given ability to ventilate. Key aspects of the program are energy conservation education (how to do a given activity at a lower level of exertion) and improved endurance. The focus is on moderate-intensity exercises with longer duration rather than on high-intensity or short-burst exercises. Isometric exercises are not recommended due to increased intrathoracic pressures. Supplemental oxygen should be used as needed to maintain saturation above 90%, with education to return supplemental oxygen to baseline resting need after exercise to prevent resting hypercarbia. Patients with COPD generally have relatively modest oxygen needs and can often exercise with 1 to 6 L of oxygen via nasal cannula. For patients with sleep apnea or ventilatory failure, programs should also concentrate on incorporation of the bilevel ventilation into their routine and look to improve compliance. Of special note, for patients being considered for LVRS, pulmonary rehabilitation is considered essential both to qualify for the surgery and after surgery to assure adequate outcomes (17).

For patients with significant secretions, airway clearance and chest physical therapy may be an important part of the rehabilitation program. External percussion devices, vibration devices, and inhalation of saline may help to mobilize secretions. Cough training and huffing can help to clear secretions, and family training is essential Finally, medication education is essential, including the appropriate use of inhaled medications and oxygen and management of equipment (18).

Interstitial Lung Disease

Pulmonary rehabilitation for ILD is similar to that for obstructive lung disease. The key differences lie in that patients with ILD often have profound hypoxemia and need to have high-flow oxygen with exercise to maintain adequate saturation for activity. Prevention of chronic hypoxemia is essential to preventing the onset of PH as this secondary pulmonary disease, when present with ILD, makes patients profoundly symptomatic and can markedly decrease life expectancy. Appropriate exercise can be more intense in this group of patients, with oxygenation the key limiting factor. Airway clearance is generally less of an issue and most patients with ILD are not on ventilatory support until the very end stages of disease when rehabilitation may no longer be possible (19).

Since many of these conditions are progressive, it is often important to either have patients referred for transplantation or start end-of-life planning to allow for achieving as many patient goals as possible.

Pulmonary Hypertension

Patients with PH are very similar to CHF patients with many similar precautions. With the onset of effective pulmonary vasodilators, patients now have much longer life expectancy and live with chronic management for decades. Because they may have experienced debility prior to the institution of effective therapy or have concern about exercise many patients could benefit from pulmonary rehabilitation. It is important to maintain oxygenation during exercise, and patients with severe PH may need to have cardiac monitoring as arrhythmias and right heart failure are issues to be considered. High-flow supplemental oxygen and education in the use of their vasodilating agents are part of the program. Patients with intravenous or continuous subcutaneous vasodilating medication infusions can be safely incorporated into exercise programs, but there need to be long warm-up and cool-down periods with an emphasis on moderate- to low-level exercise for patients with severe pulmonary vascular disease. Further research into efficacy and safety of pulmonary rehabilitation for patients with pulmonary vascular disease is still ongoing.

Ventilatory Failure

Patients with ventilatory failure who are on either invasive or noninvasive ventilation require mobilization as well and should have exercise programs. For patients with nocturnal or intermittent ventilatory support, exercise programs can improve efficiency and allow greater activity and less fatigue while off the ventilator. Detailed management for patients with need for noninvasive ventilation is beyond the scope of this chapter. Table 11.8 has an overview of the types of patients who may present with ventilatory failure.

A summary of the indications for ventilatory support is in Table 11.9 (8).

Cardiopulmonary Rehabilitation in the Physically Disabled

Finally, there are some special considerations for patients with both disability and cardiac disease. Most of the difficulties in cardiac rehabilitation in this population are due to limited mobility, which presents difficulty in both testing and exercise training. Patients with disability may also be at higher risk of cardiac and pulmonary disease, and the presence of cardiopulmonary limitations should be remembered when engaging in any standard rehabilitation program. Patients with stroke or peripheral vascular disease are at particularly high risk since these conditions often have concurrent cardiac disease, but any patient with disability may have a cardiac or pulmonary comorbidity. In cases where cardiac or pulmonary disease is overt, cardiopulmonary rehabilitation should be provided for these disabled individuals just as it would be for the able-bodied population. Cardiopulmonary primary and secondary prevention is also important for patients with physical disabilities as they are usually more sedentary and have high rates of obesity and deconditioning. Additionally, disabled individuals usually require higher energy expenditures for mobility, with a resultant need for increased work capacity and potentially more disability from a similar level of cardiopulmonary disease.

When prescribing cardiopulmonary exercise for disabled individuals, the exercise protocols need to be adapted for the individual patient. Patients with lower extremity impairment due to neurological or orthopedic conditions can perform upper extremity ergometry, and modification of lower extremity exercise equipment will allow them to exercise with their legs. Hemiplegic patients can use adapted bicycle ergometers or airdynes.

TABLE 11.8 Assessment of Ventilatory Failure

CENTRAL HYPOVENTILATION	RESPIRATORY MUSCLE FAILURE	CHRONIC RESPIRATORY DISORDERS	OTHER
Intracranial hemorrhage, Arnold-Chiari malformation, central nervous system (CNS) trauma, congenital and central failure of control of breathing, myelomeningocele, high spinal cord injury (SCI), stroke	Amyotophic lateral sclerosis (ALS), congenital myopathies, botulism, muscular dystrophies, myasthenia gravis, phrenic nerve paralysis, polio/postpolio, spinomuscular atrophy (SMA), myotonic dystrophy	COPD, bronchopulmonary dysplasia (BPD), cystic fibrosis (CF), interstitial lung disease (ILD)	Congestive heart failure, congenital heart disease, tracheomalacia, vocal cord paralysis, Pierre-Robin syndrome
Central alveolar hypoventilation		Kyphoscoliosis, thoracic wall deformities, thoracoplasty	

TABLE 11.9 The Indications for Ventilatory Support

CLINICAL SYNDROME OF VENTILATORY FAILURE	MEDICAL CONDITIONS THAT HAVE BEEN MAXIMALLY MANAGED	FOLLOWING DIAGNOSES PRESENT	INDICATIONS FOR INVASIVE VENTILATION (TRACH)
Significant daytime CO_2 retention (>50 mmHg with normalized pH)	Optimal medical treatment	Neuromuscular disease	Uncontrollable airway secretions
Mild daytime or nocturnal CO_2 retention (45–50 mmHg) with symptoms of hypoventilation	Patient can handle secretions and protect airway	Chest wall deformity	Chronic aspiration and repeated pneumonias
Significant nocturnal hypoventilation or hypoxemia	Reversible contributing factors have been treated	Central hypoventilation or obesity hypoventilation	Failure of trial of noninvasive ventilation (NIV)
		Obstructive sleep apnea (OSA) with failure to improve with continuous positive airway pressure (CPAP)	24-hr support needed, poor supports, or inability to manage noninvasive ventilation (NIV)
		COPD with severe hypoventilation	Patient preference

Since exercise protocols for stroke and other conditions incorporate upper limb exercise, the high MVO_2 requirements for upper extremity exercise should be considered when designing a cardiac rehabilitation program for disabled patients. It is essential for disabled patients to focus particularly on task-specific activities in order to improve aerobic conditioning and endurance, while seeking to lower MVO_2 needed with each task. The physiatrist is particularly suited to take a leadership role in the area of the design of cardiopulmonary rehabilitation programs for the disabled since most traditional cardiac rehabilitation programs have limited experience with the needs of physically disabled patients.

PRACTICE-BASED LEARNING AND IMPROVEMENT

GOALS

Demonstrate competence in continuously investigating and evaluating cardiopulmonary patient care practices, appraising and assimilating scientific evidence, and continuously improving patient care practices based on constant self-evaluation and lifelong learning.

OBJECTIVES

1. Describe learning opportunities for providers, patients, and caregivers with experience in cardiopulmonary rehabilitation.
2. Use methods for ongoing competency training in cardiopulmonary rehabilitation for physiatrists, including formative evaluation feedback in daily practice, evaluating current practice, and developing a systematic quality improvement and practice improvement strategy.
3. Locate some resources including available websites for continuing medical education and continuing professional development.
4. Describe some areas paramount to self-assessment and lifelong learning such as review of current guidelines, including evidence based, in treatment and management of patients with cardiac and pulmonary disorders and the role of the physiatrist as the educator of patients, families, residents, students, colleagues, and other health professionals.

In order for the physiatrist to be a competent provider of rehabilitative care for patients with cardiac and pulmonary diseases, he or she must first perform a self-assessment of his or her knowledge base to provide care. This self-assessment should focus on a few key components: (a) ability to assess for the impairments, activity limitations, and participation restrictions in the patient with a cardiac or pulmonary disease; (b) medical knowledge of the pertinent cardiac and pulmonary anatomy, normal and abnormal physiology of the heart and lungs, and principles of cardiac and pulmonary rehabilitation; (c) effectiveness of communication with other clinicians involved in the care of patients with cardiac and pulmonary disease; (d) ability to teach patients effectively about their cardiac or pulmonary disease, as well as strategies to minimize impact of the impairments associated with their disease and maximize function; and (e) ability to identify systems-wide issues relating to the safety and quality of rehabilitative care and implement interventions to improve the quality and safety of care provided to the patients living with cardiac and pulmonary disease.

This self-assessment can be accomplished in a variety of ways such as (a) reflecting on one's clinical practice, (b) self-assessment examinations in cardiac and pulmonary rehabilitation, (c) asking trusted professional colleagues for feedback on one's clinical practice of cardiac and pulmonary rehabilitation, and (d) seeking feedback from patients.

Once the self-assessment has been completed, there are several resources available to physiatrists to address the identified gaps. Resources available from the American Academy of Physical Medicine and Rehabilitation (AAPMR) include Knowledge NOW and Academe. Knowledge NOW has several short review articles on cardiac and pulmonary rehabilitation that are informative, concise, and easy to read (20). Academe at AAPMR has an online review course on cardiac rehabilitation (21). Evidence-based resources from the Cochrane Collaboration can also be very useful (22).

Other resources include the American Heart Association guidelines, the American College of Sports Medicine exercise guidelines, and the American Association of Cardiovascular and Pulmonary Rehabilitation guidelines and educational materials. Programs and individuals can seek certification from these organizations, and there are patient educational materials also available from these resources. With advances in technology and informatics, new programs of self and program assessment will become available for practitioners to use for self and program development (10, 23).

INTERPERSONAL AND COMMUNICATION SKILLS

GOALS

Demonstrate interpersonal and communication skills that result in the effective exchange of information and collaboration with patients who have cardiac and pulmonary disorders, their families, and other health professionals.

OBJECTIVES

1. Demonstrate skills used in effective communication and collaboration with patients who have cardiac and pulmonary disorders, and their caregivers, across socioeconomic and cultural backgrounds.
2. Delineate the importance of the role of the physiatrist as the interdisciplinary team leader and consultant pertinent to cardiac and pulmonary rehabilitation.
3. Demonstrate proper documentation and effective communication between health care professional team members in patient care as it applies to cardiac and pulmonary rehabilitation.

Effective communication and interpersonal skills are an essential part of the care of the patient with a cardiac or pulmonary disease. This is because clinical care for this patient is often very complex, requiring close collaboration between several medical and surgical specialties as well as nurses, physical therapists, occupational therapists, social workers, nutritionists, and psychologists. This care is provided in a variety of settings such as acute medical and surgical wards, inpatient rehabilitation facilities, skilled nursing facilities, outpatient clinics, and the patient's home, which adds an extra dimension to the complexity of the care. The patient and his family members often have a wide range of understanding about cardiac and pulmonary disease, which can also impact on care.

It is for these reasons that physiatrists should possess or strive to develop excellent communication and interpersonal skills with their patients and those caring for them. Effective communication and conflict resolution strategies are discussed in greater detail elsewhere in this book. The physiatrist should always be compassionate and empathetic to the patient's condition when communicating with him. Ample time should be allowed to fully address the patient's concerns and questions at a level of understanding that takes into account language, socioeconomic, and cultural barriers and is appropriate for the patient's level of education.

Cardiopulmonary rehabilitation lends itself to both patient and family education and relies heavily on support groups and team communication. Weekly rounds to discuss patients and to evaluate progress are carried out, and patients and families are given both individual and group education for specific aspects of their cardiopulmonary diseases. The role of physiatrist as a team leader is essential for smooth operation of the service as well as for advocacy in the medical community for utilization of cardiopulmonary services.

Proper documentation between clinicians regarding the rehabilitation of the patient with a cardiac or pulmonary disease should be based on a thorough understanding of the patient's medical condition, his or her impairments, activity limitations, and participation restrictions. Elements that should be accurately conveyed between team members include (a) medical and surgical history for cardiac and pulmonary disease, (b) pertinent comorbid conditions, (c) surgeries and procedures performed and their outcome, (d) current medications, (e) exercise prescription and precautions, and (f) contact information for key clinicians involved in care.

PROFESSIONALISM

GOALS

Reflect a commitment to carrying out professional responsibilities and an adherence to ethical principles in cardiac and pulmonary rehabilitation.

OBJECTIVES

1. Exemplify the humanistic qualities as a provider of care for patients with cardiac and pulmonary diseases.
2. Demonstrate ethical principles and responsiveness to patient needs superseding self and other interests.
3. Demonstrate sensitivity to patient population diversity, including culture, gender, age, race, religion, disabilities, and sexual orientation.
4. Respect patient beliefs and goals, privacy, confidentiality, and autonomy.

The AAPMR Code of Conduct was written "to serve as a guideline for professional and personal behavior and to promote the highest quality of physiatric care. It is a statement of ideals, commitments and responsibilities of the physiatrist to patients, their families, other health professionals, society and to themselves." It describes ethical issues relating to the patient and the patient's family, relationships between physiatrists and members of the rehabilitation team, other physicians, community, and government. It also addresses research and scholarly activities (24).

In the practice of cardiac and pulmonary rehabilitation, the physiatrist should be sensitive to the impact that the patient's cultural background, values and religious beliefs, disabilities, and sexual orientation can have on their rehabilitation.

The physiatrist ought to be respectful of the patient's wishes when making recommendations for medical care as well as his or her privacy. The patient's needs and concerns must take priority over the self-interest of the physiatrist. The physiatrist must be aware of potential conflicts of interest when providing rehabilitative care to the patient with a cardiac or pulmonary disease and minimize their occurrence.

SYSTEMS-BASED PRACTICE

GOALS

Demonstrate awareness and responsiveness to systems of rehabilitation team care delivery, and the ability to access, evaluate, recruit, and coordinate effectively resources in the system to provide optimal safe continuum of care and outcomes as it relates to cardiac and pulmonary rehabilitation.

OBJECTIVES

1. Discuss effective coordination of care for patients with cardiac and pulmonary diseases across the continuum of rehabilitative care including at transition points.
2. Describe the judicious use of diagnostic tests, treatments, and consultants in the provision of rehabilitative care to patients with cardiac and pulmonary diseases. Identify cost-saving measures in the practice of rehabilitative medicine for patients with cardiac and pulmonary diseases.
3. Examine risk–benefit analysis in the provision of rehabilitation medicine to patients with cardiac and pulmonary diseases.
4. Explain the role of the physiatrist as an advocate for quality rehabilitative care and optimal patient care systems for patients with cardiac and pulmonary diseases.
5. Identify system problems in the rehabilitation of patients with cardiac and pulmonary diseases and utilize quality improvement tools to improve patient safety.

As mentioned earlier, the care of the patient with a cardiac or pulmonary disease can be very complex and require multiple different providers in several different settings along the health care continuum. Transition points in care are particularly dangerous for the patient, and it is essential that excellent communication regarding the patient's medical and surgical history, medications, precautions, and need for further treatment are effectively transmitted from one setting to the next. Discharge summaries and verbal communication between providers using Situation Background Assessment Recommendation (SBAR) methodology and read-back techniques are an integral part of the transfer of care.

Physiatrists should be mindful of the costs of care for patients with cardiac and pulmonary disease and minimize duplication of services, tests, and procedures for the patient. Decisions regarding the location for the provision of rehabilitative services should be based on the patient's wishes, impairments, activity limitations, participation restrictions, medical stability to undergo a rehabilitation program, number of hours that the patient can tolerate therapy per day, and need for physician and nursing supervision.

Regrettably, cardiac and pulmonary rehabilitation services may not always be covered by health care insurance companies; therefore, physiatrists should strongly advocate for access to rehabilitative services for their patients whenever possible. They should also educate other clinicians about the benefits of cardiac and pulmonary rehabilitation for this subset of patients.

Since many of the patients with cardiopulmonary rehabilitation issues are dealing with life-threatening illnesses, there is a need for rehabilitation professionals to deal with issues of profound impact to the patients. There are issues of loss of autonomy, loss of career, and potentially loss of life that involve incorporation of social and cultural expectations into the interactions with patients and families. Communication with other specialties is essential as most patients have several specialists involved in their care and there is a need for patient advocacy to improve access for patients, increase referrals, and improve coverage for rehabilitation services for patients with cardiopulmonary disease (10,23).

Quality and performance issues are also important to the maintenance of cardiopulmonary services, and further studies for CHF, PH, and new treatments are needed to continue to justify the use of cardiopulmonary (CP) rehabilitation. Usual quality markers of mortality and morbidity can be augmented with assessments of cost savings and such trends as readmissions and overall quality of care. Progress reporting and self-assessment of programs will continue to improve the quality of services provided, as well as help meet future challenges with limited reimbursements and resources. New models of care with telemedicine and home-based programs continue to be developed to try to improve access and contain costs in the newer environment of cost control and new models of delivery of care.

CONCLUSION

Cardiopulmonary rehabilitation is a very broad area of expertise with many specific aspects of knowledge that need to be incorporated. Physiatry is uniquely positioned to help negotiate the issues of the multidisabled patient, needs for education and team management, and also the need for complete interdisciplinary care. Working with supporting agencies and the data on outcomes are essential for the development of effective programs. The future for cardiopulmonary rehabilitation lies in providing more services to a greater number of patients and including underserved populations in rural and urban areas, women and minority groups, and for specialized patient populations such as the physically disabled who are living longer and now experiencing more episodes of cardiac and pulmonary disability.

CASE STUDY

A 68-year-old man with a past medical history significant for emphysema of 10-year duration is referred for physiatric evaluation for rehabilitation services. He has been having increasing difficulty performing his activities of daily living (ADLs) over the past 6 months and can only ambulate about half a block with a cane due to fatigue and generalized weakness. He needs 2 L of supplemental oxygen during ambulation and is having difficulty managing secretions. He is a retired bus driver, married, and lives in a home with one flight of stairs.

CASE STUDY DISCUSSION QUESTIONS

1. Write a pulmonary rehabilitation treatment plan for this patient.
2. What are the benefits of exercise for this patient?
3. What are some safety concerns for this patient during the rehabilitation program?
4. What are the key elements of patient education for this patient?
5. What are some resources that you can use to improve your knowledge base regarding the rehabilitation of this patient?
6. Are there any ethical concerns that can arise in the care of this patient?

SELF-EXAMINATION QUESTIONS
(Answers begin on p. 367)

1. What is the percent of oxygen extraction by cardiac myocytes at all levels of activity?
    A. 35%
    B. 45%
    C. 55%
    D. 65%
    E. 75%
2. Which of the following best describes myocardial oxygen consumption with exercise?
    A. Supine exercises have a higher myocardial oxygen consumption compared with erect exercises at low-intensity exercises
    B. Supine exercises have a lower myocardial oxygen consumption compared with erect exercises at low-intensity exercises
    C. Myocardial oxygen consumption decreases in cold weather
    D. Myocardial oxygen consumption decreases after eating
    E. Myocardial oxygen consumption decreases in extreme heat
3. Exercise above what percent of the maximal HR will have a training effect?
    A. 30%
    B. 50%
    C. 60%
    D. 70%
    E. 80%
4. Which of the following best describes the effect of aerobic training?
    A. Aerobic capacity is decreased with exercise training
    B. The maximum CO decreases
    C. Resting HR increases
    D. SV is increased at rest
    E. Peripheral resistance increases in response to exercise training
5. Following cardiac transplantation, which of the following is best expected for the baseline HR?
    A. HR between 50 and 60 bpm
    B. HR between 71 and 80 bpm
    C. HR between 81 and 90 bpm
    D. HR between 100 and 110 bpm
    E. HR between 111 and 120 bpm

REFERENCES

1. Bartels MN. Cardiopulmonary assessment. In: Grabois M, ed. *Physical Medicine and Rehabilitation: The Complete Approach.* Chapter 20. Chicago, IL: Blackwell Science, Inc.; 2000:351–372.
2. Bartels MN. Cardiac rehabilitation, Chapter 41. In: Frontera WR, DeLisa JA, Gans BM, Walsh NA, Robinson L, eds. *Physical Medicine and Rehabilitation: Principles and Practice.* 5th ed. Philadelphia PA: Lippincott Williams and Wilkins, 2010:1075–1098.
3. Balady GJ, Williams MA, Ades PA, et al.; American Heart Association Exercise, Cardiac Rehabilitation, and Prevention Committee; Council on Clinical Cardiology; Councils on Cardiovascular Nursing, Epidemiology and Prevention, and Nutrition, Physical Activity, and Metabolism; American Association of Cardiovascular and Pulmonary Rehabilitation. Core components of cardiac rehabilitation/secondary prevention programs: 2007 update: a scientific statement from the American Heart Association Exercise, Cardiac Rehabilitation, and Prevention Committee, the Council on Clinical

Cardiology; the Councils on Cardiovascular Nursing, Epidemiology and Prevention, and Nutrition, Physical Activity, and Metabolism; and the American Association of Cardiovascular and Pulmonary Rehabilitation. *J Cardiopulm Rehabil Prev.* 2007;27(3):121–129.
4. Nici L, Donner C, Wouters E, et al.; ATS/ERS Pulmonary Rehabilitation Writing Committee. American Thoracic Society/European Respiratory Society statement on pulmonary rehabilitation. *Am J Respir Crit Care Med.* 2006;173(12):1390–1413.
5. Nici L, Limberg T, Hilling L, et al.; American Association of Cardiovascular and Pulmonary Rehabilitation. Clinical competency guidelines for pulmonary rehabilitation professionals: American Association of Cardiovascular and Pulmonary Rehabilitation position statement. *J Cardiopulm Rehabil Prev.* 2007;27(6):355–358.
6. Qaseem A, Wilt TJ, Weinberger SE, et al.; American College of Physicians. American College of Chest Physicians. American Thoracic Society. European Respiratory Society. Diagnosis and management of stable chronic obstructive pulmonary disease: a clinical practice guideline update from the American College of Physicians, American College of Chest Physicians, American Thoracic Society, and European Respiratory Society. *Ann Intern Med.* 2011;155(3):179–191.
7. King M, Bittner V, Josephson R, et al. Medical director responsibilities for outpatient cardiac rehabilitation/secondary prevention programs: 2012 update: a statement for health care professionals from the American Association of Cardiovascular and Pulmonary Rehabilitation and the American Heart Association. *Circulation.* 2012;126:2535–2543.
8. Bartels MN. Pulmonary rehabilitation. In: Cooper G, ed. *Essential Physical Medicine and Rehabilitation.* Totowa, NJ: Humana Press; 2006:147–174.
9. Hamm LF, Sanderson BK, Ades PA, et al. Core competencies for cardiac rehabilitation/secondary prevention professionals: 2010 update: position statement of the American Association of Cardiovascular and Pulmonary Rehabilitation. *J Cardiopulm Rehabil Prev.* 2011;31(1):2–10.
10. Thomas RJ, King M, Lui K, et al. AACVPR/ACCF/AHA 2010 update: performance measures on cardiac rehabilitation for referral to cardiac rehabilitation/secondary prevention services: a report of the American Association of Cardiovascular and Pulmonary Rehabilitation and the American College of Cardiology Foundation/American Heart Association Task Force on Performance Measures (Writing Committee to Develop Clinical Performance Measures for Cardiac Rehabilitation). *Circulation.* 2010;122(13):1342–1350.
11. Haskell WL, Lee IM, Pate RR, et al.; American College of Sports Medicine. American Heart Association. Physical activity and public health: updated recommendation for adults from the American College of Sports Medicine and the American Heart Association. *Circulation.* 2007;116(9):1081–1093.
12. Leon AS, Franklin BA, Costa F, et al; American Heart Association. Council on Clinical Cardiology (Subcommittee on Exercise, Cardiac Rehabilitation, and Prevention). Council on Nutrition, Physical Activity, and Metabolism (Subcommittee on Physical Activity). American Association of Cardiovascular and Pulmonary Rehabilitation. Cardiac rehabilitation and secondary prevention of coronary heart disease: an American Heart Association scientific statement from the Council on Clinical Cardiology (Subcommittee on Exercise, Cardiac Rehabilitation, and Prevention) and the Council on Nutrition, Physical Activity, and Metabolism (Subcommittee on Physical Activity), in collaboration with the American Association of Cardiovascular and Pulmonary Rehabilitation. *Circulation.* 2005;111(3):369–376.
13. Williams MA, Fleg JL, Ades PA, et al.; American Heart Association Council on Clinical Cardiology Subcommittee on Exercise, Cardiac Rehabilitation, and Prevention. Secondary prevention of coronary heart disease in the elderly (with emphasis on patients > or = 75 years of age): an American Heart Association scientific statement from the Council on Clinical Cardiology Subcommittee on Exercise, Cardiac Rehabilitation, and Prevention. *Circulation.* 2002;105(14):1735–1743.
14. Balady GJ, Ades PA, Comoss P, et al. Core components of cardiac rehabilitation/secondary prevention programs: a statement for healthcare professionals from the American Heart Association and the American Association of Cardiovascular and Pulmonary Rehabilitation Writing Group. *Circulation.* 2000;102(9):1069–1073.
15. Lauer M, Froelicher ES, Williams M, et al.; American Heart Association Council on Clinical Cardiology, Subcommittee on Exercise, Cardiac Rehabilitation, and Prevention. Exercise testing in asymptomatic adults: a statement for professionals from the American Heart Association Council on Clinical Cardiology, Subcommittee on Exercise, Cardiac Rehabilitation, and Prevention. *Circulation.* 2005;112(5):771–776.
16. Haskell WL, Lee IM, Pate RR, et al. Physical activity and public health: updated recommendation for adults from the American College of Sports Medicine and the American Heart Association. *Med Sci Sports Exercise.* 2007;39(8):1423–1434.
17. Bartels MN. Rehabilitation management of lung volume reduction surgery. In: Ginsburg M, ed. *Lung Volume Reduction Surgery.* St. Louis, MO: Mosby-Year Book, Inc.; 2001:97–124.
18. Parshall MB, Schwartzstein RM, Adams L, et al.; American Thoracic Society Committee on dyspnea. An official American Thoracic Society statement: update on the mechanisms, assessment, and management of dyspnea. *Am J Respir Crit Care Med.* 2012;185(4):435–452.
19. Swigris JJ, Brown KK, Make BJ, et al. Pulmonary rehabilitation in idiopathic pulmonary fibrosis: a call for continued investigation. *Respir Med.* 2008;102(12):1675–1680.
20. http://now.aapmr.org/med-rehab/Pages/default.aspx. Accessed January 25, 2014.
21. http://me.e-aapmr.org. Accessed January 25, 2014.
22. http://www.cochrane.org/cochrane-reviews). Accessed January 25, 2014.
23. Peno-Green L, Verrill D, Vitcenda M, et al.; American Association of Cardiovascular and Pulmonary Rehabilitation (AACVPR). Patient and program outcome assessment in pulmonary rehabilitation: an AACVPR statement. *J Cardiopulm Rehabil Prev.* 2009;29(6):402–410.
24. http://www.aapmr.org/about/who-we-are/Pages/aapmr-code-of-conduct.aspx. Accessed January 25, 2014.

Adrian Cristian
Julie Silver
Frances Atupulazi
Yan Li

12: Cancer Rehabilitation

PATIENT CARE

GOALS

Provide competent patient care that is compassionate, appropriate, and effective for the evaluation, treatment, education, and advocacy for patients diagnosed with cancer and associated problems all along the care continuum and survival trajectory.

OBJECTIVES

1. Describe the key components of the assessment of the patient with cancer.
2. Formulate comprehensive interdisciplinary rehabilitation treatment plans for cancer patients that also include patient safety concerns.
3. Evaluate individuals diagnosed with cancer for physical impairments, activity limitations, and participation restrictions at their preoncology treatment baseline (prehabilitation) and following the start of oncology treatments (rehabilitation) throughout the care continuum.
4. Identify ethical issues in the rehabilitation of the patient with cancer.

Cancer patients often have one or more physical impairments associated with their cancer diagnosis and its treatments. They have been identified as having poor physical and mental health as well as unmet rehabilitation needs to address these impairments (1). An impairment-driven approach to cancer rehabilitation has been described by one of the authors and should serve as a guide to the assessment and treatment of the cancer patient at various stages of the disease process (2).

This section will address a general approach to the assessment and rehabilitation treatment plan of the cancer patient as well as focus on four commonly seen conditions in cancer patients: (a) cognitive dysfunction, (b) lymphedema in breast cancer, (c) chemotherapy-induced peripheral neuropathy (CIPN), and (d) radiation fibrosis.

PATIENT ASSESSMENT

An impairment-based approach: In the data-gathering phase of the assessment of the cancer patient, the following information is important for the physiatrist to obtain.

Medical Histories and Data Gathering

A. *History of Present Illness*: This is a thorough history of the cancer presentation and its course since the time of the initial diagnosis. It includes the type of cancer and its stage. In addition, a chronology of the types of treatments that have been used to treat the cancer including chemotherapy, surgery, and radiation therapy is very helpful. It is important that the information collected be very detailed and specific. This often entails speaking with the medical oncologist, radiation oncologist, and surgeons involved in the care of the patient and obtaining records that accurately define these interventions, their success, and complications to date. Examples include (a) the names of the chemotherapeutic medications, dosages, route of administration, number of treatment cycles to date and projected for the future; (b) total irradiation doses, number of treatments to date and planned for the future, as well as parts of the body that were irradiated; and (c) description of the surgeries performed, organs that were altered or removed as a result of the surgery, as well as plans for future surgical interventions. This is important to guide the physiatrist in identifying specific impairments associated with both the disease and its treatments.

B. *Past Medical History*: Significant comorbidities such as coronary artery disease, congestive heart failure, chronic obstructive pulmonary disease, diabetes mellitus, previous cancers treated, and pertinent past surgeries are important to note as they may have an impact on the rehabilitation program.

C. *Review of Systems*: In the review of systems, a cancer-specific checklist approach can be useful. The checklist should include impairments that are associated with specific cancers as well as those generally seen in cancer patients. Table 12.1 provides a sample list.

TABLE 12.1 Examples of Prehabilitation Interventions[a]

- Smoking cessation to improve surgical outcomes
- Relaxation techniques to decrease anxiety prior to starting treatment
- Nutritional support for peri-and postoperative recovery
- Musculoskeletal screening to identify preexisting issues with appropriate referrals to physical therapy/occupational therapy
- Pelvic floor exercise training to improve postoperative urinary continence in prostate cancer
- Swallowing exercise training to improve posttreatment swallowing in head and neck cancer
- Sleep hygiene counseling to reduce fatigue
- Home safety evaluation to reduce risk of falls
- Work evaluation to recommend adaptive strategies and equipment

[a]This is not meant to be a complete list.

Specific cancers should lead physicians to pursue relevant avenues of investigation. For example:

a. Head and neck cancer patients can have limitations in range of motion of the neck and shoulders, problems opening and closing the mouth, or speech and swallowing difficulties as a result of the cancer or its treatments.
b. Breast cancer survivors may have complaints of swelling of the arm(s), restricted range of motion of the shoulder, and pain in the thorax following mastectomy surgery.
c. Brain cancer patients may complain of changes in vision, weakness in the limbs, sensory deficits, forgetfulness, poor attention, difficulty keeping up with conversations, or occupational responsibilities due to slowed mental processing speed, difficulties with multitasking, and problems with organizational skills. Patients may describe forgetfulness as difficulty recalling something they were previously told, forgetting recent events, forgetting location of items, forgetting dates and times of appointments, and forgetting names of people and locations. These neurocognitive impairments can affect an individual's ability to perform instrumental activities of daily living (IADLs) such as managing finances as well as working and driving. It is therefore important for physiatrists to ask about changes in the cancer patient's ability to successfully engage in these activities.

Unfortunately, pain is a highly prevalent symptom among those carrying a cancer diagnosis, and the physiatrist would therefore do well to spend some time assessing for possible sources of this pain with some regularity. These sources are likely to be both nociceptive and neuropathic in nature and their prompt, precise identification is an important cornerstone of any plan of care. A protocol for the investigation of pain-related complaints that can yield significant information would assess location, intensity, quality, radiation, and aggravating and alleviating factors.

D. *Social and Functional History*: Given that a primary goal of cancer rehabilitation is to maximize the level of function and quality of life, it is important to establish a baseline level of function for activities of daily living (ADLs), IADLs, and work. In addition, the physiatrist should ascertain the nature of social support available to the patient, living arrangements (e.g., house vs. apartment; stairs, etc.), and difficulties with driving. Drug (smoking) and alcohol habits are also important to factor into the development of treatment.

E. *Allergies and Medications*: An updated medication list should be documented. This should include chemotherapy medications such as platins (cisplatin, carboplatin), plant alkaloids (vinblastin, vincristine), and taxanes (paclitaxel, docetaxel), which have been associated with CIPN. It is important to also document a list of allergies and any advance directives. Medications should also be reviewed for potential drug–drug or drug–herb interactions and side effects.

Physical Examination

Using the information gathered from the review of medical records and interviewing the patient, the physiatrist performs a physical examination with focus on body systems that may have been adversely impacted by cancer and its treatment. Vital signs such as blood pressure and heart rate in the supine and sitting or standing position may indicate the presence of orthostatic changes. Respiratory rate and pulse oximetry provide an indication of pulmonary function and oxygenation, respectively.

Inspection of the patient can yield significant information such as atrophy of muscles, fibrosis of soft tissues, lymphedema, medial winging of the scapula, contractures, scars, and deformities. Palpation provides information about tender areas over the spine, extremities, and trunk.

Inspection of the skin is important to look for evidence of infection, ulcerations, or atrophy, especially in areas treated with radiation therapy. The skin and underlying soft tissues in these areas should also be palpated for evidence of loss of elasticity. An assessment of range of motion is important for the joints of the upper and lower extremities as well.

Lymphedema is generally characterized by nonpainful swelling. In patients with lymphedema it is important to determine the stage. Stage 0 is considered subclinical and not evident on physical examination, though the patient may complain of heaviness. Stage 1 is considered mild and pitting in nature. With elevation, pitting edema can usually be reversed. Stage 2 is characterized by increasing fibrosis, which on examination feels more firm than with stage 1. This firmness also means that the pitting that is seen in stage 1 is typically no longer present. In this stage, nonpitting edema is less responsive to elevation. Due to the chronic excess protein in the interstitial spaces and deposition of adipose tissue, the tissue becomes fibrotic and the skin starts to harden. Stage 3 is considered severe, and the swelling is considered cartilage like and has been described as "lymphostatic elephantiasis." In addition to stage of lymphedema, the physiatrist should also evaluate for the following: (a) evidence of erythema or warmth in the arm, suggesting possible skin infection; (b) tenderness on palpation of the arm; and (c) restriction to range of motion at the shoulder, elbow, wrist, and hand. It is also beneficial to establish circumferential measurements in the affected extremity at the time of initial assessment and then subsequently chart the changes with appropriate treatments.

As far as comorbid neurological pathologies are concerned, it is important to assess speech characteristics (e.g., dysarthria, fluency, comprehension, naming, and repetition) and swallowing function (e.g., ability to tolerate sips of water), and assess for vision or hearing loss. A brief cognitive evaluation that assesses level of alertness, orientation, attention span, immediate and delayed recall, and organizational skills is important, as is a brief evaluation for depression using a standardized instrument. In patients with a history of head and neck cancer and treatment, checking for mouth opening (*trismus* is an inability to open the mouth completely due to severe muscle spasm) is important, as is evaluating the range of motion of the neck.

Motor strength is tested and graded in major muscle groups of the trunk and extremities evaluating for localized (e.g., footdrop, scapular winging) or generalized weakness. Sensation should be tested for light touch, pinprick, temperature proprioception, and vibration. It is important to evaluate for patterns of sensory loss (e.g., glove stocking distribution, peripheral nerve or radicular distribution). Muscle stretch reflexes and tone can provide additional information that is useful in identifying upper motor or lower motor neuron involvement. Balance and gait evaluations are important to evaluate in ambulatory patients. Functional assessment tools such as functional reach, timed up and go test, and 6-minute walk tests can yield significant information as well.

Laboratory Tests and Imaging: It is helpful to review recent laboratory tests such as (a) albumin and prealbumin to assess patient's nutritional status; (b) hemoglobin levels to check for anemia; (c) platelet counts to assess for thrombocytopenia; (d) potassium, sodium, and calcium levels; (e) kidney function tests (blood urea nitrogen, creatinine, and glomerular filtration rate); and (f) liver function tests.

It is also useful to review pertinent imaging studies such as CT scan, MRI, bone scan, and x-rays, especially in patients with cancer that involves the extremities, brain, and/or spine. That information, along with pertinent laboratory studies, can be useful in determining safety parameters in the rehabilitation program.

TREATMENT PLAN

The rehabilitation treatment plan begins with identifying the impairments, activity limitation, and participation restrictions affecting the cancer patient. Once identified, appropriate and realistic goals should be determined. Based on these goals, an appropriate impairment-driven rehabilitation treatment plan should be written and communicated with the treating rehabilitation team.

Ideally, the physiatrist should be involved in the care of the cancer patient from the time of initial diagnosis; however, he or she can be of great benefit at any time during the life of the cancer patient. This includes the period of acute cancer treatment, period of cancer survivorship, or at the end of life.

A. *Acute Cancer Treatment.* During the period of acute cancer treatment, the patient is actively receiving treatment for the cancer. The treatment can include surgery, chemotherapy, and radiation therapy. There are expected and unexpected consequences associated with these treatments affecting both healthy and diseased organs. The cancer patient may experience significant side effects such as nausea, vomiting, generalized weakness, fatigue, and pain—all of which can interfere with the patient's ability to tolerate rehabilitation interventions.

The role of the physiatrist in the acute cancer treatment phase is to identify impairments associated with the cancer and/or its treatments early on and initiate appropriate rehabilitation interventions before these impairments have a significant impact on ADLs and IADLs. The physiatrist can diagnose neuromusculoskeletal impairments by performing a thorough physical examination as well as using diagnostic tests such as electromyography to diagnose peripheral nerve lesions, myopathy, and neuromuscular junction disorders. The physiatrist can then use this information to generate a treatment plan consisting of therapeutic exercise, injections, and medications to treat painful neuromusculoskeletal disorders as well as prescribe orthotics and prosthetics when necessary.

As mentioned, decisions on treatment plans should be driven by specific impairments. Some examples include:

a. A head and neck cancer patient with impaired swallowing function and restricted jaw, neck, and shoulder range of motion secondary to radiation fibrosis can benefit from speech-language pathologist evaluation and treatment, as well as physical therapy to improve neck and shoulder range of motion.
b. A neurooncology patient may have cognitive impairment, aphasia, hemiparesis, and incontinence of bowel and bladder. In this case, a neuropsychologist can identify the cognitive impairments and in conjunction with a speech pathologist identify strategies to minimize the effects of the cognitive impairment using memory aids, checklists, compensatory strategies, and role-playing. An occupational therapist can train the patient and family on strategies to improve performance of ADLs as well as recommend adaptive equipment and perform a home evaluation for safety. A rehabilitation nurse can work with the patient on establishing an effective bowel/bladder routine. A physical therapist can work on balance and gait training. If an ankle foot orthosis is needed, a physiatrist can prescribe one, and an orthotist can fabricate it.
c. A breast cancer patient may present with a combination of lymphedema and restricted range of motion in the shoulder of the affected limb and may benefit from management of the lymphedema with elevation, retrograde massage, manual lymph drainage, compression therapy with sequential graded pumps, compressive garments, therapy to improve the range of motion in that limb, and education on protection of the arm to minimize risk of infection.
d. A patient with CIPN may have a combination of neuropathic pain, impaired balance, footdrop, and altered gait, and would benefit from medications to treat the pain, physical therapy to improve balance and gait, and a prescription for an ankle foot orthosis.

Appropriate goal setting is important, as is the reality that in active treatment the patient's medical status may change quickly. If the patient's cancer diagnosis is associated with a rapid decline, it is a good idea to be proactive in anticipating possible future impairments and introducing interventions to minimize the impact of the decline in function.

Screening for depression, anxiety, and adjustment disorder during the acute treatment of cancer and treating them if present can be very beneficial for the patient.

B. *Cancer Survivorship.* Cancer survivors often have significant general as well as specific cancer- or cancer treatment-related impairments that can adversely affect the quality of their life and roles in their families, communities, work, and school settings. It is important to recognize that cancer-related impairments can have a considerable impact on individuals as they age. Impairments that were relatively well tolerated at a younger age may pose a greater functional burden on individuals as they get older.

Using an impairment-driven approach in cancer rehabilitation, physiatrists can tailor their treatment plan on the effective management of those impairments and utilize rehabilitation resources in a cost-effective manner throughout the life span of the cancer patient.

C. *End-of-Life Care.* Physiatrists can have a significant role in the care of the cancer patient in the final stages of life. In this setting, some important functions include (a) minimizing complications associated with debility such as pressure ulcers and contractures, (b) appropriate management of pain conditions through use of pharmacological and nonpharmacological interventions, and (c) providing emotional support to the family and patient.

Patient Safety and the Rehabilitation Treatment Plan

One of the most important roles of the physiatrist in the care of the cancer patient is to minimize the risk of harm while he or she is undergoing a rehabilitation program. This should ideally be addressed in a proactive manner emphasizing good communication between providers at transition points in care and recognizing the potential safety risks to the cancer patient while receiving rehabilitative treatments.

Some preventive measures to maximize safety include:

A. Appropriate prophylaxis for venous thromboembolism (VTE)
B. Advising restrictions on range of motion and weight-bearing precautions in patients with bone metastasis
C. Minimizing risk of infection by washing hands and disinfection of exercise equipment
D. Swallowing evaluation in patients at risk for aspiration-related complications
E. Cardiac and pulmonary precautions during exercise
F. Hematological precautions in patients with profound anemia and thrombocytopenia undergoing therapeutic exercise (3)

Ethical Issues During Rehabilitation and Treatment

Ethical issues and conflicts in the practice of cancer rehabilitation can arise, and the physiatrist should be able to recognize them when they come up, as well as have a strategy for dealing with them. It is important to respect the patient's wishes and autonomy in making clinical decisions regarding care and end-of-life treatments (e.g., advance directive), identify safety risk factors, and utilize interventions that will minimize the risk for harm. Lastly, given the limited use of rehabilitation services by cancer patients in need, the physiatrist must work with the patient's family, members of the oncology team, and health insurance companies to ensure that access to rehabilitation services is not restricted.

MEDICAL KNOWLEDGE

GOAL

Demonstrate knowledge of established evidence-based and evolving biomedical, clinical, epidemiological, and sociobehavioral sciences pertaining to cancer, as well as the application of this knowledge to guide the impact of physical and functional impairments and cancer treatment on survivors and society.

OBJECTIVES

1. Review important oncology principles including cancer types, stages, and grades.
2. Describe the cancer prehabilitation and rehabilitation care continuum.
3. Explain the prospective surveillance model (PSM) in cancer rehabilitation.
4. Identify opportunities to screen cancer patients for their rehabilitation needs along the care continuum.
5. Consider safety concerns in the cancer survivor population.
6. List examples of physical and/or cognitive impairments that may be amenable to cancer rehabilitation interventions.
7. Educate patients on making patient-centered decisions regarding their plans of care.

BRIEF ONCOLOGY REVIEW

Cancer is a term that describes abnormal cells dividing uncontrollably. Because these cells don't exhibit normal control, they keep dividing and begin to invade other tissues. There are more than 100 different types of cancer, but they can be divided broadly into the following:

- *Carcinomas:* These begin in the skin or in tissues that line or cover internal organs.
- *Sarcoma:* This begins in bone, cartilage, fat, muscle, blood vessels, or other connective/supportive tissues.
- *Leukemia:* This begins in tissues that form blood (e.g., bone marrow) so that large numbers of malignant cells enter the blood.
- *Lymphoma and myeloma:* These start in cells from the immune system.
- *Central nervous system cancers:* These begin in the brain or spinal cord.

The rehabilitation professional should understand cancer stage and grade, with the former generally being more important in terms of developing a rehabilitation treatment plan. Tumor grade is a description of how abnormal the cells look under the microscope. This is generally reported from G1 (low grade) to G4 (high grade). Cancer staging describes the extent or severity of a patient's malignancy and is based on the TNM system, which stands for: T = tumor (size of the primary tumor); N = nodes (whether the cancer has spread to regional lymph nodes); M = metastasis (distant spread). For example, in a woman diagnosed with breast cancer classified as T3 N2 M0, this means that she has a large tumor that has spread outside the breast to regional lymph nodes, but there is no distant spread. The TNM system is used to stage the patients from stage 0 to 4. The TNM classification system is specific to the cancer type; for example, in bladder cancer T3 N0 M0 is stage 3, whereas in colon cancer this would be stage 2. Moreover, not every cancer has a TNM classification; for example, cancers of the brain and spinal cord are classified according to their cell type and grade. Regardless of the oncology classification used, it is important for rehabilitation professionals to understand the extent of the cancer involvement, particularly if there is distant metastasis to areas such as the brain and/or bone.

UNDERSTANDING THE CANCER PREHABILITATION AND REHABILITATION CARE CONTINUUM

Prehabilitation is really the beginning of the cancer rehabilitation care continuum and has been defined as "a process on the cancer continuum of care that occurs between the time of cancer diagnosis and the beginning of acute treatment and includes physical and psychological assessments that establish a baseline functional level, identify impairments, and provide interventions that promote physical and psychological health to reduce the incidence and/or severity of future impairments" (2). The research on cancer prehabilitation is evolving, but there is often a "window of opportunity" between the diagnosis and beginning of treatment in which to better prepare patients for upcoming stressors such as surgery or chemotherapy (Table 12.1) (2). In general, treatments should not be delayed as that may adversely affect survival outcomes.

Cancer rehabilitation, though often thought of as a distinct field of medicine, may be better considered as part of the oncology care continuum. This shift in conceptualization may help to improve the delivery of cancer rehabilitation care, because it means that physiatrists and other rehabilitation health care professionals will work as part of a larger interdisciplinary oncology team. Indeed, most cancer patients are closely followed by oncologists who are more likely to refer patients and work collaboratively with rehabilitation professionals if the latter are well-integrated members of an oncology service line. This is not to say, for example, that all physiatrists who are cancer rehabilitation specialists must work in the same department or even the same institution as the referring oncologists. However, there clearly has been a significant disconnect between the evidence-based need for cancer rehabilitation services, which for some types of cancer may be over 90% of the patients, and the delivery of these services, which has been reported to be abysmally low (2).

This trend underscores the referral process as a key barrier to be overcome in the process of delivering better care. Oncologists and other key members of the oncology team, such as nurse navigators, who are responsible for the overall outcomes of these patients and/or the referral process, must be educated about cancer rehabilitation and develop close working relationships with rehabilitation professionals that they have confidence in.

Consider that there are really three ways that the rehabilitation care may take place. The first way is that the oncology and rehabilitation departments are separate entities and don't have much overlap or collaboration. This has historically been the case, and it has resulted in a significant gap in care. The second way is that the oncology health care team becomes part of the rehabilitation care continuum. This could work but is unlikely as oncologists tend to work with large well-established interdisciplinary teams already and are not likely to become very involved with another large well-established but separate interdisciplinary team. The third way, which is most likely to be successful, is for the cancer rehabilitation physiatrist and other specialists to become well integrated into the oncology care continuum—working closely with the oncologists and other key members of the team. For the physiatrist in private practice, this may mean networking with oncology colleagues and attending lectures, such as Grand Rounds, or being present when cases are discussed, such as at Tumor Board.

PROSPECTIVE SURVEILLANCE MODEL

The PSM is designed to proactively follow patients throughout the care continuum in an attempt to allow for the early identification of impairments caused by cancer or cancer treatment (4). If impairments are identified, then the goal is to refer patients for appropriate rehabilitation interventions. Although there is overlap between the definitions of PSM and cancer prehabilitation, they are not the same. However, both are important in the cancer care continuum. For the purposes of this discussion, the differences can be quickly summarized as follows:

PSM. Occurs throughout the care continuum and is primarily, though not exclusively, focused on surveillance in order to facilitate early referrals to rehabilitation once impairments develop.

Prehabilitation. Occurs only at the beginning of the care continuum and is primarily, though not exclusively, focused on interventions during this discrete time period that will reduce or eliminate current and/or future impairments.

Although prehabilitation is a discrete period of time, interventions may be conducted and assessed beyond the prehabilitation interval. For example, a prehabilitation exercise regimen that begins prior to the start of acute cancer treatments may be continued and followed during and after treatment. A recent review on cancer prehabilitation outlined many opportunities to perform baseline assessments, to provide pretreatment interventions to improve outcomes, and to potentially increase cancer treatment options (e.g., a lung cancer patient who is deemed a high-risk surgical candidate may undergo prehabilitation in order to reduce the risk of complications during the peri- and postoperative period) (5).

SCREENING CANCER SURVIVORS

The term *cancer screening* often means screening tests such as a mammogram or colonoscopy that is designed to help diagnose cancer in its early stage. However, there are other types of screening that survivors should undergo. One of the most important types of screening is screening for physical impairments and functional problems. Unfortunately, this type of screening is not consistently performed in this population, although it should be. In order for patients to be referred by oncology providers to the rehabilitation team, a screening process must take place. Therefore, this type of screening should ideally be performed by the oncology team at designated intervals throughout the care continuum (Table 12.2).

Distress screening has become an increasingly standard part of oncology care and provides a unique opportunity to perform dual screening—for physical and emotional problems—simultaneously. It makes a lot of sense to combine these screenings not only from a time management and human resource perspective but also from an evidence-based perspective. This is because physical impairments and disability are often the root causes of distress in survivors. In fact, research has shown that a leading cause of distress is physical disability (6) and that more often than not physical problems (versus emotional ones) lead to a decreased health-related quality of life in cancer survivors (7).

SAFETY CONCERNS IN CANCER SURVIVORS

There has been recent interest in establishing both effective and safe rehabilitation interventions in the cancer survivor population (3). Because exercise is known to help prevent primary cancers from developing and likely will help prevent cancer recurrence in some types of cancer, there has been a tendency to encourage patients to exercise regardless of whether they have been screened for impairments and received appropriate rehabilitation interventions. Unfortunately, the "rehabilitation" of cancer survivors too often does not include any oversight by trained rehabilitation professionals. Establishing appropriate screening protocols, identifying impairments, and referring patients to skilled rehabilitation professionals is critical. However, even when all of this is in place, there still may be safety concerns. These patients may be elderly and/or frail. They often have comorbidities and have endured one or more oncology treatments that have caused new problems in an attempt to control the cancer. They may have advanced disease with metastasis to the bone or central nervous system. Brain metastases may cause a myriad of issues that include difficulty with cognition, speech, swallowing, and mobility. Even patients without brain malignancy may be susceptible to cognitive problems due to delirium or Mild Cognitive Impairment (MCI) from chemotherapy. Safety in this population, so often prone to a complex interaction of symptoms and their triggers, is an important and evolving topic that cannot be adequately covered in this chapter. Nevertheless, it's important to note that cancer survivors should be treated by a highly skilled interdisciplinary rehabilitation team that is extremely knowledgeable about the different issues that may arise.

EXAMPLES OF REHABILITATION IN CANCER SURVIVORS

Lymphedema is a well-known and important example of cancer-related sequelae that may be treated, though not cured, by rehabilitation interventions. Poorly treated lymphedema may have devastating results and is an important condition to screen for and treat. Lymphedema most commonly occurs in the upper extremities of breast cancer survivors but may also occur in the lower extremities in other patient populations (e.g., gynecologic cancers) or in the face and neck (e.g., head and neck cancers). The mainstay of treatment is controlling the fluid collection, and this is usually accomplished with complex (also called complete) decongestive therapy (CDT)—a combination of interventions that include hands-on manual lymphatic drainage (MLD) as well as compression wraps.

CIPN is the most common neurologic sequelae in oncology patients. CIPN is frequently caused by drugs that fall into the class of taxanes. It usually begins slowly and worsens over the course of chemotherapy. Once the offending drug is discontinued, there is an opportunity for improvement. Similar to other peripheral nerve injuries, the healing usually takes place over the course of 1 year or so, and the prognosis is generally better if there is significant improvement early on. Rehabilitation interventions likely won't affect neurologic recovery but can improve functional problems, including gait and balance issues, which can be significant.

Cancer-related fatigue (CRF) is a very common problem and affects the majority of survivors. The accepted definition for CRF *is an unusual, persistent, subjective sense of tiredness related to cancer or cancer treatment that interferes with functioning* (8). Distinguishing normal fatigue from CRF is important—fatigue is deemed to be pathologic when it occurs during usual daily activities, persists for long periods of time, and does not respond to rest (9,10). Clinical guidelines for CRF have been

TABLE 12.2 Improving Cancer Rehabilitation Care

- Identify the current gap in care between the number of new cancer patients and referrals for cancer rehabilitation services (evidence-based need for rehabilitation services)
- Educate both oncology and rehabilitation professionals in evidence-based cancer rehabilitation care
- Train the oncology workforce to screen for physical impairments and functional problems amenable to rehabilitation interventions
- Train the rehabilitation workforce to evaluate and treat cancer-related impairments and functional problems
- Include both oncology and rehabilitation professionals in the formal cancer care programming, including survivorship programming
- Establish an interdisciplinary cancer rehabilitation program/service line or alternately create a referral process for rehabilitation services within the geographic area
- Document the navigation process—assessing and overcoming barriers to care
- Report outcomes across the continuum of care, beginning with a baseline assessment
- Follow-up and identify new or ongoing rehabilitation needs
- Focus on patient-centered care and encourage active participation of the patient in his or her rehabilitation care
- Refer to community-based resources to complement rehabilitation care

developed by the National Comprehensive Cancer Network (11). One of the best antidotes to CRF is exercise. However, in this potentially fragile population, it is important to consider physical impairments and functional problems before recommending any formal exercise. Traditional exercise screening protocols may not be adequate to assess safety. For example, a young breast cancer survivor may have CIPN that affects her balance, and she could potentially fall off of a treadmill. Or, this same young woman may have cardiomyopathy as a result of chemotherapy and have a cardiac event on the treadmill. There are many examples that could be given here, but the point is that prescribing exercise in cancer survivors involves a sophisticated understanding of the patient's physical and functional impairments as well as cardiopulmonary status.

Mild cognitive impairment (MCI) is often called "chemo brain." MCI generally occurs during or following chemotherapy. Chemotherapeutic drugs may cause neurotoxicity and possible mechanisms for MCI include vascular injury, oxidative damage, inflammation, and direct injury to neurons in the brain (12). CRF and MCI have some similar findings, but they are not the same. Although both conditions may have fatigue as a major patient complaint, MCI will have the additional components of *cognitive impairment,* such as memory loss and decreased attention. Rest does not seem to improve the symptoms of MCI, although lack of sleep may make it worse. Therefore, if there is a history of insomnia, sleep apnea, or some other sleep disturbance, it's important to intervene. MCI may be amenable to rehabilitation strategies that are used in other populations such as stroke or traumatic brain injury.

Radiation fibrosis syndrome (RFS) is the term used to describe a complex set of problems that may result from fibrotic sclerosis due to radiation treatment. RFS may affect any tissue including, but not limited to, skin and subcutaneous tissue, bone, nerves, muscles, lungs, gastrointestinal and genitourinary tracts, or other organs. Depending on the site of radiation therapy, radiation intensity, and individual variation in radiation sensitivity, the RFS clinical manifestation and severity vary (13). There are approximately 14 million cancer survivors in the United States. Approximately one-half of these patients will receive radiation treatment at some point during the course of their disease (14). RFS can cause both cosmetic and functional impairment. The severity of the impairment may not only reduce the quality of life but also pose significant deterioration in health and, in some cases, even be life threatening. RFS is usually progressive and irreversible (15). The most important treatment interventions are believed to be physical and occupational therapy (16). Interventions may include manual stretching, dynamic splinting, therapeutic strengthening exercises, adaptive equipment, orthotics, and modalities. Medications are often used to control pain and muscle spasms in RFS patients. A nerve stabilizer such as Pregabalin (Lyrica) is the first line for neuropathic pain of RFS patients. Tricyclic antidepressants such as Duloxetine can be considered in patients who do not respond to Pregabalin. Botulinum toxin type A has been described in the treatment of RFS-associated sequelae, including trismus, cervical dystonia, and neuralgias (17). Some trials have demonstrated that the combination of Pentoxifylline and vitamin E with hyperbaric oxygen therapy improved RFS (18–22), but their benefits are still controversial. Preventive treatment including CXCR4 inhibition by drugs such as MSX-122 may alleviate potential radiation-induced lung injury, presenting future therapeutic opportunities for patients requiring chest irradiation.

There are many physical impairments and functional problems that may result from cancer and its treatment. The problems vary widely from trismus to radiation-induced fibrosis syndrome to rotator cuff impingement. The list is far too long for this chapter. However, the basic concepts in rehabilitation remain the same. These include understanding the evidence base and evaluating and treating patients appropriately using standard of care guidelines.

SOCIOECONOMIC ISSUES IN CANCER REHABILITATION

Socioeconomic issues are very complicated and create a significant financial impact on the patient, family, and society. Although this topic is extensive, there are a few important considerations. It's important to recognize that cancer rehabilitation is generally reimbursed by third-party payers in the United States, including Medicare. However, there are opportunities to provide advocacy for more comprehensive coverage for this vulnerable population. Early research suggests that cancer rehabilitation is cost-effective. For example, one systematic review found positive cost-effectiveness ratios (23). A recent review on the effect of cancer rehabilitation and work suggested that rehabilitation interventions may reduce the financial burden of cancer to the individual and society (24). Individual patients may be struggling with significant financial concerns, and the rehabilitation team should focus on understanding whether these may present barriers to care and how best to support the patient.

PATIENT-CENTERED CARE

Patient-centered care, at its core, is about making the patient a partner in his or her care, especially the decision-making process. Patient-centered care involves educating patients and family members about treatment options while at the same time respecting their values and unique perspectives. In oncology, there is a significant focus on survivorship and patient-centered care. The Institute of Medicine released a consensus report in 2013 titled "Delivering High-Quality Cancer Care" that has a 6-part interconnected framework with the patient at the center—highlighting patient-centered oncology care (25).

PRACTICE-BASED LEARNING AND IMPROVEMENT

GOALS

Demonstrate competence in continuously investigating and evaluating cancer rehabilitation patient care practices, appraising and assimilating scientific evidence, and continuously improving patient care practices based on constant self-evaluation and lifelong learning.

OBJECTIVES

1. Describe learning opportunities for providers, patients, and caregivers with experience in cancer rehabilitation.
2. Use methods for ongoing competency training in cancer rehabilitation for physiatrists, including formative evaluation feedback in daily practice, evaluating current practice, and developing a systematic quality improvement and practice improvement strategy.
3. Locate some resources including available websites for continuing medical education and continuing professional development.
4. Describe some areas paramount to self-assessment and life-long learning such as review of current guidelines, including evidence-based, in treatment and management of patients with cancer and the role of the physiatrist as the educator of patients, families, residents, students, colleagues, and other health professionals.

Practice-based learning and improvement has been described as the competency in which the physician holds up a mirror to assess and improve his or her practice with the goal of improving the care of one's patients (26,27). Given the complexity of issues facing the cancer patient, the physiatrist caring for this population of patients has to be knowledgeable in a variety of medical and surgical subjects to fully understand the impact of the impairments and functional limitations affecting the cancer patient. He or she must be well versed in principles of oncology, radiation therapy, chemotherapy, orthopedics, pediatrics, geriatrics, and neurosurgery, just to name a few. He or she must be able to interpret imaging studies such as CT scans, MRI, x-rays, and bone scans. The physician should have a working knowledge of electrodiagnosis and its utility in diagnosing cancer-related peripheral nervous system injuries, as well as an excellent working knowledge of the musculoskeletal and nervous systems. He or she needs to be able to integrate this knowledge with data about the patient's cancer, stage of disease, and treatments rendered to diagnose neuromusculoskeletal injuries and provide appropriate treatment. Ideally, the physiatrist should also be well versed in principles of pain medicine.

In order to identify gaps in knowledge as it applies to the care of the cancer patient, it is advised that the physiatrist perform regular self-assessment of his or her knowledge base as it pertains to cancer rehabilitation. Self-assessment tools are available through the American Academy of Physical Medicine and Rehabilitation (AAPMR) (28). Reflection on the care provided to cancer patients in one's practice can be another way to identify gaps in knowledge. Some examples of topics to cover in the reflection include (a) assessment of the patient's impairments; (b) knowledge about the cancer affecting the patient, as well as its neuromusculoskeletal impairments and treatments; (c) effectiveness of treatments rendered to the patient (e.g., injections, medications, and therapies); (d) personal effectiveness in coordination of patient's care in the health care system; (e) effectiveness of communication and interpersonal skills in the care of the patient; and (f) effectiveness of the education of the patient about his cancer, complications, and treatments.

Once gaps have been identified, there are several ways in which physiatrists can address them. Some examples include (a) specialty courses in cancer rehabilitation (29,30), (b) courses offered at the annual AAPMR meeting, (c) cancer rehabilitation fellowships (31,32), (d) AAPMR resources (e.g., Maintenance of Certificate [MOC] online review course [33] and Knowledge NOW [34]), and (e) textbooks (35). It is also recommended that physiatrists periodically review pertinent sources from other clinical specialties such as oncology journals and textbooks.

Another excellent source of knowledge is through participation in the interdisciplinary team conferences involved in the care of complex cancer patients. These teams often include radiologists, medical oncologists, radiation oncologists, surgeons, and neurologists, just to name a few. A physiatrist can learn a great deal from these team members and can also teach them as well about the common impairments in cancer patients. Physiatrists can also learn by observing physical therapists, occupational therapists, speech-language pathologists, psychologists, and social workers who have specialized in the clinical practice of cancer rehabilitation as they interact with their patients.

INTERPERSONAL AND COMMUNICATION SKILLS

GOALS

Demonstrate interpersonal and communication skills that result in the effective exchange of information and collaboration with cancer patients, their families, and other health professionals.

OBJECTIVES

1. Demonstrate skills used in effective communication and collaboration with patients with cancer and their caregivers, across socioeconomic and cultural backgrounds.
2. Delineate the importance of the role of the physiatrist as the interdisciplinary team leader and consultant pertinent to cancer rehabilitation.
3. Demonstrate proper documentation and effective communication between health care professional team members in patient care as it applies to cancer rehabilitation.

Effective communication and interpersonal skills are essential in the practice of cancer rehabilitation. The care of the cancer patient is very complex, involving numerous medical and surgical specialties, nurses, therapists, social workers, and case managers across the health care system. A professional network often involves hospitals, skilled nursing facilities, home health care agencies, and outpatient facilities. This can be very overwhelming for cancer patients, who are already in a vulnerable state, as well as for their family. The problem is made even more complex when one takes into consideration the impact of cultural and socioeconomic factors on the individual with cancer.

In communicating with cancer patients and their families, physiatrists should be empathetic and compassionate in their approach. The physiatrist should be mindful of the myriad of different reactions that cancer patients often have when diagnosed with the disease as well as during their treatment. This includes understanding the evidence-based relationship between physical impairments and distress in this population. The physiatrist should allow ample time to discuss the cancer diagnosis and its impact on the affected individual's body and level of function in a language that is easy to understand and minimizes use of medical terminology.

The physiatrist should take the time to learn the patient's style of communication to identify the best way to deliver the information. Effective communication requires an appreciation for the impact of both verbal and nonverbal factors on the patient. Maintaining good eye contact and an "open" body posture in which the arms and legs are not crossed are some examples of effective nonverbal communication. The physiatrist should give the patient his or her undivided attention during the visit and be mindful of one's tone of voice as well as volume of speech. Active listening skills that include paraphrasing back to the patient what was just said and acknowledging the emotional impact of the content on the patient are important, as is checking for the patient's understanding of the content at the end of the visit.

Communication and interpersonal skills with other clinicians involved in the care of the cancer patient is also important for physiatrists in their role as rehabilitation team leaders. The physiatrist must understand the impairments, activity limitations, and participation restrictions affecting the cancer patient; integrate the input of medical and surgical specialists, nurses, therapists, psychologists, social workers, and others involved in the care of the patient; and then coordinate the team efforts through appropriate goal setting and team leadership. In addition, the physiatrist relies on effective communication and interpersonal skills to advocate for the patient with health insurance companies and administrative staff at different parts of the health care system.

Conflict resolution skills can be an added benefit in dealing with difficult situations between the patients and the clinicians involved in their care. A collaborative approach between the stakeholders at identifying the concerns and subsequently reframing the problem can be used as a foundation for identifying possible interventions.

Medical documentation is an important communication tool between providers. As mentioned earlier in the patient assessment section, the following information is important to document: (a) type and stage of cancer; (b) medical, surgical, radiation, and chemotherapy treatments that were rendered and any complications associated with them; (c) pertinent rehabilitation precautions (e.g., weight-bearing limitations and hematological precautions); (d) names and contact information of pertinent clinicians involved in the patient's care (e.g., oncologists and surgeons); and (e) treatment plan (e.g., chemotherapy, radiation, and surgery).

PROFESSIONALISM

GOALS

Reflect a commitment to carrying out professional responsibilities and an adherence to ethical principles in cancer rehabilitation.

OBJECTIVES

Exemplify the humanistic qualities as a provider of care for patients with cancer.

1. Demonstrate ethical principles and responsiveness to patient needs superseding self and other interests.
2. Demonstrate sensitivity to patient population diversity, including culture, gender, age, race, religion, disabilities, and sexual orientation.
3. Respect patient's beliefs and goals, privacy, confidentiality, and autonomy.

Professionalism in the practice of cancer rehabilitation is reflected in adherence to the principles of medical humanism. This has been described as "the relationship between physicians and their patients that are respectful and compassionate. It is reflected in attitudes and behaviors that are sensitive to the values, autonomy, cultural and ethnic backgrounds of others" (36). At its foundation, medical humanism respects the autonomy of patients to make their own decision with respect to their health care.

A principal responsibility of the physiatrist within the "shared decision making" model involves providing the patient with the necessary medical information about the risks and benefits of a particular treatment plan. This allows for the patient to make an informed decision. The physician should be sensitive to the patient's cultural background and his or her values and religious beliefs when recommending and implementing a treatment plan (37) since disparities in treatment and quality of life have been reported (38,39).

Medical professionalism is also demonstrated when physicians "align their interests with those of the ill person and be free of any self-serving motivation so that patients can trust their physician's advice" (37). To adhere to this foundational tenet of the medical profession, the physiatrist should be vigilant for the possibility of conflicts of interest when in the process of caring for patients. There is a concern that recent changes in health care reimbursement may financially incentivize physicians to pressure patients to accept a treatment that may not be consistent with their wishes (37).

SYSTEMS-BASED PRACTICE

GOALS

Demonstrate awareness and responsiveness to systems of rehabilitation team care delivery, and the ability to access, evaluate, recruit, and coordinate effectively resources in the system to provide optimal safe continuum of care and outcomes as it relates to cancer rehabilitation.

OBJECTIVES

1. Discuss effective coordination of care for cancer patients across the continuum of rehabilitative care including at transition points.
2. Describe the judicious use of diagnostic tests, treatments, and consultants in the provision of rehabilitative care to cancer patients.

3. Identify cost-saving measures in the practice of rehabilitative medicine for cancer patients.
4. Examine risk–benefit analysis in the provision of rehabilitation medicine to cancer patients.
5. Explain the role of the physiatrist as an advocate for quality rehabilitative care and optimal patient care systems for cancer patients.
6. Identify system problems in the rehabilitation of cancer patients and utilize quality improvement tools to improve patient safety.

Dietz described four categories of cancer rehabilitation interventions—preventive, restorative, supportive, and palliative. *Preventive* interventions focused on (a) improving the patient's level of function prior to the onset of the effects of the cancer and its treatment, (b) patient education, and (c) psychological support (40). *Restorative* interventions focused on returning the patient to a previous level of function and addressing impairments from the cancer and its treatments. *Supportive* interventions are meant to assist the cancer patient to function at the highest level within the context of his or her impairments, activity limitations, and participation restrictions. This would include teaching the patient to use prosthetic, orthotic, and assistive devices to help manage daily activities as well as provide emotional support. In the *palliative* stage, the interventions focus on (a) minimizing complications such as pressure ulcers, contractures, and muscle deconditioning; (b) ensuring adequate pain control; and (c) emotional support for the family.

Using the Dietz model as a guide, one can see that cancer rehabilitation services are provided in a variety of settings such as inpatient rehabilitation facilities, outpatient rehabilitation programs, skilled nursing facilities, patient's home, and hospice. The services are provided by a diverse group of rehabilitation clinicians such as physical therapists, occupational therapists, speech pathologists, rehabilitation nurses, psychologists, and social workers, depending on the types of impairments, activity limitations, and participation restrictions.

IMPROVING THE QUALITY OF CARE PROVIDED TO CANCER PATIENTS AND SURVIVORS

It has been reported that the 5-year survival rate for all cancers is 67% with a projected 18 million cancer survivors by 2022 (2,41,42). With the growing number of cancer survivors, there has been an increased awareness of the needs of survivors for rehabilitation services to address impairments, minimize activity restrictions, and maximize participation.

The Commission for Accreditation of Rehabilitation Facilities (CARF) has developed standards for organizations seeking accreditation for cancer rehabilitation specialty programs that are meant to be person centered and emphasize a holistic interdisciplinary approach to patient care. This care is meant to be provided in a variety of settings, by competent personnel who provide evidence-based care that addresses preventive, restorative, supportive, and palliative rehabilitation needs. Rehabilitation is an integral part of cancer care and emphasizes outcomes that "prevent or minimize impairments, reduce activity limitations and maximize participation." The care should be coordinated and driven by the needs of the person served and his or her families/support system to improve quality of life. There is a strong emphasis on education of the person served that is "age and culturally appropriate and fosters self-management." The cancer rehabilitation specialty program collects and analyzes outcomes data and shares that information with its stakeholders; it uses the data to improve the quality of the program. The program also acts as a resource to providers on cancer rehabilitation and to the community at large and participates in research opportunities (43).

The American College of Surgeons' Commission on Cancer (CoC) is a group of organizations that is "dedicated to improving survival and quality of life for cancer patients through standard-setting, prevention, research, education, and the monitoring of comprehensive quality care" (44).

In order for facilities providing cancer care to be accredited by the CoC, they must demonstrate compliance with standards that ensure that high-quality, comprehensive, multidisciplinary care is provided to cancer patients. Cancer rehabilitation is a current accreditation standard for the CoC. In 2012, the CoC announced new accreditation standards (3.1–3.3) that deserve mention since they are relevant to the provision of cancer rehabilitation services. These standards are (a) Patient Navigation (3.1), (b) Psychosocial Distress Screening (3.2), and (c) Survivorship Care Plan (3.3). In order to meet these standards, accredited facilities must demonstrate that (a) barriers to access to care are identified on a regular basis; (b) there is monitoring for psychosocial distress in cancer patients with appropriate services provided; and (c) cancer survivors are provided with a summary of their care as well as a survivorship care plan to assist them with navigation through the health care system and facilitate access to appropriate clinical resources. Given that cancer survivors often have significant physical impairments that require rehabilitative care, it is important that facilities providing cancer care screen for them and subsequently remove barriers to access appropriate rehabilitation resources. Resources have been developed to assist clinicians in meeting the intent of these standards from a rehabilitation perspective. The STAR Program® (Survivorship Training and Rehabilitation) offers a certification program for hospitals and cancer centers that includes tools for "evidence based assessment of methods and treatment protocols for both physical and psychosocial impairments in cancer survivors" (45).

Physiatrists are ideally suited for the management of an interdisciplinary team across the continuum of rehabilitative care for the cancer survivor. They are experts at the diagnosis and treatment of impairments of the nervous and musculoskeletal systems and can serve as clinical care coordinators and advocates for cancer patients among the various physicians involved in the care of the cancer patient. As mentioned earlier, this can often include many different providers including, but not limited to, oncologists, surgeons, neurologists, and interventional radiologists.

Patient care coordination is an essential role for the physiatrist in the care of the cancer patient. This is best accomplished by having a good understanding of the patient's underlying cancer diagnosis and stage, treatments rendered to date (e.g., surgical, chemotherapy, and radiation therapy), complications, and comorbidities, as well as their socioeconomic status and extent of family support. The physiatrist should communicate this information to the various clinicians involved in the care of the patient as the patient moves through various health care systems—especially at transition points when some information may not be relayed between providers of care. Accurate and complete documentation in discharge summaries are an essential part of patient care coordination. In addition, direct contact either by phone or in person with key team members (e.g., oncologist, surgeon, and therapist) using techniques such as SBAR (Situation, Background, Assessment, and Recommendation) can further help with communication and coordination of care (46).

At times, the patient's medical condition may fluctuate, and new impairments may arise that can have an impact on the patient's care and quality of life. For example, new lesions in the proximal femur of a cancer patient may increase his or her risk for pathological fractures. The physiatrist may be asked by therapists regarding the weight-bearing status as well as use of exercises and modalities in the care of this patient, and she in turn would need to discuss the implications of these new findings with orthopedists, radiologists, and oncologists and relay that information back to the treating therapists. Appropriate patient goals for various stages of the cancer can be useful guides for the physiatrist in his or her role of coordinating the rehabilitative care of the various care providers.

The physiatrist also bears a responsibility to identify appropriately trained and experienced therapists and other clinicians to care for the cancer patient since not all rehabilitation therapists and providers have the same level of expertise in the treatment of cancer impairments.

RISK–BENEFIT ANALYSIS AND COST AWARENESS

In risk–benefit analysis, the goal is to provide treatment in which the benefits to the patient outweigh the risks of the treatments. A recent systematic review of cancer rehabilitation found favorable cost-effectiveness ratios, but there is limited research in this area (47). Rehabilitative interventions can provide significant benefit to cancer patients such as improvement in range of motion, strength, level of function, and reduction in pain. However, there are risks associated with rehabilitative interventions such as pathological fractures with aggressive range of motion or weight bearing, falls, and theoretical potential for injury with use of certain modalities. For example, in a recent study in lung cancer patients, exercise tolerance improved at the cost of increased pain, and rehabilitation did not improve patients' quality of life (48). The physiatrist should identify the risks and benefits to the cancer patient as well as the possibility of its occurrence. These should be discussed with the patient and his or her wishes taken into consideration.

Cost of tests and treatments also needs to be taken into consideration. Given the fragility of the cancer patient, the potential for rapid changes in his or her medical condition is always present. Therefore, there is always the possible need for diagnostic tests (e.g., MRI, CT scan, and bone scan) as well as treatments (e.g., chemotherapy and radiation oncology), which can further drive up costs for the patient's care. To complicate matters further, the patient's health insurance coverage may have limitations with respect to payment for tests and treatment.

Another consideration for inpatient rehabilitation facilities is the need for the patient to be able to participate in 3 hours of therapy per day if the payer is Medicare. This can be challenging to achieve if the patient is away at tests, receiving chemotherapy, receiving radiation therapy, or not feeling well enough to fully participate in the rehabilitation program. This in turn may limit their functional gains.

ADVOCACY FOR QUALITY AND OPTIMAL PATIENT CARE

Physiatrists should advocate for the rehabilitative needs of cancer patients. There is evidence that in spite of the presence of significant physical impairments that are adversely impacting on the patient's ability to ambulate and perform ADLs, there is an underutilization of rehabilitation services by cancer patients. This is multifactorial in nature: (a) reluctance on the part of patients to tell their oncologists about their problems with ambulation, generalized weakness, impaired balance, and cognition; (b) lack of awareness and inquiring about these problems on the part of the ontological team; and (c) lack of referral for appropriate rehabilitation services (49). As the number of cancer survivors continues to grow, the need for rehabilitative services will continue to grow in importance. Physiatrists should educate oncologists, surgeons, neurologists, primary care providers, nurses, hospital administrators, and payers. The physiatrist should advocate for the right cancer rehabilitation services at the right location at the right time and by the right cancer rehabilitation providers to maximize the patient's level of function. The physiatrist should also educate cancer patients about the important role that rehabilitation medicine has in their care as well as provide strategies to best advocate for their own rehabilitation needs in the health care system.

PATIENT SAFETY AND SYSTEM ERRORS

Patient safety is an important consideration in the provision of rehabilitation care across the health care system. As mentioned earlier, cancer and its treatment can increase the risk of harm to the patient receiving medical and rehabilitative care (50). Ideally, patient-centered rehabilitative care is provided by qualified clinicians all along the care continuum. Competency of rehabilitation team members with respect to rehabilitation of the cancer patient should be assessed and gaps in knowledge base identified and addressed through education and mentoring. The site where the rehabilitative care is provided should also be assessed for potential safety risks as well as for appropriate emergency equipment should an urgent situation arise (3).

Communication and patient care coordination are important roles for the physiatrist, especially at transition points in care when the cancer patient is especially vulnerable. Use of detailed discharge summaries, checklists, and structured communication techniques can be very helpful (3).

Physiatrists providing and coordinating the care of cancer patients should have a working knowledge of patient safety precautions in the provision of rehabilitative care in various settings. In addition, they should understand principles of quality improvement methodology as well as root cause analysis and how to use them in assessing the quality of care provided to cancer patients in the rehabilitation setting as well as in various ways that the quality of care rendered can be improved. The reader is referred to the chapter on systems-based practice elsewhere in this book, as well as other available resources for additional information (3,51).

CASE STUDY

A 50-year-old female home health attendant with a history of breast cancer that was initially treated with mastectomy and axillary dissection, chemotherapy, and radiation therapy now presents with stage 4 cancer and is admitted for acute rehabilitation to an inpatient rehabilitation facility for medical debility. There is evidence of metastatic disease involving the proximal femur and humerus on the right side and to the brain. She has a past medical history of noninsulin diabetes mellitus, hypertension, and a recent seizure disorder related to metastatic disease. She lives with her husband in an apartment on the second floor of a building with no elevator. She has been gradually declining in level of function and ambulation. She complains of difficulties with memory, fatigue, pain in her left shoulder, and numbness and tingling sensation in the hands and feet. Physical examination is significant for poor attention span, impaired memory and organizational skills, generalized weakness, nonpitting lymphedema in the left upper extremity associated with restricted range of motion in the shoulder, "stocking-glove" sensory loss in the feet and hands, impaired proprioception, and poor balance. She has a history of falls with injuries that have not required medical care. Functionally, she has difficulty with transfers from bed to chair and is limited to short-distance ambulation with a walker.

CASE STUDY DISCUSSION QUESTIONS

1. Identify the impairments, activity limitations, and participation restrictions for this patient.
2. Write a rehabilitation treatment plan for her, addressing the impairments, activity limitations, and participation restrictions, that includes short- and long-term goals, precautions, and exercise.
3. Summarize the potential ethical issues involved in the patient's care.
4. Describe the medical and rehabilitative management of the impairments identified in this patient's care.
5. Identify the elements of a patient and family education program.
6. Describe effective communication strategies between the various caregivers involved in this patient's care to minimize risk of injury to the patient.
7. Cite patient safety issues in this patient's care and identify strategies to minimize them from occurring.

SELF-EXAMINATION QUESTIONS
(Answers begin on p. 367)

1. Which of the following medications has been associated with CIPN?
   A. Digitalis
   B. Cisplatin
   C. Caporal
   D. Simvastatin
   E. Aspirin

2. Which of the following is a significant and specific safety concern for the cancer patient undergoing a rehabilitation program?
   A. Weight-bearing precautions in a patient with metastatic disease to the lower extremities
   B. Blood pressure precautions in a patient with no history of hypertension
   C. Weight-bearing precautions in a patient with metastatic disease to the liver
   D. Seizure precautions in a patient with nonmetastasized colon cancer
   E. Hypoglycemic precautions in a nondiabetic patient

3. In the TNM cancer staging system, what does TNM stand for?
   A. T = tumor location; N = nodular density of tumor; M = malignancy
   B. T = type of tumor; N = name of tumor; M = membrane surrounding the tumor
   C. T = time since diagnosis of cancer; N = number of tumors; M = memory is affected by tumor
   D. T = size of the primary tumor; N = spread of cancer to regional lymph nodes; M = metastasis or distant spread of cancer
   E. T = size of the primary tumor; N = name of tumor; M = metastasis or distant spread of tumor

4. Which of the following best characterizes cancer prehabilitation?
   A. It is the period of time after the acute treatment of the cancer has been completed and onset of cancer-related impairments
   B. It is the period of time between cancer diagnosis and the end of acute treatment and includes physical and psychological assessments that establish a baseline functional level, identify impairments, and provide interventions that promote physical and psychological health to reduce the incidence and/or severity of future impairments
   C. It is the period of time between cancer diagnosis and the beginning of acute treatment and includes physical and psychological assessments that establish a baseline functional level, identify impairments, and provide interventions that promote physical and psychological health to reduce the incidence and/or severity of future impairments

D. It is the period of time between cancer diagnosis and the beginning of acute treatment that focuses on psychological assessments and interventions to promote psychological health to reduce the incidence and/or severity of future psychological impairments

E. It is the period of time when the cancer is in remission for a minimum of 10 years

5. Which of the following best describes the most likely reason for underutilization of rehabilitation services by cancer patients?
   A. Patients are reluctant to tell their friends about their difficulties with ambulation, weakness, impaired balance, and cognition
   B. Oncological team members have a very good understanding and awareness of the physical impairments facing cancer patients and refer often; however, the patients don't believe there is much benefit from rehabilitation so they don't participate
   C. There is a lack of awareness and inquiring about these problems on the part of the oncological team and lack of referral for appropriate rehabilitation services
   D. There is awareness about these problems on the part of the oncological team; however, there is a lack of referral for appropriate rehabilitation services

DISCLOSURE

Julie Silver, MD, is the cofounder of Oncology Rehabilitation Partners LLC, which developed the STAR Program (Survivorship Training and Rehabilitation).

REFERENCES

1. Cheville AL, Troxel AB, Basford JR, et al. Prevalence and treatment patterns of physical impairments in patients with metastatic breast cancer. *J Clin Oncol*. 2008;26:2621–2629.
2. Silver JK, Baima J, Mayer RS. Impairment-driven cancer rehabilitation: an essential component of quality care and survivorship. *CA Cancer J Clin*. 2013;63:295–317.
3. Cristian A, Tran A, Patel K. Patient safety in cancer rehabilitation. *Phys Med Rehabil Clin N Am*. 2012;23:441–456.
4. Stout NL, Binkley JM, Schmitz KH, et al. A prospective surveillance model for rehabilitation for women with breast cancer. *Cancer*. 2012;118(suppl 8):2191–2200.
5. Silver JK, Baima J. Cancer prehabilitation: an opportunity to decrease treatment-related morbidity, increase cancer treatment options and improve physical and psychological health outcomes. *Am J Phys Med Rehabil*. 2013;92(8):715–727.
6. Banks E, Byles JE, Gibson RE, et al. Is psychological distress in people living with cancer related to the fact of diagnosis, current treatment or level of disability? Findings from a large Australian study. *Med J Aust*. 2010;193(suppl 5):S62–S67.
7. Weaver KE, Forsythe LP, Reeve BB, et al. Mental and physical health-related quality of life among U.S. cancer survivors: population estimates from the 2010 National Health Interview Survey. *Cancer Epidemiol Biomarkers Prev*. 2012 Nov;21(11):2108–217.
8. National Comprehensive Cancer Network. *NCCN Clinical Practice Guidelines in Oncology: Cancer-Related Fatigue*. Rockledge, PA: National Comprehensive Cancer Network; 2009.
9. Dimeo FC. Effects of exercise on cancer-related fatigue. *Cancer*. 2001; 15:92(suppl 6):1689–1693.
10. Fukuda K, Straus SE, Hickie I, et al. The chronic fatigue syndrome: a comprehensive approach to its definition and study. International Chronic Fatigue Syndrome Study Group. *Ann Intern Med*. 1994;121(12):953–959.
11. Mock V, Atkinson A, Barsevick AM, et al. Cancer-related fatigue. Clinical practice guidelines in oncology. *J Natl Compr Canc Netw*. 2007;5(10):1054–1078.
12. Nelson CJ, Nandy N, Roth AJ. Chemotherapy and cognitive deficits: mechanisms, findings, and potential interventions. *Palliat Support Care*. 2007;5(3):273–280.
13. Andreassen CN. Independent prospective validation of a predictive test for risk of radiation induced fibrosis based on the gene expression pattern in fibroblasts irradiated in vitro. *Radiother Oncol*. 2013;108(3):469–472.
14. Mariotto AB, Yabroff KR, Shao Y, et al. Projections of the cost of cancer care in the United States: 2010–2020. *J Natl Cancer Inst*. 2011;103:117–128.
15. Anscher MS. The irreversibility of radiation-induced fibrosis: fact or folklore? *J Clin Oncol*. 2005;23(34):8551–8552.
16. Stubblefield MD, Odell MW, eds. Chapter 57: radiation fibrosis syndrome. In: Stubblefield MD, ed. *Cancer Rehabilitation, Principles and Practice*. New York, NY: Demos Medical Publishers; 2009:742.
17. Stubblefield MD, Levine A, Custodio CM, et al. The role of botulinum toxin type A in the radiation fibrosis syndrome: a preliminary report. *Arch Phys Med Rehabil*. 2008;89:417.
18. Magnusson M, Höglund P, Johansson K, et al. Pentoxifylline and vitamin E treatment for prevention of radiation-induced side-effects in women with breast cancer: a phase two, double-blind, placebo-controlled randomised clinical trial (Ptx-5). *Eur J Cancer*. 2009;45:2488.
19. Gothard L, Cornes P, Earl J, et al. Double-blind placebo-controlled randomised trial of vitamin E and pentoxifylline in patients with chronic arm lymphoedema and fibrosis after surgery and radiotherapy for breast cancer. *Radiother Oncol*. 2004;73:133.
20. Jacobson G, Bhatia S, Smith BJ, et al. Randomized trial of pentoxifylline and vitamin E vs standard follow-up after breast irradiation to prevent breast fibrosis, evaluated by tissue compliance meter. *Int J Radiat Oncol Biol Phys*. 2013;85:604.
21. Gothard L, Stanton A, MacLaren J, et al. Non-randomised phase II trial of hyperbaric oxygen therapy in patients with chronic arm lymphoedema and tissue fibrosis after radiotherapy for early breast cancer. *Radiother Oncol*. 2004;70:217.
22. Teas J, Cunningham JE, Cone L, et al. Can hyperbaric oxygen therapy reduce breast cancer treatment-related lymphedema? A pilot study. *J Womens Health* (Larchmt) 2004;13:1008.
23. Mewes JC, Steuten LM, Ijzerman MJ, et al. Effectiveness of multidimensional cancer survivor rehabilitation and cost-effectiveness of cancer rehabilitation in general: a systematic review. *Oncologist*. 2012;17(12):1581–1593. Epub 2012/09/18. doi:10.1634/theoncologist.2012–0151. PubMed PMID: 22982580
24. Silver JK, Baima J, Newman R, et al. Cancer rehabilitation may improve function in survivors and decrease the economic burden of cancer to society. *Work* 2013;46:455–472.
25. Ganz P, et al. *Delivering High Quality Cancer Care*. Washington, DC: Institute of Medicine. National Academies; 2013.
26. Ziegelstein RC, Fiebach NH. "The mirror" and "the village": a new method for teaching practice-based learning and improvement and systems-based practice. *Acad Med*. 2004;79(1):83–88.

27. Johnson JK, Miller SH, Horowitz SD. Systems-based practice: improving the safety and quality of patient care by recognizing and mproving the systems in which we work. In: Henriksen K, Battles JB, Keyes MA, et al., eds. *Advances in Patient Safety: New Directions and Alternative Approaches* (Vol. 2: Culture and Redesign). Rockville, MD: Agency for Healthcare Research and Quality (US); 2008.
28. www.aapmr.org. Accessed January 4, 2013.
29. http://cme.med.harvard.edu/cmeups/pdf/03314597.pdf. Accessed January 4, 2013.
30. www.mskcc.org. Accessed January 4, 2013.
31. http://www.mskcc.org/education/fellowships/fellowship/cancer-rehabilitation-. Accessed December 14, 2013.
32. http://www.mdanderson.org/education-and-research/education-and-training/schools-and-programs/graduate-medical-education/residency-and-fellowship-programs/cancer-rehabilitation-fellowship.html. Accessed December 14, 2013.
33. http://me.e-aapmr.org/moc3.aspx. Accessed December 14, 2013.
34. http://now.aapmr.org/Pages/default.aspx. Accessed December 14, 2013.
35. Stubblefield MD, Odell MW, eds. *Cancer Rehabilitation, Principles and Practice*. New York, NY: Demos Medical Publishers; 2009.
36. http://humanism-in-medicine.org/. Accessed December 14, 2013.
37. Hartzband P, Groopman J. Keeping the patient in the equation—humanism and health care reform. *N Engl J Med*. 2009; 361(6):554–555.
38. Powe BD, Hamilton J, Hancock N, et al. Quality of life of African American cancer survivors. A review of the literature. *Cancer*. 2007;109(suppl 2):435–445.
39. Payne R, Medina E, Hampton JW. Quality of life concerns in patients with breast cancer: evidence for disparity of outcomes and experiences in pain management and palliative care among African-American women. *Cancer*. 2003;97(suppl 1):311–317.
40. Dietz JH. *Rehabilitation Oncology*. New York, NY: John Wiley & Sons; 1981.
41. American Cancer Society. *Cancer Facts and Figures 2012*. Atlanta, GA: American Cancer Society; 2012.
42. Siegel R, Descants C, Virgo K, et al. Cancer treatment and survivorship statistics 2012. *CA Cancer J Clin*. 2012;62:220–241.
43. http://www.amrpa.org/uploads/docuploads/Conference%20 2013/2013presentations/Cancer%20Rehab%20Program%20Standards%20MacDonell%20-%20Roberts.pdf. Accessed December 10, 2013.
44. Commission on Cancer. *Cancer Program Standards 2012: Ensuring Patient-Centered Care, Version 1.1*. Chicago, IL: American College of Surgeons; 2012. http://www.facs.org/cancer/coc/programstandards2012.pdf. Accessed December 14, 2013.
45. http://www.oncologyrehabpartners.com/star-certifications/star-program/. Accessed January 4, 2014.
46. Leonard M, Graham S. The human factor: the critical importance of effective teamwork and communication in providing safe care. *Qual Saf Health Care*. 2004;13(suppl 1):i85–i90.
47. Mewes JC, et al. Effectiveness of multidimensional cancer survivor rehabilitation and cost-effectiveness of cancer rehabilitation in general: a systematic review. *Oncologist*. 2012.
48. Stigt JA, et al. A randomized controlled trial of postthoracotomy pulmonary rehabilitation in patients with resectable lung cancer. *J Thorac Oncol*. February 2013;8(2):214–221.
49. Black JF. Cancer rehabilitation. http://emedicine.medscape.com/article/320261-overview. Updated March 19, 2013. Accessed January 4, 2014.
50. Brown JC, et al. Safety of weightlifting among women with or at risk for breast cancer-related lymphedema: musculoskeletal injuries and health care use in a weightlifting rehabilitation trial. *Oncologist* 2012;17(8):1120–1128.
51. www.ihi.org. Accessed January 4, 2014.

Michelle Stern
Antigone Arygriou
Roshni Durgam
Jennifer Gomez
Hejab Imteyaz
Rakhi Sutaria

13: Stroke

PATIENT CARE

GOALS

Provide patient care that is compassionate, appropriate, and effective for the treatment of a patient with stroke and the promotion of health.

OBJECTIVES

1. Describe the key components of the assessment of the patient with stroke.
2. Discuss the long-term outcomes of stroke.
3. Assess the impairments, activity limitations, and participation restrictions associated with stroke.
4. Describe the psychosocial, vocational, and educational aspects of stroke.
5. Describe potential injuries associated with stroke.
6. Formulate the key components of a rehabilitation treatment plan for the patient with stroke.

Issues that are relevant to patient care involve understanding the medical management of these patients in the acute care setting and beyond. But it begins with a thorough history and physical examination for these patients.

When taking the medical history of someone with a stroke, a chronological description of the development of the condition should be included. Risk factors associated with the stroke (both nonmodifiable and modifiable risk factors) should be assessed. Any prior workup to determine the cause (ischemic vs. hemorrhagic) should be identified.

In obtaining the rehabilitation history, it is important to ascertain the prior level of functioning, interests, avocations, vocation, social supports, and living environment. Review of systems should include all the systems as they may all be affected from both the acute and late effects of stroke.

Key elements of the physical examination particularly specific to stroke include assessments of the neurological and musculoskeletal systems. Neurological assessment should include motor and sensory testing, an evaluation of limb spasticity, swallowing, language issues, visual findings, and neglect. There are different syndromes determined by the location of the stroke. Determining the location and type of stroke will help guide the rehabilitation professional to determine the type of rehabilitation needed. Patients also need to be evaluated to determine the level of rehabilitation care they will need. Depending on their current and prior level of function, patients may require outpatient, acute, subacute, or long-term care following a stroke.

Assessment of rehabilitation needs and readiness for rehabilitation participation should, at a minimum, include the following:

Medical Stability

1. Medical workup and treatment plan
2. Stable vital signs for 24 hours
3. No chest pain within the past 24 hours, with the exception of stable angina or documented noncardiac conditions
4. No significant arrhythmia
5. No evidence of deep vein thrombosis (DVT)

Rehabilitation Needs

1. Cognitive capability of participating in rehabilitation
2. Willingness to participate in rehabilitation services
3. Adequate prior functional status
4. Capacity

It is important to determine whether the patient will be able to tolerate a 3-hour rehabilitation program and whether he or she has the ability to retain information. While under a physiatrist's care, the patient's decision-making capacity should be assessed. The key components of this are multifaceted—and it revolves around the patient's understanding of his or her condition and treatment options. The patient should be able to ascertain how it affects him or her and be able to express choices made. In stroke patients, this may prove to be rather difficult, given possible cognitive deficits and/or aphasia. Ultimately, clinical judgment prevails.

The patient's medical condition should be evaluated for level or complexity to determine if he or she will require a higher level of medical monitoring. The patient's support systems including friends and family in the community should be identified to ensure that the patient will have the necessary support to enable him or her to return to the community safely. The likelihood of motor recovery in a timely fashion should also be determined. For medical monitoring the clinician needs to think about preexisting medical illnesses that necessitate ongoing care (e.g., hypertension, diabetes mellitus [DM]), secondary poststroke complications (e.g., deep venous thrombosis, pneumonia), or acute poststroke exacerbations of preexisting chronic diseases (such as angina in a patient with ischemic heart disease). Management of these conditions can constitute major portions of the rehabilitation effort. Some patients may be more disabled by certain associated comorbid diseases than by the stroke itself. Some medical problems, such as heart disease, have been found to affect the course and outcome of rehabilitation adversely following a stroke. Medical complications can limit the patient's ability to participate in therapeutic exercise programs, inhibit functional skill performance, and reduce the likelihood of achieving favorable outcomes from rehabilitation. The rehabilitation interventions might also affect the medical condition adversely, causing an exacerbation of the disease or necessitating an adjustment in the treatment program. Patients who are treated in a stroke unit have medical complications that frequently occur during the postacute phase of rehabilitation, affecting up to 60% of patients (and up to 94% of patients with severe lesions) (1). Common medical complications have varied in different reports, but the most common complications seen after a stroke include aspiration, pneumonia, urinary tract infection, depression, musculoskeletal pain, complex regional pain syndrome (CRPS), falls, malnutrition, venous thromboembolism, and pressure ulcer (1).

RETURN TO COMMUNITY

National Stroke Association guidelines estimated that 10% of stroke survivors recover almost completely, 25% recover with minor impairments, 40% experience moderate to severe impairments requiring special care, 10% require care in a nursing home or other long-term care facility, and 15% die shortly after the stroke (2). Deutsch et al. concluded that patients with stroke, mild motor disabilities, and mild to no cognitive disabilities; patients with moderate and significant motor disabilities; and older patients with severe disabilities were significantly more likely to return to community from an inpatient rehabilitation facility rather than from a skilled nursing facility (3).

Some patients after a stroke are able to return to work (RTW). Treger noted in his article "Return to Work in Stroke Patients" that the reported rate was 19% to 73% (4). Patients more likely to RTW are those aged less than 65, a high education level, and white-collar employment. A negative predictor was the severity of the stroke. The clinician needs to work with the patient and realistically look at his or her job duties to determine if the patient will be able to RTW. The physiatrist may have to work with employers for modified work schedules on RTW. Those who are of working age and who are unable to work may need to be referred for disability.

Many stroke survivors belong to the retirement age, but one-third are younger than 65 years. In stroke patients younger than 65 years who are in the workforce, returning to work is associated with a sense of independence both socially and financially, and sense of well-being. Thus, for these younger stroke patients, RTW and community is an integral part of their rehabilitation goals in stroke recovery (5). There are some factors that help in decision making to RTW such as working years until retirement, occupation, and financial status (6). Studies have shown that weakness, neurological deficit, spasticity, and cognitive and speech impairment are negative predictors of RTW (7). In addition, activities of daily living (ADLs) is a strong predictor of RTW. The estimated rate of RTW varies widely from 11% to 85% in stroke population (4,8). Thus, it is imperative to take into account the needs and limitations to RTW in stroke survivors and set rehabilitation goals to attain maximum functional independence. The assessment of the workplace to accommodate the stroke patient function is part of the goal assessment.

Another concern for the poststroke population is return to driving. Driving requires vision, cognition, and muscular strength and physical function (9). Studies have shown that in stroke patients, fatigue, strength, and motor activity play a critical role in resumption of driving. Stroke patients might need driving evaluations, training, and adaptation to vehicles in order to return to safe driving. Rehabilitation interventions should focus on achieving safe driving assessment and training.

STROKE-RELATED IMPAIRMENTS

The risk of death after stroke is greatest in the first month and less for ischemic stroke than for hemorrhagic stroke. Thirty-day mortality after ischemic stroke is approximately 20% (10).

Death is more likely to occur from medical complications than from neurological complications. Those surviving have an increased death rate than age-matched controls. Recurrent stroke is a major cause of long-term morbidity and mortality. Recurrence is highest in patients with atherosclerosis and lowest in those with lacunar infarcts. Majority of stroke recovery occurs in the first 3 to 6 months, but cognitive and language deficits may continue to improve for up to a year later. Within 3 to 6 months, more than 85% of stroke survivors walk independently, two-thirds are independent with ADLs, and more than one-third have minimal disability (11). Bard and Hirschberg asserted that if no initial motion is noticed during the first 3 weeks or if motion in one segment is not followed within a week by the appearance of motion in a second segment, the prognosis for recovery of full motion is not favorable (12).

Factors predicting poor ADL outcome include the following: advanced age, myocardial infarction, DM, severe weakness, poor sitting balance, visuospatial deficits, cognitive changes, incontinence, and low initial ADL scores. Approximately one-third of patients with acute stroke have clinical features of aphasia. At 6 months or more after stroke, only 12% to 18% of patients have identifiable aphasia (13). Skilbeck and colleagues reported that patients with aphasia continue to show some late improvement in language function even more than 1 year after onset (14).

Patients who are classified initially as having Broca aphasia have variable outcomes. In patients with large hemisphere lesions, Broca aphasia persists with little recovery. Patients with smaller lesions confined to the posterior frontal lobe often show early progressive improvement, but the impairment may evolve into a milder form of aphasia with anomia and difficulty in finding words. Patients with global aphasia tend to progress slowly, with comprehension often improving more than expressive ability does.

The communicative ability of patients who initially have global aphasia improves over a longer period of time, up to a year or more post onset. Patients with global aphasia associated with large lesions may show only minor recovery, but recovery may be quite good in patients with smaller lesions. The extent of language recovery associated with Wernicke aphasia is variable.

The Stroke Unit Trialists' Collaboration Cochrane Review (updated in 2001) concluded, "Patients receiving organized inpatient stroke unit care were more likely to survive, regain independence, and return home than those receiving a less organized service" (15). The Cochrane review further concluded, "Acute stroke patients should be offered organized inpatient stroke unit care, typically provided by a coordinated multidisciplinary team operating within a discrete stroke ward that can offer a substantial period of rehabilitation, if required; there are no firm grounds for restricting access according to a patient's age, gender, or stroke severity" (15).

Recent studies from Thailand have helped shed better light on the medical complications during inpatient stroke rehabilitation as well as long-term morbidities in stroke survivors (16). Their experience showed that 70.3% of patients experienced at least one complication (16). Poststroke depression was found most commonly, followed by musculoskeletal pain, urinary tract infection, CRPS type 1, pneumonia, cardiovascular complications, falls, upper gastrointestinal bleeding, seizure, and pressure ulcers (16). History of myocardial infarction, low Barthel scores, urinary incontinence, indwelling catheters, and dysphagia were risk factors for complications. CRPS risk factor was limited shoulder range of motion (ROM). Their follow-up report looked at patients 1 year post stroke and evaluated the morbidities encountered. In order of the complications found 1 year post discharge were musculoskeletal pain, shoulder subluxation, depression, spasticity, joint contracture, urinary incontinence, dysphagia, pressure ulcer, infection, and neuropathic pain. Patients older than 60 years were more likely to develop complications. Please see Table 13.1 for the list of complications noted to occur with strokes; these should be kept in mind when treating stroke patients. Some of these topics will be discussed in further depth in this section.

TABLE 13.1 Complications of Stroke

COMPLICATIONS OF STROKE	RISK FACTORS	MONITORING	PREVENTION	QUALITY OF CARE
Neurological				
Seizure	Subarachnoid strokes greater risk for seizures	Monitor for clinical seizure or prolonged or intermittent stages of consciousness	May start levetiracetam and lamotrigine for poststroke seizure and epilepsy. Prophylactic treatment with an anti-epileptic drug (AED) not indicated (VA/DoD clinical practice guideline)	Seizure strikes about 22% of stroke survivors (epilepsy foundation)
Infections				
Urinary tract infections (UTI)	Immobility Indwelling catheters	Monitor for change level of consciousness Obtain UA and UCx if suspicious Monitor for urinary retention with postvoid residuals (PVRs)	Avoid indwelling catheters Initiation of early mobilization	In catheterized patients, the risk of urinary tract infection (UTI) is 5% per day, approaching 100% after 30 d Early treatment of colonization decreases the risk of catheter-associated UTI, with relative risk reduction as high as 75% Prophylactic antibiotic use is not recommended due to increase of resistance

(continued)

TABLE 13.1 Complications of Stroke (*continued*)

COMPLICATIONS OF STROKE	RISK FACTORS	MONITORING	PREVENTION	QUALITY OF CARE
Aspiration pneumonia	Severe dysphagia and abnormal pharyngeal sensation	Airway and oxygenation should be monitored Structured swallowing assessment	Initiation of early mobility Efficient pulmonary toileting Assessment of dysphagia by speech pathologist	Dysphagia occurs in approximately 45% of all stroke patients admitted and is associated with higher risk of aspiration pneumonia
Immobility Related				
Falls Contractures Pressure sores Pressure palsies	Lower body mass index (BMI) Peripheral vascular disease Diabetes mellitus Dependence on mobility	Bed and wheelchair alarms Proper positioning techniques	Encourage use of a commode, bedpan, or urinal every 2 hr during waking hours and every 4 hr at night Encourage nursing staff or family member to adhere to bathroom schedule Encourage use of a bedside commode	Pressure ulcers affect approximately 9% of all hospitalized patients and 23% of all nursing home patients
Thromboembolism				
DVT PE	Immobilization	Monitor for LE swelling or calf pain Monitor oxygen saturation, heart rate, and for any dyspnea	Range-of-motion exercises can be started during the first 24 hr poststroke SQ unfractionated heparin, LMWH, and heparinoids may be considered for immobilized patients with acute ischemic stroke If hemorrhage is a concern in the acute stroke, prophylactic prevention should include the use of bilateral–sequential compression devices	International Stroke Trial demonstrates that low-dose unfractionated heparin is safe to use in ischemic patients, recommended dose is 5,000 IU twice daily
Psychological				
Depression Anxiety Emotionalism Confusion	Overt feelings of sadness Loss of previous lifestyle Chemical and physiological changes in the brain Left frontal infarcts are 70% more likely to become depressed than those who experience similar devastating injuries	Nurse should educate the patient and family to recognize signs and symptoms of depression	Supportive therapy Cognitive behavioral therapy selective serotonin reuptake inhibitor (SSRI)/ tricyclic antidepressants (TCA)	Poststroke depression is estimated to occur in between 25% and 75% of poststroke patients. It is highly underdiagnosed, and stroke patients should be screened

(*continued*)

TABLE 13.1 Complications of Stroke (*continued*)

COMPLICATIONS OF STROKE	RISK FACTORS	MONITORING	PREVENTION	QUALITY OF CARE
Bowel and Bladder				
Constipation	Decreased mobility Inadequate fluid or food intake Depression Neurogenic bowel Unable to perceive bowel signals	Assess for bowel sounds and abdominal distension and evaluate the patient's fluid intake and hydration status	Bowel program that integrates the use of stool softeners, laxatives, suppositories, digital stimulation, and enemas Increase fluid and fiber intake Toileting schedule	Constipation and fecal impaction are more common after stroke than incontinence
Urinary dysfunction	Immobility	Bladder scanner can be used to evaluate PVRs and determine whether catheterization is necessary. If the PVR is >100, intermittent catheterization is recommended	Intermittent catheterization may be necessary to retrain the bladder	Approximately half of acute stroke patients have urinary incontinence. This number decreases to 20% 6 mo poststroke aspirin (ASA)

Immobility

Immobility can lead to pressure ulcers, atelectasis, contractures, and DVT/pulmonary embolus (PE). To help reduce these risks, the patient should be mobilized as soon as medically appropriate. Patients should be evaluated for need for specialized beds and the nursing staff instructed on proper positioning of patients to reduce skin breakdown, limb edema, and contractures. Prevention of pressure ulcers depends on early identification of patients at risk and reliable implementation of prevention strategies for patients identified to be at risk. As per Berlowtiz, patients at highest risk for skin breakdown are those with (a) dependence in mobility, (b) altered sensation, (c) fecal and urinary incontinence, (d) excessively low or high body mass index, and (e) diseases associated with cachexia (17). A valid and reliable pressure ulcer risk assessment tool, such as the Braden Scale, can help predict the risk of pressure ulcer development and thus help the rehabilitation team implement interventions to prevent skin breakdown.

DVT prevention should include the use of low-molecular-weight heparin (LMWH), heparinoid, or unfractionated heparin (if not already on warfarin). Without prophylaxis, a DVT can develop in up to 50% of patients with severe stroke (18).

The PREVAIL study determined that LMWH (40 mg per day, starting between 24 and 48 hours after stroke onset) was superior to using 5,000 units of unfractionated heparin twice daily (19,20). In patients who are not ambulatory, antiembolic stocking (i.e., compression stockings) and intermittent pneumatic compression may enhance the benefit from heparin treatment to reduce the incidence of DVT and DVT complications. Prevention of PE with the use of retrievable or permanent inferior vena cava filters (IVCFs) may be considered for some patients who have contraindications to anticoagulation and are at high risk.

Dysphagia

All stroke patients should have an evaluation for their swallow function. Dysphagia along with impaired cough and gag reflex are risk factors for developing aspiration pneumonia (ASPNA). Dehydration and nutritional deficiencies can occur as well. A formal swallow evaluation with video fluoroscopy or FEEST (flexible endoscopic evaluation of swallowing with sensory testing) may be required. The clinician should also be aware of the modified textures of food and liquids that are available at their facility and order appropriately. A nasogastric tube may be needed in some patients temporarily, and severe dysphagia or cognitive impairments may necessitate a PEG (percutaneous endoscopic gastrostomy tube) placement. Patients with decreased level of consciousness, multiple infarcts, brainstem infarcts, or large infarcts are at greatest risk for aspiration. The clinician can do a water swallowing test at bedside, with coughing, choking, or a wet voice after drinking being suggestive of aspiration.

Falls

Reported rate of falls is 40% in patients (21). Depression, cognitive impairment, and sensory deficits are increased risk factors for falls. Most falls occur when trying to transfer out of a wheelchair. There is also a high risk of falls in this patient population in the community, with 14% of patients falling, with the highest incidence in the first 6 months post discharge (21). It is also important to minimize medications that may cause orthostatic hypotension (e.g., polypharmacy) as well as to maintain proper hydration.

Orthostatic Hypotension

Orthostatic hypotension is a potential adverse effect of drugs used currently in the treatment of cardiovascular conditions such as hypertension and cardiac arrhythmias. Caution must be taken in the use of these medications as many have a diuretic effect, which may induce orthostatic hypotension. However, orthostatic hypotension is more common with medications such as alpha-1 blockers, adrenergic blockers, and centrally acting drugs. Drugs used for the treatment of psychiatric illnesses are all associated with orthostatic hypotension. See Table 13.2—orthostatic medications. The table lists common medications associated with drug-induced orthostatic hypotension.

The medical conditions for which the aforementioned medications are used are very common. Appropriate screening and monitoring of orthostatic hypotension should be routinely carried out to prevent falls, injuries, and further adverse effects.

Urinary Incontinence

Forty to sixty percent of people admitted to the hospital after a stroke can have problems with urinary incontinence, with 25% of stroke survivors still having problems on hospital discharge, and 15% remaining incontinent after 1 year (22). Increased age, increased stroke severity, the presence of diabetes, prostate hypertrophy in men, preexisting impairment in urinary function, and the occurrence of other disabling diseases increase the risk of urinary incontinence in stroke. Stroke survivors usually develop a hyperreflexic bladder. The development of a urinary tract infection can occur with prolonged catheter use, alterations in bladder emptying, or reduced fluid intake.

Constipation

Constipation and fecal impaction are more common after stroke than fecal incontinence. Immobility and inactivity, inadequate fluid or food intake, depression or anxiety, a neurogenic bowel, constipating side effects of medications, the inability to perceive bowel signals, lack of transfer ability, and cognitive deficits may each contribute to this problem. Goals of management are to ensure adequate intake of fluid, bulk, and fiber and to help the patient establish a regular toileting schedule. Stool softeners and judicious use of laxatives may be helpful. Patients on tube feeds may develop diarrhea. Fecal incontinence that does not clear 2 weeks poststroke is a poor prognostic indicator (23).

Spasticity

Sixty-five percent of stroke survivors develop spasticity after a stroke (24). Treatment options include stretching, ROM, and serial casting. While oral medication for spasticity is not as effective for spasticity from cerebral causes versus those of spinal origin, medication that can be used include baclofen, tizanidine, dantrolene and benzodiazepines. For long-term patients with spasticity, there is benefit from phenol and botulinum toxin injection. For more severe cases, intrathecal baclofen pumps have been used in select cases.

Hemiplegic Shoulder Pain

Lindgren found shoulder pain to be a frequent complication after stroke and impairs potential recovery and function (25). Poduri reports pain can occur as early as 2 weeks poststroke, but typically occurs 2 to 3 months after stroke (26). Suspected factors contributing to the syndrome include subluxation, contractures, CRPS, rotator cuff injury, and spastic muscle imbalance of the glenohumeral joint.

Depression

Major depression has been reported by Robinson and Spalletta to occur in 21.7% and minor depression in 19.5% of patients following a stroke (27). It is associated with worse long-term functional outcome after stroke, and treatment with antidepressant agents such as selective serotonin reuptake inhibitors have been shown to be beneficial.

Aspiration

An observational study assessed the factors that help decide the postacute level of care for stroke patients with ASPNA (28). It concluded that patients with ASPNA and a National Institutes of Health Stroke Scale (NIHSS) value of 7.44 or greater

TABLE 13.2 Orthostatic Medications

MEDICATION CLASS	MEDICATIONS
Alpha-1 antagonists	Terazosin
	Prazosin
	Doxazosin
Antihypertensives/vasodilators	Angiotensin-converting enzyme inhibitors
	Beta-blockers
	Alpha-beta-blockers
	Calcium channel blockers
	Clonidine
	Hydralazine
	Methyldopa
	Nitrates
	Dipyridamole
	Reserpine
Diuretics	Hydrochlorothiazide
	Loop diuretics
Anticholinergics	Oxybutynin
	Ditropan
Phosphodiesterase type 5 inhibitors	Sildenafil
	Vardenafil
Antidepressants	Tricyclic antidepressants
	Trazodone
	Monoamine oxidase inhibitors
Muscle relaxants	Baclofen
	Tizanidine
	Cyclobenzaprine
	Methocarbamol
Opioids	Morphine
	Oxycodone
	Tramadol

showed the need for additional postacute care. Those patients with ASPNA and an NIHSS value of 10.93 or greater showed the need for a skilled nursing facility or subacute care. Patients older than 69 years with ASPNA had increased chances of placement in subacute care (28).

Cardiac Precautions

A useful set of cardiac precautions in patients undergoing rehabilitation was developed by Fletcher et al. (29). Activity should be terminated if any of the following develops:

- New-onset cardiopulmonary symptoms
- Heart rate decreases more than 20% of baseline
- Heart rate increases more than 50% of baseline
- Systolic blood pressure (BP) increases to 240 mmHg
- Systolic BP decreases to ≥30 mmHg from baseline or to less than 90 mmHg
- Diastolic BP increases to 120 mmHg

STROKE RECOVERY AND ROLE OF REHABILITATION

For patients further out from stroke, Pang found there is strong evidence that aerobic exercise (40%–50% heart rate reserve (HRR) progressing to 60%–80%) conducted 20 to 40 minutes and 3 to 5 days per week is beneficial for enhancing aerobic fitness, walking speed, and walking endurance in people who have had mild to moderate stroke and are deemed to have low cardiovascular risk with exercise after proper screening assessments (grade A recommendation) (30). The effects of aerobic exercise on other health outcomes require further study.

Motor pattern of recovery from stroke was discussed in the classic articles by Twitchell, who detailed stages of recovery from a flaccid state to a progressive increase in tone (31). It also details the synergy patterns that develop in the upper and lower extremities during the recovery phase. In middle cerebral artery (MCA) strokes, proximal recovery occurs before distal, lower extremity recovers before upper extremity, and synergy patterns develop before isolated voluntary movement. In a study of 188 patients with stroke, Nijland et al. found that assessment of finger extension and shoulder abduction within 72 hours after stroke can help to predict upper limb recovery (32). If, by the second day following stroke, patients in whom upper limb motor function was affected were capable of some voluntary extension of the fingers and some abduction of the hemiplegic shoulder, there was a 0.98 probability that they would regain some dexterity by 6 months. Patients with no such voluntary movement on the second day had only a 0.25 probability of regaining dexterity by 6 months. Full recovery at 6 months was achieved in 60% of patients with some early finger extension (29).

There are various different therapy techniques that have been used during the rehabilitation process. The most commonly used models consist of (a) traditional therapy, (b) Bobath concept—neurodevelopmental training (see Table 13.3), (c) proprioceptive neuromuscular facilitation (PNF) (see Table 13.4), and (d) Brunnstrom (see Table 13.5). Traditional therapy includes ROM, strengthening, mobilization, and compensatory

TABLE 13.3 Neurofacilitation Technique

Bobath's Technique:

Aims to inhibit spasticity and synergies, using inhibitory postures and movements, and to facilitate normal autonomic responses that are involved in voluntary movement

TABLE 13.4 Proprioceptive Technique

Proprioceptive Neuromuscular Facilitation Technique:

Uses quick stretching and manual resistance of muscle activation of the limbs in functional directions, which are often spiral and diagonal in direction

TABLE 13.5 Brunnstrom Stages

Stage 1	Immediately following the stroke is flaccid paralysis
Stage 2	Recovery begins with developing spasticity: At this time, development of minimal movement is seen in synergies
Stage 3	Spasticity becomes more pronounced and patient gains voluntary control through synergy pattern: Voluntary movement is synergy dependent
Stage 4	Spasticity begins to decline: Some movements come out of synergy
Stage 5	Spasticity continues to decline: Movement is almost independent of synergy
Stage 6	Normal movement with normal speed

techniques (see Table 13.3). In his article about the effectiveness of the Bobath concept, Kollen describes it as the most popular treatment approach used, but limited data to support its superiority (33). Persons with motor deficiencies following stroke are unable to direct nervous impulses to muscles in the different combinations used by persons with an intact central nervous system (CNS). The goal is to suppress abnormal muscle patterns before normal patterns are introduced. Abnormal patterns are modified at proximal key points of control, such as the neck, spine, shoulder, and pelvis. PNF stimulates nerve/muscle/sensory receptors to evoke response through manual stimuli to increase ease of movement and promote function. Brunnstrom encourages synergy patterns that develop after stroke through the use of cutaneous/proprioceptive stimuli. Other therapy protocols that are currently being evaluated include the use of constraint therapy as well as the role of robotics (see Table 13.6)

TABLE 13.6 Constraint-Induced Therapy

Forces the individual to use the impaired limb by constraining the unaffected extremity

Brunnstrom stages: Synergistic patterns that develop during recovery from a stroke. A patient can plateau at any of these stages but will generally follow this sequence if one makes it to full recovery.

MEDICAL KNOWLEDGE

GOALS

Demonstrate knowledge of established and evolving biomedical, clinical, epidemiological, and sociobehavioral sciences pertaining to stroke, as well as the application of this knowledge to guide holistic patient care.

OBJECTIVES

1. Describe the epidemiology, anatomy, physiology, and pathophysiology of stroke.
2. Identify the pertinent laboratory and imaging studies important in stroke.
3. Review the treatment and management of stroke.

Taking care of stroke patients is a challenge for the rehabilitation specialist. There is a large spectrum of symptoms and outcomes for the different stroke syndromes. This chapter will focus on issues the provider needs to understand in order to best care for patients after developing a stroke. To understand how to manage patients with stroke, the clinician must be aware of the pathophysiology of the type of stroke that person has, the likelihood of recovery, and the long-term implications for the patient. We will first start off describing the various stroke subtypes and provide insight into what the clinician should be aware of.

It is imperative that the rehabilitation specialist is aware of the stroke subtype his or her patient has, as this will lead to differences in recovery and complications. Stroke can be divided into ischemic or hemorrhagic lesions, with the ischemic lesions being the predominant subtype (see Table 13.7). Though there are many different causes of stroke, this is out of the scope of this chapter. The most common causes and those seen most often in the rehabilitation setting will be discussed in this chapter.

Stroke is one of the four leading causes of death and the number one cause of severe neurological disability in adults. In the United States, there are four million stroke survivors and more than 750,000 new strokes each year (34,35). Risk factors for stroke include both modifiable and nonmodifiable causes, which are listed in Table 13.8.

TABLE 13.7 Types of Stroke

Ischemic lesion	Hemorrhagic lesion
Thrombotic	Intracerebral
Embolic	Subarachnoid

TABLE 13.8 Stroke Risk Factors

NONMODIFIABLE RISK FACTORS FOR STROKE	MODIFIABLE RISK FACTORS FOR STROKE
Age (most important risk factor) Risk increases after age 55 and doubles after each decade after 55	Heart disease (congestive heart failure, coronary artery disease, valvular heart disease) Atrial fibrillation (increases risk of embolic stroke by 5)
Race (African Americans greater than Whites greater than Asians)	Diabetes (twofold increased risk) Hypercoagulable states
Sex (male greater than female)	Hypertension Cigarette smoking Carotid stenosis
Family history	Hyperlipidemia Alcohol and cocaine use

ISCHEMIC STROKE

An ischemic stroke is caused by focal cerebral ischemia. There are several different mechanisms that can disrupt blood flow in the brain. The neurological deficits manifested after stroke will depend on the vascular distribution affected by the stroke. Eighty-five percent of strokes are ischemic in nature (36). Ischemic strokes can be further subdivided into thrombotic or embolic.

The Trial of Org 10172 in Acute Stroke Treatment (TOAST) classification system for ischemic stroke is based on the underlying stroke mechanisms (37):

1. *Large artery atherosclerosis: Intracranial, extracranial (carotid, aortic arch)*: Usually occurs during sleep and patient awakens unaware of deficits. Deficits may have an insidious progression over the course of 24 to 48 hours.
2. *Cardioembolic*: The source of embolic strokes is most often cardiac in nature as up to 75% of all cardiac emboli travel up to the brain, causing an ischemic stroke. Cardiac conditions that can cause stroke include atrial fibrillation, segmental wall akinesis, paradoxical embolus, patent foramen ovale, and congestive heart failure. Atrial fibrillation alone is associated with a four to five times increased risk of ischemic stroke. The rapid cardiac fibrillations induce the formation of thrombi that can embolize and enter the cerebral circulation. Vegetations on heart valves in endocarditis or prosthetic heart valves can also be a cause. Embolic strokes have a sudden onset and usually occur when patients are awake.
3. *Small vessel: Lacunar infarction* Lacunes are small infarcts that may be seen in the putamen, pons, thalamus, caudate, and internal capsule. They are caused by the occlusion of small 50 to 200 mm arteries of deep penetrating branches of larger

blood vessels. Lacunar infarcts are highly associated with hypertension. Since lacunar infarcts affect smaller vessels, they usually do not involve higher cortical functions, which remain intact following stroke.

4. *Other:* Vessel dissection, venous thrombosis, drug induced
5. *Cryptogenic*

There are other rarer causes for ischemic stroke that account for less than 5%. In patients under 30, 20% of those strokes can be caused by an arterial dissection (38). There are also other causes that are related to vascular (fibromuscular dysplasia, moyamoya disease, cerebral autosomal dominant arteriopathy with subcortical infarcts and leukoencephalopathy (CADASIL) syndrome), hematological (sickle cell disease, polycythemia vera, essential thrombocytosis, thrombotic thrombocytopenic purpura (TTP), Waldenstrom macroglobulinemia, hypercoagulable states), inflammatory (vasculitis), drug related, infectious, malignant, or metabolic causes, as well as migraines. Again for the purpose of this chapter, the focus is on the most common stroke subtypes.

There are many different stroke syndromes (Table 13.9) to be aware of. Each syndrome will have important implications throughout the rehabilitation process.

These can be divided based on anatomy into (a) MCA syndrome, (b) anterior cerebral artery (ACA) syndrome, (c) internal carotid artery syndrome, (d) posterior cerebral artery (PCA) syndrome, and (e) vertebrobasilar syndrome.

ANATOMY

Anterior Circulation
Middle Cerebral Artery

- Occlusion occurs at the stem of the MCA or at one of the two main divisions (superior or inferior) of the artery in the Sylvian sulcus.

Superior division of the MCA:

- The superior division of MCA supplies the rolandic and pre-rolandic areas.
- Patients will present with sensory and motor deficits on the contralateral face and arm more than on leg.
- Head and eyes will deviate toward affected side.
- Dominant hemispheric lesions on the left side will present with global aphasia or Broca's aphasia.
- Nondominant right-sided lesion will cause visual spatial deficits, hemineglect, and apraxia.

Inferior division of the MCA:

- The inferior division of the MCA supplies the lateral temporal and inferior parietal lobes. Lesions affecting this territory will present with superior quadrantanopia or homonymous hemianopsia.
- They will also present with Wernicke aphasia if the lesion is on the left and visual neglect if the lesion is on the right.

TABLE 13.9 Ischemic Stroke Syndromes

VASCULAR SUPPLY	SYNDROME	LOCALIZATION	CLINICAL SYMPTOMS
Middle Cerebral Artery	Ataxic hemiparesis	Posterior limb external capsule Pons	Contralateral ataxia and weakness
	Gerstmann syndrome	Dominant parietal lobe	Agraphia Acalculia Finger agnosia Left–right disorientation
	Inferior division		Contralateral: homonymous Hemianopia Upper quad anopsia Constructional apraxia Receptive aphasia
	Superior division		Contralateral: Weakness—lower half face, upper and lower extremity Hemisensory loss extremities and face Hemineglect Expressive aphasia
Posterior Cerebral Artery	Alexia without agrapha	Left occipital region and Splenium of corpus collosum	Alexia Contralateral–homonymous hemianopia

(continued)

TABLE 13.9 Ischemic Stroke Syndromes (*continued*)

VASCULAR SUPPLY	SYNDROME	LOCALIZATION	CLINICAL SYMPTOMS
Posterior Cerebral Artery (cont.)	Balint syndrome	Bilateral parietal–occipital lobes	Loss of voluntary extraocular movemets (EOM) Optic ataxia Asimultagnosia
	Claude syndrome	Midbrain-Tegmentum	Ipsilateral-oculomotor nerve palsy Contralateral—extremity ataxia
	Anton-Babinski syndrome	Bilateral occipital lobes	Bilateral vision loss with unawareness of blindness
	Dejerine-Roussy syndrome (thalamic pain syndrome)	ventral posterlateral nucleus (VPL) and ventral posteromedial nucleus (VPM) nuclei of thalamus	Contralateral sensation loss followed by dysethesia or allodynia
	Weber syndrome	Midbrain-base	Contralateral weakness Ipsilateral lateral gaze weakness
	Unilateral occipital	Occipital and Inferomedial temporal lobes	Contralateral—homonymous hemianopia
	Ventral pontine syndrome	Ventral medial pons	Ipsilateral lateral rectus paresis Contralateral hemiplegia with facial sparing
Anterior Inferior Cerebellar Artery	Lateral pontine syndrome (Marie-Foix syndrome)	Lateral pons and middle cerebellar peduncle	Ipsilateral: - Ataxia - Facial pain and temperature sensory loss - Hearing loss - Facial paralysis - Nystagmus Contralateral: - Trunk and extremity pain and temperature sensory loss
Posterior Inferior Cerebellar Artery	Lateral medullary syndrome (Wallenberg syndrome)	Upper part of medulla oblongata and the inferior cerebellar peduncle	Ipsilateral: - Ataxia - Facial pain and temperature sensory loss - Horner syndrome - Dysphagia - Vertigo - Nystagmus Contralateral: - Trunk and extremity pain and temperature sensory loss - Hiccups
Basilar Artery	Ataxic hemiparesis	Posterior limb external capsule	Contralateral weakness Contralateral ataxia
	Anton-Babinski syndrome	Bilateral occipital lobes	Bilateral vision loss with unawareness of blindness

(*continued*)

TABLE 13.9 Ischemic Stroke Syndromes (continued)

VASCULAR SUPPLY	SYNDROME	LOCALIZATION	CLINICAL SYMPTOMS
Basilar artery (cont.)	Lateral pontine syndrome (Marie–Foix syndrome)	Lateral pons and middle cerebellar peduncle	Ipsilateral: - Ataxia - Facial pain and temperature sensory loss - Hearing loss - Facial paralysis - Nystagmus Contralateral: - Trunk and extremity pain and temperature sensory loss
	Inferior medial pontine syndrome (Foville syndrome)	Pons	Contralateral weakness Ipsilateral lateral gaze palsy and facial weakness
	Medial medullary syndrome (Dejerine syndrome)	Medial medulla	Contralateral weakness and loss of vibration and proprioception Ipsilateral tongue weakness and atrophy
	Ventral pontine syndrome (Raymond syndrome)	Ventral medial pons	Ipsilateral lateral gaze weakness Contralateral weakness
	Ventral pontine syndrome (Millard-Gubler syndrome)	Basis pontis Fascicles of CN VI and CN VII	Contralateral weakness Ipsilateral lateral gaze weakness
	Locked-in syndrome	Bilateral ventral pons	Preserved consciousness and sensation with paralysis Sparing of vertical gaze and eyelid opening

Anterior Cerebral Artery

Occlusion at the stem of the ACA, proximal to its connection with the anterior communicating artery, usually does not cause significant deficits because of sufficient collateral circulation available from the opposite side.

Depending on anatomical variation, both anterior cerebral arteries may originate from the same stem. An infarction of the ACA in this case can cause major disturbances such as aphasia, paraplegia, incontinence, and frontal lobe impairments.

Occlusion of one ACA distal to the anterior communicating artery will result in contralateral weakness and contralateral sensory loss with minimal involvement of the upper extremities. Urinary incontinence and gait apraxia with a contralateral grasp reflex may also be present. Transcortical motor aphasia may occur in left-sided involvement.

Internal Carotid Artery

The most common area of occlusion of the internal carotid artery (ICA) is beyond the carotid bifurcation. While these occlusions can be asymptomatic in many patients, occlusion of the ICA can manifest as a variety of syndromes with a variable presentation depending on the severity of the infarction and the degree of collateral circulation.

Distal ICA occlusion may affect part or all of the ipsilateral MCA territory as well. Patients will present with contralateral motor and/or sensory symptoms.

Complete ICA occlusion will have a variable clinical presentation. In those with sufficient collateral circulation, symptoms may not be present; however, complete occlusion of the ICA can potentially cause a massive infarction involving the ACA and MCA territory with motor and sensory symptoms found on the contralateral side.

If the retinal branch or central retinal artery is occluded, ocular infarction may occur, causing visual deficits. Transient monocular blindness, also known as amaurosis fugax, can be seen prior to the onset of stroke in a small subset of patients due to transient occlusion of the ICA. Complete infarction of the central retinal artery is extremely rare due to the ample amount of collateral circulation available in this region.

Posterior Circulation
Posterior Cerebral Artery
The PCA supplies the upper brainstem, the inferior parts of the temporal lobe, and the medial parts of the occipital lobe. Clinical presentations vary depending on the area of occlusion as well as anatomical variations.

Seventy percent of the time, both PCAs arise from the basilar artery and are connected to the internal carotids through the posterior communicating artery. Twenty to twenty-five percent of the time, one PCA comes from the basilar artery and the other PCA comes from the ICA. Five to ten percent of the time, both PCAs arise from the carotid arteries (39).

Infarcts of the PCA will present with visual field deficits, loss of ability to read (alexia), and loss of power to comprehend written or spoken words with repetition intact (transcortical sensory aphasia). The oculomotor (CN3) and trochlear (CN4) nuclei and nerves can also be involved.

Vertebrobasilar System
The vertebrobasilar arteries supply the midbrain, pons, medulla, cerebellum, and the posterior and ventral aspects of the cerebral hemispheres. Vertebral arteries originate from the subclavian arteries and are the main arteries of the medulla. At the pontomedullary junction, the two vertebral arteries join to form the basilar artery, which supply the pons and midbrain.

The cerebellum is supplied by the posterior inferior cerebellar artery (PICA) from the vertebral arteries and by branches of the basilar artery—anterior inferior cerebellar artery (AICA) and superior cerebellar artery.

Symptoms of vertebrobasilar infarction include vertigo and nystagmus, ipsilateral cranial nerve dysfunction, as well as ipsilateral motor or sensory deficits of the face and contralateral side of the body, ataxia, dysphagia, and dysarthria. Cortical involvement is spared.

Lacunar Infarcts
Pure motor stroke/hemiparesis, the most common lacunar syndrome, is located in posterior limb of the internal capsule, basis pontis, and corona radiata.

Ataxic hemiparesis, the second most frequent lacunar syndrome, is typically associated with a small deep infarction in the pons, internal capsule, or corona radiata. Dysarthria/clumsy hand syndrome is typically localized to the upper basis pontis, corona radiata, and anterior limb or genu of the internal capsule. The main symptoms are dysarthria and clumsiness of the hand. Pure sensory stroke is localized at the contralateral thalamus (VPL), pons, and posterior corona radiata.

Those who suffer lacunar strokes have a greater chance of survival beyond 30 days (96%) than those with other types of stroke (85%), and they also have better survival beyond a year (87% versus 65%–70%) (40). Between 70% and 80% with lacunar strokes are functionally independent at 1 year, compared with fewer than 50% otherwise (40).

HEMORRHAGIC STROKE

Hemorrhagic strokes are not as common as ischemic, but they have a higher rate of morbidity and mortality among the stroke population. Intracerebral hemorrhage (ICH) is bleeding directly in the brain parenchymal tissue, and subarachnoid hemorrhage (SAH) is due to a rupture of a vessel in the cerebrospinal fluid.

The most preventable risk factor is hypertension for ICH (41). Other risk factors include smoking, heavy alcohol (ETOH) use, and drugs (cocaine, amphetamines) (41,42). Secondary ICH occurs in a minority of patients in association with vascular abnormalities, tumors, or impaired coagulation (43,44). Cerebral amyloid angiopathy–associated ICH is seen in patients older than 70 years. ICH has propensity to certain brain sites such as basal ganglia (40%–50%), lobar regions (20%–50%), thalamus (10%–15%), pons (5%–12%), cerebellum (5%–10%), and other brainstem sites (1%–5%) (43,44). Herniation syndromes, which are potentially fatal, are seen as a result of increased intracranial pressure (ICP) from displacement of brain parenchyma (45). Other consequences of elevated ICP may be mass effect, intraventricular extension of hemorrhage (IVH) that may manifest as headache, nausea, vomiting, seizures, focal neurological deficits, and altered mental status requiring intubation in these patients. Consequently, these patients may need urgent evacuation of the hemorrhage to relieve the ICP, such as ventriculostomy. Age, Glasgow Coma Score (GCS), initial hematoma size, expansion and presence of IVH location of hemorrhage (supra versus infratentorial location), and patient's age are the major prognostic factors in ICH stroke (41). About 30% to 50% of patients survive, and those who do may show a better recovery than their ischemic stroke counterparts in terms of function (46).

Intracranial saccular aneurysms represent the most common etiology of nontraumatic SAH. Over the past several decades, the incidence of other types of strokes has decreased; however, the incidence of SAH has not decreased. Due to the nature of SAH, these patients are likely to be younger and have a longer ICU stay than other stroke syndromes and have different complications. Aneurysms usually occur in the terminal portion of the ICA and the branching sites on the large cerebral arteries in the anterior portion of the circle of Willis. A meta-analysis by Wermer and group showed an annual rupture risk of 0.6% to 1.3% (47). Subgroup analyses revealed that asymptomatic aneurysms were four to five times less likely to rupture than symptomatic aneurysms. Those aneurysms that were smaller than 5 mm were two to three times less likely to rupture than aneurysms larger than <space> 5 mm. The same study also showed anterior circulation aneurysms were two to three times less likely to rupture than posterior circulation aneurysms (those involving the vertebrobasilar system or posterior cerebral arteries) (47). Clipping or coiling aneurysms is the surgical approach to prevent rebleeding. The left ventricular systolic dysfunction is thought to be due to excessive release of norepinephrine from myocardial sympathetic nerves, which could damage both myocytes and nerve terminals. Though SAH can occur from childhood onward, the incidence is most common between ages 40 and 60 years (48). Prevalence is also 1.6 times higher in women than in men (48).

Cognitive deficits are present even in many patients considered to have a good outcome. Complications of SAH include the following: hydrocephalus, rebleeding, delayed cerebral ischemia from vasospasm, ICH, IVH, left ventricular systolic dysfunction, subdural hematoma, seizures, increased ICP, and myocardial infarction. Nimodipine is used to help reduce vasospasms.

STROKE WORKUP

Patients presenting with stroke will require an in-depth workup to determine the type and etiology of their stroke. See Table 13.10 for a list of diagnostic tests.

One of the main components of the stroke workup is the carotid ultrasound examination. This test evaluates the arterial blood flow for stenosis and plaques along the carotid wall. If significant stenosis is identified the clinician will often discuss interventional treatment options. Physiatrists should be familiar with the landmark Carotid Revascularization Endarterectomy versus Stenting Trial (CREST), which compared the outcomes of carotid artery stenting with those of carotid endarterectomy among patients with symptomatic or asymptomatic extracranial carotid stenosis (49). The 2010 CREST trial found no significant difference, after 4 years of follow-up, between surgery and carotid stenting (49). Overall, patients younger than 70 years had better outcomes with stenting, while the older population tended to have better outcomes with surgery. The study concluded that both carotid artery stenting and carotid endarterectomy are considerable options in the treatment of carotid stenosis and that age may be a considerable factor in determining which treatment option will have a better outcome for patients.

TABLE 13.10 Stroke Workup

Labs	1. Complete blood count, including platelets
	2. Serum electrolytes, urea nitrogen, creatinine, liver function test
	3. Prothrombin time and international normalized ratio (INR), activated partial thromboplastin time
	4. HgA1C
	5. Lipid panel
	6. Homocysteine
Cardiac studies	1. ECG (electrocardiogram)
	2. Echocardiogram: Transthoracic echocardiography (TTE)/transesophageal echocardiography (TEE) studies are used to assess heart valves and look for cardiac abnormalities that could contribute to stroke such as a mural thrombus or patent foramen ovale
	3. Holter monitor
Imaging	1. CT scans are more useful in the acute phase because they can detect the presence of a hemorrhage and guide treatment options if one is detected. In acute infarcts, CT scans are often normal. Infarcted areas appear as hypodense (black) usually after 24–48 hours after the stroke. Subtle CT changes may be seen early with large infarcts, such as obscuration of gray/white matter junction, sulcal effacement, or early hypodensity. Edema can be seen on the third or fourth day as a well-defined hypodense area
	2. MRI of the brain is more sensitive than CT scan in detecting ischemic infarcts (including small lacunes) and posterior cranial fossa infarcts, which are not visualized on CT scan. Early infarcts appear as increased (white) signal intensities on T2-weighted images, more pronounced after 24 hours up to 1 week. T1-weighted images may show mildly decreased signal. Chronic infarcts may show decreased T1- and T2-weighted signals
	3. MRA: Extracranial and intracranial arteries are also common sources of brain embolism and should be studied
	4. Angiography: Angiography may also be performed to evaluate blood vessels and check circulation. They are particularly useful in detecting vascular anomalies such as aneurysms, vascular malformations, arterial dissections, narrowed or occluded vessels, and angiitis
	5. Transcranial Doppler ultrasonography is useful for evaluating more proximal vascular anatomy through the infratemporal fossa, including the MCA, intracranial carotid artery, and vertebrobasilar artery
	6. Other imaging studies include carotid ultrasound with real-time B-mode imaging and direct Doppler examination, which can detect carotid stenosis or ulcerative plaques

(continued)

TABLE 13.10 Stroke Workup (*continued*)

Toxicology screen	In selected patients, for example, young adults toxic screen is useful 1. Blood alcohol level 2. Cocaine 3. Other toxins
Specific test	1. Lumbar puncture if subarachnoid hemorrhage is suspected and head CT scan is negative for blood 2. Electroencephalogram if seizures are suspected
Patients under the age of 50 should be worked up for hypercoagulable disorders	They will need the following laboratory tests: Lupus anticoagulant, cardiolipin Abs, protein C and protein S activity, AT III activity, factor V Leiden, prothrombin gene mutation, activated protein C resistance, beta-2, glycoprotein 1 Abs, MTHFR mutation, HIT antibodies, and serum HB electrophoresis can be considered

FUNCTIONAL EVALUATION

The physical functioning in stroke patients can be assessed by a number of measures such as the functional independence measure (FIM), NIH Stroke Scale, Barthel Index, and modified Rankin Scale (mRS). FIM is the most widely used scale in the rehabilitation field. It is an 18-item ordinal scale that is used during inpatient rehabilitation to monitor progress. FIM was created in 1996 by the Guide for Uniform Data System for Medical Rehabilitation (UDSMR) (www.udsmr.org). The Centers for Medicare and Medicaid services (CMS) use the UDSMR FIM instrument for Inpatient Rehabilitation Facility Prospective Payment System.

The Barthel Index of ADLs rates each ADL on an ordinal scale. The ADLs that are graded are as follows: feeding, bathing, grooming, dressing, bowels, bladder, toilet use, transfers (bed to chair and back), mobility, and stair negotiations. The scale ranges from 0 to 100. The highest score of 100 indicates full independence in all of these categories and 0 indicates a bedridden, fully dependent state. A higher number on the scale is associated with a greater likelihood of independence of the patient following discharge from the hospital.

The NIH Stroke Scale is used as a clinical assessment tool to evaluate acuity of stroke patients, determine appropriate treatment, and predict patient outcome. It is an abridged neurological examination that allows the clinician to evaluate consciousness, cranial nerve function, motor activity, sensation, language, and speech. Physiatrists should familiarize themselves with the scale, which can be found online at www.ninds.nih.gov/doctors/NIH_Stroke_Scale.pdf

The mRS was created in 1957 by Dr. John Rankin of Stobhill Hospital Glasgow, Scotland, and modified by Prof. C. Warlow's group at Western General Hospital in Edinburgh. The mRS measures the degree of disability or dependence in carrying out ADLs in stroke patients.

PRACTICE-BASED LEARNING AND IMPROVEMENT

GOALS

Demonstrate competence in continuously investigating and evaluating your own stroke patient care practices, appraise and assimilate scientific evidence, and continuously improving your patient care practices based on constant self-evaluation and lifelong learning.

OBJECTIVES

1. Describe learning opportunities for providers, patients, and caregivers with experience in stroke.
2. Locate some resources including available websites for continuing medical education and continuing professional development.
3. Describe some areas paramount to self-assessment and lifelong learning, such as review of current guidelines, including evidence based, in treatment and management of patients with stroke and the role of the physiatrist as the educator of patients, families, residents, students, colleagues, and other health professionals.

There is still so much that needs to be learned about stroke recovery. It is imperative for the new clinician to stay abreast on all the latest details regarding treatment and recovery from stroke. There is a wealth of material regarding stroke and new treatment protocols are being developed. Outcomes measures that should be looked at include morbidity, mortality, quality of life, functional status, patient satisfaction, access to care, and utilization of health care. Effective rehabilitation improves functional outcomes. The most widely used measure is the FIM score, and the physiatrist should be aware of scoring. This tool has been tested, but it still lacks the ability to monitor the patient's ability to carry out more complex tasks such as shopping, meal preparation, use of telephone, driving a car, and money management. New stroke-specific outcome measures such as the Stroke Impact Scale may be more comprehensive. Cochrane Reviews (www.cochrane.org) is a useful resource in obtaining the latest recommendations based on evidence decision making. The evidence-based stroke review of stroke rehabilitation (www.ebrsr.com) may serve as a resource for information as well as the VA/DoD clinical practice guidelines for management of stroke (50).

A 2010 article by Reeves looked at the development of stroke performance measures, definitions, methods, and current measures (51). Based on recommendations from the 2008 report from the American College of Cardiology/American Heart Association (ACC/AHA), Get With The Guidelines®-Stroke is an in-hospital program for improving stroke care by promoting consistent adherence to the latest scientific treatment guidelines. Ten process-based performance measures relevant to acute hospital-based stroke care have now been developed and endorsed (51). These measures include intravenous thrombolysis, DVT prophylaxis, dysphagia screening, stroke education, discharge-related medications (antithrombotic therapy, cholesterol-reducing agents), smoking cessation, and assessment for rehabilitation (51).

There are currently at least five major U.S.-based stroke quality improvement programs implementing stroke measures. Data indicate that rapid improvements in the quality of stroke care can be induced by the systematic collection and evaluation of stroke performance measures. However, current stroke measures are relatively limited, addressing only inpatient care and mostly patients with ischemic stroke. Stroke quality improvement is still in its early stages, but data suggest that large-scale improvements in stroke care can result from the implementation of stroke performance measures. Performance measures that address multidisciplinary stroke unit care, outpatient-based care, and patient-oriented outcomes such as functional recovery should be considered. Ongoing challenges relevant to stroke quality improvement include the role of public reporting and the need to link better stroke care to improved patient outcomes.

Other organizations monitoring include The Joint Commission, which identifies centers that make exceptional efforts to improve patient outcomes and comply with clinical guidelines. The CMS also has an incentive with pay reporting program for clinicians and hospitals.

INTERPERSONAL AND COMMUNICATION SKILLS

GOALS

Demonstrate interpersonal and communication skills that result in the effective exchange of information and collaboration with patients, their families, and other health professionals.

OBJECTIVES

1. Demonstrate skills used in effective communication and collaboration with patients with stroke and their caregivers, across socioeconomic and cultural backgrounds.
2. Delineate the importance of the role of the physiatrist as the interdisciplinary team leader and consultant pertinent to stroke.
3. Demonstrate proper documentation and effective communication between health care professional team members in patient care as it applies to stroke.

Physiatrists specialize in identifying the medical needs and goals of patients who have suffered strokes. They are responsible for directing the multiple teams that are involved in patient care and bridging communication between such members. Furthermore, the patient's caregivers and loved ones need to be fully educated on the patient's stroke prognosis and recovery.

Stroke is one of the foremost leading causes of disability, and the impact this has on patients and their families is immense. Stroke patients and their family members are faced with making many decisions regarding immediate medical care, as well as short-term and long-term follow-up. It is imperative to provide appropriate education and counseling to help patients and their caregivers make informed decisions about their care and to assist them in adjusting to any new roles that are emerging. Family meetings comprised of the medical team, patient, and their caregivers provide the perfect platform for open exchange of information. During these meetings, the physiatrist will be the team leader and have the responsibility of counseling and educating the patient and his or her loved ones on the treatment plan. As team leader, the physiatrist must remember to be empathetic and consider both the patient's wishes and the family's when deciding care.

A multidisciplinary approach involving occupational therapists, physical therapists, neuropsychologists, speech pathologists, nursing staff, orthotists, social workers, and physicians enables a panoramic view. To optimize care, all team members should be aware of the subset of stroke, the resultant deficits, and the prognosis for recovery. Team members should be working together in setting goals and all relaying the same information to the patient and family. Careful documentation is important in identifying the rehabilitation goals and needs of the patient. In particular, functional recoveries and motor gains should be recorded so team members may track the progress and adjust short- and long-term goals accordingly.

Together, the team can be the ultimate patient advocate. It is the role of the medical team to educate the patient and his or her family on the risks of the patient's type of stroke and the appropriate lifestyle modifications to prevent a secondary event. The patient should feel included in the rehabilitation treatment plan and should understand his or her rehabilitation potential. As providers, it is important to recognize the fears and frustrations undertaken by the patient.

The challenges presented in stroke patients run a large range. They might be losing their independence and their role in the family and have difficulty with speech and comprehension, making communication challenging or feeling frustrated over modifications needed in their diet. After a stroke, a large number of patients will likely not return to their previous baseline of function and their frustration and fear must be understood by the clinician. They must learn to adjust to their new limitations safely, and the medical team can aid this process by providing and explaining the role of adaptive equipment such as walkers, wheelchairs, or orthotics and the process of the rehabilitation program. Communication is key and patience is essential when guiding patients in their poststroke care.

The poststroke rehabilitation guideline published by the AHCPR (1995) does not address whether or not goals should be set, but rather how goals should be used (52). Best common practice is to develop comprehensive goals that cover the level of disability and include psychosocial needs. The guideline recommends that "Both short-term and longer term goals need to be realistic as relates to current levels of disability and the potential for recovery" (52). Setting patient goals has multiple utilities. Goals should be realistic targets for use by the patient, family, and staff. Goals can create an environment of treatment consistency among treating disciplines, serve as benchmarks for response and recovery, and provide a basis for team meetings.

Stroke rehabilitation is faced with the daunting task of discussing with the patient and caregivers the extent of functional limitation and guidance on the likelihood of desired rehabilitation outcomes being achieved. Many of these patients may have speech difficulties and cognitive deficits and face the frustrations of having an expressive aphasia, leading to inability to convey their needs to the medical team and their family. Thus, the rehabilitation team has a responsibility to employ patience in dealing with stroke patients and practice sensitivity in communication with the stroke population. When communicating with stroke patients, it is imperative to keep the content simple and delivered in a slow, normal, and pleasant tone. You should give them a reasonable amount of time to respond, and repeat a statement when necessary without interrupting to ensure you comprehend. Also try to avoid corrections. It has been shown that using gesture and visual aids can augment communication (53). Recommendations include that patient and family/caregiver education should be provided in an interactive and written format, family conferences are a useful tool, and patient and family education should be documented.

PROFESSIONALISM

GOALS

Reflect a commitment to carrying out professional responsibilities and an adherence to ethical principles in stroke.

OBJECTIVES

1. Exemplify the humanistic qualities as a provider of care for patients with stroke.
2. Demonstrate ethical principles and responsiveness to patient needs superseding self and other interests.
3. Demonstrate sensitivity to patient population diversity, including culture, gender, age, race, religion, disabilities, and sexual orientation.
4. Respect patient privacy and autonomy.
5. Recognize the importance of patient education in the treatment of and advocacy for persons with stroke.
6. Describe the impact of demographics on the care of persons with stroke.

The rehabilitation specialist has to be mindful of cultural barriers that may affect stroke patients. Issues of privacy are important, but many stroke patients may be cognitively impaired and aphasic and will require identification of a medical proxy to help with decision making. It is also essential to address issues of recovery for patients with severe stroke and treatment given. If necessary, DNR (do not resuscitate) and DNI (do not intubate) orders should be clarified as well as the need for a feeding tube. A living will can be suggested to cognitively intact patients to ensure their further wishes are followed.

The rehabilitation specialist must be mindful of coverage based on insurance issues for rehabilitation services and durable medical equipment. Medicare does not cover wheelchairs for patients who can walk short distances on flat surfaces in the home, even though patients may not be able to negotiate at a community level. It is important to be mindful of these restrictions that can impact your patient's quality of life and reintegration to the community. The physiatrist must be ready to advocate on the patients' behalf.

The importance of humanistic qualities including empathy and compassion are of utmost importance for the physiatrist to encompass. The physiatrist must empathize and realize the impact of the stroke on the patient and his or her life. It is also important to be mindful of cultural, diversity, gender, age, race, religion, disabilities, and sexual orientation in the care of the patient by the clinician. It has been noted in studies that minorities have a higher stroke risk with stroke occurrence at an earlier age. African-Americans and Hispanic Americans may have a stroke at a younger age, as noted by Trimble. A younger patient may not feel comfortable going to a subacute rehabilitation facility, often misunderstanding it as a long-term nursing home. The physiatrist needs to explore these issues and be sensitive to feelings their patients might have over these issues (54). Health disparity issues lead to a greater risk for stroke and the need for preventative care must be highlighted.

It is important to develop a trusting relationship with the patients and encourage them during their rehabilitation process to ensure the patients feel part of the team when developing their rehabilitation plans. Support groups may be useful for survivors of stroke. In older patients who suffered from a severe stroke, there may be ethical issues about end-of-life decisions and nutritional support. Patients with SAH are usually of a younger age, and 50% of these patients may remain permanently disabled because of cognitive dysfunction (55). These issues, as well as long-term return into the community setting and adjusting to new roles in the family, should be addressed with the patient and family.

The ethical issues pertaining to a stroke population are not limited to withdrawal of life-sustaining treatment; they also encompass poststroke rehabilitation (56). Some stroke patients might be high functioning, with cognitive deficit and lack of insight; these patients might require one-to-one observation for the risk of elopement or compliance to treatment. The use of restraint is not encouraged in stroke patients in the rehabilitation unit. The use of sedatives can impair the level of alertness. Restraint use in stroke patients with agitation, falls, impulsivity, and poor mental status interferes with medical management and therapy. The Eastwood 1999 study looked into the high-cost physical restraints have in the rehabilitation patient from direct observation (57). The Amato study in 2006, a study on quality improvement, showed that 34% of rehabilitation patients fall while they are in physical restraint (58). The alternatives of restraints are also employed to maintain patients' self-respect.

Patients with dysphagia may be frustrated by their inability to eat a regular diet and require a PEG tube placement until their dysphagia improves.

Family caregivers and friends play a critical role in a loved one's recovery from stroke, particularly as time spent in hospitals and rehabilitation facilities continues to decrease. Stroke recovery lasts for at least 2 years after stroke onset, so most of the support during this period comes from informal sources including friends and family members. Studies revealed that family support is associated with progressive improvement for rehabilitation patients (both physically and psychologically). Further, greater communication as a rehabilitation team with caregivers can reduce psychological stress and facilitate better adjustment to an illness or disability, thereby improving quality-of-life and long-term outcomes. In terms of emotional reactions, caregivers often feel one or more of the following: anxiety, guilt, depression, frustration, resentment, impatience, and fear. (Fear that a stroke may happen again, fear that the stroke survivor may be unable to accept his or her disabilities, fear that the survivor may require nursing home placement, fear that the caregiver may make mistakes, and fear that families and friends will abandon them.) Coping with these reactions is paramount to a healthy caregiver, and ultimately, to a well-adjusted patient. It is crucial for family members to take care of their own needs in addition to those of the patient.

Finally, patients must understand their risk for further stroke and the importance of lifestyle modifications to help prevent further strokes. Further intervention may be needed to let the public at large be aware of the early warning signs of stroke so that they seek medical attention early and be in the window for treatment with tissue plasminogen activator (t-PA) for ischemic stroke. With the use of t-PA there may be a reduction in the degree of disability from an ischemic stroke. Education about the importance of early intervention is important for patients and families.

Physicians can work on educating the public on stroke prevention, by making the public aware of modifiable risk factors that can help reduce the risk of developing the most common types of stroke. Education remains of key importance in instructing patients of the significance of treatment of hypertension, heart disease, diabetes, reducing cholesterol levels, and smoking cessation.

Ischemic strokes have the highest incidence in people over 65 years of age. Given the advanced age of these patients, home care services and facility settings may be appropriate for many of these patients. The physician's role is to advocate for these patients, in both having rehabilitation services available to them during their potential for maximal recovery and having resources available to them in the community to help them maintain their maximum level of independence and reduce the costs needed for caregivers.

SYSTEMS-BASED PRACTICE

GOALS

Awareness and responsiveness to systems of care delivery, and the ability to recruit and coordinate effectively resources in the system to provide optimal continuum of care as it relates to stroke.

OBJECTIVES

1. Describe key components and available services in the rehabilitation continuum of care and community rehabilitation facilities.
2. Discuss how to work effectively in various systems of care.
3. Describe optimal follow-up care.
4. Identify important markers of quality of care.
5. Discuss cost-effectiveness, utilization, and management of resources.
6. Review proper medical record keeping and documentation as the patient moves along the continuum of care.
7. Demonstrate an advocacy role that the physician should display for quality of care for their patients with stroke.
8. Participate in identifying and avoiding potential systems- and medical-related errors for stroke and strategies to minimize them.

A physiatrist must be able to assess and evaluate the resources needed for achieving optimal outcomes in all spheres for persons with a stroke. It is essential to assess the patient in order to place him or her in the proper treatment program, ranging from an acute setting, subacute setting, home, outpatient, or home exercise program. Each stroke patient may require a different approach for his or her long-term rehabilitation needs. Consideration must be given to the patient's expected recovery based on his or her functional deficits and comorbid conditions. Furthermore, the amount of family support, health insurance, and resources available must be considered as the patient goes through each stage of the rehabilitation plan.

Post stroke, the first component of the rehabilitation system begins in the acute hospital setting (59). Acute care is defined as the period immediately following the onset of an acute stroke, which usually takes place in either a medical service or a specialized stroke unit. From the medical perspective, BP monitoring is of prime importance. From a rehabilitation perspective, prevention of secondary complications such as skin breakdown, venous thromboembolism, atelectasis, ASPNA, contracture formation, depression, and bowel/bladder issues is equally important. Education of the long-term consequences of stroke in regard to activity limitations, recovery, and the rehabilitation process should begin here. When educating the family, the importance of how to avoid secondary complications through crucial interventions such as proper positioning and therapy should be emphasized. Secondary complications are minimized if the rehabilitation process is started early.

Stroke rehabilitation after discharge from acute care can be administered in an acute inpatient rehabilitation unit, subacute nursing facility, the patient's home, or an outpatient facility (60). It must be determined if the patient is more appropriately suited for an acute 3 hr/d program versus a subacute 1 hr/d program. Factors that need to be accounted for in order for proper placement include current medical status, functional deficits, predictors of recovery, and family support. Strong family support has been shown to improve outcomes, especially in patients with severe physical or cognitive deficits (61). The Stroke Unit Trialists

Collaboration concluded that patients receiving organized inpatient stroke unit care were more likely to survive, regain independence, and return home than those receiving a less organized service (15). Rehabilitation should start as early as possible, once medical stability is reached.

Patient safety issues that need to be addressed in this patient population include adequate assessment of swallowing and risk for aspiration, risk of fall, decubitus ulcer prevention, appropriate DVT prophylaxis, and concurrent cardiac issues. Patients at highest risk for skin breakdown may have impaired sensation and mobility, urinary incontinence, diabetes, peripheral vascular disease, or lower body mass index (62). More than 50% of stroke mortality is attributable to medical complications (63). The most common is infection, with pneumonia and urosepsis each occurring with a frequency of about 10% and 13%, respectively (64).

While obtaining routine workup for patients to look for DVT is not recommended, DVT prophylaxis is encouraged for all patients after a stroke unless there is a contraindication.

A patient who is not currently independent may still be able to go home with proper training and equipment if he or she is equipped with strong family support, insurance that supports home care services, and transportation benefits. Home therapy sessions can be useful to help evaluate for necessary adaptive equipment. As patients improve, they may be advanced to an outpatient setting with specialized equipment. Following good progress and advancement, an outpatient therapy setting may become more appropriate due to the specialized equipment afforded in the gym to further maximize functional capabilities. Some patients, however, require further rehabilitation prior to going home to an outpatient program. It may be a difficult choice for those patients to make the transition from an acute rehabilitation setting to a subacute rehabilitation setting instead of going home with their families. It should be explained to the patient that there is a continuum of rehabilitation services and care and the importance of transitioning to the next level should be emphasized. There is a financial consideration to being admitted to a subacute rehabilitation, and not all may have this benefit based on their insurance coverage. Others may not have the option or benefits to cover for longer-term care. These issues should be addressed as well to best help the patient and his or her plan for long-term needs. If patients were working prior to their stroke but are now unable to work, alternate insurance plans should be explored. Various health insurance plans might be available, and with the help of the patient's social worker, the optimal plan that covers the patient's current and future medical and rehabilitation needs can be chosen.

As the patient transitions between the care units, good handoffs are key. It is important to implement a process that clearly defines the transfer of responsibility from one caregiver to another. The purpose of the handoff is to provide the accepting doctor a summary of the patient's clinical course to date. Although it is often impossible and even counterproductive to include all details, certain pertinent medical information is critical and should be required (see Table 13.11). Particularly for stroke patients, this includes type of stroke, location of stroke, medical comorbidities, and medication, allergies, as well as a review of critical laboratory work and vital signs. To ensure proper patient care, good communication goes beyond the referring provider and receiving physiatrist. It should include the therapists and nursing staff as well. The therapist should have clearly written orders specifying parameters for heart rate, systolic BP, and to contact the medical team to discuss changes in vitals and occurrence of symptoms.

The physiatrist must ensure that proper transition occurs to either the accepting skilled nursing facility or the patient's home

TABLE 13.11 Information to Include in Sign-Out/Transition of Care

Patient demographic	Age, sex, past medical history (PMH), past surgical history (PSH)
Reason for admission	Chief complaint with duration of symptoms Diagnose
Hospital course	Admitting service Diagnostic tests and procedures—with dates Treatments Major events—falls, codes, emergent care received
Active problems	Infections Pending procedures
Baseline physical examination	Mental status—awake, oriented to person, place, and time Manual muscle test— upper extremity (UE) and lower extremity (LE) Aphasia—present or not
Medications	Corresponding diagnosis—what are you treating
	Parameters—when to hold or to start
	Antibiotics—start date, end date, total days of treatment
	Recent changes—if so why?
	Anticoagulation—DVT prophylaxis allowed, full treatment dose allowed, or when should be started
Medical teams	Consult services following patient
Diet	Texture/consistency liquid
Bowel/bladder	Urinary retention—bladder scans required, indwelling catheter placed? When to remove indwelling catheter?
Restrictions	Weight-bearing status Parameters of BP and HR for therapist
End-of-life goals	Health care proxy DNR/DNI status
Discharge	Follow-up appointments Level of supervision

upon discharge. When discharging a patient into the community, the physiatrist should, whenever possible, be in communication with the patient's primary care doctor, particularly in regard to medication and follow-up appointments. Written instructions on post discharge care should always be provided and must clearly outline the necessary follow-up appointments and necessary restrictions in activity, diets, and level of supervision.

Physiatrists need to be aware that when transferring patient data, the medium which they choose must comply with Health Insurance Portability and Accountability Act (HIPPA) regulations. Most often, personal e-mails and portable drives do not meet the requirements to ensure patient privacy and confidentiality. Hospitals should provide secure accessible drives that allow residents to update and transfer signoff information while maintaining compliance.

Essentially, the physiatrist must follow a transfer-of-care process, which is systematic and well defined to ensure pertinent information is correctly conveyed between caregivers. Implementing a confidential standardized flow sheet ensures that crucial information is not missed and that patient care is not compromised.

Stroke is a heterogeneous diagnosis; patients surviving from a stroke range from having no symptoms to being bedbound and severely impaired. The clinician must be mindful of the fact that a cookie cutter approach to caring for these patients will not provide optimal care. Each patient after a stroke will have his or her own set of neurological issues, medical issues, psychological issues, risk factors for recurrent stroke, and different family dynamics. The rehabilitation assessment should include evaluation to prevent complications, which includes swallowing problems, skin breakdown, risk for DVT, bowel and bladder dysfunction, malnutrition, and pain. The assessment of impairments includes communication impairment, motor impairment, cognitive deficit, visual and spatial deficiency, psychological issues, and sensory deficit. Education about stroke prevention is key. All these issues must be addressed and understood by the patient, family, and the team. An individualized plan must be developed for these patients taking into account patient wishes, realistic expectations, and medical needs that will enable the patient's function to progress to the next level of care.

CASE STUDY

Mr J, a 64-year-old African American man with a past medical history of DM2, hyperlipidemia, and hypertension, was brought into the ED by his daughter for sudden onset of right-sided weakness and slurring of his words. As per his daughter, the patient was last seen at his normal baseline 1 hour ago. CT scan revealed an acute left MCA infarct. The patient was medically stabilized and treated. A rehabilitation consult was done, which recommended admission to acute rehabilitation. On admission to rehabilitation, the patient was noted to have expressive aphasia, right hemiparesis with his arm weaker than with his leg. During his stay, his functional status improved. He was able to ambulate 150 feet with a quad cane, feed, and dress himself independently. He was also able to tolerate a mechanically soft diet with thin liquids. However, despite his motor recovery, Mr J was unable to express himself. He had difficulty communicating with others.

In preparation for his discharge, a family meeting was held to discuss with the daughter the patient's needs after discharge. During the meeting the daughter expressed concern about having her father live with her. Her father was always an independent man, who now, due to his stroke, will have to depend on others for help. The daughter was also concerned and wanted to know if she could leave her father alone while she was at work, or if he would require 24-hour care. Further, she wanted to know if his insurance would cover the cost.

After the meeting the doctor met with the patient to discuss the meeting. The doctor acknowledged the frustrations the patient may have due to his lack of speech and loss of autonomy. It should be noted that insurance usually has limited home care coverage for a patient who is able to ambulate and perform ADL independently. Due to his speech issues, he would initially need to be monitored closely at home for safety. The daughter was able to find support from neighbors and church groups that would be able to look in on him during the day while she was at work to supplement his home care services.

CASE STUDY DISCUSSION QUESTIONS

MEDICAL KNOWLEDGE: Describe the symptoms of a left MCA infarct.

PROFESSIONALISM: After this stroke, which has left the patient with aphasia, what are the important issues the physiatrist needs to discuss with the patient and family in regard to future medical decisions if the patient becomes cognitively impaired?

PATIENT CARE: In what ways can a physiatrist optimize patient care?

PRACTICE-BASED LEARNING AND IMPROVEMENT: Name 10 process-based performance measures relevant to acute hospital-based stroke care.

SYSTEMS-BASED PRACTICE: For the patient's safety, he should have a speech and swallow evaluation soon after being admitted to the hospital. What are the patient's main concerns? What are the therapist's main concerns? What should be taken into consideration when planning for discharge?

INTERPERSONAL AND COMMUNICATION SKILLS: Describe the interaction of the physiatrist with the patient and family in addressing their concerns. Was the physiatrist able to communicate effectively with the patient regarding his loss of autonomy?

SELF-EXAMINATION QUESTIONS
(Answers begin on p. 367)

1. Which of the following is a nonmodifiable risk factor for stroke?
   A. Coronary artery disease
   B. Diabetes
   C. Smoking
   D. Hypertension
   E. Age

2. Which of the following types of stroke is most commonly associated with atrial fibrillation?
   A. Large artery atherosclerosis
   B. Embolic
   C. Subarachnoid
   D. Lacunar
   E. Intracerebral hemorrhagic

3. Which of the following is considered to be the most common type of stroke?
   A. Ischemic
   B. Hemorrhagic
   C. Subarachnoid
   D. Embolic
   E. Intracerebral hemorrhagic

4. Which of the following is least likely to occur in a stroke patient?
   A. Shoulder pain
   B. DVT
   C. Heterotopic ossification
   D. Falls
   E. Depression

5. Which of the following assessment tools is commonly used in rehabilitation for the Inpatient Rehabilitation Facility Prospective Payment System?
   A. Barthel Index
   B. NIH Stroke Scale
   C. Modified Rankin Scale
   D. FIM score
   E. Short Form-36

REFERENCES

1. Kalra L, Yu G, Wilson K, et al. Medical complications during stroke rehabilitation. *Am Heart Assoc J Stroke*. 1995;26:990–994.
2. Rehabilitation Therapy After Stroke. (n.d.). *National Stroke Association*. http://www.stroke.org/site/PageServer?pagename=rehabt. Accessed January 25, 2014.
3. Deutsch A, Granger CV, Heinemann AW, et al. Poststroke rehabilitation: outcomes and reimbursement of inpatient rehabilitation facilities and subacute rehabilitation programs. *Stroke*. 2006;37(6):1477–1482.
4. Treger I, Shamea J, Giaguinto S, et al. Return to work in stroke patients. *Disabil Rehabil*. 2007;29(17):1397–1403.
5. Daniel K, Wolfe CD, Busch MA, et al. What are the social consequences of stroke for working-aged adults? A systematic review. *Stroke*. 2009;40(6):e431–e440.
6. Vestling M, Tufvesson B, Iwarsson S. Indicators for return to work after stroke and the importance of work for subjective well-being and life satisfaction. *J Rehabil Med*. 2003;35(3):127–131.
7. Miller EL, Murray L, Richards L, et al. Comprehensive overview of nursing and interdisciplinary rehabilitation care of the stroke patient: a scientific statement from the American Heart Association. *Stroke*. 2010;41(10):2402–2448.
8. Wozniak M, Kittner S. Return to work after ischemic stroke: a methodological review. *Neuroepidemiology*. 2002;21:159–166.
9. Perrier MJ, Korner-Bitensky N, Mayo NE. Patient factors associated with return to driving poststroke: findings from a multicenter cohort study. *Arch Phys Med Rehabil*. 2010;91(6):868–873.
10. Fonarow GC. Relationship of National Institutes of Health stroke scale to 30-day mortality in Medicare beneficiaries with acute ischemic stroke. *J Am Heart Assoc*. 2012;02(1):42–50.
11. Wade DF, Wood VA, Heller A, et al. Walking after stroke. Measurement and recovery over the first 3 months. *Scand J Rehabil Med*. 1987;19(1):25–30.
12. Bard G, Hirschberg GG. Recovery of voluntary motion in upper extremity following hemiplegia. *Arch Phys Med*. 1965;46:567–572.
13. Bruno-Petriina, A. (n.d.). Motor recovery in stroke. *Motor Recovery in Stroke*. http://emedicine.medscape.com/article/324386-overview. Accessed January 26, 2014.
14. Skilbeck CE, Wade DT, Hewer RL, et al. Recovery after stroke. *J Neurol Neurosurg Psychiatry*. 1983;46(1):5–8.
15. Stroke Unit Trialists' Collaboration. Organized inpatient (stroke unit) care for stroke. *Cochrane Database Syst Rev*. 2001(3):Cd000197.
16. Kitisomprayoonkul W, et al. Medical complications during inpatient stroke rehabilitation in Thailand: a prospective study. *J Med Assoc Thai*. 2010;93(5):594–600.
17. Berlowtiz DR, Wilking SY. Risk factors for pressure sores. A comparison of cross sectional and cohort derived data. *J Am Geriatr Soc*. 1989;37:1043–1050.
18. Dennis, MS. Effective prophylaxis for deep vein thrombosis after stroke: low-dose anticoagulation rather than stockings alone: against. *Stroke*. 2004;35(12):2912–2913.
19. Sherman DG, Albers GW, et al. The efficacy and safety of enoxaparin versus unfractionated heparin for the prevention of venous thromboembolism after acute ischaemic stroke (PREVAIL Study): an open-label randomized comparison. *Lancet*. 2007;369(9570):1347–1355.
20. Muir KW. The PREVAIL trial and low-molecular-weight heparin for prevention of venous thromboembolism. *Stroke*. 2008;39(7):2174–2176.
21. Tutuarima JHP, van der Meulen RJ, de Hann A, et al. Risk factors for falls of hospitalized stroke patient. *Stroke*. 1997;28(2):297–301.
22. Thomas LH. Treatment of urinary incontinence after stroke in adults. *Cochrane Database Syst Rev*. 2008;CD004462.
23. Nakayama H, Jorgensen HS, Pedersen MA, et al. Prevalence and risk factors of incontinence after stroke: the Copenhagen stroke study. *Stroke*. 1997;28:58–62.
24. Gallichio JE. Pharmacologic management of spasticity following stroke. *Phys Ther*. 2004;84(10):973–981.
25. Lindgren I, Jönsson AC, Norrving B, et al. Shoulder pain after stroke: a prospective population-based study. *Stroke*. 2007;38(2):343–348.
26. Poduri KR. Shoulder pain in stroke patients and its effect on rehabilitation. *J Stroke Cerebrovasc Dis*. 1993;3:261–266.
27. Robinson RG, Spalletta G. Poststroke depression: a review. *Can J Psychiatry*. 2010;55(6):341–349.
28. Ifejika-Jones NL, Arun N, Peng H, et al. The interaction of aspiration pneumonia with demographic and cerebrovascular disease risk factors is predictive of discharge level of care in acute stroke patient. *Am J Phys Med Rehabil*. 2012;91(2):141–147.
29. Fletcher BJ, Dunbar S, Coleman J, et al. Cardiac precautions for nonacute inpatient settings. *Am J Phys Med Rehabil*. 1993;72:140–143.
30. Pang MY, et al. Using aerobic exercise to improve health outcomes and quality of life in stroke: evidence-based exercise prescription recommendations. *Cerebrovasc Dis*. 2013;35(1):7–22.
31. Twitchell TE. The restoration of motor function following hemiplegia in man. *Brain*. 1951;74(4):443–480.

32. Nijland RH, et al. Presence of finger extension and shoulder abduction within 72 hours after stroke predicts functional recovery: early prediction of functional outcome after stroke: the EPOS cohort study. *Stroke.* 2010;41(4):745–750.
33. Kollen BJ, et al. The effectiveness of the Bobath concept in stroke rehabilitation: what is the evidence? *Stroke.* 2009;40(4):89–97.
34. American Heart Association. 1999 heart and stroke statistical update. *Am Heart Assoc.* 1998.
35. Williams GR, Jiang JG, Matchar DB, et al. Incidence and occurrence of total (First-Ever and Recurrent) stroke. *Stroke.* 1999;30:2523–2528.
36. Council on Cardiovascular Disease in the Young E. Management of stroke in infants and children: a scientific statement from a Special Writing Group of the American Heart Association Stroke Council and the Council on Cardiovascular Disease in the Young. *Stroke (1970).* September 2008;39:2644–2691.
37. Adams HP, Bendixen BH, Kappelle LJ, et al. Classification of subtype of acute ischemic stroke. Definitions for use in a multicenter clinical trial. Trial of Org 10172 in Acute Stroke Treatment. *Stroke.* 1993;24(1):35–41.
38. Stapf C, Elkind MS, Mohr JP. Carotid artery dissection. *Ann Rev Med.* 2000;51:329–347.
39. Zorowitz R, Baerga E, Cuccurullo S. Stroke. In: Cuccurullo S, ed. *Physical Medicine and Rehabilitation Board Review.* New York: Demos Medical; 2010:7.
40. Bejot Y, Catteau A, Caillier M, et al. Trends in incidence, risk factors, and survival in symptomatic lacunar stroke in Dijon, France, from 1989 to 2006. A population-based study. *Stroke.* 2008;39(7):1945–1951.
41. Manno EM. Update on intracerebral hemorrhage. *Continuum (Minneap Minn).* 2012;18(3):598–610.
42. Kase CS, Mohr JP, Caplan LR. Intracerebral hemorrhage. In: Barnett HJ, Mohr JP, Stein BM, et al. eds. *Stroke: Pathophysiology, Diagnosis, and Management.* New York, NY: Churchill Livingstone; 1998:649–700.
43. Martini SR, Flaherty ML, Brown WM, et al. Risk factors for intracerebral hemorrhage differ according to hemorrhage location. *Neurology.* 2012;79(23):2275–2282.
44. Lee SH, Koh JS, Bang JS, et al. A case of ruptured peripheral aneurysm of the anterior inferior cerebellar artery associated with an arteriovenous malformation: a less invasive image-guided transcortical approach. *J Korean Neurosurg Soc.* 2009;46(6):577–580.
45. Liebeskind D, Lutsep L. Intracranial hemorrhage. *eMedicine*, January 23, 2013; Web July 12, 2013.
46. Broderick JP, Brott TG, Duldner JE, et al. Volume of intracerebral hemorrhage. A powerful and easy-to-use predictor of 30-day mortality. *Stroke.* 1993;24(7):987–993.
47. Wermer MJ, van der Schaaf IC, Algra A, et al. Risk of rupture of unruptured intracranial aneurysms in relation to patient and aneurysm characteristics: an updated meta-analysis. *Stroke.* 2007;38(4):1404–1410.
48. Rinkel GJ, Djibuti M, Algra A, et al. Prevalence and risk of rupture of intracranial aneurysms: a systematic review. *Stroke.* 1998;29:251–256.
49. Brott TG, Hobson RW, Howard G, et al. Stenting versus endarterectomy for treatment of carotid-artery stenosis. *N Engl J Med.* 2010;363(1):11–23.
50. VA/DoD clinical practice guideline for the management of stroke rehabilitation. Department of VA. http://www.healthquality.va.gov/stroke/stroke_full_221.pdf
51. Reeves MJ, et al. Development of stroke performance measures: definitions, methods, and current measures. *Stroke.* 2010;41(7):1573–1578.
52. Post-Stroke Rehabilitation Guideline Panel. *Post-Stroke Rehabilitation.* Clinical Practice Guideline No. 16. Rockville, MD: US Department of Health and Human Services, Public Health Service, Agency for Health Care Policy and Research; 1995.
53. "Aphasia." *Effects of Stroke.* http://www.stroke.org/site/PageServer?pagename=aphasia. Accessed September 7, 2013.
54. Braun SM, Beurskens AJ, Kleynen M, et al. A multicenter randomized controlled trial to compare subacute 'treatment as usual' with and without mental practice among persons with stroke in Dutch nursing homes. *J Am Med Dir Assoc.* 2012;13(1):85, 81–87.
55. Kreiter KT, Copeland D, Bernardini GL, et al. Predictors of cognitive dysfunction after subarachnoid hemorrhage. *Stroke.* 2002;33:200–209.
56. Creutzfeldt CJ, Holloway RG. Treatment decisions after severe stroke: uncertainty and biases. *Stroke.* 2012;43(12):3405–3408.
57. Eastwood EA, Schechtman J. Direct observation nursing: adverse patient behaviors and functional outcomes. *Nurs Econ.* 1999;17(2):96–102.
58. Amato S, Salter JP, Mion LC. Physical restraint reduction in the acute rehabilitation setting: a quality improvement study. *Rehabil Nurs.* 2006;31(6):235–241.
59. Uchino K, Pary JK, Grotta JC. *Acute Stroke Care: A Manual from the University of Texas-Houston Stroke Team.* New York, NY: Cambridge University Press; 2007.
60. Gresham GE, Duncan PW, Stason WB, et al. *Post-Stroke Rehabilitation.* Clinical Practice Guideline, No. 16. Rockville, MD: US Department of Health and Human Services, Public Health Service, Agency for Health Care Policy and Research; May 1995. AHCPR Publication No. 95–0662.
61. Glass TA, Matchar DB, Belyea M, et al. Impact of social support on outcome in first stroke. *Stroke.* 1993;24:64–70.
62. Berlowitz DR, Brandeis GH, Anderson JJ, et al. Evaluation of a risk-adjustment model for pressure ulcer development using the Minimum Data Set. *J Am Geriatr Soc.* 2001;49:872–876.
63. Johnston KC, Li JY, Lyden PD, et al. Medical and neurological complications of ischemic stroke: experience from the RANTTAS trial. RANTTAS Investigators. *Stroke.* 1998;29:447.
64. California Acute Stroke Prototype Registry Investigators, B. Frequency and determinants of pneumonia and urinary tract infection during stroke hospitalization. *J Stroke Cerebrovasc Dis.* 2006;15(5):209-213.

Ajit B. Pai
Isaac Darko
William Robbins

14: Moderate and Severe Traumatic Brain Injury

PATIENT CARE

GOALS

Provide patient care that is compassionate, appropriate, and effective for the treatment of moderate to severe traumatic brain injury (TBI) and the promotion of health.

OBJECTIVES

1. Identify appropriate components of a history and physical examination for a patient with TBI.
2. Discuss impairments and complications after TBI.
3. Describe a sample rehabilitation program for a patient with TBI.

Appropriate care for the patient with TBI includes many components. In the following paragraphs, we will discuss specifics related to the assessment and treatment of the adult with moderate to severe TBI. The medical history of a patient with TBI is highly important. Much can be gleaned from details at the time of injury, triage in the emergency department, surgical interventions, and so on.

HISTORY

History of Present Illness
Understanding the mechanism of injury (e.g., fall, motor vehicle accident, sport-related, assault, and blast-related) will allow providers insight into potential complications and allow for teams to educate persons with TBI and their families about future preventative measures. Traditionally, TBI is divided into primary and secondary injuries. Primary injury is the direct result of the force being applied to the head. It can be subdivided into open or closed injuries. Open head injuries result in the brain exposed to the outside environment due to a tear in the dura mater. This results in a higher risk of infection. Certain types of open head injuries result in more focal damage to the brain, such as blunt trauma and gunshot wounds. In closed head injuries the skull remains intact, resulting in mechanical and inertial forces that shear axons and lead to diffuse axonal injury (DAI) and contact forces associated with intracranial bleeds. Secondary injuries develop over the hours and days after the initial impact and are caused by bleeding, swelling, ischemic changes, complex biochemical changes, and changes in blood supply to the brain. Concomitant injuries such as musculoskeletal injuries and internal injuries (commonly seen in high-speed crashes and active combat injuries) should also be documented. In civilians, associated injuries are linked with more disability even 1 year after the injury (1).

Blast-related injuries can be subdivided into primary, secondary, tertiary, and quaternary. Primary injury represents the transduction of blast waves that damage tissue. These waves tend to also damage the hollow organs of the body. Secondary injury results from shrapnel and other objects traveling at high speeds due to the explosion. Tertiary injury is a result of the person being thrown from the blast into a stationary object. Finally, quaternary injury is due to hypoxic or toxic damage secondary to thermal or inhalation injuries.

The severity of the brain injury should always be documented. Severity of injury (Table 14.1) is based on several measures: Glasgow Coma Scale (GCS) at time of injury, length of coma (LOC), and length of posttraumatic amnesia (PTA). If a person exhibits different grading of TBI based on the 3 measures, the severity is graded as the most severe (worst) of the measures. Mild TBI is defined as a GCS of 13 to 15; the patient is awake, may be confused, but is able to communicate and follow commands, and PTA is less than 1 hour. Moderate TBI is defined

TABLE 14.1 Severity Grading of TBI

	MILD	MODERATE	SEVERE
GCS	13–15	9–12	<8
LOC	<30	30 min–1 d	>1 d
PTA	<1 hr	1 hr–1 wk	>1 wk

as a GCS of 9 to 12, an LOC between 30 minutes and 24 hours, and PTA less than 1 week. Severe TBI is defined as GCS of 8 or less, LOC greater than 24 hours, and PTA greater than 1 week. Intoxication at the time of the accident can affect GCS, as well as sedative medications given in the field.

Review of Systems
Symptoms such as headaches, weakness, dizziness, tinnitus, change in taste or smell, dysphagia, dysarthria, aphonia, vertigo, visual field deficits, decreased or altered sensation, focal weakness, and impaired balance can direct the provider's attention to specific areas in the brain that may be injured. Understanding the symptoms allows a physiatrist to plan a treatment course.

Past Medical History
Previous TBI or stroke; previous pulmonary function and history of COPD or other lung disease; and previous psychiatric history including depression, anxiety, and personality disorders are important to understand in the treatment of persons with TBI.

Allergies and Medications
A complete list of allergies and medications is important in the care of patients with TBI. Medication reconciliation will allow the physiatrist to understand the medication of benefit and those that may be counterproductive to cognitive recovery.

Social History
Level of education and previous cognitive function, vocation and hobby history, socioeconomic status, home environment, and level of support from family should be documented and taken into consideration. The same is true for smoking, alcohol, and drug abuse history.

Functional History
Current and premorbid functional status is highly important to treatment planning. Recording both areas will allow a team to understand the baseline line of the patient and the rehabilitation potential.

PHYSICAL EXAMINATION

Cognition
Emergence from a disorder of consciousness is important early on in the treatment of TBI. Several scales are validated to monitor level of cognition in persons with disorders of consciousness, including the Coma–Near Coma and JFK Coma Recovery Scale Revised. Tests for awareness of self and environment, ability and consistency at which patient can follow simple and multistep commands, attention, concentration, memory testing of declarative and procedural memory, testing of PTA, and testing of higher cognitive function such as abstract thinking and judgment are important in the understanding of persons with cognitive disorders. Tests to help determine these areas include the Galveston Orientation and Amnesia Test, the Orientation Log, the Montreal Cognitive Assessment, and so on. The Rancho Los Amigos Scale allows standardized communication between rehabilitation team members about the person with TBI; it accounts for behavior and cognitive function.

Cognitive impairments are very common. Arousal is one of the most basic cognitive functions; it is fundamental in performing other higher levels of function and is often impaired following injury (2). Attention is commonly affected in patients with more severe TBI. Impaired attention can result in reduced information processing, impaired memory, and poor performance of multitask commands (3). Memory can be affected by many factors, but specific memory functions such as retrieval and consolidation are related to specific brain locations. Higher cognitive functions such as abstract thinking and judgment are often impaired.

Behavior
Behavioral changes are common to patients with moderate to severe TBI. These include mood disorders such as depression, anxiety disorders, and irritability. Screening for mood disorders such as depression and anxiety disorders will help in the rehabilitation of TBI. Depression after TBI can present as low mood, decreased interest, or anhedonia. Patients can complain of concentration and other cognitive issues, and certain behavioral changes might be seen, such as hyperactivity and disinhibition (4). In addition, irritability, akithesia, and restlessness are common after TBI. These symptoms may need to be treated to allow progression through the rehabilitation spectrum. Depending on the location of injury, agitation, disinhibition, and impulsivity can occur following moderate to severe TBI. Each of these problems can reduce the patient's ability to participate in a rehabilitation program.

Musculoskeletal
Range of motion (ROM), concomitant fractures or dislocation, hemiplegia, hemiparesis, and increased tone are common after TBI. Spasticity, velocity-dependent increase in tone, is commonly graded using the Modified Ashworth Scale (Table 14.2). Gait is often altered after TBI, but the patient may be too functionally impaired to test.

Concomitant musculoskeletal injuries often limit ROM. Limited ROM can affect mobility and ambulation, resulting in poor functional outcome. Upper motor neuron damage resulting

TABLE 14.2 Modified Ashworth Scale

No increase in muscle tone	0
Slight increase in muscle tone; catch and release or minimal resistance at the end of ROM	1
Slight increase in muscle tone; catch followed by minimal resistance through <50% of ROM	1+
Marked increase in muscle tone; resistance through >50% of ROM	2
Considerable increase in muscle tone; passive ROM is difficult	3
Increased muscle tone such that affected part is rigid in flexion or extension	4

in increased tone and spasticity is associated with more severe injury, spinal cord injury, anoxic injury, and older age.

Neurologic

Focal neurologic injuries are associated with the location and severity of the injury. Cranial nerve injuries resulting in facial weakness, dysphagia, dysarthria, and visual dysfunction are common, as well as vestibular dysfunction. Cranial nerve testing for nystagmus, tracking, visual field defects, blurred vision, facial weakness, facial sensation, gag reflex, hearing, taste, and smell will help determine focal nerve injury. The sense of taste and smell is often altered after TBI. Sensation to light touch, sharp touch, and proprioception can do the same. Check for increased deep tendon reflexes, as well as other tests for upper motor neuron (UMN) lesions such as Hoffman and Babinski reflex. Patients with more severe injury might show primitive and/or brainstem reflex. Romberg test, fine motor testing, and rapid alternating movements are useful in determining cerebellar involvement. Hemiplegia and hemiparesis in specific distribution can be related to the location of the brain injury. Diffuse weakness can be a result of deconditioning related to prolonged hospitalization. Autonomic dysfunction can also occur after brain injury.

General Examination

Skin breakdown and pressure ulcers are common after prolonged hospitalization. Providers should check the occiput, shoulders, sacrum, greater trochanters, elbows, and heels. Also check for skin integrity around the tracheostomy site and gastrostomy tube. Respiratory examination should include checking for amount and quality of sputum production. Abdominal distension and constipation are both common as a result of lack of mobility. Bowel incontinence is associated with more severe injury. Diarrhea can be associated with enteral feeds and infections. Check for amount and quality of urine and indwelling catheter integrity.

IMPAIRMENTS, ACTIVITY LIMITATIONS, AND PARTICIPATION RESTRICTIONS

More severe TBIs are related to increased activity limitation and participation restrictions. Activity limitation is an inability to execute a certain class of movement or cognitive function (i.e., difficulty bathing or dressing). A participation restriction is an inability to complete a task that most others are able to complete secondary to an activity limitation (i.e., maintaining employment or returning to school).

COMPLICATIONS OF MODERATE AND SEVERE TBI

There are many potential complications that can occur after TBI. Table 14.3 provides a checklist.

Autonomic dysfunction, oftentimes referred to as dysautonomia or paroxysmal autonomic instability and dystonia (PAID), is characterized by hypertension, tachycardia, and diaphoresis. This can occur any time after TBI and is due to sympathetic storming.

TABLE 14.3 Common Problems After TBI

Autonomic dysfunction
Constipation
Heterotopic ossification
Insomnia
Normal pressure hydrocephalus
Posttraumatic headaches
Posttraumatic seizure
Spasticity
Venous thromboembolism (VTE)

Constipation occurs often after TBI due to immobility. It is prevented with hydration and an aggressive bowel program with stimulants and softeners. Once a patient is on a stable bowel regimen, then a slow wean of bowel medications can start.

Heterotopic ossification (HO) occurs after TBI; it usually affects the hips, shoulders, and elbows. Preventative measures for HO include ROM exercises, nonsteroidal anti-inflammatory drug (NSAID) medication, radiation treatment, and calcium-binding chelating agents, although in TBI there is no supporting literature for any of these treatments.

After TBI, sleep disorders are common and can be managed medically and through environmental control. These problems include insomnia and obstructive sleep apnea. At times, a sleep study can assist in diagnosing issues related to sleep.

Hydrocephalus may or may not be associated with elevated pressure. It is best managed with early detection of clinical signs and symptoms (cognitive decline including altered mental status, urinary incontinence, gait instability, headaches, etc.) as well as findings on imaging or large-volume spinal tap, it is commonly treated with neurosurgical placement of a ventriculoperitoneal shunt, although shunts can drain into the heart, pleura, or pelvis.

Posttraumatic headaches develop within 1 week of trauma and are classified based on traditional headache classification. Posttraumatic headaches can be managed nonpharmacologically using relaxation, biofeedback, and avoidance of triggers. They can also be managed pharmacologically using abortive agents such as NSAIDs, acetaminophen, and serotonin receptor agonists. Prophylactic treatment includes beta-blockers, calcium channel blockers, antidepressants, and anticonvulsants. One must rule out increased intracranial pressure, vascular injury, cerebrospinal fluid (CSF) leak, infection, and other serious complications that can present as headache.

Posttraumatic seizures (PTSs) are classified as immediate, which occur within 1 day of injury; early, occurring within 1 week of injury; and late, occurring after 1 week. Prophylactic phenytoin for 7 days following injury can prevent early seizure, but not late PTS or posttraumatic epilepsy. Many acute care providers will use other antiepileptics such as levetiracetam, carbamazepine, or valproic acid. Patients who have had an early or late PTS are at higher risk for future seizures and may require longer treatment.

Early detection of spasticity can be managed with splinting devices, systemic drugs, local chemodenervation, or potentially intrathecal baclofen. Care must be taken to balance the use of systemic drugs and central nervous system (CNS) suppression. Baclofen, diazepam, and tizanidine all act centrally, but are first-line agents in spasticity management. Each of these medications can cause sedation, thus slowing cognitive recovery.

Appropriate venous thromboembolism (VTE) prophylaxis, speech therapy, and enteral feeding methods can prevent other common injuries such as blood clots and aspiration. It is important for the physiatrist to remain vigilant for these complications in order to quickly diagnose and treat appropriately.

SAMPLE REHABILITATION PROGRAM

A typical inpatient rehabilitation program for patients with TBI will include physiatrist oversight for medical management; 24-hour nursing to assist with medication management and daily care needs; physical therapy for mobility and transfer deficits; occupational therapy for activity of daily living (ADL) retraining; speech therapy for cognition, communication, and swallowing deficits; recreational therapist for community reentry; psychology for adjustment; and social work for case management. In addition, other useful team members will include a low vision therapist as TBI often creates difficulties with vision; neuropsychologist for return to work or school treatment planning; dietician for optimal caloric intake; wound care specialist; pharmacist; and patient/family educator. Most programs offer 6 or 7 days a week of therapy, and most days should consist of more than 3 hours of therapy a day. The daily schedule should be structured, as this will allow patients with cognitive or behavioral problems to adjust more quickly and help prevent agitation or irritability. Priority should be placed on sleep hygiene, stimulation reduction, and pain control. Additionally, the rehabilitation program should include a robust education program that incorporates both patients and social support.

A typical outpatient brain injury rehabilitation program includes interdisciplinary interactions with a physiatrist, case manager, physical therapist, occupational therapist, speech and language pathologist, and psychologist. If an interdisciplinary setting is not available, then the physiatrist should coordinate care between all individuals in a multidisciplinary manner. In the outpatient setting, the person with TBI may occasionally work with a recreational therapist when engaging in new activities or a neuropsychologist for testing prior to starting new schoolwork or an occupation. In addition, the physiatrist should be available for consultation for the patient's primary care physician.

MEDICAL KNOWLEDGE

GOAL

Demonstrate knowledge of established and evolving biomedical, clinical, epidemiological, and sociobehavioral sciences pertaining to the field of TBI, as well as the application of this knowledge to guide holistic patient care.

OBJECTIVES

1. Explain the anatomy, physiology, and pathophysiology of moderate to severe TBI.
2. Discuss treatment options of complications of moderate to severe TBI.
3. Discuss ethical issues involved in managing a person with moderate to severe TBI.

ANATOMY

The brain is protected by the scalp, skull, and the dura, which is made up of three layers: the dura mater, which lines the skull; the arachnoid mater, a film that covers the entire brain and contains blood vessels; and the pia mater, which contains blood vessels that reach deep into the brain. Between the arachnoid and the pia is the subarachnoid space, which contains the CSF. CSF is formed in the choroid plexus and circulates through the ventricles into the subarachnoid space and then returns to the dural veins by the arachnoid villi. The brain is a complicated structure containing many parts. The cerebrum is divided into four lobes that lie above the cerebellum. The base of the skull includes multiple bony ridges that abut the brain parenchyma of the anterior temporal and inferior frontal lobes. This predisposes those areas to injury during trauma.

PHYSIOLOGY

The brain is made up of neurons, which consist of the soma, or body; dendrites, which receive communication; the axon, which is a long slender tube that carries information away from the cell; and the terminal buttons, which branch off from the axon and secrete neurotransmitters. Each neuron synapses with another neuron within the brain, the spinal cord, or end organs (in the case of cranial nerves). Neurons are typically colocated with neurons of similar function. Pockets of neurons make nuclei.

PATHOPHYSIOLOGY

Following initial injury, the brain undergoes a complex metabolic, chemical, and neurochemical cascade. Cell death occurs as a result of both apoptosis and cellular necrosis. Secondary injury also results in cerebral edema, elevated intracranial pressure (ICP), and decreased cerebral perfusion pressure. Excitatory amino acids (EAAs) are released, resulting in an influx of sodium and an increase of intracellular calcium, resulting in cellular swelling causing delayed injury and cell death, respectively. Certain areas of the brain, like the hippocampus, have a higher distribution of EAA-sensitive receptors that contribute to injury. Elevated lactate levels are also seen post injury and are thought to be neuroprotective. Lactate is also important for metabolism in the injured state. Inflammation is characterized by cytokine release including interleukins and tumor necrosis factor which can lead to secondary injury via blood brain barrier disruption, cerebral edema, and cell death. At later time points, cytokines may support neuroprotection and neurorepair through their effects on neurotrophin production (2). Several neurotransmitters are affected after injury; dopaminergic and noradrenergic systems are disrupted. Cholinergic transmission in the hippocampus is also decreased.

BIOMECHANICS

Contact forces occur when the head is struck in a fixed position. Inertial forces occur when the head is set in motion and accelerates. Inertial forces associated with angular acceleration can cause DAI, which is a result of tensile strain causing disruption of the axons. Superficial axons and axons in the gray–white matter junction are most vulnerable. Neurons in the corpus collosum and midbrain also are susceptible to DAI. Inertial forces associated with translational acceleration result in more focal injuries, such as contusions. Contusions at the site of impact are termed coup injuries and contusions at the opposite side of impact resulting in the brain's impact with the skull are termed contrecoup injuries. As described earlier, the frontal and anterior temporal lobes are most susceptible to contusion due to their location close to skull ridges. Epidural hematomas (Figure 14.1) result from local impact and injury to dural veins and arteries. Subdural hematomas (Figure 14.2) result from inertial forces and tearing of bridging veins and are associated with falls. Subarachnoid hemorrhage (Figure 14.3) results from angular acceleration and shearing of vessels located in the subarachnoid space.

EPIDEMIOLOGY

The two age groups most at risk are 0 to 4 years and 15 to 19 years. Motor vehicle accident is the leading cause of TBI in the 15 to 19 age group. Also, younger individuals have a tendency to engage in higher-risk behaviors. Persons over the age of 65 are at the highest risk of fall-related TBI. Men are at higher risk than women, and persons of lower socioeconomic status are also at high risk. Military personnel have a higher risk of TBI related to blast injury and other combat-related injuries. Each year there are over 1.7 million occurrences of TBI in the United States (5). Only 25% of those are moderate to severe injuries (6). Two studies show that the cost of TBI in the year 2000 was upward of $75 billion in the United States; 90% of the total costs of TBI are attributed to severe injuries (7,8).

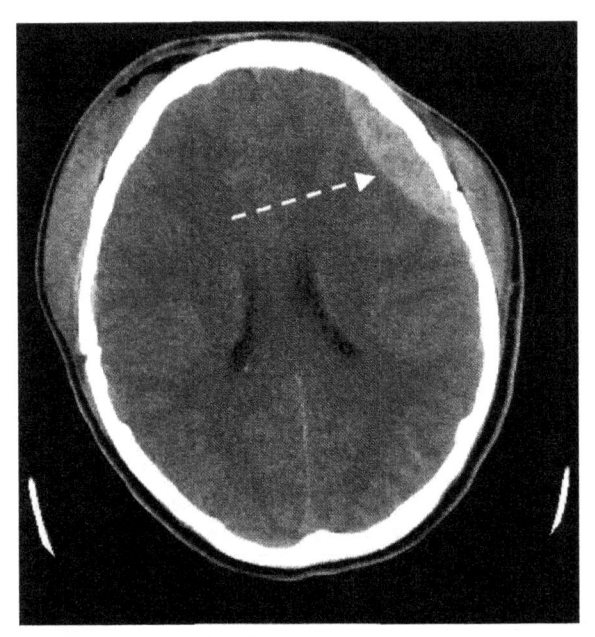

FIGURE 14.1 Epidural Hematoma

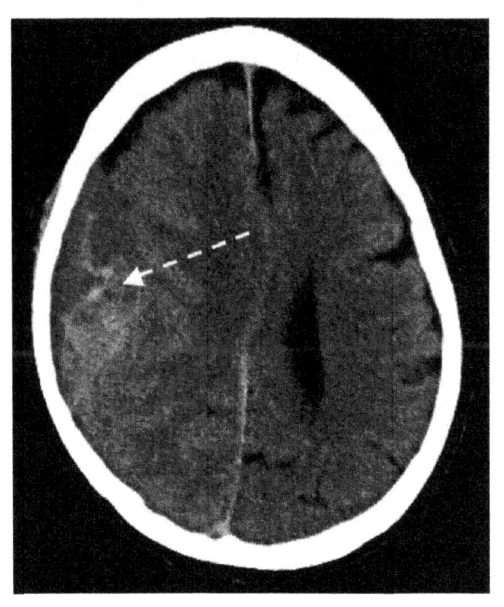

FIGURE 14.2 Subdural Hematoma

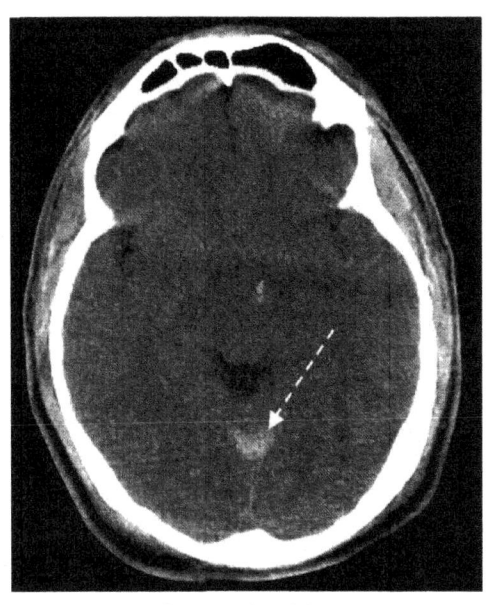

FIGURE 14.3 Subarachnoid Hematoma

TREATMENT

Although evidence for neuropharmacologic treatment is sparse, many providers choose to treat various conditions with medication. Cognitive impairment can be treated with amantadine in patients with a disorder of consciousness. Giacino et al. found that it accelerates the pace of functional recovery during active treatment (9). Although the mechanism of action is unclear, amantadine appears to act as an N-methyl-D-aspartate antagonist and indirect dopamine agonist. It also possesses noradrenergic properties that may affect a variety of cognitive domains. Additionally, it is thought to improve initiation. Side effects include a reduced seizure threshold, although, in Giacino's study, there were no significant differences in adverse events as compared to placebo. Methylphenidate can increase dopamine and norepinephrine in the cortical and subcortical areas (10,11). It is commonly used to improve processing speed and attention as reported by multiple researchers. Side effects of methylphenidate include headache, insomnia, nausea, dizziness, and anorexia.

Amphetamines and precursors to norepinephrine can minimize damage and improve cognitive function as well. Cholinesterase inhibitors can be used as a first-line agent in memory impairment, although there is no evidence they work in TBI. Selective serotonin reuptake inhibitors (SSRIs) and other similar antidepressants are commonly used in patients with depression and anxiety. Antidepressants are also used in low doses to control chronic agitation and aggression. Propranolol has also been shown to improve aggression. Care must be taken as it can result in hypotension and bradycardia. Mood stabilizers such as anticonvulsants are routinely used in the treatment of post-TBI lability, impulsivity, and/or disinhibition (12). First-generation antipsychotics such as haloperidol should be avoided because they have been shown to cause neuronal damage and decreased neuroplasticity.

Several oral medications are used to control spasticity and tone in TBI. Dantrolene acts at the sarcoplasmic reticulum to inhibit calcium activity; however, it can negatively affect the liver, so care must be taken when prescribing this medication. Baclofen, which acts at GABA B receptors, is also commonly used in the treatment of spasticity. Other agents for spasticity treatment include benzodiazepines, tizanidine, and clonidine. Oral medications, other than dantrolene, cause increased somnolence, which limit their use in TBI as they can slow recovery.

Static and dynamic splinting devices are commonly used to control spasticity. In combination with passive ROM and stretching therapies, they lengthen affected muscles and tendons. Superficial and deep heat, electrical stimulation, and cryotherapy are also used in concert with medication and splinting to control spasticity.

Chemodenervation can provide local spasticity management without systemic side effects. Phenol used in nerve blocks causes denaturation of the nerve. Botulinum toxin injection into an affected muscle can also provide good spasticity control in adjunct to physical modalities and splinting.

DIAGNOSTIC TESTING

Routine laboratory work, including monitoring of electrolytes, is important in inpatient neurorehabilitation as endocrine abnormalities, such as diabetes insipidus, are common after brain injury. Prealbumin levels and liver function should be followed to monitor nutrition status with the goal to achieve a positive nitrogen balance to meet the increased metabolic demand following brain injury.

CT scan is the standard for initial evaluation for patients with moderate to severe TBI. It can provide early detection of bleeds, contusions, and other mass lesions and can dictate neurosurgical intervention. CT is also used to monitor progression of the brain injury and to evaluate for complications such as rebleed or hydrocephalus. CT is better than MRI when used to evaluate skull fractures. MRI is more useful when evaluating for extent and location of axonal injury, imaging the posterior fossa, and visualizing cortical and subcortical hemorrhages and edema.

Somatosensory evoked potential (SSEP) is used in severe TBI to predict survival; it can also evaluate coma and vegetative state. SSEP records transmission from the scalp after stimulation of peripheral or mixed nerves. EEG (electroencephalography) can detect injury severity and depth of coma; it is also used in evaluation of seizures. Continuous EEG can evaluate for subclinical seizures that are associated with a poorer outcome.

ETHICAL ISSUES

Bioethics plays an important role in the recovery of persons with TBI. Table 14.4 describes six terms that play a role in ethical issues associated with TBI. Capacity is the person's ability to make his or her own medical decisions. It is not static and can be determined on a decision-to-decision basis. A patient may be able to make simple decisions but may not be able to make a more complex medical decision. Capacity is based on many cognitive factors including alertness, communication, orientation, and understanding and manipulating relevant medical information in regard to the consequences of medical decision making. Competency is a legal term and can only be formally determined by the legal system. If a person is deemed incompetent by a court, it may affect other legal decisions outside of the medical realm including the right to vote, marry, and enter into other legally binding agreements. At times, providers struggle with the balance of beneficence (doing good for the patient) versus autonomy (patient making an informed and voluntary decision). In the patient with TBI, these bioethical principles may be at odds. A patient with poor executive functioning and awareness may make a decision that can harm himself or herself, so it is up to the TBI provider to explain treatment options in a manner that the person with TBI can understand. At times, only the social support system can convince a person with TBI to follow the appropriate decision. Additionally, it is the duty of the physiatrist to practice with nonmaleficence (do no harm to the patient). This can be accomplished by minimizing risks of procedures or adverse effects of medications. Lastly, a physiatrist must acknowledge that there are various stakeholders in the rehabilitation unit. It is important to balance the leverage of those stakeholders with the principle of justice. Persons with TBI are a vulnerable population; the physiatrist must advocate for them by allowing equal access to care.

At times, the physiatrist is faced with the difficult task of discussing end-of-life care with social support systems. Although

TABLE 14.4 Ethical Principles in TBI Rehabilitation

Capacity	A person's ability to make his or her own decisions
Competence	A person's mental capacity to participate in legal matters
Beneficence	A provider performs an action to benefit the patient
Autonomy	A person's ability to make informed and voluntary decisions
Nonmaleficence	To not intentionally harm or injure a person
Justice	Fair and equal treatment for all

persons with TBI can have vastly different outcomes, sometimes the outcome is death. It is important to incorporate the services of mental health and/or hospice providers when discussing end-of-life matters. A team approach will provide the family with an understanding of the process. If the person with TBI has an advanced directive dictating end-of-life care or his or her wishes, this will make the conversation and decision easier on family members. Approaching the conversation with empathy and compassion is paramount. TBI providers must allow family members to grieve and make decisions in their own time.

PRACTICE-BASED LEARNING AND IMPROVEMENT

GOALS

Demonstrate competence in continuously investigating and evaluating patient care practices, appraising and assimilating scientific evidence, and continuously improving patient care practices based on constant self-evaluation and lifelong learning as it applies to the care of individuals with moderate to severe TBI.

OBJECTIVES

1. Describe learning opportunities for providers, patients, and caregivers with experience in TBI.
2. Use methods for ongoing competency training in TBI for physiatrists, including formative evaluation feedback in daily practice, evaluating current practice, and developing a systematic quality improvement and practice improvement strategy.
3. Locate some resources including available websites for continuing medical education and continuing professional development.
4. Describe some areas paramount to self-assessment and life-long learning such as review of current guidelines, including evidence-based, in treatment of patients with TBI and the role of the physiatrist as the educator of patients, families, students, colleagues, and other health professionals.

PATIENT ASSESSMENT

Ongoing competency can be found in Certified Brain Injury Specialty training, American Board of Physical Medicine and Rehabilitation Brain Injury certification, American Academy of Physical Medicine and Rehabilitation self-assessment courses, American Board of Psychiatry and Neurology, American Academy for the Certification of Brain Injury Specialists, Academy of Certified Brain Injury Specialists, and other organizations.

Information on evidence-based practice guidelines (Tables 14.5 and 14.6) can be found at the Foundation for Education in Research in Neurological Emergencies (FERNE), evidence-based guidelines by AANS/CNS for management of severe TBI, PubMed search for review articles, the Brain Trauma Foundation (BTF), the National Institute of Neurological Disorders and Stroke (NINDS), and Cochrane recommendation, as well as other published literature on management and prognosis of severe TBI. However, one must consider the limitations concerning articles on prognostic models pertaining to TBI.

TABLE 14.5 Resources for Evidence-Based Practices

Databases	Medline/PubMed, Cochrane databases, OVID, and first CONSULT, clinicaltrials.gov
Journals	*CHEST, JAMA, Journal of Head Trauma Rehabilitation, Brain Injury, PM&R*
Clinical Practice Guidelines	Best Practices Guidelines, National Guidelines Clearing House, and meta-searches such as SUMSearch

TABLE 14.6 Useful Websites for Evidence-Based Practices

Foundation for Education in Research in Neurological Emergencies	www.ferne.org
Society of Neurological Surgeons	www.neurosurgery.org
The Brain Trauma Foundation	www.braintrauma.org/coma-guidelines
National Institute of Neurological Disorders and Stroke	www.ninds.nih.gov/disorders/tbi
The Cochrane Library	www.thecochranelibrary.com

TREATMENT

Most appropriate treatment is achieved through review of current guidelines on topics, as well as recommendations that pertain to the team approach to common problems with patients with moderate to severe TBI, including pharmacology/neuroprotective agents; discomfort and pain; respiratory, cardiovascular, and sleep disorders; dysautonomia; spasticity; movement disorders; gastrointestinal and genitourinary issues; HO; neuropathic pain; endocrine dysfunction; concomitant orthopedic problems; wound care; and prosthesis-related status, if applicable. Associated mental health issues such as PTSD and depression should also be considered. These are areas that physiatrists should learn about and update throughout their professional career. This can be accomplished through the aforementioned resources.

EDUCATION

Respect and courtesy are the primary basis of appropriate etiquette when interacting with people with disabilities. The physiatrist should educate families and patients on some of the difficulties that exist (extent of impairment) or may be encountered in the patient with TBI. This will prevent the patient and family from being surprised by unanticipated deficits and able to have a tool for measuring whether an observed difficulty is within the realm of what is expected or something that warrants more attention and hence medical investigation. The difficulties can be physical, behavioral, and/or cognitive. A significant cognitive problem is with memory (especially short-term memory), concentration, processing speed, organization, and problem solving. Patients with TBI may have trouble concentrating or organizing their thoughts, so when in a public area with many distractions, move to a quiet or private location, repeat what is communicated orally or in writing, provide extra time for decision making, and present information at a level conducive for fostering understanding such as sixth-grade reading level. Educate the family against interrupting the person with TBI during conversations as he or she may relatively easily lose the train of thought; in addition, advise the family on the benefits of setting short-term attainable goals to encourage participation. In terms of physical limitations, the family has to know that offering help can be valuable; however, they should wait for the patient to accept the offer of assistance and not overassist or be patronizing. This will give the family a good gauge of the level of function of the patient both physically and cognitively, as well as allow them to recognize changes. Behavioral changes that may be prevalent include anxiety, agitation, frustration, impulsiveness, repetitiveness, depression, regression (return to childlike behavior), and disinhibition (inability to control impulsive behavior and emotions). Family has to be counseled on being patient, flexible, and supportive. Patients and family can use assistive technology to help address some of the struggles seen in patients with TBI. The natural history of TBI is that usually the patient is expected to get better with time; however, there may exist a plateau for different patients. The prognosis for recovery and resumption of life roles should also be presented to the patient and family in order to prepare for the postdischarge social, academic, and work environment. Table 14.7 provides useful resources to provide patients and caregivers.

TABLE 14.7 Useful Resources for Patient and Family Support

Brain Injury Association of America	www.biausa.org/brain-injury-family-caregivers.htm
Duke Health	www.dukehealth.org/services/speech_and_audiology/care_guides/speech_pathology_resources/traumatic-brain-injury/traumatic-brain-injury-web-sites
Department of Veterans Affairs: Polytrauma/TBI System of Care	www.polytrauma.va.gov/support/training-and-education.asp
Department of Veterans Affairs: Quality Enhancement Research Initiative	www.queri.research.va.gov/ptbri/patients.cfm
Society for Cognitive Rehabilitation	www.societyforcognitiverehab.org/patient-family-resources/tbi/tbi-resource-sites.php
Virginia Commonwealth University TBI Model System	http://model.tbinrc.com
Defense Veterans Brain Injury Center	http://dvbic.dcoe.mil
Centers for Disease Control and Prevention	www.cdc.gov/traumaticbraininjury/

It is important to provide a structured environment for patients with TBI and to establish new routines to help them relearn old skills and develop new strategies. Caregivers should be encouraged to learn nursing routines and different therapeutic strategies so they can apply new caregiving skills (i.e., positioning, transfers, feeding, bathing, toileting, and medication management). Throughout this process, the medical team should guide and support the patient and the caregiver(s).

Issues that need to be considered include impact of cognitive impairments; need for adequate rest and sleep; minimizing (or, better yet, eliminating) alcohol and substance abuse; risk of depression/suicide; need for assistance with nutrition, wound care, ADLs, and instrumental ADLs (IADLs), and assistance with mobility (bed mobility, transfers, and ambulation with assistive device). Teams should educate patients and families on strategies for appropriate behavior, side effect of medications, pain management, dysautonomia, motor agitation, and so on. The possibility of long-term placement after acute rehabilitation stay should be discussed once recognized.

For military personnel, of paramount importance is acute management of TBI from point of injury to stateside military treatment facilities. It is also important for the physiatrist to be able to describe the following: TBI assessment, treatment, and overall coordination of care, and then communicate that information to the patient and family (13). Adaptive techniques for learning and communication include repeating, reviewing, giving feedback, and using assistive technology. Caregivers should be counseled on using oral and written presentation of materials to the patient, as well as giving the patient a longer time to process information and complete tasks.

QUALITY IMPROVEMENT/PRACTICE IMPROVEMENT ACTIVITY

Patients with significant brain injuries require care that is optimized by an interdisciplinary team that understands the physiology behind the injury and achieves the goals established in each phase of the recovery. Some areas that can be used to monitor the quality of care provided to moderate to severe TBI patients include frequency of acute transfers; occurrence of VTE; development of HO, contractures, or seizures; prevalence of behavioral and emotional problems such as depression; cognitive and functional changes; and discharge to community.

Performance improvement and delivery of expected outcomes are essential throughout health care in general and in rehabilitation medicine in particular. Outcomes are selected to maximize the ability of the clinician to formulate and document the natural course of recovery of TBI, predict outcome, measure the effect of treatment, and make comparisons with comparable facilities. Using an internally generated outcome measure or benchmarking based on previous performance creates a goal for performance improvement. Ultimately, the goal is to help drive improvements in delivery and assessment of effectiveness of major aspects of patient care. This process leads to selection of treatment interventions in a skilled manner that is individualized for each patient and takes into account psychosocial, functional, and quality-of-life objectives. Improving the quality and outcomes of rehabilitation addresses all elements of the basic cycle of assessing (diagnosis and fact finding); planning; treating; measuring the result; and reassessing whether to modify, continue, or discontinue a certain intervention. A large number of outcome scales are now available in both rehabilitation and health care in general. The Center for Outcome Measurement in Brain Injury's (COMBI) website (www.tbims.org/combi/list.html) features materials on instruments or scales used in measuring outcomes. Joint Commission on the Accreditation of Healthcare Organizations (JCAHO) requires that institutions compare their process and outcomes with those known to be attainable elsewhere; the Commission on Accreditation of Rehabilitation Facilities (CARF) also expects program improvement.

Evidence-based resources that are important to the practicing physiatrist treating moderate to severe TBI are mentioned earlier, including review of outcome prediction models and development of acute care guidelines.

INTERPERSONAL SKILLS AND COMMUNICATION

GOAL

Demonstrate interpersonal and communication skills that result in the effective exchange of information and collaboration with TBI patients, their families, and other health professionals.

OBJECTIVES

1. Demonstrate skills used in effective communication and collaboration with patients with moderate to severe TBI and their caregivers, across socioeconomic and culture backgrounds.
2. Identify strategies to use in the prevention of reinjury after TBI.
3. Delineate the importance of the role of the physiatrist as the team leader and consultant.
4. Demonstrate proper documentation and effective communication between health care professionals in patient care.

COUNSELING PATIENTS AND FAMILIES

Counseling of patients and families is of paramount importance throughout all the stages of the TBI patient's recovery and rehabilitation. Patient and family have to be educated on communication strategies such as providing a quiet environment to decrease the possibility of overstimulating the patient, using noninflammatory language delivered in an even tone of voice, using calming language especially for agitated patients, allowing the patient time for processing and understanding, confirming patient understanding, and repeating to the patient as often as necessary. In moderate to severe TBI, the challenges include negative impact on cognitive impairments and need for adequate rest/sleep. It is also important for the patient to minimize or eliminate alcohol (EtOH)/substance abuse. The regular use of seat belt/air bags by drivers and wearing of helmet by motorcyclists or bicyclists are important (14). The physiatrist can help minimize risk of reinjury through education of the patient about high-risk behavior and informing the patient and family about risk of depression and suicide. The patient will benefit from assistance with nutrition, wound care, ADLs, IADLs, and mobility. In addition, strategies for appropriate behavior with family and coworkers, side effects of medications, pain management, and possibility of long-term placement after acute rehabilitation stay are also topics to discuss.

DOCUMENTATION AND EFFECTIVE COMMUNICATION

Documentation helps with improving communication between health care professionals such as social workers, therapists, nurses, physicians (including consulting teams), and all other facets of an interdisciplinary rehabilitation team. The information leads to augmented safety at transition points in patient care and planning. Appropriate documentation can reduce morbidity by informing all involved in care.

Strategies to be used by the physician when communicating with the adult with brain injury and family include allowing time for processing and understanding, confirming an understanding of the discussion, and repeating as often as necessary. Utilize the family if a cognitive deficit reduces effective transfer of information during communication. When communicating with the family, realize that the patient is the main focus of discussion; therefore, empower and instill confidence in the family by providing accurate and timely information, and keep the family informed about the medical plan, discharge options, and changes.

LEADERSHIP SKILLS

The physiatrist has the role of team leader in coordination of care for the moderate to severe TBI patient with consultants and other members of the rehabilitation team. For effective collaboration, the team will need to set a time and place for regular meetings. Some key ground rules include attendance, promptness, participation, accountability for assignments, and keeping interruptions to a minimum. Effective discussion skills include the physiatrist as the leader and coordinator or gatekeeper, formatted agenda, active listening, equal participation among members and containment of digression, requests for clarification, summarization when necessary, time management, and testing consensus when appropriate. The meeting topics should be tabulated and should include actions required to be completed. Good communication among team members augments patient care and minimizes complications, which in turn improves monitoring for changes in patient status and maximizes patient safety.

PROFESSIONALISM

GOAL

Reflect a commitment to carrying out professional responsibilities and an adherence to ethical principles in TBI.

OBJECTIVES

1. Exemplify the humanistic qualities of a TBI provider.
2. Demonstrate ethical principles and responsiveness to patient needs superseding self and other interests.

3. Demonstrate sensitivity to patient population diversity, including culture, gender, age, race, religion, disabilities, and sexual orientation.
4. Respect patient privacy and autonomy.
5. Recognize the importance of patient education in the treatment of and advocacy for persons with TBI.
6. Describe the impact of demographics on the care of persons with TBI.

Within medicine, humanistic qualities of professionals are integral to the patient–doctor relationship. Specific qualities that provide benefit in the relationship are respect, compassion, and ethics. The patient with TBI and his or her family often become experts in their own care and can provide medical providers ample historical information, symptomatology, and so on. Therefore, it is pertinent that the provider respects the patient and family by listening to their concerns throughout the recovery course. As TBI is often invisible, patients, family members, and employers at times do not understand the breadth of deficits that occur after injury. As this is the case, providers should compassionately care for their patients and advocate upon their behalf. A good procedure for inpatient rehabilitation facilities is to include advocacy groups into the educational mission; this allows patients and families to obtain information about resources to assist them throughout their recovery process.

As research on TBI continues to increase, so does the burden upon potential subjects. It is imperative for TBI experts to maintain a balance between a care provider and a researcher. The patient's best interests must be kept at heart; otherwise, he or she may be subjected to unnecessary procedures (see previously in Medical Knowledge; Ethical Issues for discussion on nonmaleficence). In addition, it is the TBI physician's responsibility to understand current and emerging research in order to answer the questions of patients and families. As research continues to evolve, so should the TBI physician's clinical repertoire.

As described earlier (see Medical Knowledge; Ethical Issues), the balance between autonomy and capacity is highly important in the recovery of persons with TBI. Again, it is the physician's responsibility to understand the balance between these two concepts in order to provide appropriate care to patients.

TBI providers have the responsibility to provide ample educational opportunities for patients and their family. It is through education that patients and caregivers start to understand the intricacies of TBI. Advocacy groups assist with the education process and should be utilized for their resources. In addition, TBI providers must utilize their expertise by educating the community, as well as national, state, and local leaders about strategies to minimize the risk of TBI. Through education, a TBI provider can advocate for the rights of individuals with TBI to allow greater access to resources.

Another aspect of professionalism requires the rehabilitation team to pay close attention to the culture, gender, age, race, and sexual orientation of individuals with TBI and their support system. Respect for an individual's experiences, worldview, learning style, and expectations will allow the team to maximally assist individuals in their recovery. It is the physiatrist's responsibility to ensure that the patient progresses; this responsibility requires that the physiatrist promote the idea of appropriate patient care by embracing the patient and family's needs, expectations, and beliefs. This includes accountability for balancing autonomy versus beneficence in situations when a patient wants to exercise his or her individual rights, which are in direct conflict with the physician's or team's recommendations.

SYSTEMS-BASED PRACTICE

GOAL

Awareness and responsiveness to systems of care delivery, and the ability to recruit and coordinate effectively resources in the system to provide optimal care as it relates to moderate to severe TBI.

OBJECTIVES

1. Identify the components, systems of care delivery, services, referral patterns, and resources in the TBI rehabilitation continuum.
2. Coordinate and recruit necessary resources in the system to provide optimal care for the TBI patient, with attention to cost awareness and risk–benefit analysis and management.
3. Describe the TBI continuum established by the Department of Veterans Affairs and the Department of Defense.
4. Introduce quality improvement as a key factor in TBI rehabilitation programs, including identification of system errors.

The TBI continuum of care includes many components, such as the acute care hospital, inpatient rehabilitation facility (IRF), long-term neurobehavioral programs, community reentry/transitional rehabilitation program, skilled nursing facility (SNF), day rehabilitation programs, outpatient rehabilitation program, and home. Each person with TBI may not necessarily move through each of those settings, but each setting must be kept in mind when considering the next step in the rehabilitation process.

In the acute care setting, the main goal is to prevent death, reduce morbidity, and stabilize the patient. If an individual with TBI has appropriate social support, resources, and potential for benefit from intensive rehabilitation, then the IRF is an appropriate next step in the recovery timeline. From the IRF or the acute care setting, a patient who progresses slowly may need care in a long-term neurobehavioral program. A physiatrist must keep in mind that these programs are mostly private pay, and not all patients qualify for treatment. For those who do not have financial resources to cover the cost of a long-term neurobehavioral program, transition to home or an SNF may be beneficial. However, if an individual with TBI progresses well in an IRF, but is not yet ready for home/community living, then transfer to a transitional rehabilitation program focusing on community reentry or even vocational rehabilitation would be beneficial. Those individuals without family support or whose family is unable to provide the necessary level of care may need to be transferred to an SNF. Many of these facilities continue the rehabilitation process by offering physical therapy, occupational therapy, and speech therapy, but at a reduced number of visits. Patients who are at home but continue to have significant basic self-care, mobility, cognitive, communication, or swallowing needs would benefit from a day rehabilitation program. These programs offer multiple therapies on a daily basis. They also allow time for family training and education. Many patients will graduate from these programs to a reduced amount of outpatient therapy visits. It is highly imperative that patients and family members continue the strategies learned during the rehabilitation process, as recovery and maintenance from TBI is a lifelong process.

It is important within each setting for patients and family members to have at hand the etiology and severity of the TBI, medication list, side effects, list of team members, and rehabilitation goals. The treating team should supply this information with encouragement for patients and family to provide their input into the recovery process.

Within each of these settings, patient safety must be addressed. Refer to the chapter Patient Safety in Rehabilitation Medicine (PM&R Clinics of NA, May 2012, Vol. 23, Number 2) for more information.

Long-term follow-up for TBI is important. In the private setting, persons with TBI can see a physiatrist who specializes in TBI. If one does not practice close to the person's home, then a TBI specialist and the patient's primary care provider, or a physiatrist practicing close to the patient's home, can coordinate care. America's Veterans can follow up in the Polytrauma System of Care (PSC). The PSC provides care for Veterans and Active Duty Service members with TBI. This system includes the full spectrum of TBI care (acute inpatient rehabilitation, residential/transitional rehabilitation, and outpatient clinics). Long-term brain injury follow-up is easily coordinated through the PSC and allows each provider within the system to access the patient's full medical record in a timely fashion. Within the Department of Defense, each military treatment facility and most military bases have brain injury clinics. Active Duty Service members can follow up with TBI specialists in these settings or in the VA's PSC.

For many years now, TBI researchers have searched for appropriate outcomes measures. As mentioned earlier, COMBI has compiled a list of outcomes measurement tools that TBI specialists can use to determine the quality of their programs. CARF looks at four key areas when evaluating quality of care in programs: (a) effectiveness, (b) efficiency, (c) access, and (d) satisfaction. It is prudent to use validated and reliable outcomes measurement tools when determining quality improvement measures in TBI programs.

At times, programs can become bogged down with systems-based errors. In the inpatient rehabilitation setting, a variety of team members will have input into the patient's care on a 24/7 basis. In this case, appropriate and consistent communication is highly beneficial. Poor communication can lead to reduced effectiveness, efficiency, and satisfaction. Implementing strategies for building a sound TBI rehabilitation program will enable a team to provide exceptional care to this population of injured persons.

As discussed earlier, the annual cost of TBI is over $75 billion. This estimate includes direct medical and indirect costs, such as lost productivity (7,8). The lifetime costs of caring for a severely injured person with TBI is between $600,000 and $1.875M. With such high costs associated with moderate and severe TBI, it is of utmost importance to focus on primary prevention.

The CDC, Defense Veterans Brain Injury Center (DVBIC), and the Brain Injury Association of America (BIAA) are a few of the organizations that provide educational material. Utilizing their resources allows a TBI provider to increase the awareness of his or her patients, their families, and the community at large (Table 14.8).

TABLE 14.8 Patient Safety Checklist

■ Motor vehicle safety
▪ Seat belts
▪ Child restraint systems
▪ Impaired or distracted driving
▪ Teen drivers
▪ Pedestrian safety
■ Fall reduction
▪ Early identification of fall-related TBI
▪ Falls in older adults
▪ Falls in children
■ Sports and recreation safety
■ Violence prevention

Source: Adapted from CDC website.

CASE STUDY

A 20-year-old man is involved in a motorcycle crash. He is found with his helmet off on the side of the road and a GCS of 5 at the scene. Upon arrival to the emergency department, his GCS is 6 and the patient is combative. He is intubated, and his urine drug screen is positive for alcohol. CT scan is completed and shows a large right subdural hematoma with midline shift of 8 mm along with numerous cerebral contusions. The patient undergoes emergent craniectomy and is transferred to the ICU. He is started on levetiracetam for seizure prophylaxis. After a few days, the patient stabilizes and is extubated. He is subsequently transferred to an IRF for further management. At the time of admission, he is noted to have poor initiation and demonstrates significant cognitive deficits.

CASE STUDY DISCUSSION QUESTIONS

1. What are the key components of the medical history and physical examination for this patient at time of admission to an IRF and what are the key issues in the medical management of this patient?
2. If the patient was to become agitated during his rehabilitation stay, what is the recommended assessment and management for agitation in a brain-injured adult?
3. Describe the current understanding of the pathophysiology of TBI and the role of rehabilitative medicine in its treatment.

4. Describe the current scientific understanding of seizure prophylaxis in a patient with a TBI and identify resources that you can consult to obtain evidence-based medicine on this topic.
5. Identify the key team members involved in this patient's care and describe effective communication, documentation, and interpersonal skills between them in the care of this patient.
6. What are some safety concerns for this patient and how would you minimize their risk of occurrence?

SELF-EXAMINATION QUESTIONS
(Answers begin on p. 367)

1. A man sustains a TBI from a motor vehicle crash. His initial GCS is 10 and he is unconscious for 29 minutes. He also exhibits memory loss for 2 days after injury. Which of the following is best characterizes the severity of his TBI?
   A. Mild
   B. Moderate
   C. Severe
   D. Unknown
   E. Extremely severe

2. Which of the following best describes characteristics of dysautonomia?
   A. Hypotension, bradycardia, and diaphoresis
   B. Hypertension, bradycardia, and diaphoresis
   C. Hypotension, tachycardia, and diaphoresis
   D. Hypertension, tachycardia, and diaphoresis
   E. Hypotension, tachycardia, and bradycardia

3. Which of the following medications cannot be used for agitation management?
   A. Propranolol
   B. Sertraline
   C. Valproic acid
   D. Acetaminophen
   E. Olanzapine

4. Which of the following antispasticity medications does not cause sedation?
   A. Dantrolene
   B. Baclofen
   C. Tizanidine
   D. Diazepam
   E. Clonazepam

5. What is the lifetime cost of a severely injured person with TBI?
   A. $100K to $600K
   B. $600K to $1.9M
   C. $2.0M to $3.4M
   D. $3.5M to $4.4M
   E. $4.5M to $5.4M

REFERENCES

1. Wagner AK, Hammond FM, Sasser HC, et al. Use of injury severity variables in determining disability and community integration after traumatic brain injury. *J Trauma*. 2000;49:411–419.
2. Wagner AK, Arenth PM, Kwasnica C, et al. Traumatic Brain Injury. In Braddom RL, ed. *Physical Medicine and Rehabilitation*. 4th ed. Philadelphia, PA: Elsevier Incorporated; 2011:1133–1175.
3. Koehler R, Wilhelm E, Shoulson I. *Cognitive Rehabilitation Therapy for Traumatic Brain Injury: Evaluating the Evidence*. Washington, DC: National Academic Press, 2011:127.
4. Jorge RE, Starkstein SE. Pathophysiologic aspects of major depression following traumatic brain injury. *J Head Trauma Rehabil*. 2005;20(6):475–487.
5. Faul M, Xu L, Wald MM, et al. *Traumatic Brain Injury in the United States: Emergency Department Visits, Hospitalizations, and Deaths*. Atlanta, GA: Centers for Disease Control and Prevention, National Center for Injury Prevention and Control; 2010.
6. Centers for Disease Control and Prevention (CDC), National Center for Injury Prevention and Control. *Report to Congress on Mild Traumatic Brain Injury in the United States: Steps to Prevent a Serious Public Health Problem*. Atlanta, GA: Centers for Disease Control and Prevention; 2003.
7. Finkelstein E, Corso P, Miller T, et al. *The Incidence and Economic Burden of Injuries in the United States*. New York, NY: Oxford University Press; 2006.
8. Coronado VG, McGuire LC, Faul M, et al. *The Epidemiology and Prevention of TBI* (in press). 2012.
9. Giacino JT, Whyte J, Bagiella E, et al. Placebo-controlled trial of amantadine for severe traumatic brain injury. *N Engl J Med*. 2012;366(9):819–826.
10. Berridge CW, Devilbiss DM, Andrzejewski ME, et al. Methylphenidate preferentially increases catecholamine neurotransmission within the prefrontal cortex at low doses that enhance cognitive function. *Biol Psychiatry*. 2006;60(10):1111-1120.
11. Tye KM, Tye LD, Cone JJ, et al. Methylphenidate facilitates learning-induced amygdala plasticity. *Nat Neurosci*. 2010;13(4):475–481.
12. Fields CD, Rao V. Rational neuropharmacology in traumatic brain injury. In: Zollman FS, ed. *Manual of Traumatic Brain Injury Management*. 1st ed. New York, NY: Demos Medical Publishing, 2011:261.
13. Jaffee MS, Helmick KM, Girard PD, et al. Acute clinical care and care coordination for traumatic brain injury within the Department of Defense. *J Rehabil Res Dev*. 2009;46(6):655–656.
14. Cradall CS, Olson LM, SKlar DP. Mortality reduction with air bag and seat belt use in head-on passenger car collisions. *Am J Epidemiol*. 2001;153:219–224.

Foluke A. Akinyemi
Shane McNamee

15: Mild Traumatic Brain Injury

PATIENT CARE

GOALS

Provide patient care that is compassionate, appropriate, and effective for the treatment of mild traumatic brain injury (MTBI) problems and the promotion of health.

OBJECTVES

1. Perform a pertinent history and physical of the MTBI adult patient.
2. Identify key impairments, functional, and activity limitations for adults with MTBI.
3. Identify the psychosocial and vocational implications of MTBI and strategies to address them.
4. Describe injuries commonly associated with MTBI.
5. Describe a sample rehabilitation treatment plan for adults with MTBI.

Key elements of the history should include at a minimum the history of present illness, past medical history, review of systems, medication review, psychosocial and vocational history, and allergies.

History of present illness should include the following:

1. Details of the injury event
2. Mechanism of injury
3. Duration and severity of alteration of consciousness
4. Length of amnesia, immediate symptoms
5. Symptom course and prior treatment
6. Other injuries (such as fractures and cervical trauma)
7. Patient's symptoms and health concerns
8. Screening for premorbid conditions, potential cooccurring conditions, or other psychosocial risk factors such as substance use disorders that may exacerbate or maintain current symptom presentation
9. Assess danger to self or others

Past medical history should include any history of past brain injury; alcohol, tobacco, or illicit or prescription drug abuse; attention deficit hyperactivity disorder (ADHD), depression, anxiety, posttraumatic stress disorder (PTSD), chronic pain, and other psychosocial risk factors; acquired or congenital brain disease/abnormalities and past head or brain surgeries.

Social/vocational history: Preinjury academic and/or employment histories and marital/social support history are essential, particularly as they influence recovery following MTBI.

Review of systems: When obtaining the review of systems, the physiatrist should review the presence or absence of somatic symptoms commonly seen after MTBI and should ask about headache, vestibular system dysfunction, sleep disturbance, dizziness/coordination/balance problems, nausea, blurred vision, sensitivity to noise and sound, fatigue, and musculoskeletal pain.

The physiatrist should also screen for common cognitive problems such as impaired memory, concentration, attention, speed of processing, judgment, and executive control. If any of these are present, he or she should inquire about the impact of any of these symptoms on school or work performance.

The patient should be asked about symptoms such as depression, anxiety, agitation, irritability, impulsivity, and aggression and, if present, inquire about the impact of these difficulties on family/work relationships.

The patient should also be asked about the course and resolution (or lack thereof) of the symptoms since the time of injury. The frequency and severity of symptoms should be documented in order to set a baseline for monitoring subsequent treatment efficacy and for establishing co-occurring conditions.

It is also important to ask patients if and how their symptoms impact their daily functions, especially how they impact their basic activities of daily living (ADLs) and instrumental ADLs (IADLs). IADLs are activities and skills that allow patients to live independently such as managing finances, shopping, preparing meals, and performing basic housework.

Medications: Review of past and current medications and drug allergies should be performed. The physician should make note of past medications tried for the patient's current symptoms, efficacy, and reason for stopping the medications, if applicable.

Screen for current medications that may worsen neurologic recovery or cause sedation, cognitive slowing, or increased risk for suicidal ideations.

After each history taking, it is imperative that the physician validate the patient's concerns and symptoms.

Physical examination should include the following:

A. Focused neurologic examination that includes the following:
   1. Mental status examination (MSE)
   2. Cranial nerve testing
   3. Sensation
   4. Extremity testing of tone
   5. Muscle stretch reflexes
   6. Motor strength testing
   7. Postural stability (Romberg test; dynamic sitting and standing)

B. Focused vision examination including gross acuity, eye movement, binocular function, and visual fields/attention testing.

C. Focused musculoskeletal examination including range of motion, focal tenderness, and palpation of the head, neck, jaw, spine, and extremities.

D. Cognitive evaluation: There are several brief screening tools available, including the Mini Mental Status Examination (MMSE) and the Montreal Cognitive Assessment (MoCA). MoCA has been validated in the setting of mild cognitive impairment associated with several clinical disorders. The test, test information, and administration instructions are accessible for clinicians at www.mocatest.org.

FUNCTIONAL IMPAIRMENTS AND ACTIVITY LIMITATIONS ASSOCIATED WITH MTBI

Impairments commonly seen in MTBI patients include impaired balance, coordination, vision, hearing, and sleep. Cognitive impairments such as memory, concentration, attention span, and speed of mental processing of information can be present. Behavioral and emotional impairments such as emotional liability and apathy can also be seen.

Patients with MTBI are typically independent in basic ADLs such as grooming, bathing, dressing, toileting, and mobility; however, a minority of patients may report that their symptoms negatively impact their abilities in IADLs, such as driving, home management, child care, financial management, and on-the-job or school performance.

KEY PSYCHOSOCIAL ASPECTS ASSOCIATED WITH MTBI AND ITS VOCATIONAL IMPLICATIONS

MTBI may create physical, social, marital, vocational, and avocational activity limitations and participation restrictions for the patient. For example, after MTBI, patients may be unable to return to work or school and have difficulty performing their role in their family or community. They may also have difficulties with relationships at home and/or work, such as problems relating to one's spouse, children, and coworkers. They may also have comorbid depression, anxiety, and PTSD.

School and/or vocational needs must be addressed, and the decision on when and how to return to school or work is based on the severity of the cognitive, physical, and emotional impairments and the type of work previously engaged in.

Work performance and abilities may be negatively impacted from the cognitive, behavioral, and physical problems mentioned earlier. An individual may have problems securing or maintaining his job due to inability to meet his or her work demands. There may be difficulties with job performance—forgetting appointments, problems completing tasks, difficulties getting along with supervisors and coworkers. Subsequently, individuals may need to change occupations/jobs frequently and some eventually become unemployed.

Immediately following a TBI episode, symptomatic patients should have a period of rest to avoid sustaining another concussion and to facilitate a prompt recovery. After the short rest period, they should be encouraged to expediently return to normal activity (work, school, duty, leisure) and a gradual resumption of activity is recommended. A period of work restriction or accommodation such as provision of additional time to complete tasks and working in a quiet environment with additional supervision may be necessary to ensure successful reintegration. If symptoms reemerge after returning to previous normal activity levels, a monitored progressive return to normal activity as tolerated should be recommended (1).

Common injuries associated with MTBI include whiplash and musculoskeletal injuries, which may be seen in patients who have sustained TBI as a result of motor vehicle accident (MVA), falls, contact sport, subtle fractures, and substance abuse. In addition, cumulative effects of MTBI may include psychiatric disorders and loss of long-term memory.

Strategies to prevent MTBI and related injuries including education of the patient, family, and caregiver is the keystone to prevention (2). Clinicians should provide information to patients, families, and caregivers about risk behaviors and activities that increase potential for TBIs of all types. Other recommendations for preventing MTBIs include the following:

1. Consistent use of seat belt
2. Never drive under the influence of alcohol, drugs, or medications that can impair cognition or cause drowsiness
3. Consistent helmet use when engaging in at-risk activities such as biking, motorcycle, snowmobile, skiing, snowboarding, skating, contact sports, baseball or softball, and horse riding
4. Always buckle small children in cars
5. Regular vision check to decrease fall risk
6. Remove household tripping hazards

Patients with MTBI often complain of concurrent physical, cognitive, and behavioral symptoms. It is important to treat the symptoms that cause the patient the most distress first. Patients should be screened for comorbid mental health disorders. Headache is one of the most common symptoms associated with MTBI (3). Assessment and management of headaches in individuals with MTBI should be comparable with those for other causes of headache (4). (See Table 15.1 for recommendations for specific symptoms.)

In patients with persistent post-concussive symptoms, who are refractory to treatment, consideration should be given to other factors such as psychiatric issues, psychosocial support and also consider extrinsic factors such as patient involved in litigation and those seeking compensation for their injuries.

TABLE 15.1 Common Postconcussive Symptoms and Management Approach

SYMPTOMS	MANAGEMENT
Physical Problems	
Headache	Prophylactic and abortive medications
	Education on stress and lifestyle management
Balance and vestibular dysfunction	Physical therapy, vestibular rehabilitation
Blurred vision/photosensitivity	Sunglasses for photosensitivity, vision therapy, referral to optometrist
Tinnitus and hearing impairment	Audiology referral for tinnitus and hearing impairment
	Education on hearing protection and environmental modifications
Musculoskeletal pain syndromes	Physical therapy, pain medication—avoid narcotics
Sleep disorder	Refer for sleep study if sleep apnea is suspected
	Educate on proper sleep hygiene to include avoidance of alcohol, caffeine products, or stimulants before sleep; establish a consistent sleep schedule, limit daytime naps, and avoid stimulating activities immediately before sleep
	Sleep medications—avoid benzodiazepines
Cognitive Problems	
Impaired memory, concentration, attention, processing speed, executive control	Neuropsychology testing
	Cognitive remediation training
	Referral to speech pathology/occupational therapy for training on compensatory strategies

(continued)

TABLE 15.1 Common Postconcussive Symptoms and Management Approach (continued)

SYMPTOMS	MANAGEMENT
	Voice recorders, use of smart phones, and/Personal Digital Assistance (PDA) for memory aid. Global positioning devices (GPS) for direction and to avoid getting lost
Behavioral Problems	
Depression	May require either psychotherapeutic or pharmacological treatment modalities, or both
Anxiety	
Irritability	
Poor impulse control	Medications include SSRIs
Aggression	Mental health referrals should be considered for management of depression, PTSD, and anxiety; referrals to substance abuse treatment specialists as needed
PTSD	

PHARMACOLOGICAL TREATMENT APPROACH TO MTBI

When considering medications to manage symptoms of MTBI, it is important to keep in mind that injured brains are sensitive to the side effects of medications. Choose medications with the least amount of negative effect on cognition, brain recovery, and minimal side effect profiles. Monitor patients closely during treatment and evaluate for potential toxicities and drug–drug interactions. Avoid medications that can lower the seizure threshold or result in drowsiness or slowed thinking. Avoid medications associated with increased risk of suicidal ideation. Examples of medications to avoid are benzodiazepines and anticholinergic and antidopaminergic agents.

SAMPLE REHABILITATION PROGRAM, MANAGEMENT, OR TREATMENT PLAN FOR MTBI

A 23-year-old man is involved in an MVA, in which he sustained mild grade 1 American Academy of Neurology (AAN) TBI. He presents to your office 3 months later with complaints of mild balance problems and dizziness, daily headaches lasting 4 hours, short-term memory impairments, light sensitivity, and mild impairment in hearing. He also reports difficulty falling and frequent awakening from sleep secondary to nightmares.

TREATMENT PLAN

Start by (a) validating the patient's experience and symptoms, (b) educating the patient regarding the natural history of MTBI, and (c) reassuring the patient that most people with MTBI have resolution of their symptoms within a few weeks.

Symptom management for this patient includes the following:

1. Physical therapy for vestibular rehabilitation to address the dizziness and balance problems.
2. Speech therapy for compensatory strategies and memory aids.
3. Vision therapist for photosensitivity. Recommend sunglasses.
4. Audiology for hearing impairments.
5. Sleep management should include review and discussion of sleep hygiene. If sleep apnea is suspected, a referral for sleep study should be done first before prescribing sleep medications. In this case study, sleep apnea was ruled out; however, he stated that he did not like taking PO medications, so he was started on trazodone 50 mg QHS and also started on a trial of prazosin for nightmares.
6. If PTSD is suspected, referral for mental health treatment is indicated.
7. Headache management should start with attempts to characterize the type of headache—tension versus migraine versus combined. If the patient has migraine headaches, both prophylactic and abortive medications are indicated. Past and present medications were reviewed, and the patient was asked about efficacy and reasons for discontinuing medications.

The patient was started on Sumatriptan for abortive therapy and topiramate for headache prophylaxis (Botox injection is another alternative).

9. Educate the patient on stress reduction and sleep management. Instruct him to avoid factors that trigger his migraines.

At the conclusion of the clinical visit, the patient was educated on how to avoid future TBI; a follow-up appointment is given and a written summary of important points and plans are provided to the patient.

Management of common symptoms in MTBI is given in Table 15.2.

MEDICAL KNOWLEDGE

GOAL

Demonstrate knowledge of established and evolving biomedical, clinical, epidemiological, and sociobehavioral sciences pertaining to the field of TBI, as well as the application of this knowledge to guide holistic patient care.

TABLE 15.2 Management of Symptoms Common in MTBI

SYMPTOMS	KEY INFORMATION AND NONPHARMACOLOGY MANAGEMENT	PHARMACOLOGICAL MANAGEMENT
Headache	Treatment is based on type of headaches (migraine vs. tension vs. mixed) ■ Treat contributory comorbid sleep, mental health disorders. ■ Educate patient on avoiding triggers. ■ Nonpharmacological treatment includes: 　■ Relaxation, biofeedback, visualization, extracranial pressure, and cold compresses. Regular exercise, maintaining regular sleep, and meal. ■ Patients with episodic tension-type headache may also benefit from physical therapy to exercise neck muscles.	■ Abortive medications should be taken at onset of headache ■ Nonnarcotic pain medication ■ NSAIDs (e.g., ibuprofen and naproxen) ■ Triptans (for migraines) ■ NSAIDs such as aspirin, ibuprofen, or choline-magnesium-trisalicylate and acetaminophen are the first-line medications for treating tension headaches ■ *Combination medications* (aspirin, acetaminophen, or both are often combined with caffeine or a sedative drug) in a single medication can be effective in treating episodic tension headache, but persistent usage can lead to rebound headaches ■ Prophylactic medications are indicated for migraines occurring more than once a week or tension-type headache occurring more than 3 times a week. ■ For headache that is disabling despite aggressive acute interventions; if the patient desires to reduce frequency of acute attacks; or when headaches compromise work attendance, societal integration, or daily life: divalproex, topiramate, and metoprolol are first-line headache prophylactic agents.
Musculoskeletal pain	■ May involve both pharmacological and nonpharmacological treatment such as physical therapy and modalities such as cold/heat, Transcutaneous electrical nerve stimulation (TENS)	■ Avoid use of narcotics as this can be detrimental to cognitive recovery

(continued)

TABLE 15.2 Management of Symptoms Common in MTBI (*continued*)

SYMPTOMS	KEY INFORMATION AND NONPHARMACOLOGY MANAGEMENT	PHARMACOLOGICAL MANAGEMENT
Insomnia/sleep dysfunction	■ Goal is to establish a regular, unbroken, nighttime sleep pattern and to improve perceptions of the quality of sleep ■ Educate on sleep hygiene, establishing regular sleep routine, limiting caffeine and alcohol before bedtime ■ Refer to sleep specialist to treat concurrent *primary* sleep disorder (e.g., sleep apnea, restless leg syndrome, or narcolepsy) if present ■ Consider training patient in behavioral techniques, such as relaxation training or meditation; this may improve the quality of sleep	■ Nonbenzodiazepene sleep medications such as trazodone may be helpful in the short term ■ Prazosin may be helpful in patients with nightmares
Cognitive impairments	■ Referral to speech and language pathology for compensatory memory strategies and memory aids may be indicated ■ Screen for comorbid medical and psychiatric conditions such as PTSD that may be contributing to memory problems and determine if the psychiatric contribution is significant; this may need to be treated first before referring for speech and language therapy ■ Patients with problems obtaining or maintaining employment may benefit from referral to vocational rehabilitation	
Dizziness and disequilibrium disorders	■ May be secondary to inner ear disorders (peripheral vestibular disorders), central nervous system disorders, psychological disorders, and musculoskeletal disorders ■ Perform a detailed medication review and ask about the temporal relationship of dizziness to the initiation or dosing of these medications; If possible, discontinue offending medication ■ Management depends on etiology and may include pharmacological and nonpharmacological treatment; it may also include referral to physical therapy for vestibular rehabilitation and/or referral to Ear, Nose and Throat specialist; referral to neurology ophthalmology, vision rehabilitation	■ Medications should only be considered if symptoms are severe enough to significantly limit functional activities ■ Trials should be limited to 2 weeks. First-line medication choice would be meclizine, followed by scopolamine and dimenhydrinate, depending upon symptom presentation
Comorbid depression/anxiety/PTSD	■ Assess suicidal/homicidal ideations ■ Refer to mental health	■ First-line antidepressant is SSRIs such as citalopram and sertraline

OBJECTIVES

1. Discuss the following as they relate to MTBI: (a) epidemiology, (b) pathophysiology, (c) diagnostic test and criteria, (d) special patient population, (e) treatment approach, and (f) ethical issues.

EPIDEMIOLOGY

Traumatic brain injury (TBI) can be defined as brain dysfunction caused by external mechanical force to the brain. The external force may be due to contact, penetration, and/or acceleration/deceleration forces. It is an important public health problem in the United States, affecting approximately 1.7 million people annually and leading to a substantial number of cases of death and disability (5). TBI most commonly affects children between 0 and 4 years, adolescents 15 and 19 years, and adults over the age of 65. TBI is more common in males than in females in all affected age groups. In the civilian population, fall is the leading cause of TBI and motor vehicle/traffic injury is the second-leading cause of TBI, although it is the leading cause of TBI-related deaths. Approximately 80% of the total incidence of TBI is classified as MTBI (6). MTBIs cost the nation nearly $17 billion each year.

DIAGNOSTIC CRITERIA FOR MTBI

In this chapter, we will use the most commonly used criteria of MTBI as set forth by the Mild Traumatic Brain Injury Committee of the Head Injury Interdisciplinary Special Interest Group of the American Congress of Rehabilitation Medicine (ACRM) (7).

According to these criteria, a patient with MTBI is a person who has had a traumatically induced physiological disruption of brain function as manifested by at least one of the following:

1. Any period of loss of consciousness (LOC)
2. Any loss of memory for events immediately before or after the accident
3. Any alteration in mental state at the time of the accident
4. Focal neurological deficits that may or may not be transient

However, the severity of the injury does not exceed the following:

1. LOC of approximately 30 minutes or less
2. After 30 minutes, an initial Glasgow Coma Scale (GCS) of 13 to 15
3. Posttraumatic amnesia (PTA) not greater than 24 hours

Mechanism of injury in the aforementioned definition includes the head being struck or the head striking an object and the brain undergoing acceleration/deceleration movement without external trauma to the head. Imaging, EEG, or neurological examination may be negative.

PATHOPHYSIOLOGY

While the underlying pathophysiology of MTBI is still heavily debated, dysfunction can occur due to cortical contusions and potential axonal damage at the time of impact or injury. There may also be disruption of axonal neurofilament organization, which leads to impaired axonal transport, axonal swelling, degeneration, and damages (20,21).

DIAGNOSTIC TEST AND IMAGING

Clinical neuroimaging findings are normal in the majority of MTBI cases. Therefore, emergency room physicians should follow a selective approach to CT scan imaging and use in high-risk patients such as those described subsequently. It is critical to rule out intracranial hemorrhage and other neurosurgical abnormalities. When clinical neuroimaging findings are present following a MTBI, the injury is classified as complicated MTBI (8).

Noncontrast CT scan is the modality of choice for the initial evaluation of acute head injury, because it is fast, widely available, and highly accurate in the detection of skull fractures and acute intracranial hemorrhage. CT scan is used primarily to identify urgent surgical conditions that can improve outcomes. Specifically, mass effect due to hemorrhage or cytotoxic edema if promptly addressed by surgical decompression can greatly mitigate secondary damage.

Noncontrast head CT is *indicated* (level A recommendations) when the patient has LOC or PTA *plus* one or more of the following: age >60 years, GCS <15, headache, vomiting, evidence of trauma above the clavicle, posttraumatic seizure, drug or alcohol intoxication, short-term memory impairment, coagulopathy, and focal neurological deficit.

Noncontrast head CT should be *considered* (level B recommendation) in patients with head trauma but no LOC of PTA *if* one or more of the following is present: age >65 years, GCS <15, severe headache, vomiting, physical signs of basilar skull fracture, coagulopathy, focal neurological deficit, or a dangerous mechanism of injury (9).

MRI is recommended for patients with TBI when the neurological findings are unexplained by CT, and it is the modality of choice for evaluation of the subacute or chronic period. It plays a more important role in the evaluation of patients with persistent posttraumatic sequelae. It is more sensitive than CT in MTBI patients (10,11), and MRI findings have been correlated with neuropsychological performance in MTBI (11).

In general, microscopic diffuse axonal injury, reported as present in autopsy studies of MTBI, is largely undetectable using traditional neuroimaging techniques (12); as a result, more sensitive imaging techniques and biological markers are being developed and investigated in the symptomatic MTBI patients with negative clinical neuroimaging. Experimental neuroimaging techniques are being developed that may positively impact clinical care in the future. These include diffusion tensor imaging (DTI), magnetization transfer imaging (MTI), magnetic resonance spectroscopy, and functional techniques such as functional MRI (fMRI), positron emission tomography (PET), and single-photon emission computed tomography (SPECT) (13).

X-rays: Skull films are not recommended in the diagnosis of MTBI (14).

Laboratory tests are not routinely used in the diagnosis of MTBI. However, laboratory tests may be ordered for exploring other differential diagnoses.

Blood alcohol level and/or urine drug screen (UDS) should be obtained in the acute setting to assist in stratification of those who may require further workup such as noncontrast CT scan.

Biomarkers: Traumatic injury results in the release of proteins. One of the most studied astrocyte proteins in TBI is the S-100B, which is found in the human serum within 30 minutes of brain injury. As of this writing, measuring S-100B has not become the standard of care in the diagnosis of TBI. Electroencephalography (EEG)—routine use of EEG in the clinical assessment of persons with MTBI—is not recommended. EEG is best reserved for posttraumatic epilepsy monitoring and predicting poor recovery in disorders of consciousness.

SPECIAL POPULATIONS

Military population and MTBI sustained in sports are 2 notable special populations of MTBI.

MTBI Epidemiology in the Military Population

TBI has been termed the signature injury of the wars in Iraq and Afghanistan; about 253,330 service members sustained TBI between 2000 and 2012, and approximately 77% of these were MTBI.

In the military, the leading causes of TBI in both deployed and nondeployed individuals are blast exposures, fragments, falls, motor vehicle-related accidents, sports, and assaults. In the deployed setting, blasts are the leading cause of TBI. Those who are at a higher risk for sustaining TBIs are young men who are performing military duties, as well as those with a history of prior concussion and/or substance abuse (15).

Civilian and military MTBI share some common symptoms; however, PTSD is more common in the military MTBI population when compared with civilians. PTSD or depression is present in more than one-third of OIF/OEF veterans with suspected postconcussion syndromes (PCSs) secondary to MTBI (16).

It is often difficult to clinically differentiate PTSD from MTBI because of their overlapping symptoms, but, in general, clinical distinction between the two disorders is usually based on the predominant symptoms. A PCS is more likely when the patient's predominant symptoms are more physical and cognitive, as opposed to PTSD where nightmares, hyperarousal, avoidance, and reexperiencing phenomena predominate (17). In addition, certain symptoms such as hearing and vestibular dysfunction and photosensitivity are more common in military populations with TBI because of the effect of pressure waves of blast and explosions on fluid/air-filled body cavities such as ears and eyes.

MTBI in Sports

The term *concussion* is often used in the medical literature, especially in sports medicine as a synonym for MTBI; the 2 most widely used guidelines for return to play after concussion are those of the American Association of Neurological Surgeons and those of Cantu. Concussion is graded as I (mild), II (moderate), and III (severe).

The AAN guidelines emphasize the qualitative importance of LOC, whereas Cantu guidelines distinguish between brief and extended LOC and draw attention to the duration of PTA.

The Quality Standards Subcommittee of the AAN defines the spectrum of concussions related to sports injuries as follows:

A. Grade I: Concussion is defined as transient confusion, no LOC, and duration of mental status abnormalities on examination that resolve in *less* than 15 minutes.
B. Grade II: Concussion consists of transient confusion, no LOC, concussion symptoms or mental status, abnormalities on examination that last *more* than 15 minutes.
C. Grade III: Concussion is defined as any LOC, either brief (seconds) or prolonged (minutes).

Return to play guidelines for athletes after a concussion have been described. The most commonly cited is the Cantu return to play guidelines, which have been revised over the years.

TREATMENT APPROACH TO MTBI

The symptoms associated with MTBI are heterogeneous and are not unique to MTBI. There are no pathognomonic symptoms or signs, and each patient tends to exhibit a different mix of symptoms. Most signs and symptoms that occur in the acute period following a single concussion resolve quickly within hours or days after the injury and most of those persisting beyond that resolve by 2 to 4 weeks. However, in a minority of patients, the symptoms persist beyond 6 months to a year. *Postconcussion syndrome* is a term frequently used to describe a constellation of symptoms (at least 2 nonfocal, neurologic symptoms) occurring at least 1 to 3 months after concussion. In a minority of persons, postconcussion symptoms persist late after injury (18).

The etiology of these symptoms is controversial, and it is unclear and debatable whether these symptoms constitute a PCS per se. Several factors have been postulated as being responsible for these symptoms, including neurobiological dysfunction in one or more areas of the central nervous system, pre- or postinjury psychological/psychiatric factors, somatization, malingering, or a combination of these. It may be accurate to describe PCS as commonly occurring symptoms rather than syndromal Sequela of TBI (18,19).

Commonly seen symptoms after MTBI can be classified into 3 broad categories: physical, cognitive, and behavioral symptoms. Approach to treatment can also be classified into 3 main groups: education, symptom management, and coordination of care.

ETHICAL ISSUES IN MTBI

Ethical issues arise frequently when treating patients with MTBI. Such ethical issues involve deciding when and how to discuss the patient's cognitive impairments with family members or supervisors at work, or legal authorities if there is reason to do this without violating Health Insurance Portability and Accountability Act (HIPAA).

Another area is the bioethical principles of justice, beneficence, nonmaleficence, and autonomy as they apply to the care of the MTBI patient, as well as some potential ethical conflicts. Some specific examples include (a) the patient's wishes (autonomy) versus the physician recommendations (beneficence); (b) the patient may work in a sensitive job (e.g., law enforcement) and issues may arise regarding potential harm to self and others due to impaired judgment.

PRACTICE-BASED LEARNING AND IMPROVEMENT

GOALS

Demonstrate competence in continuously investigating and evaluating your own MTBI patient care practices, appraising and assimilating scientific evidence, and continuously improving your patient care practices based on constant self-evaluation and lifelong learning.

OBJECTIVES

1. Describe key components of self-assessment and lifelong learning for a physiatrist with respect to continuing medical education (CME)/continuing professional development (CPD) as relating to MTBI.
2. Teach patients, families, residents, students, and other health professionals relating to MTBI.

3. Identify benchmarks/best practices, and describe key practice-related systematic quality improvement (QI) and practice performance improvement (PI) for MTBI.
4. Identify sources of evidence-based practice guidelines and information technology useful in the treatment of MTBI.

KEY COMPONENTS OF SELF-ASSESSMENT AND LIFELONG LEARNING

Physiatrists should continually engage in self-assessment of their strength and deficiencies as pertaining to gaps in patient assessment, medical knowledge, treatment, and education of patients. There is a continuous ongoing research in TBI pertaining to different aspects, and physiatrists should stay up-to-date with ongoing research through avenues such as CME and journals and familiarize themselves with evidence-based recommendations as they become available. For those interested, advanced training in TBI via fellowships is available.

KEY PATIENT AND FAMILY EDUCATION POINTS

Physiatrist should educate patients and their families about the following:

1. Natural history of MTBI
2. Impact of cognitive impairments
3. Need for adequate rest and sleep
4. Minimize risk for future TBI
5. Minimize Ethyl alcohol (ETOH)/substance abuse
6. Risk for depression/suicide
7. Strategies for appropriate behavior with family and coworkers
8. Side effects of medications
9. Provide links and references for pertinent patient/family education resources. For example, Brain Injury Association of America has valuable resources, and the site can be accessed via http://www.biausa.org/
10. Early education of patients and their families is the best available treatment for MTBI and for preventing or reducing the development of persistent symptoms

Patients and their families need to be educated on the causes, symptoms, treatments, and prognosis of MTBI. The education should start at the first contact with a health care professional and should be reinforced during each interaction with a provider. Studies show that patients who were educated on the natural history MTBI do better than those who were not (2). It is important to inform patients with MTBI that in the natural history of MTBI, symptoms often resolve quickly.

The educational materials and method of delivery must take into account the patient's cognitive and emotional impairments, cultural and religious beliefs, and preferred method of learning. The educational materials must be written at an appropriate reading level and in a language that the patient understands. Written information should be given to patients at the end of every clinical visit. Family education is also critical to the patient's recovery, and family members should be encouraged to participate in educational activities and support groups.

Education should also include avoidance of high-risk behavior that could increase the risk of additional head injuries, compensatory strategies for impaired memory and concentration; relaxation techniques; strategies for successful reintegration in work, school, and social activities; anger and stress management techniques; diet and exercise; limiting alcohol and caffeine intake; and avoidance of recreational drugs.

KEY PRACTICE-RELATED QUALITY IMPROVEMENT ACTIVITIES FOR MTBI

QI activities are important in ensuring quality outcome in the treatment of MTBI. Examples of QI activities include:

1. Reducing the incidence of MTBI in identified at-risk civilian population (e.g., men between 18 and 25 years of age) through educating patients on avoiding at-risk activities/behaviors
2. Reducing the risk of future MTBI due to high-risk behavior
3. Increasing the percentage of MTBI patients who are successfully reintegrated in school and work
4. Reducing the incidence and prevalence of MTBI patients with active substance abuse
5. Reducing the incidence and prevalence of MTBI patients who commit suicide

EVIDENCE-BASED PRACTICE GUIDELINES, BEST PRACTICES, OR BENCHMARKS IN THE ASSESSMENT AND REHABILITATION MANAGEMENT OF MTBI

It is imperative that the physiatrist treating MTBI be up-to-date with evidence-based medicine (EBM) guidelines. EBM resources that are important to the practicing physiatrist treating MTBI include the following:

1. Carroll LJ, Cassidy JD, Peloso PM, et al. Prognosis for mild traumatic brain injury: results of the WHO Collaborating Centre Task Force on Mild Traumatic Brain Injury. *J Rehabil Med.* 2004;36(Suppl 43):84–105.
2. Berrigan L, Marshall S, Velikonja D, Bayley M. Quality of clinical practice guidelines for persons who have sustained mild traumatic brain injury. *Brain Inj.* 2011;25:7–8. 742–751. Epub 2011 May 23.
3. Department of Labor and Employment Traumatic Brain Injury Medical Treatment Guidelines. *Division of Workers'Compensation.* Denver, CO: State of Colorado; 2005.
4. McCrory P, Johnston K, Meeuwisse W, et al. Summary and agreement statement of the 2nd International Conference on Concussion in Sport, Prague 2004. *Br J Sports Med.* 2005;39(4):196–204.
5. McCrory P, Meeuwisse W, Johnston K, et al. Consensus statement on concussion in sport: the 3rd international conference on concussion in sport held in Zurich, November 2008. *Br J Sports Med.* 2009;43(Suppl 1):i76–i90.
6. VA/DoD clinical practice guideline on MTBI which can be accessed via http://www.healthquality.va.gov/management_of_concussion_mtbi.asp

INTERPERSONAL AND COMMUNICATION SKILLS

GOAL

Demonstrate interpersonal and communication skills that result in the effective exchange of information and collaboration with MTBI patients, their families, and other health professionals.

OBJECTIVES

1. Discuss the key areas for physicians to counsel patients and families, across socioeconomic and cultural backgrounds.
2. Identify key elements that need to be documented in the patient's medical record.
3. Demonstrate skills for conducting effective communication and listening skills.
4. Demonstrate leadership skills and consultative role as it relates to MTBI.

The key areas for physicians to counsel patients and families specific to MTBI are as follows:

1. Minimizing the risk for future brain injuries through reducing high-risk behavior
2. Minimizing substance abuse
3. Adequate rest and sleep
4. Allowing patient adequate time to complete a task
5. Behavior strategies in communicating with family and coworkers

The key points that need to be documented in the patient's medical record that are specific to MTBI include:

1. Detailed mechanism of injury
2. Initial GCS
3. LOC
4. Altered level of consciousness
5. PTA
6. Symptoms and current management
7. History of drug or alcohol use
8. Prior history of brain injury and disease, psychiatry problems

Key points for conducting effective communication and listening skills are as follows:

1. Questioning patient and/or the caregiver closely. When possible, ask open-ended questions to elicit more details about the injury, such as "Tell me about," or "Describe...."
2. Listen carefully for information the patient or caregiver may give regarding difficulties in physical, cognitive, or behavioral status. Validate patient's concerns.
3. Provide printed, easy-to-read and understand information to patients about the condition and expectations, appropriate referrals, and available community resources.
4. Write out clear instructions for the patient and/or caregiver to take home and, as appropriate, to share with workplace supervisors or school staff.

PHYSIATRIST AS TEAM LEADER

The physiatrist is in charge of coordinating and managing the patient's medical care and therapeutic program and communicating regularly with the patient and his or her family regarding medical needs. The physiatrist directs the rehabilitation team in monitoring the patient's recovery, making needed changes in treatment plans, and consulting with other physician specialists as necessary.

PROFESSIONALISM

GOAL

Reflect a commitment to carrying out professional responsibilities and an adherence to ethical principles in MTBI.

OBJECTIVES

1. Demonstrate appropriate humanistic qualities.
2. Display sensitivity to a diverse patient population (culture, gender, age, race, religion, disabilities, sexual orientation).
3. Demonstrate respect for patient's privacy and autonomy.
4. Demonstrate advocacy, responsibility, accountability, and commitment to excellence in quality care.
5. Demonstrate responsiveness to patient needs superseding self-interests, as it relates to MTBI.

The physiatrist should possess and display integrity and honesty in dealing with the MTBI patient. This is especially important when discussing the natural history of MTBI and discussing treatment options. This will empower the patient in taking active part in his or her own care.

The physiatrist should also show respect and courtesy to the patient and family and be able to communicate in an empathetic manner the treatment plan, as doing this will facilitate treatment compliance.

The patient management approach used in MTBI requires consideration of cultural and language issues that may impact on the patient/patient's family's understanding of MTBI and recovery. This includes differences arising from other cultural and linguistic diversity. For instance, poor communication can directly or indirectly impact on the outcome for patients, particularly for those patients from a non-English-speaking background or where English is their second language.

The clinician needs to ensure that information and advice are understood; therefore, using a language interpreter might be indicated. Moreover, patients may hold cultural assumptions that can influence the presentation of symptoms or the patient/family's response to diagnosis and treatment. For example, people may differ in what they see as a symptom. The definition and concepts of pain management or self-management may differ between cultures.

Patients usually maintain their autonomy and privacy after MTBI. However, potential issues that may arise include patient's individual rights, such as privacy and autonomy versus physician disclosure to employer information regarding the extent of patient's cognitive impairment—especially in jobs that can affect the patient's health and that of others (e.g., bus driver, firefighter, and police officer).

The physiatrist's responsibilities to the patient with MTBI include education, treatment, coordination of care, and advocating for patient's needs.

The physiatrist plays an important role in advocating for the needs of the patient with MTBI at school, work, and family and in other parts of the health care system. Postconcussive cognitive impairment may cause patients to experience problems on the job, problems with school performance, and strain on family relationships. It is the role of the physiatrist to advocate for the patient to receive necessary modifications in these settings. Moreover, due to heterogeneity and diverse postconcussion symptoms, patients usually require services of different specialties, and it is the physiatrist's role to advocate for patients in these other parts of the health care system.

SYSTEMS-BASED PRACTICE

GOAL

Awareness and responsiveness to systems of care delivery, and the ability to recruit and coordinate effectively resources in the system to provide optimal care as it relates to MTBI.

OBJECTIVES

The physiatrist will understand the following issues as it relates to MTBI.

1. Describe key components and available services in the rehabilitation continuum of care and community rehabilitation facilities.
2. Discuss how to work effectively in various systems of care.
3. Identify patient safety components or checklist.
4. Describe optimal follow-up care.
5. Identify important markers of quality of care.
6. Discuss cost-effectiveness, utilization, and management of resources.
7. Review proper medical record keeping and documentation as the patient moves along the continuum of care.
8. Demonstrate the advocacy role that the physician should display for quality of care for his or her patients with MTBI.
9. Participate in identifying and avoiding potential systems- and medical-related errors for MTBI and strategies to minimize them.

1. *Key components of the rehabilitation continuum of care*

Due to a variety of symptoms present in TBI, most patients will require services across different medical specialties; therefore, effective care coordination is very important in this population. It is also important for patient's social service needs to be adequately addressed. Patients with MTBI can receive care in various locations, such as in an outpatient clinical setting. An ideal setting will be one that has the capability to provide multidisciplinary rehabilitation; however, this may not always be feasible, and patients requiring services such as physical, occupational, or speech therapies may be referred to independent therapy clinics. Other patients may receive care in the school setting, while some patients may present to the psychiatric setting for behavioral issues.

Outpatient multidisciplinary rehabilitation should include physiatry and may include the following disciplines: physical therapy, occupational therapy, vision therapy, optometry, speech and language pathology, neuropsychology, pain management, mental health, neuro-ophthalmology, vocational rehabilitation, and social work (Table 15.4).

2. *Patient safety components or checklist applicable to MTBI*

Individuals with mild brain injury are at risk for the following safety concerns: (a) risk of future brain injuries through high-risk behavior; (b) substance abuse-related patient safety concerns; (c) impact of behavior-related problems, which may lead to violence, depression, and even suicide.

In order to minimize these safety concerns, the physiatrist needs to be aware of the risk, educate patients on avoiding high-risk behavior that may lead to repeat brain injury, and educate and encourage abstaining from use of illegal substances and alcohol. Mental health conditions must also be promptly referred to mental health providers for treatment.

TABLE 15.3 Key Rehabilitation Disciplines Involved in MTBI Continuum of Care

Physiatrist	Leads the team and coordinates patient care among the other involved disciplines
Physical therapist	Provides therapy for musculoskeletal problems; a specially trained therapist may also provide vestibular rehabilitation as needed
Occupational therapist	Provides therapy for musculoskeletal needs, and also addresses any deficits in ADLs and IADL; in some settings, it provides vision rehabilitation and cognitive rehabilitation
Speech and language pathologist	Provides for cognitive remediation and compensatory mechanisms for memory and memory aids
Vision rehabilitation therapist	Addresses vision complaints and may identify and refer patients to optometrist/neuro-ophthalmologist as needed
Neuropsychologist	Provides various testing to identify areas of psychocognitive needs
Psychologist/psychiatrist/mental health	Manages and treats comorbid psychological and psychiatric problems such as PTSD, depression, and anxiety
Social worker	Addresses psychosocial issues such as homelessness and family issues
Vocational rehabilitation specialist	Assist with vocational needs

3. *Optimal follow-up care.*

The following is a recommended follow-up adapted from the Department of Defense (DOD) guidelines:

A. All patients presenting to the physiatrist after acute MTBI should be followed up in 4 to 6 weeks to confirm resolution of symptoms and address any concerns the patient may have.
B. If, on this follow-up, the patient recovers from acute symptoms, then the provider can provide contact information with instructions for available follow-up, if needed.
C. If the patient demonstrates partial improvement, then consider augmentation or adjustment of the current intervention and follow-up within 4 to 6 weeks.
D. If the patient does not improve or the status worsens, focus should be on other factors including psychiatric issues, psychosocial support, and compensatory/litigation; in addition, a referral to a specialty provider should be considered.

For patients diagnosed with concussion/MTBI and persistent symptoms beyond 4 to 6 weeks, the goal of follow-up visits is to monitor the severity of symptoms, impact of the symptoms on activities, effects of treatments, and presence of adverse effects to treatments, and to assess patients for new symptoms suggestive of other diagnoses. The amount of time between visits will vary depending on a number of factors, including the following:

1. Quality of the provider/patient relationship
2. Distress of the patient
3. Need for refinement of the treatment plan or additional support
4. Presence or absence of psychosocial stressors, and severity of the symptoms

Initially, a follow-up at 2 to 3 weeks would be appropriate, and then follow-up every 3 to 4 months would be recommended. Telephone follow-up may be sufficient to evaluate resolution of symptoms and reinforce education.

4. *Important markers of quality of care for MTBI*: rate of reinjury; rate of return to school or work, suicide rate

5. *Appropriate information that is important to document as the patient moves along the continuum of care includes the following:*

A. Detailed mechanism of injury
B. Initial site of injury
C. GCS
D. Presence or absence of LOC, alteration in consciousness, PTA. Also note the duration of any of these if present.
E. Current symptoms and their current management and response to treatment.
F. Extent of cognitive impairments and their impact on patient's role in society, school, work, family, and so on.
G. Preinjury/postinjury substance abuse, mental health problems
H. Past history of brain injury
I. Medications
J. Vision or hearing loss

6. *Advocacy role of physiatrist in ensuring quality of care for patients with MTBI.*

The physiatrist has an important role for the MTBI patient in the community and health care field. This role involves educating the community and other health care providers about risk factors, etiology, pathophysiology, symptoms, and resulting impairments in MTBI. An important part of this role is educating the public, families, and patients about prevention strategies.

7. *Potential systems-related errors for MTBI and strategies to minimize them.*

Inappropriate handoffs may occur from limited information as the patient moves through the health care system or from the health care system to work or school. Hence, the physiatrist should ensure appropriate handoff and that essential information is communicated to other parties involved in the patients, care. Another source of potential system-related error is that of patients inappropriately being diagnosed with a psychiatric condition when they have a TBI instead.

CASE STUDY

Mr. Jones is a 45-year-old man with a history of childhood ADHD and anxiety who is referred to your concussion clinic after sustaining a head trauma with 2 to 3 minutes of LOC in an MVA 2 weeks ago. His initial GCS on the scene was 13.

He was evaluated in the local emergency room immediately following the accident. It is unknown whether any imaging was done. He was released home the same day. He is married, drinks ETOH socially, and smokes marijuana recreationally.

His wife brought him back to his primary care physician 2 weeks after the accident because she reported that Mr. Jones has not quite been himself since the accident. He is having nightmares, complains of daily severe headache, is forgetful, and has not quite been himself since the accident.

CASE STUDY DISCUSSION QUESTIONS

1. How would you grade the severity of this patient's traumatic brain injury?
2. What are the risk factors for MTBI in this patient?
3. What other elements of his past medical and social history are important to elicit?
4. How would you approach the patient's current symptoms? Discuss key points in evaluation of his headache, sleep disorder, and memory impairment.
5. Is a head CT indicated in this patient? Explain your reasoning.
6. List 5 common symptoms seen in MTBI and briefly discuss the treatment approach.

SELF-EXAMINATION QUESTIONS
(Answers begin on p. 367)

1. Which of the following patients best describes sustaining a MTBI based on the American Congress of Rehabilitation Medicine (ACRM) criteria?
   A. A 40-year-old man slipped and fell while ice-skating, hit his head, sustained an epidural bleed, and lost consciousness for 1 hour
   B. A 5-year-old child dropped from a high changing table, with initial GCS on the scene of 7
   C. A 75-year-old man injured in a motor vehicle collision, no LOC, no PTA, sustained a left tibia fracture
   D. An 18-year-old marine, who fell who off his truck and hit his head, reported being dazed and confused for 10 minutes, no other neurological deficits reported
   E. A 25-year-old marine sergeant was exposed to an improvised explosive device (IED) blast; he did not lose consciousness nor was he dazed or confused, but he reported being surprised at the suddenness of the blast

2. A 25-year-old man with a history of MTBI, presents to your office with migraine headaches, occurring daily and interfering with his job. Which of the following is the best course of management at this time?
   A. Over-the-counter ibuprofen only
   B. Refer patient to a movement and relaxation class and tell him to take over-the-counter Excedrin migraine
   C. Sumatriptan and topiramate combined with stress reduction techniques
   D. Vicodin and topiramate
   E. 12 hours of sleep a night

3. A 55-year-old woman with a history of MTBI presents to your office with complaints of insomnia and waking up unrefreshed. Review of system is positive for snoring and headache upon morning awakening. Which of the following is the best next diagnostic step in the management of this patient?
   A. Brain MRI to rule out brain tumors or rebleed
   B. ENT referral to rule out nasal polyps
   C. Psychiatry referral to rule out PTSD
   D. Sleep study referral to rule out sleep apnea
   E. No further diagnostic test is indicated

4. In which of the following patients is a head CT scan indicated?
   A. A 16-year-old boy who fell and hit his head while driving a bicycle, negative neurological examination, GCS 14, no LOC or PTA
   B. A 70-year-old man who fell in the bathroom, lost consciousness for 5 seconds, and is now walking and talking
   C. A 55-year-old man involved in an MVA, no LOC. He reports being dazed for 5 seconds
   D. An 18-year-old army recruit who complained of confusion for 10 seconds after being exposed to an IED blast. Immediate GCS was 15 and normal physical examination
   E. A 22-year-old college football player with mild neck pain after a hard tackle, with no documented LOC or altered level of consciousness and normal neurologic examination

5. Which of the following is the best available treatment for MTBI and for preventing or reducing the development of persistent symptoms?
   A. Early education of patients and their families
   B. Cognitive rehabilitation
   C. Methylphenidate for brain recovery
   D. Cognitive behavioral therapy
   E. Beta-blockers for brain recovery

REFERENCES

1. VA/DoD clinical practice guideline on MTBI. http://www.healthquality.va.gov/management_of_concussion_mtbi.asp. Accessed December 26, 2012.
2. Mittenberg W, Canyock EM, Condit D, et al. Treatment of postconcussion syndrome following mild head injury [Review]. *J Clin Exp Neuropsychol.* 2001;23(6):829–836.
3. Dikmen S, Machamer J, Fann JR, et al. Rates of symptom reporting following traumatic brain injury. *J Int Neuropsychol Soc NR.* 2010;16:401–411.
4. Lane JC, Arciniegas DB. Post-traumatic headache. *Curr Treat Options Neurol.* 2002;4(1):89–104.
5. Faul M, Xu L, Wald MM, et al. *Traumatic Brain Injury in the United States: Emergency Department Visits, Hospitalizations, and Deaths.* Atlanta, GA: Centers for Disease Control and Prevention, National Center for Injury Prevention and Control; 2010.
6. Traumatic brain injury in the United States emergency department visits, hospitalizations and deaths 2002–2006 Prepared by the Division of Injury Response, National Center for Injury Prevention and Control Centers for Disease Control and Prevention, U.S. Department of Health and Human Services. http://www.cdc.gov/traumaticbraininjury/pdf/blue_book.pdf
7. American Congress of Rehabilitation Medicine: Definition of mild traumatic brain injury: Report of the Mild Traumatic Brain Injury Committee of the Head Injury Interdisciplinary Special Interest Group of the American Congress of Rehabilitation Medicine. *J Head Trauma Rehabil* 8:86–87, 1993
8. Williams DH, Levin HS, Eisenberg HM. Mild head injury classification. *Neurosurgery.* 1990;27:422–428.
9. http://www.ferne.org/Lectures/emra_saem_2008/pps/ferne_emra_2008_neuro_conf_saem_jagoda_mtbi_053108_final.pps.
10. Eisenberg HM, Levin HS. Computed tomography and magnetic resonance imaging in mild to moderate head injury. In: Levin HS, Eisenberg HM, Benton AL, eds. *Mild Head Injury.* New York, NY: Oxford University Press; 1989:133–141.
11. Levin HS, Amparo E, Eisenberg HM, et al. Magnetic resonance imaging and computerized tomography in relation to the neurobehavioral sequelae of mild and moderate head injuries. *J Neurosurg.* 1987;66:706–713.
12. Borg, J., Holm, L., Cassidy, D., et al. Diagnostic procedures in mild traumatic brain injury: Results of the WHO Collaborating Centre Task Force on mild traumatic brain injury. *Journal of Rehabilitation Medicine*, 2004;43: 61
13. Vanderploeg RD, et al. Recent neuroimaging techniques in mild traumatic brain injury. *J Neuropsychiatry Clin Neurosci.* 2007;19:5–20.
14. Jagoda AS, Bazarian JJ, Bruns JJ Jr, et al. Clinical policy: neuroimaging and decisionmaking in adult mild traumatic brain injury in the acute setting. *Ann Emerg Med.* 2008;52:714–748.
15. http://www.dvbic.org/sites/default/files/uploads/dod-tbi-worldwide-2000-2012Q2-as-of-120820.pdf

16. Elder GA, et al. Blast-induced mild traumatic brain injury. *Psychiatr Clin N Am.* 2010;33:757–781.
17. Hicks R, Fertig SJ, Desrocher R, et al. Neurological effects of blast injury [Review]. *J Trauma Injury Infection Crit Care.* 2010;68(5):769.
18. Arciniegas et al. Mild traumatic brain injury: a neuropsychiatric approach to diagnosis, evaluation, and treatment. *Neuropsychiatr Dis Treat.* 2005;1(4):311–327.
19. Alexander MP. Mild traumatic brain injury: pathophysiology, natural history, and clinical management. *Neurology.* 1995 45(7):1253–1260.
20. Goodman JC. Pathologic changes in mild head injury. *Semin Neurol.* 1994;14:19.
21. Povlishick JT, Katz DI. Update of neuropathology and neurological recovery after traumatic brain injury. *J Head Trauma Rehabil.* 2005;20:76.

Thomas N. Bryce
Vincent Huang

16: Spinal Cord Injury

PATIENT CARE

GOALS

Provide competent patient care that is compassionate, appropriate, and effective for the evaluation, treatment, education, and advocacy for persons with spinal cord injury and disease (SCI/D) across the entire spectrum of care, from the acute injury until death.

OBJECTIVES

1. Assess comprehensively persons with tetraplegia and paraplegia in both the acute and chronic settings.
   A. Evaluate the adequacy of the workup for cause of SCI/D and subsequent treatments.
   B. Perform neurologic assessments as outlined in the International Standards.
   C. Identify the actual body structure limitations by organ system caused by the SCI/D.
   D. Identify the potential complications of SCI/D as they relate to level of and completeness of injury.
   E. Identify the body function limitations caused by SCI/D.
2. Develop and carry out treatment plans for persons with tetraplegia and paraplegia in both the acute and chronic settings.
   A. Describe the management of each of the actual body structure limitations or complications by organ system caused by SCI/D.
   B. Describe preventative strategies for the potential complications of SCI/D.
   C. Develop specific therapy prescriptions addressing body function, activity, and participation limitations.
3. Identify the psychosocial and vocational implications of SCI/D problems and strategies to address them.

In taking a history of someone with SCI/D, a chronological description of the development of the condition should be included. If the cause was traumatic, the mechanism of injury should be elicited. If nontraumatic, the workup for cause should be reviewed for completeness. The adequacy of treatment should also always be determined. As SCI/D affects the person who experiences it so profoundly, a thorough inventory of the individual's prior level of functioning, interests, avocations, vocation, social supports, and living environment should be ascertained. Past medical, surgical, and psychological histories should be elicited as these may affect how someone with SCI/D copes both physically and mentally with the body changes imposed by the SCI/D. Review of systems should include all the systems, since all can be affected. Body structures located above the injury should not be neglected. Traumatic brain injury, for example, may be seen in over a quarter of those with traumatic SCI (1).

Key elements of the physical examination that are particularly specific to SCI/D include assessment of the neurologic, musculoskeletal, and integumentary systems. Neurologic assessment should include motor and sensory testing utilizing the International Standards for Neurological Classification of SCI (ISNCSCI) (2); an evaluation of limb spasticity; and an evaluation of sacral reflexes, anal sphincter tone, and anal volition. These last three elements help determine the status of the bowel and bladder, which are usually affected by SCI/D. Sensory and motor testing provides the data needed to determine the neurologic level of injury as well as completeness of injury. The sensory level is the most caudal dermatome where both light touch and pinprick are normal, whereas the motor level is indicated by the most caudal muscle having grade 3 or better strength where all muscles above are graded 5. The single neurologic level is the most rostral of the sensory and motor levels. The American Spinal Injury Association Impairment Scale (AIS) is a 5-point scale used to specify the severity of SCI (2). AIS "A" defines a complete injury. AIS "B" denotes sensory without motor function present more than three levels below the neurologic level including S4–S5. AIS "C" denotes motor function present more than three levels below the neurologic level but the majority of key muscles below the level are less than grade 3 and sensory or motor function at S4–S5 is present. AIS "D" denotes motor function present more than three levels below the neurologic level where at least half the key muscles below the level are grade 3 or better and sensory or motor function at S4–S5 is present. For AIS "E", all components of the standardized examination are normal. Musculoskeletal assessment should include measurement of range of motion (ROM) of all major joints, especially the shoulders, which often develop contractures in those with cervical injuries due to inadequate movement, and the hips, which can develop contractures due to heterotopic ossification (HO), a condition of the deposition of true bone at extraskeletal sites. Integumentary assessment is important as pressure ulcers are common over bony prominences in areas of altered sensation in persons who have impairments in functional mobility. Proper staging and assessment of pressure ulcers allow one to develop a comprehensive treatment plan (Table 16.1).

Body structures that are affected by SCI/D include the spinal cord, urinary and alimentary tracts, respiratory system for those with injuries above the lowest thoracic level, the skin, and the skeletal system. Alterations in these body structures cause body function limitations, which in turn lead to activity limitations, and ultimately participation limitations. Affected body functions can be stratified by neurologic level of injury and degree of injury completeness. Maintenance of blood pressure, dysphagia, adequacy of respiration, and motor control of the upper extremities are functions primarily affected in those with cervical injuries. Control of urination, elimination of feces, sexual function, and motor control of the lower extremities are functions that persons with injuries at all levels are affected with. Grasping and manipulating objects, dressing, self-feeding, washing oneself, and transferring oneself are affected by those with cervical SCI/D, while standing, walking, regulating urination and defecation, relationships, sexual activity, and employment are affected in persons with injuries at all levels.

All persons with SCI/D, regardless of level, are highly susceptible to developing pressure ulcers due to impaired mobility and sensation. Special air-filled or gel bed and wheelchair support surfaces as well as proper positioning can help prevent pressure ulcers from developing and help them heal if they should occur. Persons with impaired sensation and mobility are taught to completely reposition in bed every 2 hours and to perform pressure relief when sitting approximately every 20 minutes for at least 1 minute.

Musculoskeletal conditions are common; they can cause pain and reduce functional ability in persons with SCI/D. Therefore, preventive measures should be initiated early. Contractures are best prevented by proper positioning in bed, daily passive ROM exercises of all joints, and prophylactic splinting. A common cause of contractures is HO, formation of true bone in ectopic sites (3). HO often develops within 4 months of SCI and most commonly develops around the hips. Individuals with SCI/D develop osteoporosis in the lower limbs and are at increased risk of fractures with minimal trauma. Treatment for mininimally displaced fractures in those who are nonambulatory is usually nonoperative, with a goal of preserving prefracture function, avoiding complications, and assuring proper alignment for healing.

Pulmonary complications, including atelectasis, pneumonia, respiratory failure, and pulmonary embolism (PE), are the leading causes of death for persons with SCI/D. The diaphragm, innervated by the phrenic nerve (C3–C5), is the major primary muscle of inspiration. Intercostal muscles and abdominals are innervated from T1–T11 and T6–T11, respectively. Muscles of the neck and shoulder girdle that contribute to respiration are innervated from C3–C8. Injury to the spinal cord affecting these muscles can result in respiratory compromise and restrictive pulmonary disease with a decrease in all lung volumes. Strategies to maintain optimal pulmonary function include proper positioning; lung expansion; secretion mobilization with postural drainage and chest percussion; and secretion clearance with suctioning, manually assistive coughing, and insufflator-exsufflator use. Adequate hydration and use of bronchodilators and mucolytics are also often indicated.

In the past, renal failure was a leading cause of death after SCI/D. However, by implementating strategies to screen for and reduce the incidence of recurrent infections, hydronephrosis, cancer, and urinary tract stones—predisposing complications of this dreaded outcome—renal failure is now rare. Although transurethral indwelling catheters are usually appropriate during the acute postinjury period to monitor fluid and electrolyte balance, intermittent catheterization (IC) of the bladder is generally accepted as the best option for long-term bladder management for persons who can perform IC themselves (4). Reflex voiding is another viable option for males with upper motor neuron (UMN) bladders who empty (to <200 mL) spontaneously or with suprapubic tapping with low bladder pressures (<40 cm H_2O). Long-term bladder drainage with an indwelling suprapubic catheter is another reasonable option for persons who are unable to perform IC.

Neurogenic bowel is a ubiquitous consequence of SCI/D and is often categorized into UMN and lower motor neuron (LMN) subtypes. Suprasacral SCI/D leads generally to a reflexic or UMN bowel in which defecation cannot be initiated by voluntary relaxation of the external anal sphincter. In contrast, destruction of the S2–S4 anterior horn cells or cauda equina produces an areflexic or LMN bowel in which there is no reflex-mediated colonic peristalsis. The goal of a bowel program is to allow effective and efficient colonic evacuation while preventing incontinence and constipation. Evacuation of the rectum can

TABLE 16.1 Primary Myotomal Innervations for Key Muscles of ISNCSCI

KEY MUSCLE ACTION	PRIMARY MYOTOMAL INNERVATION
Elbow flexion	C5
Radial wrist extension	C6
Elbow extension	C7
Distal finger flexion	C8
Finger abduction	T1
Hip flexion	L2
Knee extension	L3
Ankle dorsiflexion	L4
Great toe extension	L5
Ankle plantar flexion	S1

ISNCSCI, International Standards for Neurological Classification of Spinal Cord Injury.

be managed by digital stimulation of the anus to trigger reflex colonic contractions for persons with an UMN-type bowel and digital removal of stool for persons with a LMN-type bowel (5).

Symptomatic autonomic dysfunction in SCI/D is common in persons with high-level paraplegia and tetraplegia. Orthostatic hypotension and relative hypotension is nearly ubiquitous in those with higher level injuries. Orthostasis occurs as a result of loss of sympathetic tone and systemic loss of vascular resistance. Management includes application of elastic stockings, abdominal binders, adequate hydration, progressive daily head-up tilt, and, at times, administration of salt tablets, midodrine, or fludrocortisone. Autonomic dysreflexia (AD) is a syndrome that affects persons with a neurologic level at T6 level or above, who are unable to vasodilate the splanchnic vascular bed in response to acute hypertension. It is caused by a noxious stimulus below the injury level leading to sudden reflex sympathetic activity. Symptoms of AD include pounding headache; bradycardia; hypertension; profuse sweating; and cutaneous vasodilatation with flushing of the face, neck, and shoulders. Delay in treatment of AD may lead to intracerebral and subarachnoid hemorrhage, stroke, retinal hemorrhage, seizure, cardiac dysrhythmias, and even death. The most important step of acute management of AD is to find and remove the noxious stimulus, of which bladder distension is the most common, causing the problem (6). Other measures include sitting the person upright, loosening tight clothing, and monitoring the blood pressure until the problem resolves. If symptoms are not relieved quickly with the above measures, which should include bladder emptying in the absence of any other easily identified cause, and the systolic blood pressure remains above 150 mmHg, treatment with a rapidly acting and preferably reversible antihypertensive such as topical nitroglycerine should be considered while searching for other sources of noxious stimuli.

Individuals with SCI/D are prone to developing deep vein thrombosis (DVT) secondary to stasis of the venous circulation, hypercoagulability of blood, and intimal vascular injuries. The greatest period of risk is during the first 2 weeks following the injury, with the incidence decreasing thereafter. The majority of persons with SCI/D do not have clinical signs or symptoms such as swelling, warmth, or pain. PE and the postphebitic syndrome are potential sequelae of DVT. Because of the high incidence of DVT and potential fatal outcomes of PE, DVT prophylaxis with low-molecular-weight heparin has been shown to be the most effective of the available options. DVT prophylaxis is typically continued for no longer than 3 months as the risk of further DVT is not thought to be greater than the risk of adverse events due to anticoagulation at that point. Warfarin is generally given for 3 to 6 months after the diagnosis of DVT or PE with a target international normalized ratio goal of between 2 and 3. Inferior vena cava filters are indicated for patients who have a contraindication to anticoagulation or have failed anticoagulation.

Spasticity after UMN SCI/D is characterized by several different features including velocity-dependent increases in tonic stretch reflexes, uninhibited spastic co-contractions of agonist and antagonist muscles, and low-threshold phasic muscle spasms occurring in either a flexor or an extensor pattern. Each of these features may be more or less present in any one person. Furthermore, although spasticity can cause difficulty with mobility, positioning, and comfort, it can also be helpful with ambulating and performing activities of daily living, maintaining muscle bulk, and increasing venous return, depending on which features predominate. Treatments include stretching of spastic muscles; proper wheelchair seating and positioning; splinting and casting; standing; keeping warm; functional electrical stimulation; and medications such as baclofen, various benzodiazepines, and tizanidine. More invasive treatment options for spasticity include intrathecal baclofen administration through an implanted pump; percutaneous nerve or muscle blocks with phenol, alcohol, or botulinum toxin; and rarely surgical rhizotomy.

Pain is a significant problem for many individuals with SCI. Approximately 80% of people with SCI report chronic pain, while approximately one-third report chronic severe pain that interferes with activity and affects quality of life (7). There are two basic types of pain, neuropathic and nociceptive pain. Neuropathic pain is pain arising as a direct consequence of an injury or disease affecting the somatosensory system, whereas nocipetive pain is pain arising from activation of peripheral nerve endings or sensory receptors that are capable of transducing and encoding noxious stimuli. The International Spinal Cord Injury Pain (ISCIP) Classification organizes SCI pain hierarchically into three tiers (7). The first tier includes the main types of nociceptive and neuropathic pain. The second tier includes subtypes for neuropathic (at level, below level, or other neuropathic pain) and nociceptive (musculoskeletal, visceral, or other nociceptive pain) types, while the third tier is used to specify the primary pain source at the organ level as well as the pathology. Medications used to treat neuropathic pain related to SCI/D include anticonvulsants, antidepressants, and opioids. A significant proportion of the chronic pain reported by persons with SCI/D is due to overuse of the upper extremities. Education, physical training, and adaptive techniques for doing activities should be primary interventions to minimize overuse nociceptive pains of the upper limbs.

Key psychological issues related to SCI/D include adjustment to body structure and function limitations as well as pain, coping, family and caregiver roles, and ultimately the assumption of a new identity. Adjustment is usually gradual and may or may not progress in a linear fashion. The influence of social supports and premorbid coping strategies can either help or hinder the adjustment process. Peers with SCI/D can be invaluable in facilitating a positive adjustment and assumption of a new identity.

MEDICAL KNOWLEDGE

GOALS

Demonstrate knowledge of established evidence-based and evolving biomedical, clinical, epidemiological, and sociobehavioral sciences pertaining to SCI/D, as well as the application of this knowledge to guide holistic patient care.

OBJECTIVES

1. Describe the epidemiology, anatomy, physiology, and pathophysiology of SCI/D.
2. Describe the different SCI syndromes.
3. Assess the expected functional outcomes by neurologic level injury after SCI/D.
4. Examine the ethical and socioeconomic issues pertinent to the care of the SCI/D patient.
5. Educate patients on making patient-centered decisions regarding their plans of care.

SCI/D results in temporary and permanent changes to motor, sensory, and/or autonomic function resulting in multibody system dysfunction. Trauma results in approximately 12,000 injuries per year in the United States, of which 4 out of 5 are experienced by men (8). Approximately 42% of the injuries result from motor vehicle crashes, 20% from falls, and 17% from violence (9). Approximately 30% of the injuries cause incomplete tetraplegia, 25% complete paraplegia, 20% incomplete paraplegia, and 20% complete tetraplegia (9). Life expectancy today remains significantly below that expected for persons without SCI. Persons acquiring paraplegia from a traumatic etiology at 20 years of age have a life expectancy shortened by 14 years, while persons acquiring an SCI with ventilator dependency at 40 years of age have a life expectancy shortened by 32 years (9). The leading causes of death after SCI are diseases of the respiratory system accounting for one-fifth of the deaths, of which four-fifths are due to pneumonia (9).

The spinal cord is organized into a series of tracts that carry motor (descending) and sensory (ascending) information; 31 pairs of nerve roots (8 cervical, 12 thoracic, 5 lumbar, 5 sacral, and 1 coccygeal) extrude from the spinal cord. Each spinal segment has a pair of ventral (motor) and dorsal (sensory) spinal nerve roots. The cervical nerves exit above the corresponding vertebrae and the thoracic and lumbar nerves exit below the corresponding numbered vertebrae.

During embryologic development, the vertebral column elongates more than the spinal cord. Therefore, the spinal cord is shorter than the spinal canal, and the individual spinal cord segments do not line up with the corresponding numbered vertebrae. The spinal cord terminates as a conical structure known as conus medullaris at the L1–L2 intervertebral disk. Below the L1–L2 intervertebral level, the nerve fibers of the cord continue as the cauda equina, named as such because it resembles a horse's tail.

A cross-sectional view of the spinal cord reveals gray and white matter. The central gray matter is subdivided into two horns on each side called the ventral (anterior) and dorsal (posterior) horns. The dorsal horns contain projections of the cell bodies of sensory fibers from dorsal root ganglia, and the ventral horn contains motor neurons. The peripheral white matter is subdivided into three columns on each side called anterior, lateral, and posterior columns. The posterior column is further subdivided into tracts: fasciculus gracilis located in the medial posterior column and fasciculus cuneatus located in the lateral posterior column relay touch, vibration, and position sense for T7–S5 dermatome and above T7, respectively. This posterior column ascends ipsilaterally and decussates at the medulla. The anterolateral spinothalamic tract, located peripherally in the lateral column, contains fibers that carry information for pain and temperature (laterally) and touch and pressure (anteriorly). This tract decussates within three segments of their origin and ascends contralaterally to the thalamus. The corticospinal tract is located centrally and posteriorly in the lateral column and carries information for voluntary and reflexive movement.

UMNs are corticospinal neurons originating in the cerebral cortex and synapsing in the anterior horn with LMNs. LMNs originate in the anterior horn of the spinal cord and exit via spinal nerves to target muscles. Damage to UMNs leads to spasticity, while damage to the anterior horn cell or nerve roots (LMNs) leads to decreased muscle tone, absent muscle stretch reflexes, and flaccid paralysis.

A subset of incomplete SCI/D has been grouped by clinical presentation into six SCI syndromes: Brown-Séquard syndrome (BSS), central cord syndrome (CCS), anterior cord syndrome (ACS), posterior cord syndrome (PCS), conus medullaris syndrome (CMS), and cauda equina syndrome (CES). BSS is defined by ipsilateral proprioceptive and motor loss and contralateral pain and temperature sensation loss below the level of the lesion due to injury to the spinal cord in which one side is damaged more than the other. Of all the SCI clinical syndromes, BSS has the best prognosis for ambulation. CSS is characterized by disproportionately more motor impairment of the upper than the lower extremities with varying degrees of neurogenic bowel and bladder and sensory loss below the level of the lesion. It is the most common of the SCI syndromes, usually the result of falls, especially in older individuals with cervical spondylosis who experience a hyperextension injury. ACS is characterized by paralysis and dysesthesia below the level of lesion, with preservation of touch, position, and two-point discrimination. It is associated with flexion injuries or vascular insufficiency produced by occlusion of the anterior spinal artery. PCS is the least common of the SCI clinical syndromes and is characterized by selective injury to the posterior columns, resulting in a loss of proprioceptive and vibratory sense below the level of lesion. CMS is an injury of the sacral cord (conus) and lumbar nerve roots within the spinal canal characterized by a combination of UMN and LMN signs (Table 16.2).

PRACTICE-BASED LEARNING AND IMPROVEMENT

GOALS

Demonstrate competence in continuously investigating and evaluating your own SCI/D patient care practices, appraising and assimilating scientific evidence, and continuously improving your patient care practices based on progressive self-evaluation and lifelong learning.

OBJECTIVES

1. Describe learning opportunities for providers, patients, and caregivers with experience in SCI/D.
2. Use methods for ongoing competency training in SCI/D for physiatrists, including formative evaluation feedback in daily

TABLE 16.2 Expected Functional Outcomes by Neurologic Level of Injury

ACTIVITY	C4	C5	C6	C7	C8–T12
Self-feeding	D	IA	IA	IA	I
Upper body dressing	D	A	I	I	I
Lower body dressing	D	D	A	I or A	I
Level transfers	D	A	I	I	I
Bed mobility	D	A	A	I	I
Wheelchair mobility	IP	IP	IM	IM	IM

Abbreviations: D, dependent; I, independent; IA, independent with adaptive equipment; IP, independent power wheelchair; IM, independent manual wheelchair; A, assistance needed.
Source: From Whiteneck et al.

practice, evaluating current practice, and developing a QI and Practice Performance Improvement activity strategy.
3. Locate some resources including available websites and professional organizations for continuing medical education and continuing professional development in SCI/D.
4. Describe some areas paramount to self-assessment and lifelong learning such as review of quality care markers; current guidelines, including evidence-based, in treatment and management of patients with SCI/D; and the role of the physiatrist as the educator of patients, families, residents, students, colleagues, and other health professionals.

Continuous systematic self-assessment, lifelong learning, and implementation of changes to one's practice are the hallmarks of this competentcy. By monitoring rehabilitation, medical, and patient satisfaction outcomes of persons with SCI/D who are being cared for in a rigorous fashion by collecting outcome data and comparing these data to national and local benchmarks, one can see at least if minimal standards of care are being met. There are numerous third-party vendors who provide this service, and more and more indicators are being mandated to be collected by insurers, of which the Centers for Medicare and Medicaid Services (CMS) in the United States is the vanguard. On an institutional level, incorporating formative evaluation feedback provided by senior physicians, coworkers, and patients into daily practice is also important.

By analyzing the various outcomes as they relate to national and local benchmarks, certain deficiencies will become apparent. The first step to addressing the deficiences specifically, whether they relate to rehabilitation, medical, or patient satisfaction outcomes, is to find out what other providers who are performing better are doing in order to achieve these outcomes. Modeling these others who have better outcomes is one way of improving one's own scores.

Identification, development, and implementation of a practice-related quality and performance improvement project is an excellent way of improving patient care and outcomes. The specific project chosen should be based on an identified deficiency, safety concern, or regulatory necessity. Obvious choices include those which address accepted markers of quality of care for SCI/D including unscheduled discharges from the inpatient setting and the incidence and prevalence of common complications such as falls, pressure ulcers, urinary tract infections, urinary reflux, pneumonia, contractures of limbs, and pain.

With regard to maintaining competancy in the care of those with SCI/D, one should read related published literature of the major journals; attend local and national conferences on SCI/D; be familiar with teaching and learning materials produced often with the impetus of national and international professional organizations; and be aware of clinical practice guidelines (CPGs) related to SCI/D. Two major SCI/D journals are the *Journal of Spinal Cord Medicine* and *Spinal Cord*. Three major SCI/D professional organizations with a strong US presence are the American Spinal Injury Association (ASIA), the International Spinal Cord Society (ISCoS), and the Academy of Spinal Cord Injury Professionals (ASCIP), all of which host annual educational and scientific conferences. Familiarity with and use of up-to-date evidence-based CPGs not only can allow one to practice medicine with confidence that what one is doing is not out of date but is also essential in protecting oneself in case of legal action. The Consortium for Spinal Cord Medicine—composed of representatives of major professional organizations including various physician specialities, physical therapy, occupational therapy, nursing, psychology, consumer groups, and the insurance industry—has produced several CPGs and consumer guides that are freely available on the website of its major sponsor, the Paralyzed Veterans of America (www.pva.org). With regard to freely available online educational materials in several different formats, there are 3 major organizations that maintain specific dedicated educational sites. ISCoS maintains a comprehensive e-learning site on all aspects of SCI/D care (www.elearnsci.org). ASIA maintains a site called the ASIA Learning Center, that contains several interactive modules that relate to learning the ISNCSCI (www.asialearningcenter.org), while Spinal Cord Injury Rehabilitation Evidence (SCIRE) is a Canadian research collaboration that maintains a site that includes evidence-based reviews of SCI/D-related topics (www.scireproject.com).

Education of individuals with SCI/D includes teaching about the body structure changes caused by the SCI/D and ways that body function changes can be overcome in order to ultimately achieve maximal participation in all wanted interests, avocations, vocations, and social interactions. This includes promoting healthly behaviors, maintaining physical and mental health, and preventing secondary complications. As SCI/D doesn't just affect the person with SCI/D but everyone around him or her, it is essential that family members and significant others be involved as well. As persons with SCI/D are treated and managed by an interdisciplinary team, all members of the team should participate in the educational process, each to his or her strengths. For example, education on available community and government resources, benefits, and services may be best provided by a social worker, while a vocational therapist may best facilitate return to education and work, with the physician providing information about prognosis, current regenerative research, and sexual functioning.

INTERPERSONAL AND COMMUNICATION SKILLS

GOALS

Demonstrate interpersonal and communication skills that result in the effective exchange of information and collaboration with SCI/D patients, their families, and the rest of the rehabilitation team.

OBJECTIVES

1. Describe and demonstrate the principles and importance of effective communication between physiatrists, rehabilitation team providers, and patients with SCI/D across socioeconomic and cultural backgrounds.
2. Discuss the indications for a family meeting and describe how to guide one effectively.
3. Identify key areas for physicians to counsel patients and families specific to SCI/D.
4. Identify key points to be documented in patient records to provide effective communication between team members with respect to SCI/D.
5. Delineate the importance of the role of the physiatrist as the interdisciplinary team leader and consultant for the SCI/D patient.

> **BOX 16.1 Indications for a Family Meeting**
> - *Proactive prophylactic (routine) meetings*
> - *Reactive (initiated in response to problems)*
> - *Need for family input for major care decisions and discharge planning*
> - *Conflict (or concerns about conflict) over goals and rehabilitation or medical care*
> - *After a long length of stay especially if the initially discussed goals have changed*

As a SCI/D can be so life altering and affect so many bodily functions, it is imperative that the physician and team caring for a person with newly diagnosed SCI/D explain these changes to both the injured individual and his or her designated significant others and/or family; both those changes that have already occurred and those that are expected to happen in the future, including prognosis for functional recovery. The most effective way of disseminating this information is through a formal scheduled meeting that includes all affected parties: patient, family, significant others, and treatment team, henceforth called a family meeting. This can be done more than once with fewer team members present as long as all team members convey the same message.

Optimally family meetings should first occur within a few days after injury in the acute care hospital or arrival to the rehabilitation unit. A second meeting should be held depending on the length of stay and complexity of the injury closer to discharge. Since SCI is relatively uncommon, with only approximately 12,000 newly diagnosed traumatic SCIs occurring each year, leading to a total of approximately 200,000 persons in the United States who experience deficits consistent with SCI on a daily basis, it is safe to assume that most people are unfamiliar with the specifics of the effects of SCI/D on an individual's life (8). Furthermore, families, patients, and clinicians differ in both their understanding of the patient's condition and prognosis (neurologic, functional, and vocational) and the emotional impact of the illness, especially before a meeting.

During a family meeting, physicians should not just focus on the medical aspects of care and prognosis but also address empathetically the emotional and quality-of-life issues related to SCI/D (Box 16.1). This could be done simply by acknowledging the difficulty for the family when a loved one is challenged with multiple life-altering functional impairments. Information provided to patients and families must be straightforward, jargon free, and with vocabulary of an appropriate educational level for the target audience. Physicians should not avoid sensitive topics such as sexuality and reproduction. Physicians should avoid dominating the discussion both in terms of taking up the most time speaking and in how they direct which topics are addressed. All team members as well as the patient and family members should be given the opportunity to speak. Patient/family satisfaction with family meetings has been associated in other specialties with supportive physician behaviors such as allowing the patient and family to participate actively. When dealing with patients and families who do not fluently speak the same language as the treatment team, use of trained interpreters is essential, but clinicians should recognize that inaccuracies in translation are common.

Occasionally, some family members and patients want to avoid the truth with regard to neurologic or functional prognosis (e.g., prognosis for walking) and will collude with the clinician to avoid discussing upsetting information regarding prognosis. However in general, the literature seems to support the notion that provision of information about prognosis promotes patient and family peace of mind and trust. Families are more satisfied after longer family meetings and when they sense they are being given complete information. This being said, the process of sharing unwelcome prognostic information is laden with psychological concerns for families, patients, and staff. Steering between brutal frankness and unrealistic hopefulness can be a delicate task for the physician, who always seeks to be kind and truthful but is fearful that the news may set back any progress that has been made in rehabilitation by eliminating the drive to improve if the sole stated goal of that person is to just walk again. This can often be tempered by a discussion of "cure" research or by taking into consideration some of the coping strategies of the patient and family.

Finally, trust is a basic need that is hard to measure but that is painfully evident when it is absent. It is a marker for conflict and difficulty arriving at mutually agreeable decisions with regard to participation in care. It is familiar to all clinicians who have found themselves at odds with a patient or family regarding recommended treatments. In skillfully orchestrated family meetings and patient interactions, clinicians demonstrate that they deserve confidence by exhibiting a caring, respectful, reliable, self-assured manner and excellent clinical and communication skills (Box 16.2).

In addition to communication with patients, the physician must be facile in communication with other physicians, on the primary treatment team as well as with consultants and primary care providers; other health professionals, such as physical therapists (PTs) and occupational therapists (OTs), speech and respiratory therapists, psychologists and recreational therapists, vocational therapists and peer counselors, nurses and personal care attendants; as well as with insurance company medical reviewers. In order to communicate with other health professionals effectively, it is necessary to know in depth the role each plays. In communicating with medical reviewers in order to obtain approval for a service or to have a denial of medical necessity for a service (e.g., coverage for acute inpatient rehabilitation) overturned, it is important to know the current medical and functional status (body structure and function limitations) of a person as well as the expected trajectory with regard to both velocity and degree of change and ultimate prognosis of said individual. This includes knowledge of the skills of the treatment team and confidence in their abilities to facilitate achievement of expected goals within the constraints of the therapeutic environment. It is important to have a good grasp of the specific environmental barriers (e.g., at home) and social supports (e.g., who will be at home) that are associated with and can lead to actual and potential activity limitations and participation limitations for the individual in question. Finally, it is necessary to know the details of the individual's health care coverage and the limits to coverage. Only if all these details are known can a solid case be built to justify approval for a service or to have a denial of medical necessity decision for a service overturned.

Learning these communication skills can occur by shadowing and modeling other providers, creating simulations, and practicing during family meetings, team conferences, and during communications with consultants and primary care providers. Physicians in training should gradually acquire increasing responsibility by participating in and eventually taking leadership roles in the team conferences and family meetings. Learning about the activities of other key team members (e.g., PTs and OTs) involved with the care of those with SCI/D can be facilitated by frequently visiting and observing therapy sessions and participating in-services with these other disciplines.

PROFESSIONALISM

GOALS

Reflect a commitment to carrying out professional responsibilities and an adherence to ethical principles in the approach to SCI/D.

OBJECTIVES

1. Describe and demonstrate *People First Language*.
2. Exemplify the humanistic qualities in patient-centered care.
3. Demonstrate ethical principles, responsibilities, and responsiveness to patient needs superseding self and other interests.
4. Demonstrate sensitivity to patient population diversity, cultural competence, gender, age, race, religion, disabilities, and sexual orientation.
5. Respect patient privacy, confidentiality, autonomy, and shared decision making.

Although persons with SCI/D may have profound body function limitations, activity limitations, and participation limitations that may color how they are perceived by others, they are still people, foremost, with the same motivations, coping strategies, fears, and desires as those without these limitations. It is important to recognize the underlying person and not perceive the individual as his or her diagnosis. One key step to doing this is to not label people by their diagnoses by using *people first language*, which puts the person before the diagnosis and describes what a person *has*, not who a person *is* (e.g., use "person with paraplegia" rather than "paraplegic"). In addition, adjectives that connote emotional responses should also be avoided (e.g., use "sustained an injury" rather than "suffered an injury" and "wheelchair user" rather than "wheelchair bound"). Like gender or ethnicity or sexual orientation, body function limitations, whether congenital or acquired, are characteristics of being human. Every human being has unique and individual strengths, and physicians need to be wary of falling into the trap of defining a person's value and potential by his or her diagnosis. By recognizing individual body function limitations and activity limitations and by knowing what someone with these limitations with the appropriate supports and therapies can achieve, one can help an individual overcome these limitations to achieve maximal participation with regard to interests, avocations, vocations, and social interactions, the hallmark of a successful rehabilitation after SCI/D.

The recognition of someone with SCI/D as a person foremost is important and often difficult for the physician in training to incorporate due to the severity of the functional and activity limitations; the muting of characterizing aspects of one's underlying personality by the stress of the injury, loss of autonomy, and secondary depressed mood; and the importance of attention to the medical complications for which medical attention is primarily sought and to which the bulk of medical training is directed to

---

BOX 16.2 Principles of Effective Communication Between Physicians and Patients

- *Allow extra time for interactions*
- *Avoid distractions*
- *Sit face to face*
- *Maintain eye contact*
- *Listen*
- *Speak slowly, clearly, and loudly*
- *Use short, simple words and sentences*
- *Use charts, anatomic models, and pictures*
- *Frequently summarize important points*
- *Give patients and families an opportunity to ask questions and express themselves*

addressing. Learning about the person can be gleaned by a thorough discussion of his or her hobbies, vocations, education, family, home environment, and personal history. This history is best obtained using open-ended-type questions. The physician needs to use open positive body language, appear unrushed, and listen and convey understanding without judgment. This is particularly relevant as many persons with SCI may have been injured in activities related to violence (17% in North America) or alcohol use related to falls or motor vehicle crashes, the two major causes of traumatic SCI, and may be less than forthcoming about their experiences and background to someone they are meeting for the first time. Victims of violence are often of a lower socioeconomic status than the physician, and predominantly young, male, and often of different race/ethnicity, all of which may influence the physician–patient relationship due to lack of common experiences and beliefs. Nevertheless, by acknowledging the differences and by making a concerted effort to learn about the person with SCI/D through a thorough social history, the physician can make a strong first impression that can go a long way in establishing a productive trusting relationship.

A person who has just sustained an SCI/D is vulnerable both physically and emotionally. As such, it is imperative that the physician who is in charge of his or her care is dependable and accountable in preventing physical and emotional complications from occurring. The physician should be humble enough to ask for help when it is needed from mentors, colleagues, consultants, family members, and other treatment team members and utilize all the resources available in order to avoid adverse outcomes. This often includes recruiting the help of peer mentors for persons who are having difficulties adapting to their new body and activity impairments. Sometimes a plan to prevent adverse outcomes from occurring is at variance with the wishes of the person with SCI/D. For example, it is standard in many SCI/D rehabilitation units to facilitate turning persons with motor and sensory impairments who are unable to turn themselves from one side to the other every 2 hours while in bed in order to prevent skin breakdown. The person with SCI/D, however, may not want to turn at night as it interrupts his or her sleep. The person may also refuse other things that the physician and treatment team have prescribed such as therapy participation, bathing, or even suctioning. Now an ethical dilemma presents itself. The person with SCI/D is a person foremost with needs, wants, and rights not to be forced to do something he or she does not wish to do. The physician and treatment team who purport to practice patient-centered care, if nothing is done, feel helpless as the individual deteriorates both physically and mentally before their eyes. One practical approach is to insist that certain life-preserving treatments be done such as turning in bed and suctioning if needed while letting the individual refuse non-life-sustaining treatments. All social supports and resources should be accessed in order to help convince the individual that perhaps the choices he or she is making may not be in his or her best interest for survival, much less adapting to the body and activity limitations that he or she is presented with. It is useful in these situations for the treatment team and the family to provide a consistent message of support. Development of a behavior plan with positive reinforcement for participation in activities and essential care can often be helpful.

Acknowledging the psychodynamics of the refusal can provide a basis for cognitive restructuring of the situation into a more productive one. For example, for a person who was previously independent in all activities and constantly making decisions and choices who now has a high-level SCI/D with profound body and activity limitations, the ability to make an important decision may seem absent lying in bed attached to a ventilator in a controlled hospital setting but a decision to say no is a decision nevertheless (subconscious or conscious), even if it may not seem logical to the team. Getting the person to see that there are other positive decisions to be made and directions of care to be learned is the first step of rehabilitation. The next step is outlining, interpreting, and providing resources to implement a plan to address overcoming the body function and activity limitations in order to ultimately achieve maximal participation in all wanted interests, avocations, vocations, and social interactions. Once this is completed, one presumably will have achieved a positive adjustment and assumption of a new identity that has incorporated the body function and activity limitations caused by the SCI/D.

SYSTEMS-BASED PRACTICE

GOALS

Demonstrate awareness and responsiveness to systems of care delivery, and the ability to access, evaluate, recruit, and coordinate effectively resources in the system to provide optimal continuity of care and foster outcomes as it relates to SCI/D.

OBJECTIVES

1. Identify the key components in the spectrum of rehabilitation continuum of care settings for patients with SCI/D.
2. Coordinate and recruit necessary resources in the system to provide optimal care options available for the person with SCI/D with attention to safety, cost considerations, and risk–benefit analysis, as well as management. Identify the components, systems of care delivery, services, referral patterns, and resources.
3. Describe optimal long-term follow-up for persons with SCI/D, markers of quality of care and improvement metrics, and use of documentation in SCI/D rehabilitation programs.

As a result of the lifelong involvement in the care of persons with SCI, physicians are in a unique position to be involved in prevention of SCI with regard to both organizing and giving talks to schools and local and national organizations and working with legislators, usually as a representative of a professional organization, to develop laws that aim to decrease the incidence of traumatic SCI.

Post injury, the first component of the rehabilitation system of care as it relates to traumatic SCI begins in the acute hospital soon after injury. Here on seeing a newly injured individual, the physician should ensure that measures are implemented to prevent secondary complications such as skin breakdown, venous thromboembolism, urinary retention, atelectasis, bowel impaction, and joint contractures. Education of the individual with SCI as well as the family about SCI and what can be expected with regard to body function and activity limitations, recovery, the rehabilitation process, and participation should begin here, optimally via a family meeting.

Secondary complications are minimized if a person with traumatic SCI is transferred early to an acute inpatient rehabilitation unit, specifically one that is experienced in the care of persons with SCI. One mark of quality for inpatient SCI/D care is accreditation of the facility by the Commission on Accreditation of Rehabilitation Facilities (CARF). It is within an acute SCI/D rehabilitation program that most of the physical skills are acquired in order to adapt to body function and activity limitations. In addition to learning how to do things differently, individuals with SCI/D learn how to direct the care that they need if they are no longer able to do such care by themselves.

Several secondary conditions commonly encountered after SCI/D are eminently preventable yet cause significant morbidity, mortality, and health care resource use. Hospital-acquired pressure ulcers and pneumonia are two such conditions that can be designated as patient safety issues. Impaired sensation and mobility as well as lack of volitional bowel and bladder control seen after SCI/D predispose one to developing pressure ulcers. Near constant monitoring of skin integrity and intervention if breakdown is detected needs to be a primary concern of both the individual with SCI and the staff caring for that person. This task should not be viewed as the sole responsibility of any one individual, but of every member of the team: the physician, nurse, therapist, nutritionist, and most importantly, the person with SCI/D and his or her family. Valid risk assessments should be performed on a regular basis and specific prevention measures implemented, as described in the Patient Care section, depending on the determined stratified risk. Pulmonary complications, specifically pneumonia, are the leading cause of death for persons with SCI/D. Atelectasis is the most common respiratory complication and predisposes one to develop pneumonia. Strategies to maintain optimal pulmonary function and minimize the risk of developing atelectasis and pneumonia are described in the Patient Care section. In addition, strategies to promote safe swallowing and ensure good oral hygiene help prevent aspiration of bacteria. Prevention of pneumonia in the long term may include regular pulmonary percussion and drainage, sputum clearance, smoking cessation, sleep apnea detection and management, maintenance of general fitness and activity, and immunization to both pneumococcus and influenza.

Optimally after undergoing a program of acute inpatient rehabilitation, someone with SCI/D should be ready to return to the community utilizing available resources and social supports. Once in the community, a person with SCI/D typically requires ongoing therapy, initially at home and ultimately in an outpatient setting. Ultimately depending on his or her success in overcoming the body function limitations caused by the SCI/D he or she will return to being a productive and adjusted member of society.

As few will argue that health care resources are unlimited, efficient management of these resources is of paramount importance in achieving optimal outcomes with regard to maintenance of health, recovery of function, and societal participation. As the cost of health resources has increased in the United States over time, limited resources have more and more been a driver of the length of time a person with SCI/D spends in any one of the components of the rehabilitation continuum of care, if at all. The traditional components include acute hospital care, acute inpatient rehabilitation, subacute rehabilitation (rehabilitation in a nursing home or extended care setting), home care, and outpatient care. Nominally the cost of medical care is borne by medical insurers for those who have it, which include in the United States: CMS, private insurance companies, state worker's compensation programs, the US Department of Veteran's Affairs, and in some states no-fault automobile insurers. Each insurer has different ways of covering the costs, prescribing coverage limits, and defining medical necessity, which vary widely by state and system.

As SCI/D affects a person so completely, affecting profound body structure and function limitations, it is important to realize that the medical and emotional needs cannot be provided by any one person. Thus, the physician trained in physical medicine and rehabilitation (PM&R) should be able to competently evaluate, care, educate, and advocate for individuals with SCI/D along the entire spectrum of care from the acute injury until death and needs to recognize that they will need assistance. Optimal lifelong care should include regular follow-up with the PM&R physician, competent in the care of those with SCI/D and optimally Board certified in the specialty of SCI medicine, and a primary care physician, as well as with specialists as needed, including a psychologist, a wheelchair seating specialist, a wound care specialist, a neurourologist, and a spinal surgeon, among others.

CASE STUDY

Ms. Smith is a thin 32-year-old woman who experienced C8–T1 bilateral jumped facets resulting in tetraplegia during a motor vehicle crash. She underwent emergent spinal surgery for stabilization. She was then sent to a nursing home where she has resided for the past 6 months. She is sent by the facility to you for an evaluation. She is noted to need significant assistance with changing her diaper several times per day, lower body dressing, transferring into and out of bed, and moving about in bed. She also does not have a wheelchair. She is incontinent of bowel and bladder. When the idea of a bowel routine is brought up, she refuses to entertain the idea of a bowel routine, noting only that no one "is going to put anything up my anus." Prior to her injury, she resided in a single-level home with her purported supportive family to which she would like to return if she didn't need so much help with her activities of daily living. She has not let her family visit her for the last 5 months, however, as she doesn't wish them to see her in her current condition.

On physical examination she has normal strength in her shoulders, elbow flexors, wrist extensors, and elbow extensors. Her finger flexor strength is 4/5 bilaterally. She has 1/5 strength in her finger abductors. She has no voluntary motor function in any myotomes below the T1 level. Her sensation is intact for pinprick and light touch at the C8 dermatomes bilaterally, impaired in the T1 dermatomes bilaterally, and absent in all those dermatomes distal. She is cognitively intact on screening and has no significant tone or ROM limitations. She has a 2 cm × 2 cm

× 2 cm wound over her sacrum. There is 2 cm of undermining from 11 o'clock to 1 o'clock. The base of the wound is 20% pink granulation and 80% necrotic tissue and slough. The wound is classified as an unstageable pressure ulcer.

CASE STUDY DISCUSSION QUESTIONS

1. What are the components of a comprehensive wound care plan that need to be addressed to promote healing of the ulcer?
2. What is her potential for gaining functional independence in core physical skills given her body structure limitations?
3. What are some resources that may be accessed to determine the most appropriate evidence-based treatment approach to help manage her bowel incontinence?
4. What is one strategy that may be particularly effective in helping Ms. Smith to see the benefits of performing a bowel routine?
5. How has strict patient autonomy adversely affected her outcome thus far?
6. What are the potential options for facilitating a return to home with functional independence for Ms. Smith?

SELF-EXAMINATION QUESTIONS
(Answers begin on p. 367)

1. An individual experiences a SCI and her motor strength on motor examination is graded as 5/5 in both elbow flexors; 4/5 in the right radial wrist extensor and 2/5 in the left radial wrist extensor; and 0/5 for all distally innervated myotomes. Her sensation is graded as intact through the C7 dermatome on the right and the C6 dermatome on the left for both pinprick and light touch and absent in all distal dermatomes. Of the following, which best represents the right and left motor levels as described by the ISNCSCI?
   A. C5 right and C5 left
   B. C6 right and C5 left
   C. C6 right and C6 left
   D. C7 right and C6 left
   E. C8 right and T1 left

2. For persons with SCI, HO develops most commonly in what joint?
   A. Hip
   B. Knee
   C. Shoulder
   D. Elbow
   E. Wrist

3. Of the following procedures, which best describes digital removal of stool as opposed to triggering of a reflex evacuation of stool by digital stimulation, often required for evacuation of the rectum in order to prevent unanticipated uncontrolled evacuations?
   A. C5 AIS B due to automobile crash
   B. T8 AIS C due to transverse myelitis
   C. T6 AIS A status post fall from height
   D. CCS
   E. CES

4. A 76-year-old man with a history of cervical spondylosis presents to the emergency department complaining of weakness and decreased sensation more in the arms than in the legs after sustaining a fall. Which of the following syndromes below best describes the type of injury this gentleman most likely sustained?
   A. BSS
   B. CCS
   C. ACS
   D. PCS
   E. CMS
   F. CES

5. What is the most common cause of death for persons with SCI?
   A. Myocardial infarction
   B. Cancer of the bladder
   C. Urinary tract infection causing sepsis
   D. Respiratory failure from pneumonia
   E. Infected pressure ulcer

REFERENCES

1. Sommer JL, Witkiewicz PM. The therapeutic challenges of dual diagnosis: TBI/SCI. *Brain Inj.* 2004;18:1297–1308.
2. Kirshblum SC, Waring W, Biering-Sorensen F, et al. Reference for the 2011 revision of the International Standards for Neurological Classification of Spinal Cord Injury. *J Spinal Cord Med.* 2011;34:547–554.
3. Banovac K, Sherman AL, Estores IM, et al. Prevention and treatment of heterotopic ossification after spinal cord injury. *J Spinal Cord Med.* 2004;27:376–382.
4. Consortium for Spinal Cord Medicine. Bladder management for adults with spinal cord injury: a clinical practice guideline for health-care providers. *J Spinal Cord Med.* 2006;29:527–573.
5. Clinical practice guidelines: Neurogenic bowel management in adults with spinal cord injury. Spinal Cord Medicine Consortium. *J Spinal Cord Med.* 1998;21:248–293.
6. Acute management of autonomic dysreflexia: adults with spinal cord injury presenting to health-care facilities. Consortium for spinal cord. *J Spinal Cord Med.* 1997;20:284–308.
7. Bryce TN, Biering-Sorensen F, Finnerup NB, et al. International Spinal Cord Injury Pain Classification: part I. Background and description. *Spinal Cord.* 2012;50:413–417.
8. Devivo MJ. Epidemiology of traumatic spinal cord injury: trends and future implications. *Spinal Cord.* 2012;50:365–372.
9. National Spinal Cord Injury Statistical Center. 2013 Annual Statistical Report for the Spinal Cord Injury Model Systems-Complete Public Version. University of Alabama at Birmingham: Birmingham, Alabama. https://www.nscisc.uab.edu
10. Whiteneck G, Adler C, Biddle AK, et al., eds. *Outcomes Following Traumatic Spinal Cord Injury: Clinical Practice Guidelines for Health-Care Professionals.* Washington, DC: Paralyzed Veterans of America; 1999. Consortium for Spinal Cord Medicine Clinical Practice Guidelines.

Mohammed Zaman
Neil Patel
Marc Ross
Miksha Patel

17: Parkinson Disease

PATIENT CARE

GOALS

Provide competent patient care that is compassionate, appropriate, and effective for the evaluation, treatment, education, and advocacy for patients with Parkinson disease (PD) across the continuum of care and the promotion of health.

OBJECTIVES

1. Describe the key components of the assessment of the adult with PD.
2. Define the impairments, activity limitations, and participation restrictions for the adult with PD.
3. Identify the psychosocial and vocational implications of the adult with PD and strategies to address them.
4. Identify potential injuries to the adult living with PD.
5. Formulate a sample rehabilitation treatment plan for the adult with PD.

Diagnosis of PD is primarily clinical. The cardinal features of PD are bradykinesia, resting tremor, rigidity, and gait disturbance/postural instability. However, the symptoms of PD can vary from person to person. Early signs may be very subtle and can go unnoticed. Symptoms typically begin on one side of the body and usually remain worse on that side.

Resting tremor is the most common presenting symptom. It typically begins in the hands at 3 to 5 Hz frequency and is classically described as a pill rolling (back and forth rubbing of thumb and forefinger) movement. Rigidity in PD is described as a "lead pipe" or "cog wheel rigidity." In early PD, cogwheel rigidity can be enhanced by using attention distraction technique. For instance while examining for cogwheel rigidity in one arm, the examiner may ask the patient to make circles with the other arm or to extend knees and ankles. Cogwheel rigidity is caused by subtle tremor with superimposed rigidity. Bradykinesia (slowed motion) is described as the reduced ability to initiate voluntary movement, making the simplest task difficult and time consuming, for example, feeding, dressing, and grooming activities.

PD gait is a slow, shuffling gait with a tendency to freeze in motion, making it hard to continue to walk. To make a 180° turn, the patient usually takes five to six steps or more. The patient may have difficulty with transfers, turning, walking around objects, and changing direction. The assessment of gait and balance can be accomplished with a variety of clinical instruments such as the 6-minute walk test (1), Timed Up and Go Test (2), Functional Reach Test—step length (3), and Berg Balance Scale (4,5).

This can predispose the individual with PD to falls. Most falls in PD are intrinsic in nature, that is, they are caused primarily by the underlying balance disorder and not by an obvious environmental cause such as a collision or loose rug on the floor. Two-thirds of the people living in the community with PD will have fallen in the previous 12 months. Beyond the acute trauma that they may cause, falls may lead to "fear of falling," self-imposed restrictions in activities of daily living (ADLs), wheelchair confinement, and nursing home admission.

Energy expenditure for ambulation is also increased. Fatigue may also be seen in many patients. Posture is usually "stooped forward" or "slumped over," causing instability. Blinking, smiling, and swinging of arms while walking are all unconscious movements that can diminish or disappear in the patient with PD. Some individuals develop a fixed staring expression with an inability to blink. Others present with a masked facies.

Speech impairment and communication impairment are very common in persons with PD (6). Some characteristics include (a) slurred speech, (b) low volume, (c) hesitation before speaking, (d) rapid speech, (e) monotonous tone, (f) stuttering, (g) palilalia, and (h) extended pauses.

Patients with PD can have problems in all three phases of swallowing. The videofluoroscopic swallow study is the standard for the diagnostic evaluation of dysphagia. Many patients report difficulty in attaining appropriate oral intake because of prolonged chewing. Other oral-phase abnormalities observed in these patients include excessive postswallow residuals, poor bolus control, repetitive tongue motions, delayed triggering of the swallow reflex, and delayed laryngeal elevation. Dysphagia training including mechanically altered food consistency (chopped or pureed) with thickened liquids (honey/nectar thick), chin-down positioning, double swallow, oral-motor exercises, biofeedback, and verbal prompting can be helpful. Clinicians might also choose to administer antiparkinsonian medications before meals, so that the maximal benefit of drugs occurs during mastication. Patients with severe or rapidly progressive dysphagia should be counseled on the use of enteral feedings in advance of the need for them. This allows the patient to make an informed decision before the onset of a swallow-related medical emergency.

Individuals with PD can present with cognitive impairment, memory loss, apathy, and confusion, as well as psychiatric manifestations such as major depression, anxiety disorders, and hallucinations. The person with PD can present with reduced self-esteem and lack of confidence. Approximately 24% to 31% of patients develop dementia (7). Interestingly, early PD can be mistaken for depression (8). The cognitive and psychiatric manifestations of PD can place additional stress on the patients and their families. The behavioral impairments in PD can lead to negative thoughts and adverse psychological effects in the patient's life.

Other features of PD include micrographia; anosmia; sensory disturbances (e.g., pain); sleep disturbances; autonomic disturbances; orthostatic hypotension; gastrointestinal disturbances such as constipation, incontinence, and altered visceral sensitivity (9); genitourinary disturbances (10); and sexual dysfunction (11,12).

Myerson sign or glabellar sign is often present and can be tested by tapping the glabella and observing blinking of the eyes. The blinking should normally stop after tapping a few times in the non-PD individual; however, it does not in those with PD.

There are several scales available to assist the clinician in the staging of PD. The modified Hoehn and Yahr and the Unified Parkinson's Disease Rating Scale (UPDRS) are the two commonly used (13,14). The impact of PD on ADLs can be evaluated using the Schwab and England Activities of Daily Living rating scale. In this scale the individual's ability to perform daily activities and the extent of dependency for completion of these tasks on others is rated on a scale of 0% to 100%. The lower the percentage, the higher the level of dependency on others (15).

As mentioned earlier, there is an increased risk of falls in the person with PD. This is often due to characteristics intrinsically associated with the disease such as rigidity, bradykinesia, postural instability, orthostatic hypotension, festinating gait, shuffling gait, stooped forward posture, and freezing of gait (FOG)—a late feature of the disease. FOG may present as an inability to initiate walking, or a failure to continue to move forward. When FOG is present, a patient should not be pulled or pushed to continue to walk, but should be allowed to wait until he or she is able to ambulate to minimize the risk of falling. FOG is generally short in duration, usually lasts less than 10 seconds, and is seen mainly in the form of start or turning hesitation. FOG may be minimized by asking the person to focus on each step, and using external cues. By providing visual cues for each step, patients can achieve a better cadence. One such example is spaced lines on the floor, adjusted for their stride length based on their age, height, and sex (16). Another external cue like auditory stimulation, such as rhythmic music or a metronome, would also be effective (17).

The medications commonly used to treat PD can pose their own problems due to side effects; in addition, their efficacy often decreases as the disease progresses. Side effects of anti-PD medications include increased confusion, clumsiness, dizziness, and agitation, all of which can predispose to a fall. Levodopa (L-dopa) is the most effective medical treatment for PD. However, motor complications uniquely related to L-dopa treatment may emerge that may be difficult to manage. These include fluctuating L-dopa responses and involuntary movements and postures known as dyskinesia and dystonia (18).

Additional safety risks of concern for the person with PD include aspiration-related complications and decubitus ulcers. A person with PD has a 3.7 times higher risk of developing aspiration-related complications compared to non-PD patients (19). The incidence of pressure sores is markedly increased when PD and dementia coexist (20). In severe cases, persons with PD can also develop contractures (21).

A key characteristic in persons with PD is their gradual reduction in ability to move. There are limited and controversial studies with respect to the role of physical therapy in improvement of gait in PD. One single-blind study documented improvement in UPDRS, ADLs, and motor function, but not their mentation. However, 6 months following physical therapy patients did not exercise regularly and their UPDRS regressed to the baseline (22). Another study studied flexibility/balance/functional (FBF) exercise versus aerobic exercise (AE) and home-based exercise (control) and documented outcome measures at 4, 10, and 16 months. This trial showed overall functional improvement at 4 weeks in the FBF group and increased walking economy in the AE group. There was no significant difference in overall functional improvement in either group at 10 months and 16 months compared to the control group (23). There was no true control in this study. Another trial showed that home-based therapy was beneficial for PD patients (24). Results were similar in other studies. A large meta-analysis showed only short-term benefit of physical therapy in patients with PD (25).

Strength training (26) alone does not appear to be enough to improve gait. Tactile, auditory, or visual external sensory cues that are timed with step initiation or step maintenance may be of benefit as is training in how to successfully navigate around obstacles. Other areas of focus in the rehabilitation program include strength, flexibility, balance, and endurance training. Training is also provided for ADLs such as transfers, bed mobility, dressing, grooming, and hygiene, and appropriate assistive devices are provided as needed. Since orthostatic hypotension can be common in patients with PD, pressure garment, stockings, and abdominal binders can be of help. Speech/swallow evaluation and treatment and a rehabilitation nursing program in neurogenic bowel and bladder management are also very useful. Social work and psychological interventions are also an important part of the treatment plan.

The above-mentioned impairments can significantly limit ADLs in PD. Activities such as dressing, grooming, feeding, bathing, rising from a chair, and ambulation and executive functioning can be difficult to perform. These in turn can affect the individual's role in the family and community. Activities such as work, leisure, and driving may be limited, making it difficult for the person to function in activities important to him or her. Social circles can become smaller and more fragmented for the person with PD and his or her immediate caregiver and family members. There is potential for social isolation.

MEDICAL KNOWLEDGE

GOALS

Demonstrate knowledge of established and evolving biomedical, clinical epidemiological, and sociobehavioral sciences pertaining to PD, as well as the application of this knowledge to guide holistic patient-centered care.

OBJECTIVES

1. Describe the epidemiology, anatomy, physiology, and pathophysiology of PD.
2. Identify the role of any pertinent diagnostic, laboratory, and imaging studies important in PD.
3. Review the treatment and management of PD.
4. Recognize the complications and red flags associated with PD.
5. Examine the ethical and socioeconomic issues pertinent to the care of the adult with PD.

About one-fifth of the patients with a diagnosis of PD live in the United States, surpassing over a million cases. From the 1994 U.S. government census 1% of Americans over 50 and 2.5% of Americans over 70 had PD, leading to an additional $20 billion increase in societal cost. The earlier the onset of disease, the greater the vocational impact for this group of patients.

Although onset of the disease may be in early adulthood, typical age of onset is in the 60s. About 10% of the PD population is below the age of 40. Juvenile PD has been found in patients as young as 10 years of age, and has been linked with LRRK-2 gene (Parkin 9 gene) in 50% of these cases (27).

PD is more common in elderly men than women and more in African Americans than Caucasian, Asian, or Hispanic populations. Loss of dopaminergic receptors in substantia nigra seems cause loss of motor function (28). In the vast majority of cases, the etiology of parkinsonism is unknown. Genetic influence in PD has not been conclusively proven by twin studies. Environmental factors play an important role in the older population, while genetic factors do so in the younger population. An NIH-funded twin study published in 2011 finds occupational solvent exposure, trichloroethylene (TCE), perchloroethylene (PERC), and carbon tetrachloride (CCl4) can increase risk of PD (29). Some chemical and infectious exposure has been associated with PD. These include toxic exposures (pesticides/herbicides, solvents, wood preservatives, mercury, industrial residue), infectious exposures (influenza, whooping cough), and other miscellaneous exposures (head trauma, dietary vitamin C, introvert personality, dietary vitamin E, rural living, well water) (30).

The basal ganglia are part of a neuronal network organized in parallel circuits. The "motor circuit" is most relevant to the pathophysiology of movement. Abnormal increment or reduction in the inhibitory output activity of basal ganglia gives rise, respectively, to poverty and slowness of movement (i.e., PD) or to dyskinesias (31). Inputs from the cerebral cortex, especially the primary motor strip and primary somatosensory cortex, are received in the basal ganglia and the substantia nigra. The outputs of these two areas are the primary motor cortex, supplementary motor area, the motor nuclei of the brainstem, and (via the thalamus) the premotor cortex. The location of these nuclei and pathway for movement is a circular loop that enables the basal ganglia to receive information about planned movements and motion that is performed by the primary motor cortex. With this knowledge, the basal ganglia control the motor cortex (32). The inputs from the primary motor cortex and the primary somatosensory cortex are projected to the putamen. Next, the signal is sent to the caudate and then to globus pallidus, which has two different outputs: the motor nuclei of the brainstem and the subthalamic nucleus. From the globus pallidus, the signal is then projected to the motor cortex via the ventrolateral thalamus. The feedback loop is complete when information from the primary motor and primary somatosensory cortex is sent to the putamen (33).

Specifically, the loop is maintained by two neurotransmitters: glutamate and gamma-aminobutyric acid (GABA). The substantia nigra via dopamine sends both excitatory and inhibitory signals to the caudate, which innervates different areas of the putamen. The inhibitory signal is received in the putamen and relayed to the external globus pallidus. As a result, an inhibitory postsynaptic potential (IPSP) is produced at the subthalamic nucleus. This inhibition results in an excitatory postsynaptic potential (EPSP) at the internal globus pallidus. Consequently, an inhibitory signal is sent to the thalamus, which produces an EPSP. This excitatory message is then projected to the motor cortex, which results in motor movement. The excitatory input from the substantia nigra has a somewhat similar pathway. Like the inhibitory pathway, an IPSP is produced at the globus pallidus, but at a different location, in the internal globus pallidus (33).

Many aspects of the pathophysiology of symptoms in PD remain to be unraveled. It is at present unclear why some patients develop symptoms that do not occur in others. This suggests the presence of subgroups of PD, perhaps related to difference in progression rate and prognosis. The view on the pathophysiology of PD symptoms is evolving into a modified one, in which different aspects of connectivity, plasticity, neurophysiology, and molecular biology are to be integrated. Present evidence suggests that basal ganglia are important in the spatiotemporal organization of motor cortex output. Dopamine deficiency causes electrophysiological changes in the basal ganglia and leads to biochemical alterations that ultimately result in altered gene transcription, further modified by pharmacological therapy. An important characteristic of dopamine deficiency in the basal ganglia is the loss of segregation, causing increased coherence of neurons that normally act independently. Further pathophysiological studies on coherence within basal ganglia and coherence with cortical and muscular activity might enhance our knowledge of bradykinesia and tremor. Finally, brainstem reticular nuclei seem to be involved in the generation of rigidity and axial symptomatology. These nuclei are awaiting further exploration to define their exact pathophysiological role in PD.

Pathophysiology of gait: The underlying pathophysiology leading to fall in a person with PD is complex. The basal ganglia play an important role in regulating muscle contraction, muscle force, and multijoint movement. The ability to maintain a steady gait rhythm and a stable, steady walking pattern with minimal stride to stride changes is impaired in persons with PD.

Indeed, a clinical diagnosis of resting tremor, rigidity, movement, and postural deficiencies usually reflect greater than 50% loss of the nigrostriatal system in disease. Imaging of the brain dopamine system in PD with positron emission tomography (PET) or single-photon emission computed tomography (SPECT) shows reduced uptake of striatal dopaminergic markers, particularly in the posterior putamen. Imaging can be useful in difficult cases or research studies but is rarely necessary in routine practice, as the diagnosis can usually be established on clinical criteria alone.

Medical management of PD intervenes with three components: (a) slowing of disease progression, (b) symptomatic relief of motor symptoms, and (c) amelioration of nonmotor manifestations. Additional medications may be needed to address the adverse effects of anti-PD medications. Several agents have been identified as neuroprotective agents in PD. The American Academy of Neurology recommends the following initial therapies for the initial treatment of PD:

- *Levodopa (L-dopa):* L-dopa is a keystone of PD treatment.
- *Mechanism of action:* It is decarboxylated to dopamine, thereby increasing brain levels of dopamine. L-dopa is typically administered with a peripheral decarboxylase inhibitor such as carbidopa. This combination therapy results in less peripheral availability of dopamine and therefore increases central nervous system dopamine penetration with a concomitant decrease in peripherally based side effects such as nausea.
- *Side effects and pitfalls:* Levodopa improves the motor problems of PD; however, it increases the risk of involuntary movements (dyskinesia). Also effectiveness tends to decrease after 4 to 5 years.
- *Dopamine agonist:* This group of drugs mimics dopamine to stimulate the dopamine system in the brain. These drugs include pramipexole (Mirapex), ropinirole (Requip), and bromocriptine (Parlodel).

Some monoamine oxidase B (MAO-B) inhibitors are also shown to have some mild benefit in the treatment of PD including selegiline (Eldepryl) and rasagiline (Azilect). Unlike L-dopa, these medications do not slow the progression of PD. At a certain point during the day, the effect of L-dopa wears off and symptoms can return. Azilect will slow the breakdown of dopamine, and is recommended for use for off-time treatment for PD. Similarly, a catechol-*O*-methyltransferase (COMT) inhibitor entacapone (Comtan) helps prolong the effects of L-dopa by blocking an enzyme that breaks down dopamine. Entacapone is also recommended for off-time treatment.

Large, well-designed, randomized controlled trials are needed to judge the effect of physiotherapy in PD. A meta-analysis that included 39 trials of 1,827 participants reported physiotherapy has short-term benefits in PD. Clinically significant outcomes were seen in 9 of 18 areas including speed, balance, PD rating, ADLs, and motor subscore (34).

The treatment of advanced PD is difficult, but can be systematically approached to provide the best course of action for the patient. Treatment can incorporate both medical and surgical treatments to work in concert together to provide the optimal alleviation of symptoms. Deep brain stimulation (DBS) is a surgical treatment in which a mechanical neurostimulator is planted in the thalamus, subthalamic nucleus, and globus pallidus that delivers electrical stimulation; this blocks the abnormal nerve signals that cause PD symptoms (35). DBS may help improve the motor fluctuations in some patients with PD. Other surgical procedures such as pallidotomies, thalamotomies, and subthalamotomies are also done in treating PD after other treatments fail. Although symptoms of PD are somewhat improved after the surgery, they are very expensive and may have a multitude of complications. These include bleeding in the brain, infection, behavioral and personality changes, trouble speaking and swallowing, facial paralysis, and visual abnormalities. Weight gain and depression after surgery are also common.

A clinical research study evaluated the impact of DBS in patients with PD on their quality of life using the Parkinson Disease Questionnaire (PDQ-39). This questionnaire evaluates eight domains: mobility, ADLs, emotional well-being, stigma, social support, cognition, communication, and bodily discomfort. Responses are interpreted numerically from 0 (best) to 100 (worst). Overall QOL index was worse in patients who had DBS. Difficulties were reported with mobility and communication; however, cognition was slightly improved (36).

A few studies used 36-item Short-Form Health Survey (SF-36) to monitor quality of life in patients with PD. SF-36 evaluates the physical and mental health of the patient and found depression was most significantly associated with the patient's quality of life. They have recommended taking every effort to recognize and treat depression early on in the disease process (37, 38).

Some treatments currently being studied involve fetal cell transplantation, the use of stem cells, and gene therapy. There are various ethical issues to consider in this kind of research. There is still ongoing research about various PD treatments. Medical scientists are now investigating the effect of scope of stem cell implantation and genetic engineering with the use of a virus. These novel ideas are still preliminary.

Rehabilitation plays a very important role in the treatment of PD, along with pharmacological management. It significantly improves the quality of life and helps reduce the burden on the caregivers. Rehabilitation can help individuals with PD with selected problems such as gait, voice disorders, tremors, rigidity, cognitive decline, and depression. Patients with PD will need expert help from the physical therapist (PT), occupational therapist (OT), speech language pathologist (SLP) (speech and swallow evaluation and treatment), and neuropsychologist. Vocational therapy consult in younger patients with PD may also be warranted. Physiotherapy is very important for management of PD. People with PD usually have mobility problems and are often at high risk for falls. Changes to the home environment to increase independence and safety are recommended. As a result, patients with PD will be able to cope better day to day and maintain their independence.

The role of physical therapy in the treatment of PD patients is widespread. Patients benefit from therapeutic exercises, range of motion (ROM), biofeedback, functional electrical stimulation, balance training, transfer training, progressive ambulation with assistive devices, and stair climbing. PT will also emphasize on proper gait sequence and posture stability.

Gait retraining is one of the most important concerns in the rehabilitation of patients with PD. In advance cases with gait disturbance, patients also have FOG. Physical activity and exercise can result in some measurable improvement in postural instability and balance task performance measures (39). Sufficient evidence is yet not available in regard to therapy schedules and components at different stages of the disease. Also, longer-term tier one studies need to be performed. A patient with PD usually gets 10 days to 2 weeks of patient rehabilitation from his or her insurance.

Exercise is an important component of rehabilitation. Physical therapy may help with physical function and quality of life. It usually includes active and passive exercises, gait training, and practice of normal activities. To date, no specific approach has been proven better than others. Speed-dependent treadmill training has shown to improve mobility and reduce postural instability and fear of falling in PD patients (40).

Occupational therapy helps patients with PD who can benefit from ROM of upper extremities, therapeutic exercises, fine and gross motor coordination, weights to their wrist to reduce tremor, ADLs and self-care, transfers, bed and wheelchair mobility, and posture/balance training. Patients may also benefit from adaptive devices like weighted feeding utensils, drinking cups, plate guards, and so on.

To improve the quality of speech and swallow, speech therapy is also a part of the medical treatment. Other areas that they assist in are content by specific therapies such as oropharyngeal exercises. Dysphagia treatment consisting of smaller bolus size, mechanically altered food consistency, thickened liquids, chin tuck, and head tilt techniques may be of help. Such treatment can help reduce potential aspiration; in addition, improved speech will help prevent social isolation and make their needs known, which will help direct the health care provider. They may need to coordinate with nutritionists to determine food consistency and caloric intake. Dysphagia may require use of modified barium swallow (MBS) and/or fiberoptic endoscopic evaluation of swallow studies (FEES).

Neuropsychology evaluation and treatment may be helpful and needed in patients with cognitive decline, depression, and agitation management. Patients and relatives should receive psychological counseling and learn new coping strategies for their ADLs and instrumental ADLs (IADLs). Patients and caregivers need to learn the basics of the disease and need training to cope adequately with difficult caring situations (41).

Specific rehabilitation nursing can continue to provide help in ADLs, self-care, and transfer activities that have been introduced in OT. Bedside ROM during a.m./p.m. care is important to prevent any contractures. In addition to monitoring for any skin breakdown, frequent changes in position while in bed with relief of pressure areas are important to prevent the development of decubitus ulcers. Monitoring bowel and bladder function is required to prevent urinary retention, incontinence, or constipation.

Patients with PD face a multitude of challenges as their disease progresses. Taking a simple step becomes a big hurdle. The physical activity limitation early in the disease process will prevent patients from being gainfully employed, causing financial difficulty. This may lead to difficulty obtaining medications, outpatient therapy, transportation, home care services, and medical supervision. As the patient has further functional decline, the patient becomes homebound, leading to increased assistance from family and caregivers. Patients will require constant supervision to prevent falls, aspirations, and contractures.

Patients and their families/caregivers have to be educated about the disease process, health care proxy, living will, and do not resuscitate/do not intubate (DNR/DNI), especially when patients are still cognitively intact. Emphasis is to be made on tube feeding and other end-of-life care methods.

Exceptions to the standard of care have been made in special situations where a patient has been allowed to dictate his medical care for quality of life reasons. For example, continuing oral feeds despite the risk for aspiration, allowing patients to ambulate ad lib, even though they are at a risk for falls.

Timing of the medications seems to be very important in the treatment of patients with PD. Following consideration should be prioritized (42):

Initial Diagnosis and Treatment	Management of Motor Complications
• Assessment of functional status • Timing of L-dopa • Initial titration of dopamine agonists • MAO-B inhibitor vs. dopamine agonist as initial therapy	• Initial treatment wearing off • Management of dyskinesias • Using COMT inhibitors with L-dopa • Using entacapone before tolcapone

Management of Nonmotor Complications	Management of Dementia, Depression, and Psychosis
• Treatment of orthostatic hypotension • Treatment of swallowing difficulty, daytime sleepiness, and constipation • Sildenafil for erectile dysfunction	• Assessment for depression • Quetiapine, clozapine for hallucinations • Monitoring of white blood cells in patients on clozapine

A French study done in 2005 looked at cost effectiveness of bilateral subthalamic nucleus stimulation in PD. It documented relatively low risk and little cost burden on the patient population with a total cost of $50,215 per patient for the surgery and 12-month follow-up. In this study, the UPDRS motor score improved by 51% at 3-month follow-up and 57% at 12-month follow-up (43).

PRACTICE-BASED LEARNING AND IMPROVEMENT

GOALS

Demonstrate competence in continuously investigating and evaluating your PD patient care practices, appraising and assimilating scientific evidence, and continuously improving your patient care practices based on constant self-evaluation and lifelong learning.

OBJECTIVES

1. Describe learning opportunities for providers, patients, and caregivers with experience in PD.
2. Use methods for ongoing competency training in PD for physiatrists, including formative evaluation feedback in daily practice, evaluating current practice, and developing a systematic QI and practice improvement strategy.
3. Locate some resources including available websites for continuing medical education and continuing professional development.
4. Describe some areas paramount to self-assessment and lifelong learning, such as review of current guidelines, including evidence-based, in treatment and management of patients with PD and the role of the physiatrist as the educator of patients, families, residents, students, colleagues, and other health professionals.

Physiatrists providing care for patients with PD should have a working knowledge of the key elements of the medical history and physical examination of the patient with PD. They should be able to identify impairments, activity limitations, participation restrictions, and then, in conjunction with members of the rehabilitation team, develop rehabilitation programs to address them. They should be able to recognize patient safety concerns in this population and implement strategies to minimize them from occurring. Physiatrists should be up-to-date on advances in the understanding of the pathophysiology of PD and its treatment and have a working knowledge of side effects or adverse events associated with treatments. They should also be aware of community resources available for patients with PD in their communities. Lastly, it is equally important that physiatrists have the necessary interpersonal and communication skills to effectively provide care for their patients with PD.

There are several strategies that physiatrists can use to identify gaps in their knowledge base about PD and the medical and rehabilitative care of the patient with PD. Self-reflection on their clinical practice, self-assessment examinations, asking trusted colleagues to provide feedback to them on their practice, and asking patients with PD under their care for their feedback on the care provided by the physiatrist are just some examples.

There are existing resources that physiatrists can use to keep up-to-date on the assessment, medical, and rehabilitative treatments for PD. Some examples include: AAPM&R: Knowledge Now (44), American Academy of Neurology (45), and Cochrane Database (46).

INTERPERSONAL AND COMMUNICATION SKILLS

GOALS

Demonstrate interpersonal and communication skills that result in the effective exchange of information and collaboration with PD patients, their families, and the rest of the rehabilitation team.

OBJECTIVES

1. Describe the importance of effective communication between physiatrists, rehabilitation team providers, neurologists, and patients with PD across socioeconomic and cultural backgrounds.
2. Identify key points to be documented in patient records to provide effective communication between team members with respect to PD.
3. Delineate the importance of the role of the physiatrist as the interdisciplinary team leader and consultant for the PD patient.
4. Identify key areas for physicians to counsel patients and families specific to PD.

Communication is one of the most important practices in good patient care with people with PD. It is important for all members of the team to communicate effectively with each other to provide the best care for the patient. These members include the primary care provider, physiatrist, neurologist, neuropsychologists, PTs, OTs, speech pathologists, nutritionists, social workers, and all of the nurses.

Effective communication between all parts of the team can help maximize function and minimize any possible safety risks to the patient. Areas that should be thoroughly discussed between team members include information relevant to the PD such as stage of the disease, impairments, treatments to date, adverse reactions to treatments, comorbidities, key providers involved in the care of the person with PD, rehabilitation interventions to date and their level of success, key components of the physical examination, precautions to be followed during the rehabilitation program, and advance directives.

Communication is especially important at transition points in care such as home to hospital, medical ward to acute inpatient rehabilitation facility, and rehabilitation facility to community since there are many different clinicians involved in the care of the person with PD. The SBAR (situation, background, assessment, and recommendation) method of communicating patient information across the medical team is an effective method of sharing important information (47). This method of sharing important information is meant to minimize miscommunication. It should be checked for accuracy of understanding by asking the recipient of the information to repeat the information back to the person providing the information. This acts as a double check that corrects information is being relayed at the transition point in care.

Physicians should counsel the person with PD and his or her caregivers on the diagnosis, its clinical presentation, rationale for treatment plan, side effects of medications, and strategies to minimize complications such as aspiration-related complications, falls, contractures, and pressure ulcers.

Patients should be equally educated about the latest information about the disease process. They should understand the difficulties they will face in their day-to-day activities, such as their personal hygiene, feeding, negotiating obstacles when ambulating in-house or outdoors, and managing personal finances. PT/OT/SLP can educate and train for proper techniques of ADLs, self-care, transfers, ambulation, feeding, and communication skills to maintain the patient's highest quality of life.

Patients can benefit from support groups and the PD foundation website. In addition to the previous websites, patients can visit the following websites as well to educate themselves about the disease process:

Parkinson's Disease Foundation (PDF) (48): The Parkinson's Disease Foundation (PDF) is a leading national presence in PD research, education, and public advocacy. It funds promising scientific research to find the causes of and a cure for PD while supporting people with PD, their families, and caregivers through educational programs and support services.

National Parkinson Foundation (NPF) (49): The National Parkinson Foundation (NPF) works to address the unmet needs in Parkinson's care and treatment, and to improve the quality of Parkinson's care through research, education, and outreach.

The American Parkinson Disease Association (APDA) (50): The American Parkinson Disease Association (APDA) is the country's largest grass roots organization serving the Parkinson's community. Its goal is to "ease the burden and find a cure" for PD. The organization focuses its energies on research, patient support, education and raising public awareness of the disease.

Parkinson Study Group (PSG) (51): The Parkinson Study Group (PSG) is a nonprofit, cooperative group of PD experts from medical centers in the United States and Canada who are dedicated to improving treatment for persons affected by PD.

Parkinson's Action Network (PAN) (52): Parkinson's Action Network (PAN) is the unified voice of the Parkinson's community advocating for better treatments and a cure. In partnership with other Parkinson's organizations, PAN educate the public and government leaders on better policies for research and an improved quality of life for people living with PD.

PROFESSIONALISM

GOALS

Reflect a commitment to carrying out professional responsibilities and an adherence to ethical principles in caring for patients with PD.

OBJECTIVES

1. Demonstrate humanistic qualities of integrity, respect, compassion, ethics, and courtesy in the care of patients with PD.
2. Describe the importance of patient-centered care, informed consent, and maintaining patient confidentiality in PD.
3. Respect patient's beliefs and goals, privacy, autonomy, and shared decision making as it applies to PD.
4. Describe sensitivity to culture, diversity, gender, age, race, religion, disabilities, and sexual orientation as it may apply to PD.
5. Recognize the socioeconomic factors and importance of patient education in the treatment of and advocacy for persons with PD.

The physiatrist caring for the person with PD should provide high-quality patient-centered clinical care in a compassionate, respectful, and ethical manner. The care should be delivered in a manner that is sensitive to the person's cultural, ethnic, and religious beliefs. The patient's wishes regarding his or her care should be at the center of discussions whenever medical decisions are being made. The physiatrist should be sensitive to issues such as culture, gender, age, race, religion, and sexual orientation whenever they may arise. Discussions regarding sensitive matters such as end-of-life directives should be carried out in strict confidence in an appropriate setting.

When thinking about the responsibility and accountability of the rehabilitation of a person with PD, it is important to take into consideration every member of the caregiver team. The physiatrist should have the overall responsibility of the patient across the rehabilitative care. These components include inpatient rehabilitation, subacute facilities, home therapy, and outpatient rehabilitation. By taking ownership and responsibility it is important to be an active member in organizing and communicating between all of the providers, such as PT, OT, and SLP.

The physiatrist is also an important advocate for the person with PD. Examples of advocacy include (a) coordination of clinical care with the various clinicians involved in the patient's care, (b) advocating for rehabilitative services and equipment in communications with health insurance companies, and (c) providing documentation for work accommodations.

SYSTEMS-BASED PRACTICE

GOALS

Awareness and responsiveness to systems of care delivery, and the ability to access, evaluate, recruit, and coordinate effectively resources in the system to provide optimal continuum of care and outcomes as it relates to PD.

OBJECTIVES

1. Identify the key components, systems of care delivery, services, referral patterns, and resources in the rehabilitation continuum or care for the patient with PD.
2. Identify patient safety components or checklist as they apply to PD.
3. Describe optimal follow-up care for the patient with PD.

4. Describe markers of quality in the care of the patient with PD.
5. Describe cost/risk–benefit analysis, utilization, and management of resources as they apply to PD.

Participate in identifying and avoiding potential systems- and medical-related errors in the care of PD and strategies to minimize them.

The continuum of rehabilitative care for the person with PD spans several components of the health care system such as medical wards in acute care hospitals, acute inpatient rehabilitation facilities, subacute rehabilitation facilities, outpatient facilities, and even the patient's home. A multidisciplinary coordinated rehabilitative program can help prevent secondary complications commonly encountered in the person with PD across this system, and the physiatrist, by virtue of his/her training, is an excellent leader of this effort. Typical rehabilitative services provided on medical wards in acute hospitals include bedside physical and occupational therapy and speech pathology services. Once the person with PD is medically stabilized and deemed a good candidate for further inpatient rehabilitation services, a decision is made regarding an acute inpatient rehabilitation facility (IRF) versus a subacute rehabilitation facility. Factors that should be considered in this decision include (a) a person's ability to tolerate an intensive program of 3 hours per day, (b) medical stability to tolerate a rehabilitation program, (c) need for close medical monitoring, and (d) person's health insurance coverage for rehabilitative services. Services typically provided in the IRF include physiatry, physical therapy, occupational therapy, speech pathology, neuropsychology, social work, and vocational counseling. Usually, a subacute rehabilitation facility would provide shorter daily duration of therapy and would thus be more appropriate for those who could not tolerate a more intensive program.

Following an acute inpatient rehabilitation program at an IRF, a patient may either go home or may need to go to a skilled nursing facility due to inability to return home. If the person with PD returns home and is in need of continued rehabilitative care, visiting home services may be initiated. Home care typically includes physical and occupational therapy, visiting nursing, and home attendant services. These services are typically less frequent and less intense; however, these are more convenient for the patient if he or she cannot attend outpatient services. Outpatient rehabilitative services can be obtained for physical and occupational therapy as well as speech pathology, depending on specific need.

Optimal follow-up for the person with PD moving along this continuum of care should be provided by a physiatrist who is knowledgeable about the person's condition and can best serve as an advocate for his or her needs. Ideally, the physiatrist should be in close contact with the various providers involved in the person's care and help ensure that appropriate follow-up with these specialists occurs on a timely basis.

High-quality care for the person with PD would have both preventative and restorative features. It is important to minimize the risk of aspiration-related complications, pressure ulcers, contractures, falls, medication-related side effects, malnutrition, and urinary tract infections in the inpatient, outpatient, and home settings through a preventative and proactive approach. Some examples include (a) regularly scheduled environmental rounds for fall risk in an inpatient setting, (b) environmental review in the home for fall risk modification, (c) medication review for potentially harmful medications, (d) feeding schedule of small boluses and "double swallow" technique, (e) timely removal of intravenous and indwelling catheters, and (f) nutritional evaluations and interventions for those at risk for malnutrition. Facilities should develop a data-driven approach with appropriate benchmarks to quantify the presence of these complications and should set up policies and procedures to minimize them from occurring in the first place.

Physiatrists should be particularly sensitive to transition points in care as times when medication errors can be made or propagated. Family caregiver education regarding patient medications including side effects must be addressed. Proper dosing and timing of medications must be spelled out clearly to patient and caregiver as patients with PD often exhibit cognitive deficits. Taking multiple medications requires executive decision-making capacity that a patient with PD may not have. The caregiver must be able to identify when a PD patient exhibits a change in mental status, including lethargy or confusion. Identifying which medications may be contributing to this and reporting this information to the health care provider may prevent unnecessary visits to the physician's office or to the ED, thus avoiding unwarranted diagnostic workup, including hospitalization due to confusion. Restorative interventions to maximize ambulation, endurance, and performance of ADLs are equally important and both the person with PD and his or her families should be actively engaged in them under the direction of the treating physiatrist.

CASE STUDY

A 68-year-old man, who was diagnosed with PD 15 years ago, is brought to the office by his daughter as his symptoms were worsening over the past several months. He is taking multiple medications to help with the symptoms of PD. He has fallen several times over the last 3 to 4 years. One of the falls resulted in a Colles fracture of his right hand that was treated 6 months ago. After that episode he became more fearful ; he is unwilling to ambulate, and his cognition has declined. He has constipation and bladder incontinence. He also has several side effects of the medication including involuntary movements, confusion, and agitation. He is increasingly difficult to approach, being suspicious toward his daughter and the home health aide, and at times forgetting simple things. Possibility of DBS was also entertained and a definitive decision was not taken. The daughter states it is becoming impossible to manage him at home. Today his blood pressure was 115/78 sitting and 90/60 standing, pulse 84, respiration 19, and temperature 99.8. On examination, he was oriented to self and close family member only, had a flat face, fine resting tremor that was somewhat less on finger to nose maneuver. He had a slow festinating gait, took 13 steps for a 180° turn, and was very nervous of falling. His muscle tone was increased and had cogwheel rigidity in upper extremity. There was a bruise and abrasion on both knees from a fall 2 days ago and there was a stage one sacral decubitus ulcer (measuring 2 cm × 2 cm) that was not present 2 months ago.

CASE STUDY DISCUSSION QUESTIONS

1. Identify the key medical and rehabilitative issues for this patient and describe your treatment plan to address them.
2. What are some potential ethical issues that can arise in this patient's care?
3. Describe the current understanding of the pathophysiology of PD and the role of levodopa (L-dopa) therapy in its treatment. What are some side effects of L-dopa therapy?
4. Explain the role of rehabilitation in the treatment of PD.
5. What information should be discussed with the patient and his family/support team in regard to living with PD?
6. Identify the clinical disciplines involved in the treatment of the patient with PD and describe the elements of good communication and documentation between the clinicians involved in the patient's care.
7. Identify some resources where you would get information that would help you manage this patient's medical and rehabilitative issues.
8. Identify some patient safety concerns that can arise in the care of the patient with PD and describe some strategies to minimize their risk of occurrence.

SELF-EXAMINATION QUESTIONS
(Answers begin on p. 367)

1. Which of the following are the cardinal features of PD?
   A. Masked facies, athetosis, bradykinesia, spasticity, and gait disturbance/postural instability
   B. Bradykinesia, intension tremor, spasticity, and gait disturbance/postural instability
   C. Bradykinesia, resting tremor, rigidity, and gait disturbance/postural instability
   D. Hyperkinesia, intension tremor, reduced tone, hyporeflexia, and postural instability
   E. Hyperkinesia, rigidity, reduced tone, hemiplegia, and postural instability

2. Which of the following best captures the epidemiology of PD?
   A. From the 1994 U.S. government census: 11% of Americans over 50 and 19% of Americans over 70 had PD
   B. PD leads to an additional $200 billion increase in societal cost
   C. The later the onset of disease, the greater the vocational impact for this group of patients
   D. Although onset of the disease may be in early adulthood, typical age of onset is in the 40s; about 10% of the PD population is below the age of 15
   E. Although onset of the disease may be in early adulthood, typical age of onset is in the 30s; about 20% of the PD population is below the age of 15

3. Which of the following neurotransmitters is decreased in patients with PD?
   A. Noradrenaline
   B. Dopamine
   C. Serotonin
   D. Somatostatin
   E. Substance P

4. Which of the following pairs are considered the gold standard drug(s) for the treatment of PD and mechanism of action? (55)
   A. L-dopa; increasing the amount of dopamine available
   B. The benzodiazepines; increasing the amount of dopamine available
   C. L-dopa; increasing the amount of serotonin available
   D. Prozac; increasing the amount of serotonin available
   E. L-dopa; decreasing the amount of Substance P

5. Which of the following is the major side effect and pitfall of treatment with L-dopa?
   A. Dyskinesia
   B. Apraxia
   C. Hemiballismus
   D. Dementia
   E. Urinary incontinence

6. Which of the following best describes rehabilitation of the adult with PD?
   A. Rehabilitation can help individuals with PD who have such selected problems as gait, voice disorders, tremors, rigidity, cognitive decline, and depression
   B. Changes to the home environment to reduce independence and safety are recommended
   C. The patients will not benefit from therapeutic exercises, ROM, biofeedback, functional electrical stimulation, balance training, transfer training, progressive ambulation with assistive devices, and stair climbing
   D. Physical activity and exercise does not result in measurable improvement in postural instability and balance task performance measures
   E. Speed-dependent treadmill training has shown to worsen mobility, reduce postural instability, and create fear of falling in PD patients

REFERENCES

1. Crapo RO, Casaburi, R, Coates AL et al. ATS statement: guidelines for the Six-Minute Walk test. *Am J Respir Crit Care Med.* 2002;166:111–117.
2. Bohannon RW. Reference values for the Timed Up and Go Test: a descriptive meta-analysis. *J Geriatr Phys Ther.* 2006;29(2):64–68.
3. Katz-Leurer M, Fisher I, Neeb, M, et al. Reliability and validity of the modified functional reach test at the sub-acute stage post-stroke. *Disabil Rehabil.* 2009;31(3):243–248.
4. Frazzitta G, Bertotti G, Uccellini D, et al. Short- and long-term efficacy of intensive rehabilitation treatment on balance and gait in parkinsonian patients: a preliminary study with a 1-year followup. *Parkinsons Dis.* 2013;2013:583278. doi:10.1155/2013/583278. Epub May 26, 2013.
5. Scalzo PL, Flores CR, Marques JR, et al. Impact of changes in balance and walking capacity on the quality of life in patients with Parkinson's disease. *Arq Neuropsiquiatr.* February 2012; 70(2):119–124.

6. Ho AK, Iansek R, Marigliani C, et al. Speech impairment in a large sample of patients with Parkinson's disease. *Behav Neurol.* 1998;11(3):131–137.
7. Aarsland D, Zaccai J, Brayne C. A systematic review of prevalence studies of dementia in Parkinson's disease. *Mov Disord.* October 2005;20(10):1255–1263.
8. Marsh L. Neuropsychiatric aspects of Parkinson's disease. *Psychosomatics.* 2000;41:15–23.
9. Awad RA. Neurogenic bowel dysfunction in patients with spinal cord injury, myelomeningocele, multiple sclerosis and Parkinson's disease. *World J Gastroenterol.* 2011;17(46):5035–5048.
10. Bonnet AM, Pichon J, Vidailhet M, et al. Urinary disturbances in striatonigral degeneration and Parkinson's disease: clinical andurodynamic aspects. *Mov Disord.* July 1997;12(4):509–513.
11. Bronner G. Sexual problems in Parkinson's disease: the multidimensional nature of the problem and of the intervention. *J Neurol Sci.* November 15, 2011;310(1–2):139–143.
12. Bronner G, Royter V, Korczyn AD, et al. Sexual dysfunction in Parkinson's disease. *J Sex Marital Ther.* March–April 2004;30(2):95–105.
13. Bhidayasiri R, Tarsy D. Parkinson's disease: Hoehn and Yahr scale, *Movement Disorders: A Video Atlas. Curr Clin Neurol.* 2012:4–5.
14. Factor SA, Weiner WJ, eds. Movement Disorder Society Task Force on Rating Scales for Parkinson's Disease. The Unified Parkinson's Disease Rating Scale (UPDRS): status and recommendations. *Mov Disord.* 2003 Jul;18(7):738–750.
15. Schwab RS, England AC Jr. Projection techniques for evaluating surgery in Parkinson's disease (Table 1, page 153). In: *Third Symposium on Parkinson's Disease, Royal College of Surgeons in Edinburgh, May 20–22, 1968.* Edinburgh: E. & S. Livingstone Ltd. 1969:152–157.
16. Morris ME, Iansek R, Matyas TA, et al. Ability to modulate walking cadence remains intact in Parkinson's disease. *J Neurol Neurosurg Psychiatry.* 1994;57:1532–1534. http://jnnp.bmj.com/content/57/12/1532.full.pdf+html.
17. Morris ME, Iansek R. Characteristics of motor disturbance in Parkinson's disease and strategies for movement rehabilitation. *Hum Mov Sci.* 1996;15:649–669.
18. Tarsy D. Treatment of Parkinson Disease—a 64-year-old man with motor complications of advanced Parkinson disease. *JAMA.* 2012;307(21):2305–2314.
19. Akbar U, Dham B, Okun M. A long-term analysis of aspiration pneumonia in patients with Parkinson's disease. *Neurology.* 2013;80(Meeting Abstracts 1):P04.144.
20. Nicholson PW, Leeman AL, O'Neill CJ, et al. Pressure sores: effect of Parkinson's disease and cognitive function on spontaneous movement in bed. *Age Aging.* March 1988;17(2):111–115.
21. Kyriakides T, Hewer RL. Hand contractures in Parkinson's disease. *J Neurol Neurosurg Psychiatry.* September 1988;51(9):1221–1223.
22. Comella CL, Stebbins GT, Brown-Toms N, et al. Physical therapy and Parkinson's disease: a controlled clinical trial. *Neurology.* March 1994;44(3, pt 1):376–378.
23. Schenkman M, Hall DA, Barton AE, et al. Exercise for people in early- or mid-stage Parkinson disease: a 16-month randomized controlled trial. *Phys Ther.* November 2012;92(11):1395–1410.
24. Morris ME, Martin C, McGinley JL, et al. Protocol for a home-based integrated physical therapy program to reduce falls and improve mobility in people with Parkinson's disease. *BMC Neurol.* July 16, 2012;12:54.
25. Tomlinson CL, Patel S, Meek C, et al. Physiotherapy intervention in Parkinson's disease: systematic review and meta-analysis. *BMJ.* August 6, 2012;345:11.
26. Lima LO, Scianni A, Rodrigues-de-Paula F. Progressive resistance exercise improves strength and physical performance in people with mild to moderate Parkinson's disease: a systematic review. *J Physiother.* March 2013;59(1):7–13.
27. Young-Onset Parkinson's. National Parkinson Foundation. http://www.parkinson.org/Parkinson-s-Disease/Young-Onset-Parkinsons. Accessed February 14, 2013.
28. Chakresh Kumar Jain, Nisha Vishwanathan. Parkinson's disease: a perilous magic of nature. *Sci Res Essay.* July 2007;2(7):251–255.
29. Goldman SM, Quinlan PJ, Ross GW, et al. Solvent exposures and Parkinson disease risk in twins. *Ann Neurol.* June 2012;71(6):776–784. doi:10.1002/ana.22629. Epub November 14, 2011.
30. Dick FD, De Palma G, Ahmadi A, et al.; Geoparkinson study group. Environmental risk factors for Parkinson's disease and parkinsonism: the Geoparkinson study. *Occup Environ Med.* October 2007;64(10):666–672. Epub March 1, 2007.
31. Obeso JA, Rodríguez-Oroz MC, Rodríguez M, et al. The basal ganglia and disorders of movement: pathophysiological mechanisms. *News Physiol Sci.* 2002;17:51–55.
32. Darbin O, Dees D, Martino A, et al. An entropy-based model for basal ganglia dysfunctions in movement disorders. *Biomed Res Int.* 2013;2013:742671. doi:10.1155/2013/742671. Epub May 16, 2013.
33. Wichmann T, Delong MR. Neurocircuitry of Parkinson's disease. In: *Neuropsychopharmacology: The Fifth Generation of Progress.* :1761–1779. Lippincott Williams & Wilkins; 2002.
34. Tomlinson CL, Patel S, Meek C, et al. Physiotherapy intervention in Parkinson's disease: systematic review and meta-analysis. *BMJ.* August 6, 2012;345:e5004. doi:10.1136/bmj.e5004. Review.
35. Goiss SJ, Wojtecki L, Südmeyer M, et al. Deep brain stimulation in Parkinson's disease. *Ther Adv Neurol Disord.*
36. http://www.dbs4pd.org/.
37. Kuopio AM, Marttila RJ, Helenius H, et al. The quality of life in Parkinson's disease. *Source Mov Disord.* March 2000;15(2):216–223.
38. Martinez-Martin P, Jeukens-Visser M, Lyons KE, et al. Health-related quality-of-life scales in Parkinson's disease: critique and recommendations. *Mov Disord.* November 2011;26(13):2371–2380. doi:10.1002/mds.23834. Epub July 6, 2011.
39. Dibble LE, Addison O, Papa E. The effects of exercise on balance in persons with Parkinson's disease: a systematic review across the disability spectrum. *J Neurol Phys Ther.* March 2009;33(1):14–26.
40. Cakit BD, Saracoglu M, Genc H, et al. Effects of incremental speed-dependent treadmill training on postural instability and fear of falling in Parkinson's disease. *Clin Rehabil.* August 2007;21(8):698–705.
41. Ellgring H, Seiler S, Perleth B, et al. Psychosocial aspects of Parkinson's disease. *Neurology.* December 1993;43(12, suppl 6):S41–S44.
42. Cheng EM, Siderowf A, Swarztrauber K, et al. Development of quality of care indicators for Parkinson's disease. *Mov Disord.* 2004;19(2):136–150.
43. Pollak P, Fraix V, Houeto J-L, et al. Clinical and economic results of bilateral subtha- lamic nucleus stimulation in Parkinson's disease. On behalf of the SPARK Study Group. *J Neurol Neurosurg Psychiatry.* April 2006;77(4):443–449.
44. AAPM&R: Knowledge Now. Available at: http://now.aapmr.org/table-of-contents/Pages/default.aspx. Accessed January 29, 2014.
45. American Academy of Neurology. Available at: https://www.aan.com/. Accessed January 29, 2014.
46. Cochrane Database. Available at: www.cochrane.org. Accessed January 29, 2014.
47. "Situation Background Assessment Recommendation—NHS Institute for Innovation and Improvement." Situation Background Assessment Recommendation—NHS Institute for Innovation and Improvement. NHS (n.d.) Web. May 23, 2013. http://www.institute.nhs.uk/safer_care/safer_care/Situation_Background_Assessment_Recommendation.html.
48. Parkinson's Disease Foundation. http://www.pdf.org/. Accessed January 29, 2014.

49. National Parkinson Foundation. http://www.parkinson.org/. Accessed January 29, 2014.
50. The American Parkinson Disease Association. http://www.apdaparkinson.org. Accessed January 29, 2014.
51. Parkinson Study Group. http://www.parkinson-study-group.org/. Accessed January 29, 2014.
52. Parkinson's Action Network. http://www.parkinsonsaction.org/. Accessed January 29, 2014.
53. NINDS Parkinson's Disease information page. National Institute of Neurological Disorders and Stroke. http://www.ninds.nih.gov/disorders/parkinsons_disease/parkinsons_disease.htm Updated on January 28, 2014. Accessed January 30, 2014.
54. Parkinson's disease cause. The Michael J. Fox Foundation for Parkinson's Research. https://www.michaeljfox.org/understanding-parkinsons/living-with-pd/topic.php?causes. Accessed January 21, 2014.
55. Carbidopa/Levodopa. National Parkinson Foundation. http://www.parkinson.org/Parkinson-s-Disease/Treatment/Medications-for-Motor-Symptoms-of-PD/Carbidopa-levodopa. Accessed January 21, 2014.

C. David Lin
Grigory Syrkin
Marwa A. Ahmed

18: Neuromuscular Diseases

PATIENT CARE

GOALS

Evaluate and develop a rehabilitative plan of care for patients with neuromuscular diseases (NMDs) that is compassionate, appropriate, and effective for the treatment of neuromuscular problems and the promotion of health.

OBJECTIVES

1. Discuss common rehabilitation problems in patients with neuromuscular disorders.
2. Perform a thorough neurological assessment in patients with neuromuscular disorders.
3. Identify systemic complications and management of complications in patients with neuromuscular disease.
4. Identify functional limitations caused by NMD.
5. Identify the psychosocial and vocational implications of neuromuscular problems and strategies to address them.
6. Develop and implement a treatment plan for patients with neuromuscular disorders.

The evaluation of patients with neuromuscular disorders should begin with a detailed medical and family history. NMDs oftentimes affect infants and children; thus, information should be obtained on the prenatal and peripartum periods. In children, the developmental milestones should be recorded.

Muscle weakness is a common symptom in neuromuscular disorders. In some cases the progression is rapid, such as in Guillain-Barré syndrome or myopathies with rhabdomyolysis. However, in disorders of muscular transmissions such as myasthenia gravis, the weakness can fluctuate throughout the day or with exercise. Weakness may progress in a subacute or chronic fashion as in patients with certain muscular dystrophies. The distribution of weakness is also important as it is more proximal in most myopathies and spinal muscular atrophies. In neuropathies, the weakness usually begins distally as in the feet or hands. Weakness can also be manifested by dysphagia, diplopia, and ptosis as in certain neuromuscular transmission disorders (myasthenia gravis). Sometimes respiratory difficulty is encountered and should be treated aggressively as seen in Guillain-Barré syndrome, amyotrophic lateral sclerosis (ALS), and myasthenia gravis.

It is important to assess the patient's functional level in both mobility and self-care. Difficulty combing the hair and doing overhead movements occurs in patients with shoulder girdle weakness (facioscapulohumeral dystrophy), whereas patients with difficulty writing and holding onto things indicate weakness of the forearm and hand muscles that are more prevalent with ALS and inclusion body myositis. Weakness in mobility, as in getting up from a chair, usually indicates hip extensor weakness, whereas weakness in the hip flexors and quadriceps may affect the ability to go up and down stairs. Inclusion body myositis often causes severe weakness of the quadriceps, limiting stair negotiation. When the distal muscles of the legs are affected a footdrop may occur, causing a steppage gait often seen in neuropathies.

Upper motor neuron (UMN) diseases may cause problems with muscle stiffness and spasms, as seen in spasticity. Motor unit hyperactivity resulting in spasticity is often seen in patients with stiff-person syndromes and myotonias. Patients with inflammatory myopathies may also complain of stiffness of the limbs. Fatigue is also common in patients with neuromuscular disorders and is the hallmark of the neuromuscular junction (NMJ) disorders such as myasthenia gravis. It should be noted that patients with Eaton-Lambert syndrome may have a temporary improvement in strength after brief exercise.

Decreased sensation, numbness, and tingling are common in patients with neuropathies. Oftentimes, these paresthesias are associated with pain. Usually, the area of sensory impairments is localized to specific areas of nerve innervation as in a radiculopathy or plexopathy. Sometimes the autonomic nervous system is affected and could alter blood pressure and bowel or bladder function.

Physical examination is essential to arrive at a diagnosis and also to identify functional impairments. In addition to the neurological examination, the cardiopulmonary system should be assessed as certain neuromuscular disorders, such as ALS and spinal muscular atrophies, can lead to respiratory compromise. Other organ systems should also be assessed as enlarged organs are seen in patients with neuropathies with POEMS (polyneuropathy, organomegaly, endocrinopathy, monoclonal gammopathy, and skin changes). Intellectual and cognitive function should also be assessed as it could be affected in patients with myotonic dystrophy.

The muscle examination and assessment of posture is very important. Manual muscle testing can help determine the distribution and degree of weakness and also help track progression of disease. Hyperlordosis with proximal muscle weakness is seen in myopathies. Distal muscle atrophy and weakness is more common in neuropathies. Muscle hypertrophy, especially in the calves, is common in muscular dystrophies. It is also important to assess general muscular tone to determine whether there is focal or global hypotonia, especially in infants. Gait assessment is also important as there is the waddling gait of myopathies, the steppage gait of neuropathies with footdrops, the ataxic gaits in neuropathies with proprioceptive involvement, and the circumducted gait in spasticity.

Assessment of eye and eyelid movements is important in diagnosing the ophthalmoplegia with Miller-Fisher syndrome. Paralysis of the eyes and eyelids is often seen in diabetic ophthalmoplegia and in certain oculopharyngeal dystrophies. Fluctuating ptosis and eye tracking problems may be seen in myasthenia gravis. Facial weakness can occur in various diseases as in Guillain-Barré syndrome and myasthenia gravis. Tongue atrophy and fasciculations are seen in motor neuron disease as in ALS. Weakness in the truncal muscles, especially the neck, can cause a head drop secondary to cervical extensor weakness.

Sensory examination is important to assess the type and distribution of sensory deficits and can be categorized as symmetric or focal. It is also important to assess the reflexes as these will be diminished or absent in neuropathies, as well as in some neuromuscular transmission disorders. Generally, reflexes are preserved until the late stages of myopathies. Slow relaxation of reflexes is seen in patients with myotonias and hypothyroidism (Table 18.1).

Neuromuscular pathology can often be obtained through a thorough past medical history. A prenatal and birth history is important including if there were decreased fetal movements, scoliosis, and hip dislocations. A delay in motor developmental milestones is also important. Other clues to neuromuscular issues include exposure to toxins such as alcohol, nutritional deficits, and poor tolerance to general anesthesia.

NMDs are often hereditary, so a good family history may reveal subtle pathology. Especially with congenital myopathies and hereditary neuropathies, some family members may be mildly affected. Talking to or examining a family member may also be helpful.

Social history including educational background, living situation, the number of dependents, employment, and recreational activities may help in setting a rehabilitation plan. Functional history includes the patient's level of independence, use of an assist device, and accessibility of both work and home.

A thorough review of systems in addition to the history, physical examination, and plan should be documented. Practitioners

TABLE 18.1 Key History and Physical Findings for Selected Neuromuscular Diseases

KEY HISTORY AND PHYSICAL FINDINGS	NEUROMUSCULAR DISEASE
Rapid weakness	Guillain-Barré syndrome Myopathies with rhabdomyolysis
Fluctuating weakness	Myasthenia gravis
Slow progressive weakness	Muscular dystrophies
Proximal weakness	Myopathies Spinal muscular atrophies
Distal weakness	Neuropathies
Shoulder girdle weakness	Facioscapulohumeral dystrophy
Difficulty writing/holding onto things	ALS Inclusion body myositis
Steppage gait	Neuropathies
Temporary improvement in strength after exercise	Eaton-Lambert syndrome
Ophthalmoplegia	Miller-Fisher syndrome
Paralysis of eyes and eyelids	Oculopharyngeal dystrophies Diabetic ophthalmoplegia
Muscle hypertrophy	Muscular dystrophies
Tongue atrophy or fasciculations	ALS
Facial weakness	Guillain-Barré syndrome Myasthenia gravis
Slow relaxation of reflexes	Myotonias Hypothyroidism

should routinely inquire about mood and screen for signs of depression. The social history should be expanded to incorporate current level of function and use of assistive devices, as well as activities reflecting level of endurance. Key psychological issues related to neuromuscular disease include the adjustment to an oftentimes progressive deterioration in function. ALS and muscular dystrophies require adjustment to a gradual decline in function. Social supports and coping strategies may help mitigate the ongoing adjustment process. Besides motor weakness, some NMDs can affect breathing, swallowing, and bowel/bladder function. The psychological implications of using feeding tubes and mechanical ventilation to support life are overwhelming at times. Many patients will require psychiatric consultation for depression and anxiety related to their diagnosis. Patients with similar diagnosis may help by sharing concerns in support groups.

Not being able to work secondary to a progressive neuromuscular disease can also have significant psychological implications. Vocational adaptive strategies can be incorporated in the workplace to help patients with motor deficits. With improved computer technology, patients are even able to work from home and have alternate ways of communicating, from touchpads to head control units. Financial strains coupled with the cost of medical treatment may force many patients into governmental assistance programs.

Aggressive rehabilitation and symptom management can help prolong life and improve quality of life for patients with neuromuscular disorders. Rehabilitation needs are best addressed in a multidisciplinary setting as rehabilitation is important in the management of musculoskeletal dysfunction, pulmonary complications, dysarthria, pain, psychiatric issues, and cognition. One of the goals in rehabilitation is to predict or stay ahead of the disease process and recommend corrective interventions in a timely fashion.

Rehabilitation and management of symptoms are approached in a problem-oriented manner. Prescribing exercise is important in the management of deficits related to mobility and activities of daily living. Therapies include strengthening exercises, stretching or flexibility exercises, aerobic conditioning, and balance training. Most studies of exercise in patients with neuromuscular disorders result in strength gains. However, it is not clear if these strength gains translate into a functional improvement (1).

An exercise prescription should include intensity, duration, and frequency of training sessions. Flexibility and range of motion (ROM) exercises will help prevent or reduce contractures from immobility. Strength training appears safe with a moderate-resistance strengthening program. The goal of a resistance program is to maximize the strength of the unaffected muscles and delay the onset of weakness in minimally affected muscles. With regard to aerobic training, most patients with neuromuscular disorders will have a normal cardiopulmonary response to aerobic training. Use of a treadmill or exercise bicycle is sufficient. The American College of Sports Medicine (ACSM) currently recommends 150 minutes of aerobic exercise per week (2). Balance training is important, especially in patients with neuropathy, and will help reduce falls. An exercise bicycle can be used as a mode of exercise in patients with poor balance.

Pain is common in patients with neuromuscular disease. With the exception of some neuropathic syndromes, pain is not inherent to the disease itself but rather to the effects of the disease on the neuromuscular system. Pain can arise from improper positioning, contractures, joint instability, and overuse injuries. Deconditioning, depression, and other concomitant health conditions can affect pain. Pain should be assessed and can be treated with various medications, physical therapy, acupuncture, massage, biofeedback, and modalities.

Progressive respiratory failure can not only impair quality of life but also decrease the life expectancy in many neuromuscular disorders including anterior horn cell disease, Guillain-Barré syndrome, and certain forms of muscular dystrophies and myopathies. Understanding the patient's respiratory status is important as it will affect the patient's ability to participate in rehabilitation programs. Using noninvasive ventilatory techniques (such as noninvasive positive pressure ventilation) may be part of the rehabilitation plan. Some patients may need an insufflator–exsufflator machine or manually assisted coughing devices to help clear secretions. Pulmonary management along with respiratory therapy services is important in a comprehensive rehabilitation program.

Dysarthria is a motor speech disorder that reduces speech intelligibility and can interfere with verbal communication. The goal of the rehabilitation program is to focus on independent communication and communication strategies. Techniques such as slowing speech rate, overarticulating consonants, and energy conservation may help. Palatal lifts and palatal augmentation prosthesis may help address hypophonia and hypernasality. If the dysarthria progresses, augmentative and alternate communication systems may be used. Patients with severe dysarthria and concomitant severe motor weakness may benefit from brain–computer interfaces.

Dysphagia results from weakness and incoordination of swallowing muscles. This can result in aspiration of food and water resulting in pneumonia, weight loss, and malnutrition. Identifying dysphagia is an integral part of the rehabilitation plan. Changes in the quality of speech ("wet voice"), drooling and leaking of fluids, choking, and recurrent pneumonias are signs of dysphagia. When dysphagia is present, a program of interventions and compensatory techniques can be employed to allow safe oral intake. Positional changes such as chin tucks, head turning to the side of weakness, or double swallowing may help. Dietary changes by thickening liquids and altering food consistencies may also help. Behavioral strategies include eating during times of maximal arousal and minimizing distractions. Using modified utensils such as built-up handles, universal cuffs, or balanced forearm orthoses can help in patients with weakness in the extremities, limiting the ability to bring the food to their mouth. As a last resort, if oral intake remains inadequate, then a gastrostomy tube can be used to allow adequate nutrition. The American Academy of Neurology recommends the placement of gastrostomy tubes for individuals with ALS while they can still tolerate oral intake and before the forced vital capacity (FVC) falls below 50% of predicted to reduce the complications associated with the procedure, compared to patients without severe respiratory compromise (3).

Cognitive dysfunction is common in certain NMDs such as in congenital muscular dystrophies, myotonic dystrophies, and mitochondrial myopathies. Rehabilitation management is important in identifying cognitive dysfunction and treating reversible contributors to cognitive impairments. Management should address medication management, sleep-awake cycle, and nutritional deficiencies. Multidisciplinary services such as speech-language therapy and psychology for patients and family may help with adjustment and long-term planning.

MEDICAL KNOWLEDGE

GOALS

Demonstrate knowledge of established and evolving biomedical, clinical, epidemiological, and sociobehavioral sciences pertaining to NMDs, as well as the application of this knowledge to guide holistic patient care.

OBJECTIVES

1. Describe the epidemiology, anatomy, physiology, and pathophysiology of NMDs.
2. Identify the types of NMDs (motor neuron disease, NMJ disorder, neuropathies, myopathies).
3. Describe the common NMDs.
4. Discuss how to diagnose common NMDs.
5. Formulate basic rehabilitation treatment plans for NMD.

NMD describes any intrinsic disease to the nerves or muscles. The motor unit is considered the smallest functional unit of the neuromuscular system. The motor unit is composed of a motor neuron and the skeletal muscle fibers innervated by that axon. Groups of motor units often work together to coordinate the contraction of a single muscle. Diseases of the neuromuscular system can be divided into diseases of the motor neuron itself, the peripheral nervous system, the NMJ, or the muscle itself.

MOTOR NEURON DISEASE

ALS is the most common adult-onset motor neuron disease, affecting 1.8 per 100,000 with the average age of onset around 60 years of age. It is usually a progressive and fatal disease with an average survival of 3 to 5 years. Most cases of ALS are sporadic (90%), where a small percentage are familial and usually inherited in an autosomal dominant fashion (4). ALS results from progressive deterioration of motor neurons involving mainly anterior horn cells of the spinal cord and certain motor neurons in the brain and brainstem. The result is a mix of UMN and lower motor neuron (LMN) involvement causing weakness, spasticity, cramps, and atrophy. Usually patients with ALS present with focal weakness or problems with fine motor skills. Weakness usually progresses and can result in respiratory failure. Bulbar involvement may result in dysarthria, hypophonia, and dysphagia. Extraocular motions, bowel and bladder function, sensation, and cognition are generally spared.

Diagnosis of ALS is based on the El Escorial criteria which require both UMN and LMN signs. Clinically definite ALS is defined by the presence of UMN as well as LMN signs in three regions (bulbar, cervical, thoracic, or lumbosacral). Clinically probable ALS is defined by the presence of UMN and LMN signs in at least two regions, with some UMN signs rostral to the LMN signs (5). However, approximately 25% of patients who die from an idiopathic, rapidly progressive motor neuron disease will never achieve a probable or definite diagnosis of ALS by the El Escorial criteria despite postmortem confirmation of UMN and LMN degenerations (4).

Currently there are no effective treatments that can reverse or stop the progression of ALS. The major goals in ALS are to slow down disease progression and maintain patient function. Riluzole has been shown to be the only disease-specific treatment that positively affects the natural history of the disease. At a dose of 50 mg twice a day, there was a modest benefit resulting in an approximate 10% slowing of disease progression. Approximately one-quarter of the patients do not tolerate the gastrointestinal side effects and the medication is extremely expensive. Median survival benefit was 60 days and no functional benefit was derived (6).

Spinal muscular atrophy (SMA) is an autosomal-recessive disorder that is linked to the abnormality of the survival motor neuron (SMN) gene on chromosome 5. SMA is characterized by diffuse weakness secondary to atrophy of the anterior horn cells/ventral nerve roots. Patients will have more truncal and proximal weakness. In general, there is no sensory or cognitive involvement. SMA is generally divided into three types depending on the severity and age of onset. Type I is known as Werdnig-Hoffmann disease where patients present with weakness before 6 months of age and are unable to sit anytime during their life. Infants often have difficulty moving against gravity and there may be a bell shape to the chest secondary to intercostal muscle weakness. Bulbar muscles are involved and infants may have difficulty with sucking and maintaining a patent airway. Life span is approximately 2 years. SMA Type II is a milder form of the disease with onset between 6 and 18 months. Depending on the severity of disease, patients may live into their adult years. Patients with SMA Type III, known as Kugelberg-Welander disease, can eventually stand and walk but still have profound weakness (7). Usually these patients require a wheelchair by 20 to 30 years of age. Some with Type III SMA can have near-normal life expectancies.

Postpolio syndrome (PPS) affects individuals with history of polio. Poliomyelitis is a viral infection that affects the anterior horn cells in the spinal cord. Patients who recover from the initial infection of polio may continue to have residual motor weakness. In PPS patients, previously affected muscles may present with new-onset weakness or pain after decades of stability. The current theory is that normal aging causes natural cell attrition resulting in dropout of large LMN units that have been working over their normal capacity for years (8).

NEUROPATHIES

Charcot-Marie-Tooth (CMT) disease is the most common genetically inherited neuropathy. It is also known as hereditary motor and sensory neuropathy and more than 300 genetic mutations have been described. CMT is generally initially painless with symmetric distal neuropathy. Onset is usually in the teenage to early adult years. Patients often present with a high arched foot with the toes flexed. Symptoms can progress to atrophy of the muscles below the knee described as looking like a stork or inverted champagne bottle. Weakness can also cause a claw hand, intrinsic wasting of the hands, and decreased fine motor skills. As the disease progresses, pain and paresthesias may become evident in the distal extremities. Genetic testing is available for some subtypes of CMT. Diagnosis is usually made by physical examination, family history, and electromyography (EMG) testing.

CMT1 and CMT2 are the most common subtypes. CMT1 is autosomal dominant and generally demyelinating. Hypertrophic nerves may be palpated. CMT2 is also usually autosomal dominant, shows axonal degeneration, and may have more distal weakness. CMT3, also known as Dejerine-Sottas disease, is a severe demyelinating and axonal neuropathy that begins in infancy and results in severe weakness and muscle atrophy (8). There are also X-linked types of CMT. Hereditary neuropathy with predisposition to pressure palsy (HNPP) is similar to CMT1 except that there is a deletion of the peripheral myelin protein (PMP) gene rather than a duplication. Patients with HNPP will have recurrent mononeuropathies at sites prone to nerve compression such as in the elbow (cubital tunnel), wrist (carpal tunnel), or knee (fibular head).

Acute inflammatory demyelinating neuropathy (AIDP), also known as Guillain-Barré syndrome, causes an acute generalized weakness with initial symptoms of distal numbness and areflexia/hyporeflexia. Usually a patient will experience an ascending paralysis and some patients may have respiratory compromise. Autonomic dysfunction is also common in some patients resulting in hypotension/hypertension and bowel/bladder dysfunction. Patients often will report a viral prodrome 2 to 3 weeks prior to onset of weakness. *Campylobacter jejuni* enteritis has been implicated as a trigger for AIDP. Cerebrospinal fluid (CSF) of AIDP patients shows increased proteins and low white blood cell counts (cytoalbumino-disassociation). Nerve conduction studies may show prolonged or absent F reflexes. Treatment includes medical stabilization and then treatment with plasmapheresis or intravenous immunoglobulin (IVIG). Chronic inflammatory demyelinating neuropathy (CIDP) manifests over weeks to months with weakness, loss of balance, and numbness. Similar to AIDP, CIDP patients will have reduced reflexes. Steroids and immunosuppressive medications may help with symptoms. Plasmapheresis and IVIG may be used if CIDP patients fail oral therapies.

Diabetic patients may present with a distal, symmetric sensory neuropathy usually resulting in decreased sensation and sometimes pain. Other nerve damages that may occur in diabetes include autonomic neuropathies, radiculopathies, and diabetic amyotrophy (lumbosacral plexitis). Medical treatment includes aggressive glycemic control and neuropathic pain medications.

Numerous other conditions can also cause neuropathies including drugs and occupational exposure. Alcohol abuse has also been linked to distal sensory loss, especially in the feet, with resulting balance deficits. HIV infection and related drug therapies along with coinfections may also result in numerous neuropathies. In the late stages of HIV, infection with the cytomegalovirus (CMV) may cause a rapidly progressive and often fatal polyradiculopathy (9).

NEUROMUSCULAR JUNCTION DISORDERS

Myasthenia gravis is an autoimmune disorder in which autoantibodies to the acetylcholine receptor at the postsynaptic NMJ cause destruction of the receptors. As a result, there are a reduced number of receptors and neuromuscular transmission is slowed. Use of medications that inhibit acetylcholinesterase (physostigmine, pyridostigmine) can increase concentrations of acetylcholine at the NMJ and help overcome this deficit.

Patients with myasthenia gravis experience slowed or failing NMJ transmission. This may result in weakness and fatigue of all muscles, especially with the ocular muscles. The disease can be fatal if respiratory muscles fail; thus, pulmonary function should be assessed during exacerbations (10). Early symptoms of myasthenia include ptosis and double vision secondary to ocular muscle weakness. As the muscles are activated, they tend to fatigue over a period of time. For example, patients may be able to enunciate well at first and then, as they talk more, the muscles weaken, resulting in worsening voice intelligibility. Approximately 10% of patients will have a thymoma; thus, imaging with chest x-ray (CXR) or CT scan is often indicated. Acetylcholine receptor antibodies can be identified in most patients. Specialized EMG testing with increased jitter on single-fiber EMG or a decremental response on repetitive stimulation at slow rates help confirm myasthenia gravis. Acute therapies include IVIG and plasmapheresis. Long-term management involves use of steroids, immunomodulators, and thymectomy.

Lambert-Eaton myasthenic syndrome (LEMS) is an autoimmune antibody mediated disease that prevents the presynaptic NMJ transmission by blocking the voltage-gated calcium channels needed for acetylcholine to release from the presynaptic junction. LEMS is often associated with small-cell lung cancer and other cancers and may appear years before clinically diagnosable cancer. Symptoms of LEMS usually involve weakness of the proximal legs and trunk, usually manifested by the inability to get out of a chair or negotiating stairs. Weakness is usually worse in the morning and gradually improves as the day progresses. This can also be seen on physical examination when initial muscle testing may show profound weakness, but with continued testing the muscles may gradually strengthen even to near-normal strength. This is called facilitation phenomenon and is seen in EMG when repetitive stimulation at high frequency produces a supramaximal response which is not seen in myasthenia gravis. Ocular findings such as double vision and ptosis are uncommon in LEMS patients but are common in myasthenia gravis patients. Treatment of LEMS revolves around treating the underlying neoplastic syndrome. IVIG and plasmapheresis are also used as adjunctive treatments (4).

DISEASES OF MUSCLES

Duchenne muscular dystrophy (DMD) is an X-linked recessive disorder involving the dystrophin gene. The incidence is approximately 1 per 3,500 male births with a prevalence of about 1 per 18,000 men. Dystrophin is important in the sarcolemmal cytoskeletal protein structure. Muscle biopsy usually demonstrates reduced or absent dystrophin on the sarcolemma. Serum creatine kinase (CK) levels are markedly elevated (50–100 times normal) at birth and peak at around 3 years of age. The serum CK levels decline approximately 20% per year as a result of decreasing muscle bulk (11).

Most male children with DMD appear normal at birth and attain milestones of sitting and standing with little or only slight delay. A wide-based waddling gait is noted by about 2 to 6 years of age. There may be clumsiness and falls when the child starts to walk. A classic sign is Gowers sign when the child will need to rise off the floor with a hand on the knee. Weakness is worse proximally than distally and more in the lower extremities. Ambulation becomes progressively difficult and many are confined to a wheelchair by 12 years of age. Worsening kyphoscoliosis ensues and contractures develop. Enlarged calf muscles (pseudohypertrophy) and tight heel cords result in toe walking. Respiratory function gradually declines and leads to death in most patients by the early 20s. Cardiac muscles may also be involved and echocardiograms can show dilation and/or hypokinesis of the ventricular walls. The central nervous system is also involved in DMD with affected children approximately 1 standard deviation below the normal mean.

Becker muscular dystrophy (BMD) is a less severe mutation to the dystrophin gene and can be distinguished from DMD by its slower rate of progression. The incidence of BMD is approximately 5 per 100,000. Children with BMD can have onset of disease at 5 to 15 years of age or even later. Patients usually are ambulatory past the age of 15 years. Approximately 50% of affected patients lose the ability to walk independently by the fourth decade. Cardiac abnormalities are similar to DMD. Life expectancy is reduced compared to the general population (4).

Limb-girdle muscular dystrophy (LGMD) is a group of muscular dystrophies that clinically resembles the dystrophinopathies except for the equal occurrence in men and women. The prevalence of LGMD ranges from 8 to 70 per million. Onset and severity of LGMD is variable and characteristically involves weakness of the hips and shoulders. The facial muscles, swallowing, and cognition are usually spared.

Facioscapulohumeral dystrophy (FSH) is an autosomal dominant disorder with an incidence of approximately 4 per million. It is generally a benign, autosomal dominant progressive disease that causes weakness in the face, shoulders, and upper arms. Weakness usually occurs between 3 and 44 years and can occur even later in life. The muscles of facial expression are usually affected early and FSH patients may have a horizontal smile and weak puckering of lips. Winging of the scapula with weakness of the triceps and biceps is common but with relative sparing of the deltoids. Life expectancy is near normal but some patients may require a wheelchair later in life. FSH muscular dystrophy is linked to the telomeric region of chromosome 4q35 (4).

Myotonic dystrophy type I (DM1) is an autosomal dominant disease that is linked to chromosome 19. The incidence is approximately 13.5 per 100,000 live births. DM1 can present at any age including infancy and results in limb weakness that begins in the distal extremities and can progress slowly to affect the proximal extremities. The neck flexors are affected early and atrophy and weakness of the facial and jaw muscles results in a "hatchet face" appearance. Many patients are not aware of their myotonia, but usually on examination there is delayed relaxation of the fingers after forceful hand grip. Percussion of muscle groups gives rise to a delayed relaxation. Associated manifestations include cataract, mild mental retardation, infertility, and cardiac arrhythmias/cardiomyopathy (12). Myotonic dystrophy type II (DM2) has also been described with more proximal weakness and less pronounced myotonia. Myotonic dystrophy is a multisystem, autosomal dominant disorder with associated cataract, testicular failure, glucose intolerance, and cardiac conduction defects.

Myositis includes polymyositis (PM) and dermatomyositis (DM). PM is a T-cell-mediated autoimmune disease that causes direct destruction of muscle. PM usually presents over weeks to months with a progressing fluctuating weakness of proximal muscles. In addition to fatigue, patients may have muscle pains, cramps, and dysphagia. PM can be confirmed with muscle biopsy and the treatment is usually with corticosteroid therapy. DM is an antibody-mediated autoimmune process that targets the small blood vessels, leading to necrosis and microinfarctions of muscles. DM manifests with a heliotropic discoloration of the upper eyelids. Gottron lesions, scaly erythematous eruptions, or red patches overlying the knuckles, elbow, and knees are characteristic for DM. Associated symptoms include fever, arthralgias, pain and tenderness, cardiac abnormalities, and gastrointestinal ulcers. Malignancy has been linked with patients diagnosed with dermatomyositis. Treatment is with corticosteroid and immunomodulatory therapy.

Inclusion body myositis is a slowly progressive weakness of the arms and legs. Weakness comes on over a period of months to years. It is an age-related disease with its incidence increasing with age and symptoms usually beginning after 50 years of age. Although rare, it is the most common acquired muscle disorder seen in people over 50. Muscle biopsy may show inflammatory cells invading muscle cells, vacuolar degeneration, or inclusions/plaques of abnormal proteins.

Metabolic myopathies are a group of rare hereditary disorders of deficient enzymes that results in impaired muscle energy metabolism. Metabolic myopathies include abnormalities in carbohydrate, lipid, and adenosine nucleotide metabolism. Acid maltase deficiency and McArdle disease (myophosphorlyase enzyme defect) are the common syndromes. Biochemical muscle testing can confirm the diagnosis. A deficiency in muscle enzyme can cause cramping, pain, and myoglobinuria with exercise (13).

Congenital myopathies occur at birth, usually result in hypotonia, and are usually nonprogressive. Examples of congenital myopathies include central core myopathy, nemaline rod myopathy, and centronuclear myopathy. The diagnosis is usually made by muscle biopsy.

REHABILITATION

The goal of neuromuscular rehabilitation is to maintain or improve strength, ROM, mobility, and activities of daily living. Educating both the family and patient is important. Rehabilitation is beyond just attending physical and occupational therapy sessions. Ideally, rehabilitation takes place daily and will require not only motivation from the patient but sometimes active participation of caregivers.

Rehabilitation is a team or holistic effort and will require multiple team players including the physical therapist, occupational therapist, recreational therapist, speech and language pathologist, psychologist, social worker, orthotist, nutritionist, and consult physicians. The physiatrist is responsible for designing a rehabilitation program that is accessible to the patient. The therapy prescription should include the diagnosis, frequency, and duration of therapy; description of treatments to be utilized; goals; and precautions. Part of the therapy is to train caregivers in providing continued care at home.

Rehabilitation interventions include exercise and use of appropriate braces such as ankle foot orthotics. Resting hand splints may help stretch tight fingers and hands. Mobility aids such as walkers and canes may help with mobility. Adaptive devices such as built-up utensils, raised toilet seats, and long-handled reachers can help with self-care. As fatigue and muscle weakness become more problematic, use of a seated mobility system such as a motorized wheelchair or scooter may be necessary. Patients may also require noninvasive positive pressure ventilation to help maintain breathing as they tend to fatigue. Respiratory therapy is also important in clearing secretions. Speech therapy is important to help patients maintain communication and develop compensatory strategies. Some patients will require alternative nutritional means (gastrostomy) secondary to aspiration risks from dysphagia. Surgical intervention to improve ROM and positioning may be needed for patients with severe deformities or contractures. Pain management with medications and modalities are often used to treat musculoskeletal and neuropathic complaints.

NMDs are often characterized by a gradual decline in motor function that can lead to severe respiratory compromise or even death. Caring for such patients involves the use of life-sustaining interventions. There are ethical challenges with regard to decisions to withhold and withdraw care. In providing care for patients the physician should follow the ethical principles of autonomy, beneficence, nonmaleficence, and justice (14). Autonomy is the basis for informed consent, allowing the patient to act without controlling influences. Beneficence is the duty of health care providers to be a benefit to the patient. Nonmaleficence is the duty that health care providers do not create needless harm or injury to the patient. Justice is a form of fairness that can involve allocation of limited resources. It is important to anticipate end-of-life issues early in order to allow the patient and family ample time to prepare. The physician should help the patient set up advance directives, designate a durable power of attorney, and plan end-of-life care. Some patients may refuse life-sustaining therapies such as a ventilator and these requests should be honored. Patient comfort and dignity are important, especially in a palliative care setting.

PRACTICE-BASED LEARNING AND IMPROVEMENT

GOALS

Demonstrate competence in continuously investigating and evaluating your own NMD patient care practices, appraising and assimilating scientific evidence, and continuously improving your patient care practices based on constant self-evaluation and lifelong learning.

OBJECTIVES

1. Identify learning opportunities for providers, patients, and caregivers with experience in NMD, including professional NMD organizations.
2. Appraise the evidence-based guidelines and literature for treating NMD.
3. Use methods for ongoing competency training in NMD for physiatrists, including feedback from colleagues and patients in daily practice, evaluating current practice, and developing a systematic QI and practice improvement project strategy.
4. Locate some resources including available websites for continuing medical education and continuing professional development.
5. Conduct self-assessment and lifelong learning such as review of current quality of care markers, including evidence-based, in treatment of patients with NMD and the role of the physiatrist as the educator of patients, families, residents, students, colleagues, and other health professionals.

Initially called "reflective practice," practice-based learning (PBL) refers to a process where a physician identifies areas of improvement by regular self-assessment (15). The physician will then acquire the necessary knowledge and skills with the purpose of providing better patient care. Outcomes data provide one important way to compare personal results with national benchmarks. Continued self-improvement is an intrinsic part of the Hippocratic Oath. Physicians who do not perform on par with the national quality standards will be penalized under the Affordable Care Act. Quality indicators, such as adherence to practice guidelines and complication and readmission rates, are some of the data that are collected by payers/insurances, including The Centers for Medicare and Medicaid Services (CMS). Other important areas for improvement can be identified by feedback from colleagues, health care professionals, and patients. Once a search for deficiencies is initiated, it usually will yield something that can be improved upon. Brainstorming ideas with colleagues can provide helpful tips on how to improve the delivery of quality of care.

The specific practice improvement project chosen should be based upon either an identified deficiency and/or safety concern. Obvious choices include those that address accepted markers of quality of care for NMDs, including acute care readmission rates and occurrence of common complications (such as joint contractures, falls, and pressure ulcers). Patients who are dependent on wheelchairs can have complications related to respiratory and cardiac events. Other complications in NMDs can be related to neurogenic bowel or bladder and pain.

With the ongoing research efforts and advances in medical genetics, it is very important to stay attuned to current developments. Peer-reviewed publications, such as the *Annals of Neurology*, *Neuromuscular Disorders*, *Muscle and Nerve*, and *Amyotrophic Lateral Sclerosis* are some of the major journals covering the broad topic of NMDs. There are several professional organizations that provide Maintenance of Certification (MOC) related to caring for people with NMDs and host annual educational and scientific conferences. The American Academy of Neurology, American Academy of Physical Medicine and Rehabilitation, and the American Academy of Neuromuscular and Electrodiagnostic Medicine are involved in funding programs for both patient and physician education. In addition to broadcasting results of research, these organizations regularly release clinical guidelines relevant to managing NMDs. One excellent resource is the website of the Muscular Dystrophy Association (www.mda.org), which is the largest nongovernmental entity that funds research, promotes awareness of NMDs, and provides educational materials for both patients and health care professionals.

Presentation of NMD symptoms varies widely, from mild cases of muscular dystrophy that have little effect on a patient's functional capacity to uniformly lethal, rapidly progressive conditions, such as ALS. While no two patients with the same disease are exactly alike, the knowledge that exists regarding the course of a condition can help patients and their families prepare for the obstacles that may lie ahead. Many of the family members of people affected by NMDs will experience increasing burden of care, changing roles and responsibilities, and learning new skills. Education of individuals with NMDs and their family members can alleviate some anxiety that will inevitably arise (16). Physiatrists are uniquely positioned in that they are able to manage both the disease process and maximize functional outcome. Rehabilitation specialists can help patients and their family members achieve the maximum participation in vocational as well as recreational activities. A holistic and multidisciplinary approach is needed in order to help coordinate care. For example, social workers can help improve available home/assistance services. Physical therapists can help improve a patient's mobility. Occupational therapists can help patients with functional tasks and activities of daily living.

INTERPERSONAL AND COMMUNICATION SKILLS

GOALS

Demonstrate interpersonal and communication skills that result in the effective exchange of information and collaboration with NMD patients, their families, and the rest of the rehabilitation team.

OBJECTIVES

1. Demonstrate skills used in effective communication, counseling, and collaboration methods with NMD patients and their caregivers and families across socioeconomic and cultural backgrounds.
2. Discuss appropriate documentation strategies in a patient's medical records for NMD.
3. Delineate and demonstrate the importance of the role of the physiatrist as the interdisciplinary team leader and consultant for the patient with NMD.

The diagnosis of an NMD can change the lives of patients and their family members dramatically. One of the most important tasks for a physician is to provide as much information as clearly as possible. Explaining complex disease processes in easy-to-understand everyday language will help patients and their families make informed decisions. Setting realistic and attainable goals is also important, as is asking the patients and family members about their goals and expectations (17). As most NMDs are rare and hard to predict, this will bring an element of the unknown into the planning process. Oftentimes the fear of the unknown can have a significant impact on the patient's quality of life. Additionally, no matter the severity of the diagnosis, patients and their families still need to maintain physical and mental well-being, which includes physical exercise, emotional support, sexual health, and regular rest for the caretakers.

Medical record documentation serves as a repository of interventions, treatments, and plans of care. NMDs often have many systemic complications and thus will require the interventions of multiple physicians and health care workers. Use of an integrated electronic medical record system will allow easy access and review of medical information. Common tests include electrocardiograms (ECGs) to assess for conduction defects or arrhythmias, renal ultrasounds to look out for complications of neurogenic bladder, and pulmonary function tests to assess breathing. Oftentimes these tests are done regularly and should be documented and retrieved easily as patients may need to see various specialists. Clear and meaningful record keeping facilitates interaction between multiple team members and serves to promote the best possible outcome. Medical records are also important in billing to determine the level of service. Accurate and appropriate documentation can serve as a legal safeguard in the event of litigation.

Poor communication is often cited as the main reason for dissatisfaction with the medical care received. Information regarding life-altering diagnoses may not be the easiest to digest, particularly during the initial encounter. Information should be straightforward, as we as appropriate for the educational background and current knowledge base. Asking open-ended questions invites a meaningful discussion. Everyone should have the opportunity to contribute to the conversation including family members and caregivers. Additionally there are basic techniques that facilitate an open exchange of information, such as removing distractions (pagers, cell phones), allowing ample time for the discussion, and employing open body language. Effective communication with patients involves the use of verbal, nonverbal, and written skills. By instilling feelings of trust, honesty, open communication, rapport, and comfort in the physician–patient relationship, the physician can develop and maintain a therapeutic alliance with the patient.

Leadership skills are important in directing a multidisciplinary team of professionals. The physiatrist should have a broad scope of knowledge and be able to integrate the ideas of multiple disciplines and then formulate an interdisciplinary plan of care. Leadership is the ability to motivate others toward a common goal. While ultimately all members of the team work toward the same goal, conflicts may arise and it is up to the team leader, the physician, to keep the team moving forward. Leadership skills are also important in family meetings as it will help the rehabilitation team not only communicate with the patient and family but also provide a way to solve problems in a dynamic and interdisciplinary format. Resident physiatrists have a unique opportunity to learn necessary leadership skills by first participating and later presiding over team and family meetings for patients admitted to rehabilitation units.

PROFESSIONALISM

GOALS

Reflect a commitment to carrying out professional responsibilities and an adherence to ethical principles in caring for patients with NMD.

OBJECTIVES

1. Exemplify the humanistic qualities in patient-centered care.
2. Demonstrate ethical principles and responsiveness to patient needs superseding self and other interests.
3. Demonstrate sensitivity to patient population diversity, cultural competence, gender, age, race, religion, disabilities, and sexual orientation.
4. Respect patient privacy, confidentiality, autonomy, and shared decision making.
5. Recognize the socioeconomic factors and importance of patient education in the treatment of and advocacy for persons with NMD.

Most NMDs remain largely incurable and some are progressive in nature. As a result, carrying an NMD diagnosis can have a profound emotional impact on the patient as well as family and friends. Displaying honesty and integrity as a practitioner is essential in the difficult task of informing affected individuals of their diagnosis, prognosis, and realistic treatment goals. It is also of upmost importance that physicians perceive their patients as individuals and not as their diagnoses. Previously strong, healthy individuals are often devastated with fear as well as feelings of confusion and helplessness. The physician should always display compassion, courtesy, and respect in this vulnerable setting where an individual's autonomy is challenged by disease. The chronic and often lifelong nature of neuromuscular diseases allows the physician and therapist to establish long-term follow-up care for these individuals. It is important to not only listen but also understand patients. Part of understanding is nonverbal communication such as body gestures, attitude, and personality.

As with other medical conditions, treating individuals with neuromuscular diseases requires a balance between medical management and sensitivity to the patient's social and cultural background, including religion, socioeconomic status, gender, and age. Different societies carry different stigmas or culturally influenced attitudes toward disability. These attitudes can have a profound effect on a patient's emotional health, feelings of self-worth, and ultimate quality of life. Additionally, there is a fear and uncertainty with neuromuscular diseases, leaving patients and caregivers often unsure of how to react to such a serious diagnosis. A lack of education about the disease and its course can make it difficult for patients and their families to respond appropriately. Thus, early recognition of these influential factors that may pose a threat to the patient's well-being is crucial. Addressing issues respectfully without judgment and providing education is the physician's responsibility.

Caring for patients with NMD is a multidisciplinary team effort. Besides the importance of accurate and regular communication between the different members of the team, which can include physicians of different disciplines, physical and occupational therapists, speech therapists, and social workers, it is crucial that care remain patient-centered with preserved patient autonomy. With several health care providers involved, the focus of care may deviate at times and providers can lose sight of what the patient wants versus what the medical professionals think is best for the patient. Some neuromuscular clinics have now been organized into a center where multiple disciplines are available during one clinic visit. Many hospitals that provide care for ALS patients are now providing care in a centralized fashion. Coordinated care means easier access for the patient as the patient can go to one outpatient appointment for checkups rather than setting aside time to make all the appointments at different locations and times.

Physicians are responsible and accountable for their patients with NMD. Confirmation of the diagnosis usually is the primary responsibility of the NMD specialist. Diagnosis confirmation can be critical in shaping a patient's future and oftentimes a confirmatory second opinion or even third opinion should be sought. Once the diagnosis is established, the patient should be thoroughly educated regarding the etiology, expected clinical outcome, and risk of certain medical complications. A rehabilitative program should be designed in order to maintain or maximize functional outcome. Sometimes in the later stages of disease, a palliative program may be needed for patient comfort and quality of life. Palliative care programs emphasize pain control, seating and positioning, nutrition, and pulmonary support.

The physician should be humble enough to ask for help when it is needed from mentors, colleagues, consultants, family members, and other treatment team members. Educating the family, caregivers, and other health care professionals about the different medical, psychosocial, and behavioral issues that may arise is also the physician's responsibility. Information should always be transmitted in a clear, meaningful, and respectful fashion, geared to the recipient's educational level to ensure understanding. Physicians need to be an advocate for their patients. Providing the patient with community resources such as available support/awareness groups paves the way by which persons with NMD can meet other people living with similar challenges.

Physician advocacy is important in the care of patients with NMD. Since many patients with neuromuscular disorders are children, it is important for the physician to work with school officials in developing an individual education plan. Children with NMDs have special needs and will often need therapy services or medical intervention during the school day. By working with the school nurse and teachers, the physician is crucial in making the school life of these children as normal as possible. In the community setting, the physician should support the patient's right to access various community activities and be involved in educating the general public about neuromuscular disease. Involvement in national organizations such as the MDA can help leverage funding for research from both governmental and private sources. The MDA is a nonprofit health organization dedicated to curing muscular dystrophy, ALS, and related diseases by funding worldwide research. Being part of a large nonprofit health agency can help the physician provide comprehensive health care and support services while networking with other health care leaders.

SYSTEMS-BASED PRACTICE

GOAL

Awareness and responsiveness to systems of care delivery, and the ability to recruit and coordinate effectively resources in the system to provide optimal care as it relates to NMD.

OBJECTIVES

1. Identify the components, systems of care delivery, services, referral patterns, and resources in the rehabilitation continuum of care for patients with NMD.
2. Coordinate and recruit necessary resources in the system to provide optimal care for the NMD patient, with attention to safety, cost awareness, and risk–benefit analysis and management.
3. Describe optimal follow-up, quality improvement measures, and use of documentation in NMD rehabilitation programs.

Most NMDs are lifelong and largely incurable at this time. Although NMDs are not curable they are mostly treatable. Comprehensive management of these diseases is an arduous task and best achieved through an interdisciplinary approach, taking advantage of the expertise of many clinicians. Teams commonly include physicians spanning the fields of Physical Medicine and Rehabilitation (PM&R), Neurology, Cardiology, Pulmonology, and Orthopedic Surgery. Physical therapists, occupational therapists, speech therapists, nutritionists, social workers, vocational counselors, and psychologists are also an integral part of the interdisciplinary team. The physiatrist is well suited to direct this multidisciplinary team and oversee a comprehensive, goal-oriented health care management plan. Because of the insidious onset, persons with NMD are often diagnosed in the outpatient clinic setting. Depending on the disease course and their compliance with outpatient/home exercise programs, they may intermittently benefit from inpatient rehabilitation especially after acute hospitalization.

During follow-up care, the physician should ensure that measures are taken to prevent secondary complications such as skin breakdown (pressure ulcers), joint contractures, scoliosis, atelectasis/hypoxemia, venous thromboembolism, urinary retention, and bowel impaction. Follow-up visits should occur on a regular basis and readdress the patient's goals and concerns during each visit. Prevention of secondary complications should be reinforced. Family meetings should be set up as necessary to facilitate communication between the patient, family, and other members of the rehabilitation team.

The American Board of Medical Specialties now offers a certificate of added qualification (board certification) in Neuromuscular Medicine. Physicians having board certification in neuromuscular medicine have additional training beyond primary board certification (Neurology or Physical Medicine and Rehabilitation) in the management of NMDs. One mark of quality for inpatient NMD care is accreditation of the facility by the Commission on Accreditation of Rehabilitation Facilities (CARF). Inpatient rehabilitation is often beneficial after an acute hospitalization (i.e., pneumonia) in order to counter the effects of deconditioning and to maximize functional outcome. Sometimes patients with motor neuron disorders may have paradoxical worsening with aggressive therapy, so aggressive physical therapy is not always the best way to manage these patients. Individuals with NMD may also need to learn how to direct care that they need if they are no longer able to accomplish such care by themselves.

Documentation through an electronic medical record system allows for the maintenance of up-to-date medical records/reports of diagnostic testing, which can be easily accessed by and used by other members of the multidisciplinary team. These records should capture the essential patient information while simultaneously respecting patient privacy. Language that is understandable to other providers should be used.

Health care resources are often limited and management of resources is important. NMDs can progress and health care needs become more demanding, yet health care coverage is often less generous. The long-term goal of medical care for patients with NMDs is to maintain function and quality of life in the most cost-beneficial manner possible. For example, in ALS, as the disease rapidly advances, so health care providers are faced with meeting the medical needs of the patients in the context of restrictions on resource utilization. The physician must learn how to work within the current health care system to meet the needs of patients within a short period of time. Therefore, it is imperative to start planning well in advance in order to make the medical resources available when patients are most likely to need them. In patients with ALS, costs associated with late-stage and end-of-life care are enormous, coming from numerous medical interventions including percutaneous endoscopic gastrostomy (PEG), noninvasive positive pressure ventilation (NIPPV), mechanical ventilation, drug therapies, and emergency room visits. It should be noted that the cost of drug therapy for ALS with riluzole is considerable and only modestly prolongs survival, so from a societal perspective the benefits of the medication may not exceed the cost of the medication (18).

The physician has a responsibility to advocate for the quality of care for his or her patients. The goals of rehabilitation and palliative care are to maximize functional capabilities, prolong or maintain independent function and mobility, inhibit or prevent physical deformity and medical complications, provide access for integration into the community, and ensure a good quality of life.

Rehabilitation services are important in patients with NMDs. For patients with impaired mobility or those who are homebound, therapy services can be delivered in the home setting. Home therapy is important, especially for patients who are unable to travel to a facility for therapy. There may be limitations to home therapy; for example, there may be limited access to equipment because it is too cumbersome to bring to the home setting. Most patients can receive therapy in an outpatient facility or even in the school. The patient would need to be able to travel in order to get to an outpatient facility, but the benefit would be access to specialized equipment. Patients with severe functional limitations may need acute inpatient rehabilitation if they need daily physician management, aggressive physical and occupational therapy (3 hours/day), and have rehabilitation nursing needs. Generally, acute inpatient rehabilitation is of shorter stay in the range of no more than a few weeks with the goal of getting the patient home at an independent or modified independent level. In a subacute rehabilitation facility, patients tend to stay longer but the intensity of rehabilitation is less, usually 1 to 2 hours per day. Patients with NMDs will often need inpatient rehabilitation services after an acute hospitalization if there is a deterioration of function.

NMD patients are complex and have multiple organ systems that are involved. As most NMDs are relatively rare, many doctors may not be familiar with the management of these patients. It is important for doctors to communicate with other consultants and caregivers as these patients are transferred from one point of care to another. Taking the time to go over the medical records and the discharge summaries is important in order to minimize the risk to these patients. Especially in the rehabilitation setting, it is important to integrate the recommendations of multiple disciplines including speech therapy, physical therapy, occupational therapy, and nutrition along with those of other medical consultants.

The physician should also help the patient minimize risks by helping him or her prepare for an emergency. The patient should be educated on when symptoms should be taken seriously. He or she should have a folder that can be quickly grabbed in an emergency containing all necessary insurance information, medical diagnosis, and health care provider's name and contact information along with current medications and test results. If possible, bringing a family member or a friend during a hospital visit will not only provide companionship, but also can advocate for the patient in discussions with the medical staff and help take notes on medical procedures and tests.

CASE STUDY

Jackson is a 20-year-old man who has been nonambulatory for several years. He has a long history of progressive weakness that started with not being able to walk until 17 months. However, he reached many of his motor milestones prior to this, including sitting and standing at normal times. Around the age of 2 years, he developed a more lordotic position while standing. A Gowers sign and Trendelenburg gait were noted at age 4 and the following years he continued to have progressive weakness, mainly involving the proximal muscles. By age 10 he needed braces to help him walk and by age 12 he needed a wheelchair for basic mobility.

Two years ago he was admitted to the hospital for bronchitis and improved with antibiotic treatments. He has a mild learning disability but was able to complete high school with the help of tutors. He was recently admitted to the hospital with a fever of 103.2°F and a respiratory rate of 30 breaths/minute. He had reduced breath sounds along with inspiratory rales bilaterally. He also had a weak cough. Chest x-ray confirmed bilateral infiltrates and he was subsequently treated with intravenous antibiotics and breathing treatments. He is weak and deconditioned from pneumonia and is no longer able to manage the use of his wheelchair. He also is now unable to transfer in and out of the wheelchair along with decreased bed mobility. Physiatric consultation was called for further evaluation during his acute inpatient hospitalization for pneumonia.

CASE STUDY DISCUSSION QUESTIONS

PATIENT CARE: Describe the key elements of the assessment of this patient and a multidisciplinary care plan including a rehabilitation prescription. Describe the importance of orthotic management and seating/positioning for this patient.

MEDICAL KNOWLEDGE: Describe the current medical knowledge about the epidemiology, pathophysiology, and treatment of Duchenne muscular dystrophy. Describe Gowers sign and Trendelenburg gait. Describe the role of pulmonary function tests and respiratory management in patients with NMD.

PRACTICE-BASED LEARNING AND IMPROVEMENT: Identify two to three key areas that physiatrists should demonstrate knowledge about this condition and resources where they can obtain additional information. Review the developmental milestones usually achieved in Duchenne muscular dystrophy.

INTERPERSONAL AND COMMUNICATION SKILLS: Describe how to effectively communicate prognosis and implement a treatment plan in the management of patients with Duchenne muscular dystrophy. Demonstrate how a family meeting may be utilized in order to effectively communicate discharge planning.

PROFESSIONALISM: Describe and demonstrate elements of professional behavior that the physiatrist should display in the care of patients with progressive neuromuscular disorders.

SYSTEMS-BASED PRACTICE: Describe the rehabilitation continuum of care and systems-based patient safety concerns in the care of this patient. Describe appropriateness for acute inpatient rehabilitation, subacute inpatient rehabilitation, or home discharge with home services.

SELF-EXAMINATION QUESTIONS
(Answers begin on p. 367)

1. The American Academy of Neurology recommends the placement of gastrostomy tubes for individuals with ALS while they can still tolerate oral intake and before the forced vital capacity (FVC) falls below what percentage of predicted value to reduce the complications associated with the procedure?
   A. 20%
   B. 30%
   C. 50%
   D. 60%
   E. 70%

2. Of the following, which is the most common adult-onset motor neuron disease?
   A. Amyotrophic lateral sclerosis (ALS)
   B. Spinal muscular atrophy
   C. Postpolio syndrome
   D. Charcot-Marie-Tooth disease
   E. Muscular dystrophy

3. Which of the following is NOT a characteristic of Guillain-Barré syndrome (AIDP)?
   A. *Campylobacter jejuni* enteritis has been implicated as a trigger
   B. Nerve conduction studies show prolonged or absent F reflexes

C. Areflexia or hyporeflexia is present.
D. CSF shows increased white blood cells and increased proteins
E. Treatment is with IVIG or plasmapheresis

4. Which of the following is associated with weakness of the facial and jaw muscles resulting in a "hatchet face" appearance?
   A. Facioscapulohumeral dystrophy (FSH)
   B. Becker muscular dystrophy
   C. Duchenne muscular dystrophy
   D. Myotonic dystrophy
   E. Inclusion body myositis

5. Myasthenia gravis is associated with all the following *except*:
   A. Weakness and fatigue of all muscles especially the ocular muscles
   B. Approximately 10% of patients will have a thymoma
   C. Increased jitter on single-fiber electromyography (EMG)
   D. Autoimmune antibodies that block the presynaptic neuromuscular junction
   E. Decremental response on repetitive stimulation at slow rates

REFERENCES

1. Krivickas LS. Exercise in neuromuscular disease. *J Clin Neuromuscul Dis*. 2003;5(1):29–39.
2. Garber CE, Blissmer B, Deschenes MR, et al. Quantity and quality of exercise for developing and maintaining cardiorespiratory, musculoskeletal, and neuromotor fitness in apparently healthy adults: guidance for prescribing exercise. *Med Sci Sports Exerc*. 2011;43(7):1334–1359.
3. Miller RG, Jackson CE, Kasarkskis EJ, et al. Practice parameter update: the care of the patient with amyotrophic lateral sclerosis: drug, nutritional, and respiratory therapies (an evidence-based review). *Neurology*. 2009;73(15):1218–1226.
4. Amato AA, Russell JA. *Neuromuscular Disorders*. New York, NY: McGraw Medical; 2008.
5. Brooks BR. El Escorial World Federation of Neurology criteria for the diagnosis of amyotrophic lateral sclerosis. Subcommittee on Motor Neuron Diseases/Amyotrophic Lateral Sclerosis of the World Federation of Neurology Research Group on Neuromuscular Diseases and the El Escorial "Clinical limits of amyotrophic lateral sclerosis" workshop contributors. *J Neurol Sci*. 1994;124(suppl):96–107.
6. Wokke J. Riluzole. *Lancet*. 1996;348:795–799.
7. Bertorini TE, ed. *Neuromuscular Disorders: Treatment and Management*. Philadelphia, PA: Saunders; 2011.
8. Selzer ME, Clarke S, Cohen LG, et al., eds. *Textbook of Neural Repair and Rehabilitation: Volume II Medical Neurorehabilitation*. Boston, MA: Cambridge University Press; 2006.
9. Dyck PJ, Thomas PK, eds. *Peripheral Neuropathy*. 3rd ed. Philadelphia, PA: Saunders; 2005.
10. Bach JR. *Guide to the Evaluation and Management of Neuromuscular Disease*. Philadelphia, PA: Hanley and Belfus; 1999.
11. Bertorini TE, ed. *Neuromuscular Disorders: Treatment and Management*. Philadelphia, PA: Saunders; 2011.
12. Harper PS. *Myotonic Dystrophy: Present Management and Future Therapy*. New York, NY: Oxford University Press; 2004.
13. Younger DS. *Motor Disorders*. Philadelphia, PA: Lippincott, Williams and Wilkins; 1999.
14. Vaszar LT, Weinacker AB, Henig NR, et al. Ethical issues in the long-term management of progressive degenerative neuromuscular disease. *Semin Respir Crit Care Med*. 2002;23(3):307–314.
15. Mcclure, P. *Reflection on Practice*; 2005. http://cw.routledge.com/textbooks/9780415537902/data/learning/8_Reflection%20in%20Practice.pdf. Accessed May 29, 2013.
16. Hughes RA, Sinha A, Higginson I, et al. Living with motor neuron disease: lives, experiences of services and suggestions for change. *Health Soc Care Community*. 2005;13(1):64–74.
17. Hugel H, Grundy N, Rigby S, et al. How does current care practice influence the experience of a new diagnosis of motor neuron disease? A qualitative study of current guidelines-based practice. *Amyotroph Lateral Scler*. 2006;7(3):161–166.
18. Mitsumoto H. Diagnosis and progression of ALS. *Neurology*. 1997;48(S4):2S–8S.

Chauncy Eakins
Debra Brathwaite*
Adrian Cristian

19: Multiple Sclerosis

PATIENT CARE

GOALS
Provide patient care that is compassionate, appropriate, and effective for the treatment of a patient with multiple sclerosis (MS) and the promotion of health.

OBJECTIVES
1. Describe the key components of the assessment of the patient with MS.
2. Assess the impairments, activity limitations, and participation restrictions associated with MS.
3. Describe the psychosocial, vocational, and educational aspects of MS.
4. Formulate the key components of a rehabilitation treatment plan for the patient with MS.

MEDICAL HISTORY

History of Present Illness
A thorough and comprehensive documentation of the history of present illness will provide the clinician with valuable information to make a diagnosis of MS and determine associated impairments. Attacks or exacerbations of MS are characterized by symptoms that mirror central nervous system (CNS) involvement. The sine qua non of MS is that symptomatic episodes are "separated in time and space"—that is, episodes occur months or years apart and affect different neuroanatomic locations. As an example, a patient may present with paresthesias of a hand that resolve, followed a few months later by weakness in a leg or visual disturbances. In addition, the duration of the attack should be longer than 24 hours. Presentation of MS often varies among patients. Some patients have a predominance of cognitive changes, while others present with prominent ataxia, hemiparesis or paraparesis, depression, or visual symptoms. Additionally, it is important to recognize that the progression of physical and cognitive disability in MS may occur in the absence of clinical exacerbations (1). The diagnosis of MS is challenging due to its diverse presentation. Symptoms of disorders such as cerebrovascular disorders, tumors of the CNS, myelopathy, spinal cord injury, peripheral neuropathy, collagen vascular disease, and neurodegenerative disorders can mimic those of MS, making the diagnosis difficult to establish. However, the contrary also exists. Trojano reported that 5% to 10% of individuals are misdiagnosed with MS. Diseases that can be mistaken for MS include those of inflammatory, metabolic, genetic, infectious, neoplastic, and spinal origin (2).

Past Medical and Surgical History
These include spinal surgery and dates, as well as ophthalmologic procedures.

Allergies and Medications
These should be reviewed.

Family, Social, and Functional Histories
It is important to obtain a family history since an increased incidence of MS among the offspring of individuals with MS has been reported (3). The location where the patient spent the first 15 years of his or her life is valuable information since migration studies indicate that the likelihood of developing the disease depends on where a person spent the first 15 years of life (3). These data suggest that either a causative factor was acquired in the more temperate latitudes or a protective factor was acquired in the less temperate climates. Smoking, alcohol, and drug usage are important. Work history, travel history, home environment, family support, and level of independence with regard to self-care and ambulation should be evaluated.

Review of Systems
MS is a disease that can lead to focal as well as diffuse symptomatology; therefore, the clinician should rely on a comprehensive review of symptoms which can uncover related problems that the patient might have otherwise overlooked or thought insignificant.

*Deceased.

1. *General*: Weakness, fatigue, heat intolerance.
2. *Cognitive dysfunction:* Memory loss, impaired attention, difficulties in problem solving, slowed information processing.
3. *HEENT*: Facial weakness resembling Bell palsy not associated with ipsilateral loss of taste sensation or retroauricular pain. *Eyes*: Decreased visual acuity, decreased color perception, periorbital pain aggravated by movement, blurry vision, and diplopia (4).
4. *Cardiovascular*: Autonomic alterations might relate to clinical signs such as orthostatic intolerance (5).
5. *Gastrointestinal*: Constipation occurs in greater than 30% of patients with MS. Fecal urgency or bowel incontinence is less common (4).
6. *Genitourinary*: Urinary frequency, urgency, nocturia, and uncontrolled bladder emptying. This can be due to detrusor hyperreflexia secondary to impairment of suprasegmental inhibition (4).
7. *Neuromuscular*: Weakness of the limbs, gait disturbance, or painful muscle spasms associated with spasticity.
8. *Sexuality*: Decreased libido, impaired genital sensation, impotence in men, and diminished vaginal lubrication or adductor spasms in women (4).
9. *Neurological*: Diplopia, internuclear ophthalmoplegia, or vertigo as a result of brainstem lesion, superficially resembling acute labyrinthitis; hearing loss may also occur but is uncommon; painful tingling, burning, or electrical sensations in extremities.
10. *Psychiatric*: Depression experienced by approximately half of the patients; can be reactive, endogenous, or part of the illness itself, and can contribute to fatigue. Suicide in MS patients is 7.5-fold more common than in age-matched controls (4). Euphoria was once thought to be characteristic of MS but is uncommon, occurring in less than 20% of patients (4).
11. *Musculoskeletal*: Pain in limbs, spine.

Physical Examination

A comprehensive physical examination is vital to the identification of impairments related to the disease process. A neurological examination will provide clues to the various neuroanatomic locations of lesions. MS is primarily an upper motor neuron disease. The physical examination should assess the integrity of the following:

1. Corticospinal tracts (upper motor neuron signs: Babinski, clonus, Hoffmann signs, spasticity, hyperreflexia)
2. Spinocerebellar tracts (balance and coordination including rapid alternating movements)
3. Oculomotor function (i.e., nystagmus)
4. Spinothalamic tracts (pain and temperature)
5. Bulbospinal tracts (bulbar signs)
6. Dorsal columns (fine touch, proprioception, vibration)
7. Corticocortical connections (cognition: memory, alertness, orientation, attention, executive functioning, mental processing, visual spatial deficits, and communication)

Cranial nerves II, III, IV, and VI should be examined, especially if the patient complains of visual symptoms. Diplopia may be due to an internuclear ophthalmoplegia or an ocular motor cranial neuropathy, typically a sixth nerve palsy. The occurrence of bilateral internuclear ophthalmoplegia is considered to be highly suggestive of MS, especially in young patients. Third and fourth cranial neuropathies are uncommon in MS (6).

Spasticity is defined as a velocity-dependent increase in tone associated with upper motor neuron disease, which results in muscle stiffness, pain, loss of joint range, and function. The severity of spasticity is commonly evaluated using the Modified Ashworth Scale. Complications associated with spasticity include contractures, pain, loss of function, and skin breakdown.

Musculoskeletal examination should include inspection, palpation, and range of motion of the upper and lower extremities and spine, searching for possible causes of musculoskeletal pain in the MS patient. Motor strength should also be assessed in the extremities. Functional assessment should include an evaluation of the patient's bed mobility, transfers, and gait. If the patient uses an orthotic, it is important to check for proper fit and for areas of skin breakdown. In nonambulatory patients confined to a wheelchair, it is important to check for proper positioning in the wheelchair.

There are several scales that can be used in the assessment of the MS patient. The extent of neurologic disability can be evaluated using the Kurtzke Expanded Disability Status Scale. This is a scale that grades the type and extent of disability on a scale from 1 to 10. It assesses eight functional systems—the higher the score, the more disabled the individual. A score of 10 represents death secondary to MS (7). Fatigue in MS can be assessed using the Modified Fatigue Impact Scale, Visual Analog Scale, Fatigue Severity Scales, and MS Specific Fatigue Severity Scale (8,9).

Impairments, Activity Limitations, and Participation Restrictions in MS

In order to monitor the natural history of MS and the impact it has on a patient's life, impairments, activity limitations, and participation restrictions should be assessed. As defined by the World Health Organization, impairment is a problem in body function or structure; an activity limitation is a difficulty encountered by an individual in executing a task or action; while a participation restriction is a problem experienced by an individual in involvement in life situations (10).

An impairment is a loss of or abnormality in anatomical, physiological, or psychological structures or function. These abnormalities can vary widely in MS patients. Examples include short-term memory loss, impaired concentration, depression, fatigue, visual loss, paresis, paresthesias, impaired sensation, spasticity, footdrop, bladder/bowel incontinence, sexual dysfunction, and impaired balance and coordination.

MS patients have activity limitations as a result of their neuromuscular, psychological, and cognitive impairments. Paresis and increased tone leads to decrease in ambulation, transfers, activities of daily living (ADLs), and instrumental activities of daily living (IADLs). Spasticity can lead to pain and alterations in gait pattern that can increase the risk for falls. Depression is a common impairment that can be associated with sleep disturbances and poor concentration that can adversely affect IADLs and safety in the home. It is now recognized that impaired cognition can lead to impaired working memory, judgment, and processing speed. These can lead to difficulties in planning and organizing, cooking, balancing a checkbook, safely taking medications, and difficulties with reading. Without modifications in the workplace or at home to address certain functional limitations, problems can develop with the patient's ability to participate.

Psychosocial, Vocational, and Educational Issues Affecting the MS Patient

MS has a significant impact on families, work, community, and educational activities. Fatigue, mobility impairments, and cognitive impairments were reported as the main drivers of job-related difficulties. MS has been shown to have an impact on the cessation of relationships and marriages compared to the general population. Interviews with some spouses who become caregivers to patients with MS express discontent with this new role or idea and express the desire to be loved as a spouse rather than as a caregiver (11). Onset of MS before 36 years of age and having children are good prognosticators for maintaining relationships or marriages compared to the opposite.

Participation restrictions can be especially devastating for productive young healthy individuals who depend on their physical, mental, and psychological capacity to care for themselves, family, and work. Studies have shown MS to have a strong impact on employment status, as the mean unemployment rate of those with MS was 59% (12). The rate of unemployment increases consistently with age and disease duration. Fatigue, mobility impairments, and cognitive impairments were reported as the main drivers of job-related difficulties, whereas employer's lack of support and accommodations were identified as the causes of perceived discriminations (12). Loss of income is a significant concern for MS patients, who are typically affected by the disease during their peak financially productive years and can also face increased medically related costs.

Parenting is another important limitation that is often faced by patients with MS on a relatively large scale. MS is a disease of young adults in their reproductive and parenting age. During periods of MS exacerbation, patients are rendered physically and cognitively unable to care for their children and will often require hospitalization for treatment and rehabilitation.

Children of parents with MS can experience a shift to the role of caregiver, which can be overwhelming. It is important to provide early family counseling and intervention to maintain a healthy family unit and at the same time maintain a safe environment for the patient suffering from MS.

Individuals living with MS may have been active members of social or athletic clubs, which require a certain level of physical and cognitive functional capacity, and may face increasing challenges in continuing their roles in these activities as the disease progresses.

Rehabilitation Treatment Plan for the MS Patient

The rehabilitation treatment plan for the individual with MS should be driven by the impairments, activity limitations, and participation restrictions facing that person. Given the variety of different impairments associated with the disease, a team approach to care is recommended. For example,

1. Abnormal gait can be addressed through a physical therapy program that strengthens key muscle groups used in ambulation and provides gait training using an appropriate assistive device.
2. Spasticity management can be accomplished through a combination of medications, stretching, and use of modalities.
3. Swallow dysfunction can be addressed by speech pathologists following a formal assessment by recommending specific diet modifications and strategies.
4. Difficulties performing ADLs can be addressed by occupational therapists through appropriate training and recommended modifications to home environment.
5. Several members of the rehabilitation team such as neuropsychologists, occupational therapists, and speech pathologists can evaluate cognitive impairments with compensatory strategies provided to the patient and his or her family.
6. Vocational counselors can assist the patient with return to work issues.
7. Recreational therapists can provide information and strategies specific to return to leisure activities.
8. Driving rehabilitation can be useful for the individual with MS who needs to drive but is found to need training, as well as modifications to the vehicle.
9. The role of the social worker can be vital in identifying community resources for the patient, as well as for providing emotional support and counseling.
10. A psychologist and/or psychiatrist can evaluate for depression and provide treatment as needed.
11. Rehabilitation nursing can provide education and training regarding bowel and bladder care and medication use.
12. Medical and surgical subspecialties such as neuro-ophthalmology and neurology are also commonly involved in the care of the MS patient.

The exercise prescription for the MS patient should take into consideration the patient's impairments so that exercise can be carried out safely. For example, risk of falls should be clearly communicated to the treating therapists. Fatigue and heat intolerance are additional concerns; hence, an exercise program should provide for adequate rest periods and minimize exposure to excessive heat environments.

MEDICAL KNOWLEDGE

GOALS

Demonstrate knowledge of established and evolving biomedical, clinical epidemiological, and sociobehavioral sciences pertaining to MS, as well as the application of this knowledge to guide holistic patient care.

OBJECTIVES

1. Describe the epidemiology, anatomy, physiology, and pathophysiology of MS.
2. Identify the pertinent laboratory and imaging studies important in MS.
3. Review the treatment and management of MS.
4. Examine the socioeconomic and ethical issues in MS.

MS is the most common cause of nontraumatic disability affecting young people in the Northern Hemisphere. There are about 400,000 persons in the United States living with MS, and the prevalence range is 40 to 220 per 100,000 people. The incidence of MS is 171/100,000 persons, with females accounting for approximately 70% of cases (3). Therefore, when a patient between the ages of 20 and 40 presents with these symptoms the clinician should be prompted to consider the diagnosis of MS. Patients may not seek medical attention if the impairment is not disabling. In addition, patients may experience symptoms that are nondebilitating that may not necessarily be indicative of MS.

MS is multifactorial in its causality. Environmental factors are thought to act as triggers in people who have a genetic predisposition to developing the disease (13). Investigators have shown an association between infection with Epstein-Barr virus (EBV) and patients with MS, implying that viruses may serve as triggers to manifesting the disease (14). MS also appears to involve genetic factors with HLA-DR2 in DR-positive families having a greater chance of developing the disease (13). Twin studies from different populations consistently indicate pairwise concordance (20%–30% in identical twin pairs compared to 2%–5% in like-sex fraternal twin pairs), providing additional evidence for a genetic etiology in MS (15).

MS pathology is marked by the presence of multifocal plaques of demyelination in the cerebral hemispheres, optic nerves, brainstem, and spinal cord (16). Myelin destruction is an essential element of the plaque. The plaque forming lesions in the brain has a temporal progression, based on stages of inflammatory destruction. Accordingly, acute, chronic active, and chronic silent lesions have a gradual progression, eventually producing the scarred and hardened areas within the CNS that can be appreciated via gross examination (17). The acute stage is typified by strong inflammatory infiltration combined with demyelination distributed throughout the lesion. The acute plaques include ill-defined margins of myelin loss, infiltration of immune cells, and parenchymal edema. A region of hypocellularity with loss of myelin and glial scarring characterizes the chronic plaque. In chronic active lesions, inflammation continues along the outer border comparable to acute lesions. Areas of remyelination are often observed on the edge of lesions. Chronic silent lesions are characterized by loss of the inflammation and inflammatory mediators along the border of chronic active lesions (17).

The chronic inflammatory process in MS patients is not confined to the white matter (18). Gray matter lesions are detected by MRI and by examination of pathologic specimens (17). As might be expected, inflammatory lesions within the gray matter are associated with neuronal loss and transected axons, which are more common in active lesions (17). The inflammatory process destroys myelin, oligodendrocytes, neurons, and axons. Active demyelinating lesions lead to high density of axonal transections that are persistent with low-level axonal damage in active plaque (19). In addition, there is diffuse axonal and neuronal loss throughout the nervous system. Macrophages are the most prominent inflammatory cells in the lesion and many are filled with myelin debris. MS pathogenesis has linked the disease process to myelin-specific CD4þ T lymphocytes, which upon activation by unknown factors migrate through the blood–brain barrier (BBB) and exert cytotoxic attacks on oligodendrocytes and myelin. EBV, a B-lymphotropic microorganism, has been implicated in the development of the disease by epidemiological, immune, serological, and histological studies (20).

There are several different types of MS:

- Relapsing remitting MS is the most common and is characterized by periods of disease activity followed by periods of disease inactivity.
- Secondary progressive MS is characterized by a relapsing and remitting course until the disease enters a phase of steady decline.
- Primary progressive MS is characterized by a steady worsening of the disease without episodes of relapses.
- Progressive relapsing MS in which there is a steady worsening of the disease with episodic relapses (21). Both primary progressive and relapsing and remitting MS were found to have an onset to progression at the ages of 40.2 and 38.6, respectively (22).

Diagnostic Testing in MS

The diagnosis of MS is primarily a clinical one with supporting evidence drawn from MRI, CSF analysis, and evoked potentials as needed.

1. MRI: MRI is currently the preferred imaging technique to support the diagnosis of MS. It is more sensitive than CT and may also identify subclinical lesions (23).

Multifocal areas of increased intensity on T2-weighted images are abnormal in 85% of cases. These are ovoid appearing plaques located in the periventricular white matter. Lesions are enhanced with gadolinium and may precede the onset of deficits and identify active disease. Subclinical lesions may be visualized. MRI will demonstrate disseminated lesions in space, replacing examination findings in two areas. Repeat MRIs over time showing new lesion formation can also be substituted for further attacks in making a diagnosis. The McDonald criteria (24) (Table 19.1) allow for consistent diagnostic criteria to be applied and are helpful in epidemiological studies as well as patient recruitment into clinical trials (16).

2. CSF analysis: Before MRI, this was the mainstay of study in MS. Cerebral spinal fluid: CSF protein and glucose is normal. There is an increase in oligoclonal IgG bands, IgG and WBCs.

3. Electrodiagnostic testing: Evoked potential responses: Visual evoked potentials (VEPs), brainstem auditory evoked potential responses (BAERs), and somatosensory evoked

TABLE 19.1 McDonald Criteria

CLINICAL PRESENTATION	ADDITIONAL DATA NEEDED FOR DIAGNOSIS	COMMENT
Two or more attacks; objective clinical evidence of two or more lesions	None	If MRI or CSF analysis is negative, caution must be taken before making a diagnosis of MS
Two or more attacks; objective clinical evidence of one lesion	Dissemination in space and demonstrated by MRI Two or more MRI-detected lesions consistent with MS plus positive CSF Evidence of further attacks implicating a different site	MRI scan must fulfill criteria for brain abnormality Positive CSF: Oligoclonal bands detected by established methods, preferably isoelectric focusing, different from any such bands in serum; or by a raised IgG index
One attack; objective clinical evidence of two or more lesions	Dissemination in time demonstrated by MRI or second clinical attack	MRI scan must fulfill criteria for dissemination of lesions in time
One attack; objective clinical evidence of one lesion (monosymptomatic presentation; clinically isolated syndrome)	Dissemination in space demonstrated by MRI Two or more MRI-detected lesions consistent with MS plus positive CSF and dissemination in space, demonstrated by MRI scan or second clinical attack	MRI scan must fulfill criteria for brain abnormality Positive CSF: Oligoclonal bands detected by established methods, preferably isoelectric focusing, different from any such bands in serum; or by a raised IgG index
Insidious neurological progression suggestive of MS	Positive CSF and dissemination in space, demonstrated by nine or more T2 lesions in the brain *or* two or more lesions in the spinal cord, *or* four to eight brain plus one spinal cord lesion Continued progression for 1 year	Positive CSF: Oligoclonal bands detected by established methods, preferably isoelectric focusing, different from any such bands in serum; or by a raised IgG index Scan must fulfill criteria for brain abnormality

potentials (SEPs) have been used to aid in the diagnosis of MS (25). Absence or prolonged latency of responses has been noted.

4. Visual evoked potentials: Abnormalities are most consistently seen in MS and optic neuritis (1) and there is a high sensitivity along with MRI. A study by P. Asselman found that the latency of the VEPs was prolonged in one or both eyes in 84% of those with definite MS, in 83% of those with probable MS, and in 21% of those with possible MS (26). Electromyography (EMG) findings in MS have also been described (25).

TREATMENT

Medication
May be used to decrease inflammation and also suppress the immune system.

Corticosteroids
Used in the treatment of acute attacks or exacerbations. A systematic review found a sufficient body of evidence to support the use of IV methylprednisolone in acute exacerbations of MS (23). Symptoms most responsive to this treatment include optic neuritis, brainstem involvement, acute pain, and bowel and bladder dysfunction. The least responsive symptoms involved cerebellar and sensory dysfunction (23).

Immunomodulator Agents
Used to prevent disability caused by disease progression and decrease the severity, frequency, and exacerbations of the disease. These include (a) Interferon beta-1a (Avonex), (b) Interferon beta-1a (Rebif) (25), (c) Interferon beta-1b (Betaseron), (d) glatiramer acetate (Copaxone), and (e) natalizumab (Tysabri).

Immunosuppressive Agents
Used as second-line therapies. They are reserved for patients with unresponsive disabling MS. These include cyclosporine, cyclophosphamide, azathioprine, plasmapheresis, methotrexate, and mitoxantrone (27).

Rehabilitation Program in MS
During an acute exacerbation, treatment should include a comprehensive rehabilitation program, which includes the following: relative rest, hydration, bladder and bowel management, physical therapy, occupational therapy, speech therapy, neuropsychological treatment for cognitive retraining, and dietary management.

Prescriptions for physical therapy should be tailored to address specific impairments and safety concerns. Specific muscle training is recommended for improving focal weaknesses. Since weakness is a significant problem in MS, it is very important that generalized conditioning be maintained as long as possible. Fatigue management should also be implemented. Focused muscle strengthening that incorporates progressive resistive exercises, range of motion, balance, coordination, and bed mobility and transfers can be effective in motivated individuals with mild or even severe impairments. Passive and active training should be complemented by comprehensive instructions and advice to the patients and caregivers. A systematic review found that exercise training can help improve aerobic capacity, fatigue, health-related quality of life, strength, and mobility (28).

Treatment for spasticity is also very important, especially if the patient has issues with positioning or complains of pain. Treatment should include positioning, stretching, splinting, icing, and oral medications such as baclofen, dantrolene, tizanidine, and injections such as botulinum toxin. Home exercises should also be taught.

Balance and gait disturbances must be addressed. For those whose primary goal is gait improvement, exercise must include standing and walking. Gait evaluation should be made on level surfaces, rough terrain, stairs, and elevation. A systematic review found some evidence that ambulation training with robotic assistance may be of benefit to MS patients (29). Similarly, a systematic review of the evidence for physiotherapy on balance revealed a modest benefit for patients with mild to moderate MS (30).

Aquatic exercise (swimming, water aerobics, and water walking) has been recommended to improve aerobic endurance, strength, balance, and flexibility in a safe environment while avoiding potentially detrimental increases in body temperature. Care should be taken to find a pool that is not too hot (>29°C, 84°F) for those who are sensitive to heat.

Cooling therapy has been shown to reduce fatigue, improving postural stability and muscle strength in 10 heat-sensitive MS patients when wearing a cold vest with active cooling (7°C, 60 min). Postintervention pain intensity was significantly reduced in the experimental group compared to their counterparts who had nonaquatic exercise therapy ($P < .028$), and was maintained for up to 10 weeks (31).

Occupational therapy: Restoration and maintenance of functional independence skills in everyday activities is a key goal for managing the disease. Task reacquisition; performance of ADLs and IADLs; transfers; sensory/perceptual compensation; use of adaptive equipment; modification of environment for personal, domestic, and community tasks; and driving evaluation are key components of occupational therapy.

The occupational therapists should also teach the principles of "energy conservation" referred to as the "4 Ps" to these individuals. These include planning, prioritizing, pacing (budget energy throughout the day and week), and positioning (proper body mechanics, workplace ergonomics) (3). In addition, work simplification and ergometric techniques should be taught. Referral to a work hardening program is helpful. A systematic review of the scientific literature reported an improvement in arm and hand function with motor training programs in MS (32).

Speech therapy is rarely necessary for patients with MS but may be utilized in rare cases of aphasia. In patients with dysarthrophonia, speech training together with respiratory exercises may help to improve articulation (31). In the most severely disabled patients, impaired swallowing may be a risk for respiratory infections due to insufficient respiratory function and reduced coughing. In these cases, respiratory training may help in improving respiratory functions and cough reflexes (31).

Cognitive impairment is common in persons with MS and areas of strength and weakness should be defined. Various aspects of cognitive functioning, including attention, information processing efficiency, executive functioning, processing speed, and long-term memory, should be addressed. Cognitive testing should be included as part of the neurological evaluation, on account of the psychosocial implications of a cognitively impaired young productive adult with MS. Cognitive retraining will help the patient adapt to the disease and improve quality of life.

The physician as well as the nursing team should also address and teach patients who may have bladder dysfunctions secondary to MS. The type of bladder dysfunctions can be determined by urodynamic testing and with input from physicians who have expertise in the assessment and management of neurogenic bladder dysfunction. Urinary infection should be treated if present. Depending on the type of bladder dysfunction, the patient should be treated with medications and intermittent catheterization as needed. MS patients with neurogenic bowel dysfunction can be treated with the implementation of a bowel program.

ETHICAL ISSUES IN THE CARE OF MS

It is important that physiatrists providing rehabilitative care to individuals with MS understand the ethical principles of autonomy, beneficence, nonmaleficence, and justice (33). It is equally important to realize when ethical conflicts arise in the course of physician–patient relationships.

The principle of autonomy requires that patients with MS be fully informed of the risks, benefits, and alternatives regarding their care and can make decisions that are consistent with their beliefs and wishes that are free of intimidation. Facing increasingly complex decisions, patients need up-to-date evidence-based information and decision support systems in order to make informed decisions together with their physicians (34). The principle of autonomy can be challenging when the individual with MS does not have intact cognitive abilities, but insists on a particular course of action.

The principle of beneficence requires that physicians do their best to provide high-quality care to the patient with MS. This implies that they keep their level of competence and knowledge on MS up-to-date and always have the best interest in mind for the patient's well-being. The principle of nonmaleficence refers to not harming the patient. Harm can come to the MS patient as a result of adverse reactions or side effects from treatments. In performing a benefit versus risk analysis, the physiatrist assesses beneficence versus nonmaleficence (33).

In the principle of justice, an important concept is the fair distribution of scarce resources such as medications, rehabilitation services, and mobility aids. Socioeconomic and racial disparities can serve as a challenge with the ethical principle of justice in the field of rehabilitation medicine. For example, there is some literature that more African Americans than whites experience pyramidal system involvement early in MS, leading to greater disability as measured by the ambulation-sensitive Expanded Disability Status Scale (35). This in turn can lead to limited access to these scarce resources by members of minority groups.

There are times when there can be an ethical conflict such as when a patient's wishes are contrary to the best advice of the treating physiatrist (e.g., autonomy vs. beneficence). In addressing ethical conflicts it is always important to first determine which ethical principles are involved, determine the patient's wishes, understand his or her belief system, identify any applicable laws or regulations that can provide guidance, and then seek common ground.

PRACTICE-BASED LEARNING AND IMPROVEMENT

GOALS

Demonstrate competence in continuously investigating and evaluating your own MS patient care practices, appraising and assimilating scientific evidence, and continuously improving your patient care practices based on constant self-evaluation and lifelong learning.

OBJECTIVES

1. Describe learning opportunities for providers, patients, and caregivers with experience in MS.
2. Use methods for ongoing competency training in MS for physiatrists, including formative evaluation feedback in daily practice, evaluating current practice, and developing a systematic quality improvement (QI) and practice improvement strategy.
3. Locate resources both digital and in print for continuing medical education and professional development.
4. Describe some areas paramount to self-assessment and lifelong learning such as review of current guidelines, including evidence-based, in treatment and management of patients with MS and the role of the physiatrist as the educator of patients, families, residents, students, colleagues, and other health professionals.

Practice-based learning and improvement is a core competency meant to encourage continuous self-assessment, learning, and improvement of one's own practice in the management of patients with MS. Physicians manage patients with MS based on current literature and experience.

Physiatrists should be knowledgeable about the epidemiology, neuroanatomy, pathophysiology, physical examination, and treatment of MS. In addition, they should be aware of community resources available to individuals living with MS and patient safety concerns as applicable to this population. Physiatrists should assess their current knowledge base as it pertains to the care of the patient with MS on a regular basis and, if gaps are identified, proceed to locate resources that can be used to improve their knowledge base. They can use a variety of tools to assess their current practice of patient care and medical knowledge as it pertains to MS:

- They can reflect on the care they are providing to current patients or have provided to past patients with a diagnosis of MS. Narrative-based medicine aims not only to validate the experience of the patient, but also to encourage creativity and self-reflection in the physician. It complements evidence-based medicine in that it creates a better balance between the science and the art of caring for patients with MS (36).
- They can take self-assessment examinations.
- They can ask patients and colleagues to give them honest feedback on the care provided.

A foundation built on good communication skills when dealing with patients, family, and rehabilitation team members is vital to effective timely treatment.

In the age of the Internet, there are many online resources available to physiatrists to improve their knowledge base about MS. The American Academy of Physical Medicine and Rehabilitation (AAPMR) has MS-specific content available through "Knowledge NOW." Other online resources include the Cochrane Reviews database, PubMed reviews, and "Up to Date." Attendance at national meetings that are pertinent to the care of MS patients is another resource. Fellowship training programs are also available for physiatrists interested in advancing their education in the assessment and management of MS patients.

The physiatrist providing care to MS patients should identify areas in their practice that are important to the provision of high-quality care to this population, including (a) timely access to rehabilitative care; (b) incidence of patient safety issues such as catheter-related urinary tract infections, pressure ulcers, and falls; (c) functional gains in inpatient rehabilitation facilities; and (d) patient satisfaction with care provided. These data can be compared against internal or external benchmarks and, if significant deviation exists, a QI project can be developed and recommendations to improve care implemented.

INTERPERSONAL AND COMMUNICATION SKILLS

GOALS

Demonstrate interpersonal and communication skills that result in the effective exchange of information and collaboration with MS patients, their families, and other health professionals.

OBJECTIVES

1. Demonstrate skills used in effective communication and collaboration with patients with MS and their caregivers, across socioeconomic and cultural backgrounds.
2. Delineate the importance of the role of the physiatrist as the interdisciplinary team leader and consultant pertinent to MS.
3. Demonstrate proper documentation and effective communication between health care professional team members in patient care as it applies to MS.

PATIENT AND FAMILY COUNSELING

When a patient is diagnosed with MS, the entire family is affected; therefore, the physician should identify and address key issues affecting both the patient and his or her families. The patient's spouse or partner can be put in a position of assuming multiple responsibilities such as caregiver, primary source of income, primary parent, and homemaker.

The partner can then experience feelings of depression, stress, anxiety, fear, or sleep disturbances and may find it difficult to cope, therefore putting the family dynamics in jeopardy. The physician should find out how the partner is coping emotionally and physically; suggest support groups that may be beneficial to the partner; make the partner aware of the disease progression;

address sexual dysfunction issues, which may be difficult for the couple to discuss; and make appropriate referral to the providers for care. The physician should also help children and adolescents understand and cope with the parent's disability. Anxiety problems, low self-esteem, fear of death, behavioral problems, or embarrassment should be identified and managed appropriately.

In situations where the child may now become the primary caregiver, appropriate support systems should be implemented. The children's well-being should be assessed and the physician should make himself or herself available to talk about the parent's illness. The physician should also make recommendations to the patient if the child is experiencing emotional problems. Extended family members should also be encouraged to play a role in the care of the patient where the children cannot be expected to.

The medical and rehabilitative treatment of the individual with MS is best handled using a collaborative multidisciplinary approach. The physiatrist by virtue of his or her training has experience in the team approach to patient care and is thus well suited for the role of leading a team in providing the highest level of care possible for the patient.

Communication between team members occurs in a variety of ways and in different settings. Informal verbal communication regarding patient care can occur over the phone, at the patient's bedside, or in therapy treatment areas. Formal channels of communication can occur at regularly held team conferences between team members in inpatient settings such as inpatient rehabilitation facilities and skilled nursing facilities.

The patient's medical record is an important tool of communication between team members and physicians involved in the care of the patient. To begin with, the documentation should be legible and the writer clearly identified. The content should include the date, pertinent medical history and physical examination, laboratory and imaging studies reviewed, education provided to the patient and family, and the recommended plan of care. If this is a follow-up visit, the patient's progress with treatment and any adverse reactions or side effects should be clearly noted. Changes in treatment plan as well as names of consultants and pertinent diagnostic tests ordered should also be recorded.

PROFESSIONALISM

GOALS

Reflect a commitment to carrying out professional responsibilities and an adherence to ethical principles in MS.

OBJECTIVES

1. Exemplify the humanistic qualities as a provider of care for patients with MS.
2. Demonstrate ethical principles and responsiveness to patient needs superseding self and other interests.
3. Demonstrate sensitivity to patient population diversity, including culture, gender, age, race, religion, disabilities, and sexual orientation.
4. Respect patient privacy and autonomy.
5. Recognize the importance of patient education in the treatment of and advocacy for persons with MS.

MS can have a significant effect on all aspects of the patient's personal life, self-confidence, relationships, self-esteem, employment, family goals, and future dreams. This can cause great psychological stress endangering the patient's well-being. The physician should be sensitive to this and thus provide care that is in the best interest of the patient.

Patients with MS should be part of the decision-making process in order to choose the most effective treatment plan for the disease as early as possible. Patient information should be kept confidential and it should be the patient's decision as to how this information should be shared if the patient is cognitively intact. If cognition is impaired, then the health care proxy or next of kin should make such a decision.

Patients with newly diagnosed MS can be quite vulnerable. Since MS affects the younger population, these individuals can become very self-conscious about the illness and how friends, family, colleagues, and society see them. It is very important to help them understand the disease and its treatment and assist them to function at the highest possible level.

The physiatrist caring for adults living with MS should be sensitive to the impact of culture, diversity, gender, age, race, religion, disabilities, and sexual orientation in the care of these individuals. Most young individuals may see themselves as healthy, motivated, full of energy, vibrant, and invincible. MS can cause them to become vulnerable, and can produce great denial about the disease. It is therefore imperative that disease progression is discussed and appropriate resources obtained to minimize the impact of impairments, activity limitations, and participation restrictions.

As the team leader, the physiatrist is responsible for the overall management of the individual with MS and must place the patient's well-being and needs above his or her own. The physiatrist should be aware of potential sources of conflict in the care of the patient with MS and minimize their occurrence. For example, one possible financial conflict of interest is referring the patient for rehabilitative services and durable medical equipment to companies in which the physiatrist has ownership and failing to disclose this to the patient.

The physiatrist has an important leadership role in coordination of care for the patient across the rehabilitation continuum of care and managing appropriate use of resources and therapy services. The physiatrist must use his or her knowledge about the patient's impairments, activity limitations, and participation restrictions as well as general knowledge about MS to advocate on behalf of the patient to obtain the necessary resources and services so that the patient can function at the highest possible level. One example of this level of advocacy includes working with the patient's health insurance company to obtain necessary equipment such as wheelchairs, orthotics, home modifications, and rehabilitation therapy. Other examples include (a) advocating for wheelchair accessibility in the workplace, school, home, and community and (b) advocating for air conditioning in the patient's apartment. In addition, the physiatrist can use his or her knowledge about the disease to advocate for the rights and needs of individuals with MS in the legislative branches of government or through organizations that support the rights of individuals with MS. The physiatrist should also educate the patient on how to self-advocate when dealing with community programs or agencies.

Patient Counseling and Patient Resources in MS

Educating the patient and family about the disease process in MS is an important component of practice-based medicine and improvement. Educating the patient on recognizing various symptoms of MS, the onset of an exacerbation, and progression of disease empowers the patient to be his or her own advocate. In addition, this helps to develop an effective dialogue between the physician and patient leading to earlier intervention. Physicians caring for patients with MS should be aware of resources that are dedicated to educating patients and family members. Some resources are detailed below:

1. American Academy of Neurology (AAN) (aan.com) is a resource dedicated to helping people understand neurology and the available treatment for neurologic disorders (http://www.msonetoone.com/helpful-resources).
2. The National Multiple Sclerosis Society (nationalmssociety.org) is a 50-state network that helps people with the challenges of living with MS.
3. National Family Caregivers Association (NFCA), www.familycaregiver.org, strives to educate, support, and empower those who care for a loved one with chronic illness, disability, or the frailties of old age. Multiple Sclerosis Foundation (MSF), msfocus.org, offers a wide range of free services including national toll-free support, homecare, support groups, assistive technology, and more.
4. Multiple Sclerosis Association of America (MSAA), msassociation.org, is a national, nonprofit organization dedicated to enriching the quality of life for everyone affected by MS through free programs such as a helpline, equipment distribution, MRI funding, award-winning publications and videos, and tools to help individuals better manage their MS (http://www.msonetoone.com/helpful-resources).

SYSTEMS-BASED PRACTICE

GOALS

Awareness and responsiveness to systems of care delivery, and the ability to recruit and coordinate effectively resources in the system to provide optimal continuum of care as it relates to MS.

OBJECTIVES

1. Describe key components and available services in the rehabilitation continuum of care and community rehabilitation facilities.
2. Discuss how to work effectively in various systems of care.
3. Identify patient safety risks for the patient with MS at the systems level and strategies to minimize their occurrence.
4. Describe optimal follow-up care.
5. Identify important markers of quality of care.
6. Discuss cost-effectiveness, utilization, and management of resources.
7. Review proper medical record keeping and documentation as the patient moves along the continuum of care.
8. Demonstrate advocacy role that the physician should display for quality of care for patients with MS.

Rehabilitation Continuum of Care for MS Patients

Rehabilitation services for the individual with MS are provided in inpatient, outpatient, and home settings. If the patient is admitted to an acute medical center for an MS-related complication or to receive treatment, rehabilitation services such as physical and occupational therapy can be provided either at the bedside or in acute care gyms. If the patient requires more comprehensive care for the impairments associated with the disease, referral to an inpatient rehabilitation facility (IRF) should be considered. Typical criteria for admission to an IRF include (a) need for close physician monitoring, (b) need for rehabilitation nursing for bowel/bladder training and wound care management, (c) ability to tolerate 3 hours of therapy/day, (d) realistic and achievable goals during the inpatient rehabilitation period, and (e) high patient motivation. In the IRF, the MS patient typically receives physical therapy, occupational therapy, speech therapy, neuropsychology, social work services, and vocational rehabilitation in a coordinated team approach.

For patients who do not meet criteria for acute inpatient rehabilitation in an IRF setting, rehabilitation services can be provided in subacute rehabilitation and/or skilled nursing facilities. In these settings, there may be less direct physician monitoring of the patient and less intensity of therapy services per day in comparison to IRF settings.

Outpatient rehabilitation services are typically provided in hospital-based outpatient clinics or private clinic settings. In some settings, the rehabilitation care is coordinated among a coalition of team members that can include the physiatrist, physical therapist, occupational therapist, speech pathologist, and vocational counselor, whereas in others it is based on the patient's primary impairment and recommended treatment (e.g., referral to physical therapy for gait training).

Home-based rehabilitation services can be very helpful for patients unable to attend therapy in an outpatient setting and/or who need additional rehabilitation once discharged from an IRF setting.

It is important for members of the rehabilitation team to work effectively across the rehabilitation continuum of care to ensure that there is a coordinated effort in providing optimal rehabilitation interventions to address the impairments, activity limitations, and participation restrictions for the patient with MS. Ideally, the physiatrist should be an active participant of this coordinated effort to ensure that the patient receives the right rehabilitative interventions at the right time and the right place. Coordination of care requires excellent communication skills and documentation among team members to minimize duplication of tests and services and to identify MS-related complications early as the patient moves through the continuum.

Patient Safety in Rehabilitation of the MS Patient

The physiatrist should have a proactive approach to minimizing the occurrence of injuries and maximizing safety for the MS patient as he or she moves through the rehabilitation care continuum. The MS patient is at risk for falls, contractures, pressure ulcers, medication-related side effects, and infections (e.g., catheter-related urinary tract infections, aspiration pneumonia), just to name a few.

The most common reasons for falls include trips or slips while walking, and being tired or fatigued. Falls are the most important consequences of gait and balance disturbances in patients with MS. Studies reveal that about 50% to 60% of patients report at least one fall in the community within the past 2 to 6 months (37). Common activities in which falls occur are transfers and ambulation (3). Strategies to minimize the incidence of falls include:

- Educating the patient about the risk of falls and how to avoid them from occurring
- Environmental review of home and institutional setting
- Review of medications for possible side effects that can affect cognition
- Muscle strengthening and gait training

A cross-sectional study by Hoang found that 56% of participants randomly selected were found to have a contracture in at least one major joint (38). Spasticity, muscle weakness, and decreased mobility can all contribute to the development of contractures. Strategies such as range of motion exercises for those joints at risk for contracture, treatment of spasticity, and exercises to improve muscle strength can all be beneficial.

Measures to prevent pressure ulcers include frequent position changes in bed and the wheelchair if the patient has limited mobility, minimizing incontinence, maximizing nutrition, ensuring appropriate seating surface for wheelchairs, and minimizing shearing forces across areas at risk for developing pressure ulcers.

Optimal follow-up care involves the collaborative work of various members of the rehabilitation team mentioned earlier as well as the patient's neurologist and internist at various stages of the disease. The follow-up care should ideally be provided in a multidisciplinary inpatient and outpatient setting by competent providers knowledgeable about the patient's impairments, activity limitations, and participation restrictions, as well as their management to maximize the patient's level of function and minimize complications such as falls, contractures, pressure ulcers, and infections.

Cost–Benefit Considerations in MS

The National Collaborating Centre for Chronic Conditions (NCCC) produced the national clinical guidelines for the diagnosis and management of primary and secondary care for patients with MS in Europe. It describes best practice for the health care management of this complex disease. The need remains for a comprehensive, U.S.-oriented guideline for the treatment of MS.

Until that time, payers will struggle to make management decisions for patients with MS without the benefit of a clinical consensus. New therapeutic agents and mounting cost containment pressures further complicate management decisions. Due to lack of a true consensus on how to manage patients with this disease, physicians must collaborate with the patient, caregivers, and payers. The consensus statements produced by a modified Delphi process involving management care experts provide a reference for health plans in designing their benefits and coverage policies for MS and should be used in conjunction with clinical evidence (39).

Whereas the use of disease-modifying therapies has been shown to reduce relapses and slow down the disease process, these come at a very high cost that prohibits some patients from receiving them. This is especially problematic for low-income patients, who may not have even received adequate education, particularly about immunomodulating drugs (40). This is important in light of the fact that starting disease-modifying treatment earlier in the disease process before signs of disability start results in less cost per quality-adjusted year and improvements in long-term effects of MS.

CASE STUDY

A 35-year-old woman with diagnosed MS of 1-year duration is admitted to an IRF for rehabilitation to address weakness in her legs, impaired balance, and ambulation, as well as difficulty controlling bowel and bladder function. She has received treatment with disease-modifying medications under the care of a neurologist. She denies any past medical or surgical history.

A review of systems is significant for depression, visual disturbances, and painful tingling sensations in hands and feet. She is married with 2 young children and lives in a 2-storied home in a suburb of a large metropolitan area.

Prior to the onset of MS, she had been working full time as an attorney; however, during the past year, she has had to reduce her hours to part-time status and work from home. Family finances have declined due to the increased medical costs and her loss of income. Physical examination is significant for mildly impaired attention span, short- and long-term memory, impaired vision, weakness, and spasticity in the lower extremities. There are no pressure ulcers or contractures and swallow function is intact. Transfers from bed to chair are completed with moderate assistance of one person.

CASE STUDY DISCUSSION QUESTIONS

1. Identify the impairments, activity limitations, and participation restrictions relevant to this patient and write a rehabilitation treatment plan for her.
2. Describe the current understanding of the pathophysiology of MS and the role of rehabilitative interventions and medications in its treatment.
3. What should the patient and her family be educated about with respect to her diagnosis, treatment, and return to work?
4. Identify the team members involved in this patient's care and the role of the physiatrist in coordinating the care across the health care continuum.
5. Identify safety risks for this patient and describe strategies to minimize their occurrence.
6. You find out that the patient's health care insurance has limited coverage for rehabilitative services. How would you best advocate for this patient's rehabilitation needs?

SELF-EXAMINATION QUESTIONS
(Answers begin on p. 367)

1. Which of the following best characterizes MS?
   A. Symptomatic episodes are "separated in time and space"
   B. Symptomatic episodes typically only occur in one neuroanatomic location
   C. Symptomatic episodes typically only occur once in the life of the MS patient
   D. The duration of an MS-related symptom typically should last less than 1 hour
   E. The symptomatic presentation of MS is usually the same for all patients

2. Migration studies indicated that the likelihood of developing the disease depends on where a person spent the first
   A. 5 years of life
   B. 10 years of life
   C. 15 years of life
   D. 20 years of life
   E. 25 years of life

3. Which of the following best characterizes the epidemiology of MS?
   A. MS is the least common cause of nontraumatic disability affecting young people in the Northern Hemisphere
   B. There are about 4,000,000 persons in the United States with MS
   C. The prevalence of MS ranges from 40 to 220/100,000 persons
   D. The incidence of MS is 1,710/100,000 persons
   E. Males account for approximately 70% of MS cases

4. Which of the following best describes falls in the patient with MS?
   A. An infrequent reason for falls is tripping during ambulation
   B. Fatigue is rarely a reason for falls in MS patients
   C. Falls are only rarely associated with gait or balance problems in MS patients
   D. 50% to 60% of patients report at least one fall in the community
   E. Falls rarely occur during transfers and ambulation in MS patients

5. Which of the following is true with respect to low-income minorities and MS?
   A. Low-income minorities with MS don't have difficulty accessing appropriate health care, but choose not to obtain it
   B. Low-income minorities with MS don't have difficulty accessing appropriate health care
   C. Major issue is the lack of education about surgical options for MS
   D. Major issue is the lack of education about immunomodulating drugs
   E. Major issue is the lack of education about diet

REFERENCES

1. Lin VW, and Associates. *Spinal Cord Medicine—Principles and Practice*. 2nd ed. New York, NY: Demos Medical Publishing; 2010:486.
2. Trojano M, Paolicelli D. The differential diagnosis of multiple sclerosis: classification and clinical features of relapsing and progressive neurological syndromes. *Neurol Sci*. November 2001;22(suppl 2):S98–102.
3. Braddom RL, Chan L, Harrast MA, et al. *Physical Medicine & Rehabilitation*. 4th ed. Philadelphia, PA: Elsevier Saunders; 2011:1233–1248.
4. Hauser SL, Goodin DS. Multiple sclerosis and other demyelinating diseases. In: Kasper DL, Fauci AS, Longo DL, et al. *Harrison's Principles of Internal Medicine*. 17th ed. New York, NY: McGraw-Hill; 2008:2613.
5. Merkelbach S, Haensch CA, Hemmer B, et al. Multiple sclerosis and the autonomic nervous system. *J Neurol*. February 2006;253(suppl 1):121–125.
6. Karatas M. Intranuclear and supranuclear disorders of eye movement. *Eur J Neurol*. December 2009;16(12):1265–1277.
7. Kurtzke JF. Rating neurologic impairment in multiple sclerosis: an expanded disability status scale (EDSS). *Neurology*. November 1983;33(11):1444–1452.
8. Fisk JD, Pontefract A, Ritvo PG, et al. The impact of fatigue on patients with multiple sclerosis. *Can J Neurol Sci*. 1994;21:9–14.
9. Flachenecker P, Kümpfel T, Kallmann B, et al. Fatigue in multiple sclerosis: a comparison of different rating scales and correlation to clinical parameters. *Mult Scler*. December 2002;8(6):523–526.
10. World Health Organization. http://www.who.int/topics/disabilities/en/. Accessed July 26, 2013.
11. Bowen C, MacLehose A, Beaumont JG. Advanced multiple sclerosis and the psychosocial impact on families. *Psychol Health*. January 2011;26(1):113–127.
12. Schiavolin S, Leonardi M, Giovannetti AM, et al. Factors related to difficulties with employment in patients with multiple sclerosis: a review of 2002–2011 literature. *Int J Rehabil Res*. December 12, 2012.
13. Kakalacheva K, Münz C, Lünemann JD. Viral trigger of multiple sclerosis. *Biochim Biophys Acta*. February 2011;1812(2):132–140.
14. Owens GP, Bennett JL. Trigger, pathogen, or bystander: the complex nexus linking Epstein-Barr virus and multiple sclerosis. *Mult Scler*. September 2012;18(9):1204–1208.
15. Hauser SL, Goodin DS. Multiple sclerosis and other demyelinating diseases. In: Kasper DL, Fauci AS, Longo DL, et al. *Harrison's Principles of Internal Medicine*. 17th ed. New York, NY: McGraw-Hill; 2008:2613.
16. Frontera WR, & Associates. *Delisa's Physical Medicine & Rehabilitation*. 5th ed. Philadelphia, PA: Lippincott William & Wilkins; 2010:625–637.
17. Wu GF, Alvarez E. The immuno-pathophysiology of multiple sclerosis. *Neurol Clin*. May 2011;29(2):257–278.
18. Gomi G. Is it clinically relevant to repair focal multiple sclerosis? *J Neurol Sci*. 2008;265:17–20.
19. Bjartmar JC, Wujek R, Trapp BD. Axonal loss in the pathology of multiple sclerosis: consequences for understanding the progressive phase of the diseases. *J Neurol Sci*. February 15, 2003;206(2):165–171.
20. Dutta R, Trapp BD. Mechanisms of neuronal dysfunction and degeneration in multiple sclerosis. *Prog Neurobiol*. January 2011;93(1):1–12.

21. http://www.uptodate.com/contents/epidemiology-and-clinical-features-of-multiple-sclerosis-in-adults?source=search_result&search=multiple+sclerosis&selectedTitle=2%7E150#H28.
22. Scalfari A, Neuhaus A, Daumer M, et al. Age and disability accumulation in multiple sclerosis. *Neurology*. September 27, 2011;77(13):1246–1252.
23. Grabois M, Garrison SJ, Hart KA, et al. *Physical Medicine & Rehabilitation—The Complete Approach*. Malden, MA: Blackwell Science; 2000:1378.
24. National Collaborating Centre for Chronic Conditions (UK). *Multiple Sclerosis: National Clinical Guideline for Diagnosis and Management in Primary and Secondary Care*. London: Royal College of Physicians (UK); 2004. (NICE Clinical Guidelines, No. 8.) Appendix G, The McDonald Criteria. http://www.ncbi.nlm.nih.gov/books/NBK48930/.
25. Cuccurullo, SJ. *Physical Medicine and Rehabilitation Board Review*. 2nd ed. New York, NY: Demos Medical Publishing; 2010:853.
26. Asselman P, Chadwick DW, Marsden DC. Visual evoked responses in the diagnosis and management of patients suspected of multiple sclerosis. *Brain*. June 1975;98(2):261–282.
27. Cuccurullo, SJ. *Physical Medicine and Rehabilitation Board Review*. 2nd ed. New York, NY: Demos Medical Publishing; 2010:855.
28. Latimer-Cheung AE, Pilutti LA, Hicks AL, et al. Effects of exercise training on fitness, mobility, fatigue, and health-related quality of life among adults with multiple sclerosis: a systematic review to inform guideline development. *Arch Phys Med Rehabil*. September 2013;94(9):1800-1828.e3. doi:10.1016/j.apmr.2013.04.020. Epub May 10, 2013.
29. Tefertiller C, Pharo B, Evans N, et al. Efficacy of rehabilitation robotics for walking training in neurological disorders: a review. *J Rehabil Res Dev*. 2011;48(4):387–416.
30. Paltamaa J, Sjögren T, Peurala SH, et al. Effects of physiotherapy interventions on balance in multiple sclerosis: a systematic review and meta-analysis of randomized controlled trials. *J Rehabil Med*. October 2012;44(10):811–823. doi:10.2340/16501977–1047.
31. Beer S, Khan F, Kesselring J. Rehabilitation interventions in multiple sclerosis: an overview. *J Neurol*. September 2012;259(9):1994–2008.
32. Spooren AI, Timmermans AA, Seelen HA. Motor training programs of arm and hand in patients with MS according to different levels of the ICF: a systematic review. *BMC Neurol*. July 2, 2012;12:49. doi:10.1186/1471-2377-12-49.
33. Gillon R. Medical ethics: four principles plus attention to scope. *BMJ*. July 16, 1994;309(6948):184–188.
34. Kasper J, Kopke S, Fischer K, et al. Applying the theory of planned behavior to multiple sclerosis patients' decisions on disease modifying therapy—questionnaire concept and validation. *BMC Med Inform Decis Mak*. 2012;12:60.
35. Kaufman MD, Johnson SK, Moyer D, et al. Multiple sclerosis: severity and progression rate in African Americans compared with whites. *Am J Phys Med Rehabil*. August 2003;82(8):582–590.
36. Greenhalgh T. Why study narrative? *BMJ*. January 2, 1999; 318(7175):48–50.
37. Cameron MH, Asano M, Bourdette D, et al. People with multiple sclerosis use many fall prevention strategies but still fall frequently. *Arch Phys Med Rehabil*. February 4, 2013;(13):00106–00108.
38. Hoang PD, Gandevia SC, Herbert RD. Prevalence of joint contractures and muscle weakness in people with multiple sclerosis. *Disabil Rehabil*. November 18, 2013. doi:10.3109/09638288.2013.854841.
39. Miller RM, Happe LI, Meyer KL, et al. Approaches to the management of agents used for the treatment of multiple sclerosis: consensus statements from a panel of U.S. managed care pharmacists and physicians. *J Manag Care Pharm*. 2012;18(1):54–62.
40. Shabas B, Heffner M. Multiple sclerosis for low income minorities. *Mult Scler*. December 2005;11(6):635–640.

Christine Hinke
Travis R. von Tobel
Brandon Von Tobel

20: Osteoarthritis

PATIENT CARE

GOALS

Evaluate and develop a comprehensive rehabilitative plan of care for a patient with osteoarthritis that is compassionate, appropriate, and effective for the treatment and management of osteoarthritic problems and the promotion of health.

OBJECTIVES

1. Perform a pertinent history and physical examination of the patient presenting with joint pain.
2. Identify and assess key impairments, as well as functional and activity limitations, for the patient with osteoarthritis.
3. Describe the psychosocial aspects, vocational aspects, long-term consequences, and potential injuries associated with osteoarthritis.
4. Describe the treatment plan for the patient with osteoarthritis.
5. Describe ethical issues as they apply to the patient with osteoarthritis.

The medical history and the physical examination of the adult with osteoarthritis serve as the foundation of the care plan for that individual. Most, if not all, patients with osteoarthritis present with joint pain as a chief complaint. In order to effectively address pain complaints, it is important to accurately assess the pain in a systematic fashion. The PQRST approach is ideal to assess the key components of the pain including its location, description, intensity, duration, and alleviating and aggravating factors. The components of this assessment are as follows: **P**rovokes and **P**alliates, **Q**uality, **R**egion and **R**adiation, **S**everity, and **T**emporal (1).

In further evaluating the pain complaint, it is important to question the patient regarding any history of trauma, whether recent or remote, and to inquire about a potential precipitating factor such as a fall, injury, or activity that may have contributed to the development of the pain. If identified, obtain as much detail about the event as possible in an attempt to understand the potential mechanism of injury. Fracture history, including information regarding treatment of the fracture, as well as history of musculoskeletal injuries and the treatment rendered, is important as risk for the development of osteoarthritis is increased with these types of injuries (2). The clinician should ask about the functional limitations that the joint pain is causing, as it relates to both vocational and avocational activities. It is often useful to ask the patient about activities that are avoided due to the pain.

In obtaining the past medical history, the clinician should specifically ask about hypertension, abdominal obesity, hyperglycemia, and elevated triglycerides, as patients with osteoarthritis have a higher prevalence of these conditions than the general population (3). Since a history of depression or anxiety has been associated with greater functional decline secondary to osteoarthritis (4), it is important for the physician to inquire about these conditions as well. A history of neoplasm should be documented and information regarding staging and treatments including chemotherapy, radiation, and/or surgery are important in the evaluation of patients presenting with joint pain. Any surgery to the joints, nerves, or musculature should be clearly documented since these procedures, or the injuries that required the intervention, have likely contributed to the development of osteoarthritis in this individual. Other surgeries, such as abdominal or pelvic procedures, which may have impacted core muscle strength, or any other types of surgeries that resulted in protracted courses of immobility or activity reduction should also be documented.

Information in social history regarding the patient's occupational and recreational activities are most important when screening for potential injuries that occurred during activity performance, as joint injury is a powerful risk factor for the development of osteoarthritis (4). Repetitive joint use has been shown in multiple studies to be associated with the development of radiological osteoarthritis, but not symptomatic osteoarthritis (5). Inclusion of this information can be helpful in screening for potential sites of osteoarthritis and can be targeted in a prevention program.

As in all conditions, a review of systems is essential in exploring the possibility of a systemic condition that could be contributing to arthritis type symptoms or in detecting "red flags" that could point to more ominous conditions that can mimic the presentation of osteoarthritis, such as joint tumors or infections.

Key elements of the physical examination of patients with osteoarthritis incorporate the general principles of inspection, palpation, range of motion, muscle testing, and motor and sensory evaluation (6). For each joint or region of the body, there are also special tests that should be part of the evaluation and give additional information regarding specific structures that may be involved in the patient's condition (6).

The examination should begin with asking the patient to identify, preferably by pointing to or touching, the area of pain (6). This area should then be inspected for any abnormal findings such as edema, erythema, evidence of trauma, skin abnormalities, joint deformity, or muscle atrophy. The joint structures should be palpated in a systematic way to assess for discrete areas of anatomic abnormality, tenderness, or temperature changes. For unilateral pain involving the upper or lower limbs, it is also good practice to examine the asymptomatic side to provide a basis of comparison to identify subtle differences. The joint should be examined for any malalignment and lower limb joints should be examined in both a supine and standing position.

Range of motion of the affected joint should be measured, preferably using a goniometer, and should include comparison to the opposite side if applicable. It is important to evaluate the range of motion of the joint in a lax position, so as not to confuse a reduction in range of motion with a reduction in flexibility of muscles that cross two joints. Pain with a particular motion or at a particular position during ranging should be documented as well (6).

Manual muscle testing is used to assess individual muscle strength and is always part of the joint examination. Patient participation is required for full evaluation, and any indication of reduced participation should be documented. Pain can impact the patient's ability to tolerate testing; therefore, it is important to document the presence of pain with certain motions or resistance. The motor and sensory examination is an essential part of the evaluation of a patient with osteoarthritis. These patients must be screened for evidence of nerve root dysfunction that could suggest the presence of cervical or lumbar spine pathology (6).

In addition to examining the site of pain, the clinician should examine the joint above and below the painful joint, as certain joint pathology can radiate pain to proximal and distal areas. For example, medial knee pain can be a symptom of hip osteoarthritis. The examiner should also include some evaluation of the corresponding spinal segment, such as the cervical spine in upper limb joint pain and the lumbar spine in lower limb joint pain.

General observations including body habitus, obesity, posture, and resting joint positions should be documented as part of the comprehensive evaluation. A patient should be observed from the moment he walks into the room and throughout the examination. The patient should be asked to walk during the course of the examination to note any gait deviations, painful movements, or overt manifestations of weakness such as footdrop.

Lastly, special testing, which is either joint or condition specific, should be included in the evaluation of the patient with osteoarthritis, both to elicit the possibility of a different diagnosis and to screen for evidence of injuries that can predispose the patient to the development of osteoarthritis. Table 20.1 shows examples of special testing for specific body parts.

Impairment, as defined by the World Health Organization, is the loss or abnormality of a body structure or of a physiological or psychological function. Osteoarthritis can result in the following impairments: painful joint motion, restricted joint motion, absence of joint motion, joint soft-tissue swelling, joint effusion, joint deformity, abnormal alignment, joint instability, reduced proprioception, abnormal balance, muscle inhibition, muscle weakness, and muscle atrophy. Impairments are detected via physical examination and diagnostic testing.

Functional and activity limitations are the results of impairments and may be temporary or permanent, can be reversible or irreversible, and can progress or regress. In osteoarthritis, the functional limitations will be defined by the joint(s) involved and the degree of involvement. Osteoarthritis of the upper limbs is most likely to interfere with activities of daily living. The patient should be asked about the performance of these activities and whether or not assistance is required to complete these activities. Osteoarthritis of the lower limbs is most likely to interfere with walking and other mobility activities, such as transfers and stair climbing. A complete evaluation of the patient presenting with lower limb osteoarthritis must include information regarding these activities to fully understand the impact on the patient's functioning. Limitations are detected via patient questioning based on the impairments detected by the clinician.

Coping with the pain and physical limitations of osteoarthritis requires individuals to alter their approaches to activities of daily living. The patient should be asked about the performance of these activities and whether they impact work, familial, and leisure activities. Identifying and recognizing psychological stress related to the osteoarthritis patient is important to successful treatment.

Employment is a positive influence on the perceived quality of life of human beings and can be jeopardized by the development of osteoarthritis and its associated impairments. Job loss is associated with a reduction in life satisfaction, increased symptoms of depression, and increased pain. There is not a clear relationship between pain intensity and ability to work, so pain is not a reliable indicator of ability to work. Rather, research has shown that maladaptive coping styles, such as pain catastrophizing, are more predictive of work loss (7).

Osteoarthritis can impact family life and relationships in a negative way. Parents with osteoarthritis frequently report difficulty with childcare activities and report increased psychological distress regarding parenting skills. Effective social support from family has been associated with more efficient household management and less psychological distress. In contrast, effective spousal support has not been shown to have a positive impact on psychological stress; however, poor spousal support has been shown to have a clear negative effect on psychological stress (7).

Leisure activities are essentially voluntary and rates of participation have been expected to be lower in patients with symptomatic osteoarthritis. This has not been demonstrated in research studies, except in patients with lower educational levels. Loss of participation in leisure activities has been linked to increased pain and increased fatigue (7).

TABLE 20.1 Examples of Specialty Testing for the Joints of the Upper and Lower Limb

	NAME OF TEST	EVALUATES FOR POSSIBLE
Shoulder (8)	Neer impingement sign	Rotator cuff tear, rotator cuff impingement
	Hawkins impingement sign	Rotator cuff tear, rotator cuff impingement
	Cross body adduction	Acromioclavicular joint osteoarthritis
	Apprehension sign	Anterior shoulder instability
	Sulcus sign	Inferior shoulder laxity
	Jerk test	Posterior shoulder instability
Elbow (9)	Valgus stress test	Instability of ulnar collateral ligament
	Varus stress test	Instability of the lateral collateral ligament
Wrist and Hand (10)	Finkelstein test	De Quervain tenosynovitis
	Phalen maneuver	Carpal tunnel syndrome
	Froment sign	Ulnar nerve injury
	Grind test	CMC joint osteoarthritis
	CMC joint relocation test	CMC joint osteoarthritis
Hip (11)	Trendelenburg test	Hip abduction weakness
	FABER test	Hip and sacroiliac joint pathology
JOINT	NAME OF TEST	EVALUATES FOR POSSIBLE
Knee (12)	Patellar apprehension test	Patellar instability
	Patellar grind test	Patellofemoral chondromalacia
	McMurray test	Meniscus tear
	Valgus stress test	Medial collateral ligament tear
	Varus stress test	Lateral collateral ligament tear
	Lachman test	Anterior cruciate ligament tear
	Pivot shift test	Anterior cruciate ligament dysfunction
	Anterior draw test	Anterior cruciate ligament instability
	Posterior draw test	Posterior cruciate ligament instability
	Noble test	ITB syndrome
	Ober test	ITB inflexibility
	Wilson test	Osteochondritis dissecans
Foot and Ankle (13)	Anterior draw test	Anterior talofibular ligament instability
	Varus stress test	Calcaneofibular ligament instability
	MTP instability	Acute or chronic synovitis

Since osteoarthritis is by definition a progressive disease, there is a misconception that treatment is not likely to result in any real benefit to the patient. While it is true that there are currently no treatments available that are capable of achieving structural modification or disease modification, the currently available treatments aimed at symptom modification have been shown to be effective in decreasing pain, impairment, and functional limitations (14). Prevention of osteoarthritis and educating patients in its prevention are important roles for the clinician treating these patients. Osteoarthritis has been linked to increased mortality in a number of studies, and seems to be related to the functional decline that is often a consequence of reduced mobility (4).

Injuries associated with patient falls are potential sequelae for the patient with osteoarthritis. Fall risk is increased with the diagnosis of osteoarthritis. Weakness, pain, reduced flexibility, joint deformity, and reduced proprioception can contribute to instability during standing and ambulation. All of these impairments have been shown to contribute to the increased fall risk in the geriatric population. Also, the resultant abnormal gait, reduced endurance, and impaired balance also increase the risk of falls. Treatment programs aimed at reducing these impairments and functional limitations have resulted in reduced fall risks (15).

Treatment for the patient with osteoarthritis should be individualized for each patient and should consist of a combination of interventions to be most effective (14). Nonpharmacologic treatment options include patient education, weight loss, modalities, exercise, orthoses, and activity modification (14). The 2012 ACR guidelines strongly recommend exercise and weight loss if necessary for patient with knee or hip osteoarthritis (16). There are multiple pharmacological options available including topical, systemic, and intraarticular agents. The risks and benefits of each must be explored in collaboration with the patient (14). The 2012 ACR guidelines do not have strong recommendations for any particular agent, except for the use of opioid analgesics in the treatment of refractory osteoarthritis of the knee in patients who are unable or unwilling to consider joint replacement (16). Surgical intervention should be considered when pain is refractory to nonsurgical treatment and the impairments from the osteoarthritis have resulted in significant functional and activity limitations (14).

ETHICAL ISSUES

The basic principles of medical ethics apply to the evaluation and treatment of patients with osteoarthritis. To preserve autonomy, a patient with the diagnosis of osteoarthritis should be given a complete set of appropriate treatment options by his or her physician, which includes discussion of the risks and benefits of the proposed treatments and the risks and benefits of refusing those treatments. Patients have the right to choose all, some, or none of the proposed treatments, and the physician must accept those choices even if he or she disagrees with the patient's choice. Since osteoarthritis is a chronic disease process, the physician can continue to offer previously refused treatment options, or if there are changes in the patient's condition he or she may offer additional treatment options during subsequent encounters. The principle of beneficence requires that the clinician individualize treatment options for each patient based on clinical presentation and examination findings. Physicians must consider religious and cultural differences that may affect understanding of the diagnosis and treatment options, and potentially the choice of treatment options. Nonmaleficence refers to the concept of "do no harm," and requires the clinician to discuss the diagnosis and treatment options in the context of its effects on the whole person. Certain treatments may have increased risks for individuals with certain comorbid conditions and these increased risks need to be anticipated and discussed with the patient. Lastly, the principle of justice requires the clinician to discuss all relevant treatment options, the role of diagnostic testing, and the opportunities and risks of participation in medical research conducted for osteoarthritis, as well as provide referral for expensive and high-level interventions whenever clinically indicated.

MEDICAL KNOWLEDGE

GOALS

Demonstrate knowledge of established evidence-based and evolving biomedical, clinical epidemiological, and sociobehavioral sciences pertaining to osteoarthritis, as well as the application of this knowledge to guide holistic patient care.

OBJECTIVES

1. Discuss the epidemiology of osteoarthritis, its risk factors, and its morbidity and mortality.
2. Describe the relevant normal anatomy and physiology of the synovial joint.
3. Review the pathogenesis and pathophysiology of osteoarthritis.
4. Assess the appropriate role of diagnostic testing.
5. Evaluate the treatment and management options for osteoarthritis and the evidence behind those recommendations.
6. Educate patients on making patient-centered decisions regarding their plans of care.

EPIDEMIOLOGY

According to CDC data from 2005, approximately 26.9 million U.S. adults are affected by osteoarthritis (17). These data have been obtained largely from population-based studies and have been shown to be increasing in both prevalence and incidence. Most of the increase has been attributed to the increased longevity, resulting in aging of the population and also to the increasing prevalence of obesity to epidemic proportions (4). The prevalence of the most common forms of symptomatic osteoarthritis is the following: knee (9.5%–16%), hand (8%), and hip (4.4%). The incidence of the development of these most common forms of osteoarthritis is as follows, expressed per 100,000 person years: knee (240), hand (100), and hip (88) (17).

The incidence of the development of osteoarthritis is based on systemic and local risk factors that result in the development of osteoarthritis and ultimately its progression. Once symptomatic, osteoarthritis is associated with functional decline and is the most common cause of walking-related disability and a leading cause of upper limb disability (4).

Systemic risk factors for the development of osteoarthritis include advancing age, female gender, certain types of ethnicity, genetic predisposition, obesity, bone mineral density, and nutrition. Advancing age is associated with the increased incidence and prevalence of osteoarthritis, but not its progression. Women have a higher prevalence for symptomatic development of knee, hip, and hand osteoarthritis, but there is no clear evidence that the disease progresses more rapidly in women. Ethnic differences were noted in prevalence of the development of certain types of osteoarthritis and the development of specific radiographic features. Relatively recently, genetic factors have been studied for evidence of inherited susceptibility for the development of osteoarthritis. A large number of specific genes have been identified as possible clues to the pathogenesis of osteoarthritis, but further study is necessary to more clearly define their contributions to its development and progression. Obesity is a strong risk factor, both systemically and locally, for the development of osteoarthritis; unlike the others noted, it is modifiable. Prevention and education programs surrounding modification of this risk is considered very likely to have the greatest impact at a population level. High bone mineral density has been associated with increased prevalence and incidence of osteoarthritis. Various dietary factors, such as intake of vitamin D, vitamin C, vitamin E, and vitamin K, have been implicated in the development and progression of osteoarthritis, but none consistently or clearly enough to warrant specific recommendations regarding daily intake (4).

Local risk factors for the development of osteoarthritis include joint injury, occupational exposure, physical activity, leg-length discrepancy, neuromuscular factors, joint alignment and force abnormalities, and joint bony characteristics. Especially at the knee joint, a history of joint injury is correlated with the subsequent development of osteoarthritis of that joint. Exposure to repetitive joint motion at work has long been thought to play a pivotal role in the development of osteoarthritis, but study limitations have called this into question, because most studies did not adjust for joint injury. Similarly, exercise and participation in specific sports have also been hypothesized to result in the increased likelihood of developing osteoarthritis. Proving a direct correlation has been difficult due to the association of increased injury rates in participating individuals. Leg-length discrepancies can be present before or can occur as the result of osteoarthritis of the lower limb joints. Some studies have shown knee osteoarthritis and its progression to correlate to a leg-length discrepancy, but similar findings have not been seen in other joints of the lower limb. Muscle weakness has been implicated in affecting the development of osteoarthritis; however, only one study found knee extensor weakness to correlate with the radiographic development of knee osteoarthritis in women. Sensation and proprioception have not been proven to be independent risk factors for the development of osteoarthritis. Joint malalignment, whether primary or secondary, has been shown to correlate with a greater risk of radiographic development and progression of osteoarthritis of the knee. Bony characteristics, such as hip joint dysplasias, have been shown to correlate with the development of osteoarthritis of the hip in young adults; however, this does not account for the prevalence of hip osteoarthritis in the general population (4).

Once symptomatic, osteoarthritis contributes to functional decline; however, this has not been as well studied. Like in most painful conditions, advancing age, increasing pain, obesity, depression, anxiety, and reduced physical activity are risk factors for the development of functional decline in patients with osteoarthritis. There is limited evidence that joint laxity, impaired proprioception, and reduced balance are osteoarthritis-specific factors that can contribute to functional decline and that cognitive decline and visual decline are independent predictors of functional decline in patients with osteoarthritis (17).

RELEVANT ANATOMY AND PATHOPHYSIOLOGY

Normal joint function is dependent upon the smooth articulation of the involved bones to facilitate motion when force is applied to that joint. Articular cartilage is a thin, shock-absorbing interface that, combined with the effects of synovial fluid, provides an essentially frictionless surface on which joint motion can occur. The loads to articular cartilage are primarily imposed by muscle contraction and are further increased by weight bearing during motion. Subchondral bone is highly elastic and serves as a major shock absorber during the application of higher loads. Further joint protection is offered by the periarticular muscles, which provide dynamic shock absorption by adjusting muscle length and force generation to absorb large amounts of energy (18).

Normal chondrocytes produce the collagen and ground substance that become cartilage and function to maintain the cartilage matrix. In normal cartilage, these cells do not divide. In the development of osteoarthritis, cartilage damage and degradation stimulates an inflammatory response with the proliferation of chondrocytes in an attempt to repair. Unfortunately, these proliferative cells also release matrix-degrading enzymes, growth factors, and inflammatory cytokines, which lead to further cartilage degradation. Changes in the synovial fluid, water content of the cartilage, and changes in the collagen matrix produce an inferior matrix, which leads to further cartilage loss. Destruction of articular cartilage damages the underlying bone, and attempts to repair this damage result in new bone formation. These are seen as osteophytes at the joint margins at the interface of the cartilage and periosteum and as subchondral sclerosis at the base of cartilage lesions. The progression of cartilage breakdown can result in cartilage fragments, capsular thickening, joint effusion, and bone cyst formation. Muscle weakness and atrophy near the involved joint occur via a variety of mechanisms including muscle inhibition due to pain, decreased activity levels due to pain, and altered joint biomechanics. Loss of the muscular support needed for joint protection during activities results in increased forces distributed to the already compromised articular surface and contributes to progression (14,19).

DIAGNOSTIC TESTING

Imaging studies and laboratory testing are of limited use in the diagnosis of osteoarthritis, and are more frequently used to rule out other conditions that present similar to osteoarthritis, such as rheumatoid arthritis. Several techniques are available for imaging of synovial joints, but none are useful without correlation of the clinical presentation and findings.

Plain radiography is the least expensive and most common choice for imaging a joint in a patient with a suspected diagnosis of osteoarthritis. This technique is insensitive for the detection of early osteoarthritic changes, so normal joint plain radiographs do not rule out a diagnosis of osteoarthritis. In the early stages of osteoarthritis, plain radiography is most useful for ruling out other diagnoses in the differential. Because changes on plain radiographs do not correlate with joint symptoms or pain, it is also not possible to definitively identify the causes of the symptoms to any changes that are present on imaging. Limitations in the grading system for plain radiological findings also limit its use to monitor the progress of disease (20).

MRI can visualize and provide excellent detail of articular cartilage, subchondral bone, and soft tissues of the joint. Its clinical utility in the diagnosis and management of osteoarthritis is limited due to its relatively high cost and lack of clear correlation between MRI findings and clinical presentation. Again, it is useful to rule out other causes of joint pain that can mimic osteoarthritis, such as avascular necrosis or osteochondritis dissecans. Its greatest value at present is in the research setting, where it is a useful tool in the monitoring of disease progression. This may make it useful in demonstrating the potential effectiveness of disease-modifying treatments as they are developed (20).

Musculoskeletal ultrasound may play a role in imaging the joints of patients suspected to have osteoarthritis. It is relatively inexpensive, does not expose the patient to ionizing radiation, and does not require the use of any contrast agents. It can be used to assess synovial blood flow and can therefore assess patients for synovial pathology. Its major limitation is that its utility is user dependent (20).

CT is a superior method for imaging bony morphology, but its use in the assessment of osteoarthritis is limited by several factors. It is a high-cost modality that requires relatively high radiation exposure compared to the other techniques. Additionally, soft-tissue visualization requires the use of contrast and is still inferior to MRI in many ways (20).

TREATMENT OPTIONS

Treatment options for osteoarthritis are broadly categorized as nonpharmacological interventions, medications, and surgery. Often a combination of treatment options offers a comprehensive plan for the patient that is individualized and incorporates the patient into the treatment team.

Nonpharmacologic Interventions

Patient education should be considered an important part of the treatment of osteoarthritis; it should be provided starting at the first visit and refined throughout the treatment course of this chronic condition. Reassurance and access to information detailing the expected outcomes for specific interventions will assist the patient in choosing and complying with treatment guidelines. Patients should be referred to reputable organizations and websites as alternate sources of information. Screening and discussion of the potential for associated mood disturbances should be part of this process and referral for psychiatric intervention should be pursued when necessary (14).

Obesity is a major risk factor for the development of osteoarthritis and its progression. This has been consistently demonstrated in knee osteoarthritis and is often attributed to excess forces during weight-bearing activity. However, there is also evidence that obesity contributes to the systemic development of osteoarthritis, such as in the hand (21). Weight loss is considered a major intervention in the treatment of osteoarthritis and has been shown to reduce both development and progression in knee osteoarthritis (4). Patients with osteoarthritis and obesity have several options for treatment of the obesity; these include weight-loss medications, exercise, dietary changes, and bariatric surgery. The choices again need to be individualized for each patient (22).

Exercise in the treatment of osteoarthritis has several benefits. Exercise increases caloric expenditure and can assist in weight reduction. It also strengthens muscles supporting and acting on the involved joints, which helps to further reduce joint stresses. Many patients with osteoarthritis have pain with certain activities and develop kinesiophobia, which is the fear of movement in response to the pain. Supervised programs, including physical therapy interventions, can be cost effective and useful in patients with kinesiophobia. Additionally, when exercise is combined with other weight-loss strategies, the combination is more effective than either intervention alone. Lastly, exercise has been shown to reduce pain over time and results in the reduction of self-reported disability (22).

Pain-relieving modalities can be a useful adjunct in the treatment of osteoarthritis. No one modality has been proven to have any long-term benefit, as the primary purpose of modality use is to reduce pain and enhance the patient's ability to participate in exercise. Each of the modalities has specific contraindications, and recommendations for usage must take these into account. Cold and heat modalities can be applied to painful joints, as long as the patient is aware of the purpose, safe usage, and risks and benefits of thermal agents. The use of transcutaneous electrical nerve stimulation (TENS) has not been studied extensively in the osteoarthritis population, but has been shown to be of some benefit in the short term in one study (14). Recent systemic review has not shown TENS to be of any benefit over sham stimulation (23). Pulsed electromagnetic fields and magnets have not been shown to be effective in randomized controlled studies (14).

Orthoses can be used in osteoarthritis to limit painful range of motion, allow relative rest, adjust joint alignment, reduce abnormal joint forces, accommodate deformities, and provide shock absorption. While some studies have shown benefit of specific orthoses in the treatment of osteoarthritis (14), systematic review of the evidence for their use is a conditional recommendation in the 2012 ACR guidelines (16). The use of durable medical equipment may play a role in the treatment of osteoarthritis. The cane has been demonstrated to be useful in decreasing forces across the hip and knee, when used in the contralateral hand (14). No other ambulatory devices have been studied effectively in the treatment of osteoarthritis.

Complementary and alternative medicine (CAM) usage has become increasingly popular in the treatment of osteoarthritis. Population-based studies have shown that a large majority of patients have tried CAM interventions for symptoms of osteoarthritis. Acupuncture is widely used and available and has been shown in numerous studies to have statistically significant benefits for reduction of pain and improvement of function. Electroacupuncture, or the combination of acupuncture and the application of small electric currents to the needles, has shown promise in recent studies. Other types of acupuncture combined with herbal medications and laser treatment have not shown sufficient efficacy to warrant routine usage. Other CAM treatments studied in osteoarthritis include moxibustion, a form of heat treatment, laser therapy using red-beam or near-infrared lasers, and massage. The techniques of application are not standardized and have thus not been amenable to comprehensive study; therefore, insufficient evidence exists to support their use in the treatment of osteoarthritis (23).

Medications

Pharmacological options in the treatment of osteoarthritis include topical medications, systemic medications, and injectable medications. All of the available agents are used for symptomatic relief. There are currently no available agents that prevent the development or progression of osteoarthritis (24).

There are several topical analgesics available for the treatment of pain related to osteoarthritis. Topical nonsteroidal anti-inflammatory drugs (NSAIDs) have been shown to have similar efficacy to oral NSAIDs, but have reduced GI and renal toxicity. Diclofenac is available in gel form, and specifically has an FDA indication for the treatment of osteoarthritis. It is also available in a patch form; however, it only has an FDA indication for acute pain related to sprains, strains, and contusions (24). Topical lidocaine is available in gel and patch forms as well, and has been used in the treatment of osteoarthritis; however, neither form has an FDA indication for pain secondary to osteoarthritis (14). Capsaicin is derived from chili peppers and is used topically in the treatment of pain. Its effectiveness in osteoarthritis has been demonstrated in randomized, double-blinded, placebo-controlled studies, but its usage is limited by the local burning sensation associated with its application (24).

Acetaminophen is considered the first-line systemic agent in the treatment of osteoarthritis. Early studies of its efficacy showed that therapeutic doses ranging from 2,600 to 4,000 mg/day were effective in decreasing pain at rest and with motion, and had the analgesic equivalence to 1,200 mg/day of ibuprofen. Acetaminophen at these doses had reduced GI side effects compared to oral NSAIDs. Patients using this medication regularly must be cautioned about the potential for accidental overdose, due to the abundance of over-the-counter products that include acetaminophen as an ingredient, as well as opioid combination preparations with acetaminophen.

The second-line systemic agents used in the treatment of osteoarthritis are the nonselective NSAIDs, which inhibit both cyclooxygenase (COX) 1 and 2. The inhibition of COX-2 results in the analgesia of osteoarthritis pain (24), but this is also partially responsible for potential renal toxicity, as COX-2 is also expressed in the kidney (14). Inhibition of COX-1 decreases platelet aggregation, increases GI vulnerability to gastritis and ulceration, and alters renal vascular regulation that can result in toxicity. Medications in this group can be prescribed as part of a daily regimen or can be prescribed as needed. In general, the lowest effective dose should be prescribed, as GI side effects are largely dose dependent. To avoid the renal complications of chronic use, the clinician should attempt to use intermittent, short courses of nonselective NSAIDs to manage flare-ups of osteoarthritis pain. Well-designed studies have shown the efficacy of nonselective NSAIDs in reducing pain and improving function using objective measures. There are numerous available NSAIDs, and none have been shown to be superior to any other. Therefore, choice of a particular agent is essentially up to the clinician, and failure of, or intolerance to, one agent should not preclude trial of other agents (24). The clinician should consider the concomitant prescription of misoprostol, proton pump inhibitors, or H2 blockers to reduce toxicity to the GI tract (14).

COX-2-selective NSAIDs preferentially inhibit COX-2 over COX-1 and have similar efficacy to nonselective NSAIDs for the reduction of osteoarthritis-related pain and improvements in function. These agents have considerably less GI toxicity, but still have the potential for significant renal toxicity. Additionally, these agents increase the risk of cardiothrombic events and should be used with caution in patients with cardiac risk factors. COX-2-selective NSAIDs are considered second-line treatment for patients with osteoarthritis that have increased GI risk factors and low cardiac risk factors (24).

Opioid analgesics are indicated in the treatment of osteoarthritic pain in patients who have failed treatment with acetaminophen and NSAIDs, have contraindications to the use of these agents, or have inadequate pain relief with these agents alone. Tramadol is a weak mu opioid agonist and also inhibits norepinephrine and serotonin reuptake. It is a good first-line opioid for patients without increased seizure risk or epilepsy and who are not taking any medications with significant potential for interaction (24). Other, more potent opioids can be considered for patients who have failed treatment with tramadol or have contraindications to its usage. No one agent or preparation is specifically recommended, nor is there any consensus on the use of extended-release or immediate-release opioid preparations. Patients should be maintained on the lowest effective dose and should be followed up frequently during dose adjustment. Due to the potential risks of addiction and diversion (14), responsible prescribers must screen patients for potential for abuse and diversion, discuss risks and benefits of opioid usage, provide close follow-up, and clarify patient responsibilities when using these medications. Additionally, due to the potential side effects of sedation, confusion, and constipation, these agents should be used with caution in the geriatric population (24).

Intraarticular injections should be considered in patients who have failed or could not tolerate less invasive treatment and in patients who are potentially considering surgical intervention. Because of the invasive nature of injections, these types of treatments have risks associated with the medication injected and risks that are independent of the agent injected. Joint injections are associated with the risk of injury to the skin and other soft tissues, bleeding, and infection. Injections are specifically contraindicated in patients with systemic infections, local skin infections, high risk of bleeding, and symptomatic prosthetic joints.

Corticosteroid injections have historically been used in the treatment of osteoarthritis, despite the lack of clear research to warrant their widespread use (14). Most studies have looked at the efficacy of intraarticular steroid injections of the knee and found them to be effective in relieving pain for 2 to 3 weeks. There are concerns about potential harm of repeated injections, including the possibility of causing disease progression and direct cartilage damage, but this has not been clearly demonstrated in research either (25). In general, no more than four steroid injections per year are recommended in a particular joint (14).

Viscosupplementation, or the injection of hyaluronic acid derivatives, was initially developed in an attempt to slow the progression of osteoarthritis; however, these agents have only been shown to reduce the symptoms of osteoarthritis (14). Since hyaluronic acid is decreased in the synovial fluid, these agents were thought to restore the hyaluronic acid. However, most of the agents have a short half-life in the joint, and therefore the actual mechanism of action is unknown. There is evidence to support several mechanisms of action, including an anti-inflammatory effect, a lubricating effect, an antinociceptive effect, and a synovial cell stimulation effect (14,25). At present, there are several products that are approved for the treatment of osteoarthritis of the knee. Clinical trials of viscosupplementation in other joints have shown some reduction in pain, but there is insufficient evidence to gain FDA approval for its use.

Surgery

Surgical options for the treatment of osteoarthritis should be considered only for patients who have failed nonsurgical treatment. For younger patients, osteotomies are done to improve alignment and redistribute joint forces with the goal of delaying the need for joint replacement surgery. In older patients, joint arthroplasty is appropriate for the treatment of refractory osteoarthritis. The timing of the surgery is largely patient-driven and based on the severity of the pain and its impact on the patient's quality of life. The primary purposes of these procedures are to reduce pain and increase function. Operative candidates must be willing and able to participate in postoperative rehabilitation to maximize attainment of these goals (14). Total hip arthroplasty and total knee arthroplasty are the most common joint replacement procedures performed. Both procedures have high rates of success with predictable and proven long-term results. Total shoulder arthroplasty is also associated with good outcomes for reduction of pain and resultant improvements in functional status (26).

PRACTICE-BASED LEARNING AND IMPROVEMENT

GOALS

Demonstrate competence in continuously investigating and evaluating your osteoarthritic patient care practices, appraising and assimilating scientific evidence, and continuously improving your patient care practices based on constant self-evaluation and lifelong learning.

OBJECTIVES

1. Describe learning opportunities for providers, patients, and caregivers with experience in osteoarthritis.
2. Use methods for ongoing competency training in osteoarthritis for physiatrists, including objectively measuring patient outcomes, evaluating current practice, and developing a systematic QI and practice improvement strategy.
3. Locate some resources including available websites for continuing medical education and professional development.
4. Describe some areas paramount to self-assessment and lifelong learning such as identification and access of current evidence-based treatment guidelines for osteoarthritis, and the role of the physiatrist as the educator of patients, families, residents, students, colleagues, and other health professionals.

There are a variety of resources available to physiatrists, which provide evidence-based information regarding the treatment of osteoarthritis. The Agency for Healthcare Research and Quality (AHRQ) is one of the 12 agencies within the Department of Health and Human Services. It is dedicated to the improvement in the quality, safety, efficacy, and effectiveness of health care for all Americans. The AHRQ has developed an initiative called the National Guidelines Clearinghouse (NGC), which is dedicated to providing physicians and other health care providers access to clinical practice guidelines. The NGC can be accessed via the AHRQ website at www.ahrq.gov. There are currently several guidelines available regarding osteoarthritis from various professional societies and taskforces.

The American Academy of Physical Medicine and Rehabilitation (AAPMR) is an important resource for physiatrists and has numerous online resources related to the practice of physiatry. The website gives members access to PM&R, Knowledge NOW, which is an online resource devoted to clinical topics relevant to PM&R. *PM&R*, the official journal of the AAPMR, is a monthly peer-reviewed journal geared for this specialty. In May 2012, *PM&R* published a supplement dedicated to the topic of osteoarthritis. Additionally in 2013, AAPMR has recently established a Clinical Practice Guidelines Committee that was created for the purpose of developing, endorsing, and advocating for key guidelines applicable to the practice of PM&R. During its first year, the committee reviewed existing clinical guidelines relevant to PM&R practice to either endorse or affirm their use in clinical practice. At present, there are no guidelines in review regarding osteoarthritis; however, this may be an important resource in the future.

Other specialty societies have developed osteoarthritis-specific guidelines that may be of use to physiatrists. The American College of Rheumatology (ACR) recently published the 2012 ACR Recommendations for the Use of Nonpharmacologic and Pharmacologic Therapies in Osteoarthritis of the Hand, Hip, and Knee. This guideline can be accessed on the ACR website at www.rheumatology.org. The American Academy of Orthopedic Surgeons (AAOS) currently has the following 2 clinical guidelines, which can be accessed at www.aaos.org: Treatment of Glenohumeral Joint Osteoarthritis and Treatment of Osteoarthritis of the Knee.

The Cochrane Collaboration is an independent, international network of people dedicated to promotion of evidence-based health care. The published Cochrane Reviews are systematic and comprehensive reviews compiled and made accessible to help health care practitioners, patients, and other stakeholders make well-informed decisions about health care.

Patient education regarding osteoarthritis, for both prevention and treatment, should center on weight reduction, avoidance of joint injury, and importance of regular exercise. Obesity is a primary risk factor for osteoarthritis. Obese patients without any symptoms of osteoarthritis should be informed about the increased risk of developing symptomatic osteoarthritis and should be encouraged to reduce their weight. Obese patients with symptomatic osteoarthritis also benefit from weight reduction, so weight loss should be encouraged in these patients as well (4).

Joint injury is a known risk factor for the subsequent development of osteoarthritis. Soft-tissue injuries can alter joint mechanics and have been linked to the development of osteoarthritis (4). Injury prevention programs have been studied to prevent anterior cruciate ligament (ACL) injuries, hamstring strain injuries, and ankle instability injuries. The prevention programs utilized a variety of strategies including balance and proprioceptive training, avoidance of high-risk behaviors, use of standardized warm-ups and practices, eccentric training programs, and training in sports-specific agility skills. Overall, incorporation of injury prevention strategies into routine training programs resulted in significant declines in injury rates (27). Joint injury is also a potential consequence of work-related activities such as overuse syndromes and repetitive stress syndromes. Attention to ergonomic design of workstations and employee education programs have been shown to lower risks of injury (4).

Regular exercise has been proven to be beneficial in a variety of ways. Current exercise guidelines recommend "at least 150 minutes of moderate-intensity aerobic activity, 75 minutes of vigorous-intensity aerobic activity, or an equivalent combination of each weekly" (3). Regular exercise assists with weight management and reduces obesity. Maintaining muscle strength is joint protective, both as a preventative measure against osteoarthritis and for its treatment. Regular exercise is also protective against functional decline (4).

In regard to treatment of osteoarthritis, it is most important to emphasize that osteoarthritis is not part of the natural aging process. It is a preventable and treatable condition. At present, none of the interventions modify the disease process; however, evidence-based treatments are successful at relieving pain, minimizing disability, or both (28).

Quantification of functional improvement is useful for patients undergoing treatment for osteoarthritis. The Western Ontario and McMaster Universities Osteoarthritis Index (WOMAC) uses a self-administered 24-item questionnaire assessing pain, stiffness, and physical function in patients with hip or knee osteoarthritis. The responses are scored from 0 (none) to 4 (extreme). The final score is the sum of all 24 items. A reduction in the score is evidence of improvement. The Lower Extremity Functional Scale (LEFS) is a 20-item questionnaire, which is designed to assess function in patients with lower limb impairments. The responses are scored from 0 (extreme difficulty/cannot perform) to 4 (no difficulty). The final score is the sum of all 20 items and higher scores indicated higher functional abilities. An increase in score is evidence of improvement. Both these tools can be used to objectively measure improvement in response to treatment of lower limb osteoarthritis.

INTERPERSONAL AND COMMUNICATION SKILLS

GOALS

Demonstrate interpersonal and communication skills that result in the effective exchange of information and collaboration with osteoarthritic patients, their families, and the rest of the rehabilitation team.

OBJECTIVES

1. Demonstrate skills used in effective communication, counseling, and collaboration with patients with osteoarthritis and their caregivers and families across socioeconomic and cultural backgrounds.
2. Discuss how effective communication with patients results in better treatment options.
3. Discuss appropriate documentation strategies in a patient's medical records for osteoarthritis.
4. Delineate the importance of the role of the physiatrist as the interdisciplinary team leader and consultant in the care of the osteoarthritic patient.

Good communication between the physician and the patient and his family is important in all clinical situations, and research has confirmed effective communication improves patient compliance and clinical outcomes (29). Treatment of osteoarthritis is organized in a multimodal plan, often including lifestyle changes, medications, and nonpharmacological interventions. Explanation of the diagnosis, including basic relevant anatomy, correlation with symptoms, and reassurance that treatment is likely to improve those symptoms, is important for the patient to start to understand from the first visit. Second, the physician must provide a detailed discussion regarding the initial plan, the rationale for the components of the plan, and expected responses to each component of the plan. This discussion should include the risks and benefits of each component of the plan and should provide choices if possible. On subsequent visits, the diagnosis should be reviewed with the patient to reinforce understanding of the disease process. It is important to review the initial treatment plan after discussing the initial responses to treatment. Based on the response to treatment, the plan should be reaffirmed as appropriate or adjusted as needed. The modified plan should be discussed at each visit with patient and family, complete with rationale for the options chosen and discussions of risks and benefits.

Communication with the patient should be explicitly documented in the patient record. Documentation in the medical record should reflect the diagnosis as specifically as possible and that the diagnosis was discussed with the patient. The clinician should allow the patient to ask questions and document that the patient was asked and that the questions were answered. Each treatment in the plan should be documented clearly with a brief explanation of the rationale for choosing that particular treatment; in addition, the discussion of risks and benefits should be documented when initiating a new treatment modality. Detailed therapy prescriptions should be used to communicate with any treating therapists and plans of care initiated by the therapist should be reviewed, signed, and sent back to the therapist. Copies of relevant treatment plans from other clinicians should also be placed in the chart. Many of the medications used in the treatment of osteoarthritis have associated risks; it is of particular importance to document the emergence of any adverse drug reactions (ADRs) and the plan to address them.

Traditional approaches to the treatment of osteoarthritis have not been multidisciplinary or offered in a collaborative fashion, and have failed at minimizing disability. The multimodal approach to the treatment of osteoarthritis often requires the collaboration of multiple types of health care providers and requires commitment to communication among team members. The team consists of the patient, usually several physicians, and other allied health professionals. The most important member of the team is the patient, and all the other team members should emphasize this role. Physician team members include the primary care physician and potentially specialists in physiatry, rheumatology, orthopedics, and pain management. Physical therapists and occupational therapists may also be part of the treatment team, depending on the patient's needs. If bracing is necessary, a certified orthotist may also be added to the team. For patients with comorbid mood disorders, the inclusion of a psychiatrist, psychologist, or other mental health specialists may be of benefit. Several large health systems have developed centers that provide a comprehensive and integrated approach that also includes patient education, complementary and alternative modalities, and on-site musculoskeletal imaging (30).

PROFESSIONALISM

GOALS

Reflect a commitment to carrying out professional responsibilities and an adherence to ethical principles in caring for patients with osteoarthritis.

OBJECTIVES

1. Exemplify the humanistic qualities in patient-centered care.
2. Demonstrate ethical principles, responsibilities, and responsiveness to patient needs superseding self and other interests.
3. Demonstrate sensitivity to patient population diversity, cultural competence, gender, age, race, religion, disabilities, and sexual orientation.
4. Respect patient privacy, confidentiality, autonomy, and shared decision making.
5. Recognize the socioeconomic factors and importance of patient education in the treatment of and advocacy for persons with osteoarthritis.

The physician should exhibit compassion during encounters with patients with symptomatic osteoarthritis, as the primary manifestations are pain and functional loss, which are clearly distressing to the patient. Expressing empathy toward the patient has been shown to improve patient satisfaction and compliance with treatment, and in general strengthens the physician–patient relationship (23). Physician integrity and ethics in treating patients with osteoarthritis is partially based in providing treatment options that are evidence based and reviewing the risks and benefits of each treatment. Respect and courtesy is provided to the patient by maintaining open communication, acknowledgment of the patient's beliefs and concerns, and understanding that despite good evidence and adequate explanation, patients have the right to refuse any and all recommended treatments.

Patient-centered care is especially important in the treatment of osteoarthritis. Treatment programs are individually tailored for each patient and the active role of the patient in the treatment team is emphasized. Risks and benefits are discussed and reviewed whenever necessary to empower the patient to make treatment decisions (23). Proper procedures for obtaining informed consent are appropriate for any invasive procedure and should include discussion of noninvasive options and the risks of refusal of the proposed procedure.

Patients with the capacity to make decisions have the autonomy to accept or refuse any and all treatments. Osteoarthritis is not a life-threatening disease, so treatment refusals are rarely grounds to breach patient confidentiality in the interest of patient safety. The goals of the treatment for osteoarthritis should be clear and reviewed with the patient. It is the physician's responsibility to redirect patients with unrealistic goals and to realign those goals with realistic ones. Patients' beliefs regarding their diagnosis of osteoarthritis and its potential effects on quality of life should be explored during treatment. Specific education to correct misconceptions should be provided to the patient on an ongoing basis as these can change as the patient's understanding improves (9). It then may be appropriate to discuss previously refused treatment options.

Physicians must be sensitive to sociocultural factors that can impact the physician–patient relationship and ultimately the successful treatment of diagnoses such as osteoarthritis. Since age, gender, and ethnicity are all not modifiable risk factors for osteoarthritis, it is important to screen patients for pain, regardless of the purpose of the visit, in an attempt to screen for early signs of osteoarthritis. At present, there is no valid screening tool for early symptomatic osteoarthritis, so screening for pain and careful joint examination in patients with pain may be helpful in identifying patients earlier in the disease course. Counseling patients about weight loss for obesity, avoidance of joint injury, and the role of exercise in maintaining joint health should be part of preventative care (4). Cultural and gender differences can result in differences in presentation, complaints, tendency to ask questions, compliance, and perceptions about the physician. Disparities in the treatment of osteoarthritis have been identified in racial and ethnic minorities, patients with reduced literacy and low education, and in patients with low socioeconomic status. These disparities result in greater pain, greater functional decline, and more significant earnings losses (31).

The practice of physiatry focuses on both the treatment of disease and its resultant disability. Since osteoarthritis is the most common cause of disability, physiatrists are uniquely qualified to act as team leaders in the coordination of care in patients with osteoarthritis. They are capable of treating the pain associated with osteoarthritis and are trained to provide many of the nonsurgical interventions as well. Additionally, they understand the indications for referrals for physical therapy, occupational therapy, orthotic fabrication and fitting, and some of the CAM therapies. Because of the nature of the specialty, they are natural advocates for the rights of the disabled, including those with osteoarthritis.

SYSTEMS-BASED PRACTICE

GOALS

Awareness and responsiveness to systems of care delivery, and the ability to recruit and coordinate effectively resources in the system to provide optimal continuum of care as it relates to osteoarthritis.

OBJECTIVES

1. Identify the components, systems of care delivery, services, referral patterns, and resources in the rehabilitation continuum of care for patients with osteoarthritis.
2. Coordinate and recruit necessary resources in the system to provide optimal care for the osteoarthritic patient, with attention to safety, cost awareness, and risk–benefit analysis and management.
3. Describe optimal follow-up, quality improvement markers, and use of documentation in osteoarthritis rehabilitation programs.

Patients with osteoarthritis are encountered throughout the rehabilitation continuum of care and there are treatment options available in each setting. In acute inpatient rehabilitation, osteoarthritis is one of the most common comorbidities affecting function. As a primary diagnosis, joint replacement patients can be admitted for acute rehabilitation postoperatively to facilitate rapid and safe community discharges. Acute inpatient rehabilitation provides short-term aggressive multidisciplinary treatment at an intensity of at least 3 hours/day for at least 5 days/week. There has been a recent shift of some of the joint replacement patients to receiving rehabilitation in a subacute rehabilitation setting. This type of setting provides a less expensive, longer term, lower-intensity rehabilitation program, defined as at least one type of therapy at an intensity of at least 1 hour/day for at least 5 days a week.

After discharge from the hospital, acute rehabilitation, or subacute rehabilitation, most joint replacement patients do require continued therapy in either a home or outpatient setting to achieve their maximal goals. The intensity and duration in this setting are variable and largely dependent on insurance benefits.

The majority of the patients with osteoarthritis in physiatry practice are encountered in an outpatient setting. Most of the patients who require therapy as part of their treatment are referred for outpatient therapy. The prescribed intensity is variable, but usually two to three times/week. The duration of treatment is dependent upon functional improvement, but again is largely dependent on insurance benefits and authorization. Homebound patients with osteoarthritis can undergo home therapy and, if possible, transition to an outpatient therapy setting. Again, the intensity and duration are variable. Patients with a primary diagnosis of osteoarthritis can potentially be treated in an acute rehabilitation setting, but only in the case of significant disability from osteoarthritis with failure of an aggressive course of outpatient physical therapy.

Falls are an important safety concern in patients with osteoarthritis due to increased functional decline, reduced balance, and muscle weakness. Fall prevention programs focus on patient education, home modifications, and exercises to improve strength and balance (15).

Risks associated with the use of NSAIDs are significant in patients with osteoarthritis. GI bleeding and renal toxicity are known potential risks with the use of NSAIDs, and must be used with caution in patients with increased risks of GI bleeding and kidney dysfunction. In patients on selective NSAIDs, the risk of cardiothrombotic events is increased; therefore, selective NSAIDs should be used with caution in patients with increased cardiovascular risk factors (24).

The prescription of opioid analgesics has substantial risks as well. Patients need to be screened for risk factors of abuse and diversion prior to starting the medications and must be monitored closely for development of these risk factors. Caution is necessary in the use of opioids in the geriatric population as these patients have a higher tendency to develop sedation, confusion, and constipation (24).

Regular contact with the physician who is monitoring the care of the patient with osteoarthritis is recommended based on research in integrated care systems. These patients are seen at least once every 6 months if stable, and more frequently if pain is uncontrolled, disability increases, or comorbidities warrant more frequent follow-up (30).

The Center for Medicare and Medicaid Services (CMS) will be requiring physicians to report disease-specific quality measures in order to obtain full reimbursement for office visits. The following list contains examples of these measures: (a) assessment for use of anti-inflammatory or analgesic over-the-counter medications, (b) function and pain assessment, (c) percentage of patients over age 20 with a diagnosis of osteoarthritis for whom a physical examination of the involved joint was performed during the initial visit, (d) percentage of patients over age 20 with a diagnosis of osteoarthritis on prescribed or over-the-counter NSAIDs who were assessed for GI and renal risk factors, (e) percentage of patients over age 20 with a diagnosis of osteoarthritis during which an anti-inflammatory agent or analgesic was considered, (f) percentage of patients over age 20 with a diagnosis of osteoarthritis with an assessment for use of anti-inflammatory or analgesic over-the-counter medications, and (g) percentage of patients over age 20 with a diagnosis of osteoarthritis of the hip or knee during which therapeutic exercise for the hip or knee (therapeutic exercise instructed or physical therapy prescribed) was considered.

CASE STUDY

A 55-year-old obese woman comes to your office with right knee pain that has progressed over the past 15 to 20 years. The pain is worse in the morning and gets better after she moves around for about an hour. The patient describes the pain as achy and rates the pain 6/10 to 7/10 at its worst. The pain bothers her when she goes up and down stairs and has gotten to the point that she is scared to take the stairs because she feels her knee might buckle. The knee pain is also worse when it rains and the knee seems to her to swell. She denies any past medical history for diabetes, hypertension, rheumatoid arthritis, cancer, hypothyroidism, or any autoimmune disorders. The patient has pertinent surgical history for right ACL reconstruction and partial right medial meniscectomy during college after a soccer injury in her sophomore year of division I sport 34 years ago. She claims to have recovered fully and was able to return to her prior level of function post surgery. She competed all 4 of her college years in division I soccer as a striker. The patient has intermittently tried over-the-counter ibuprofen and acetaminophen with some relief.

The patient has not had therapy since college. She has a sedentary job and rarely exercises. She does not smoke and drinks in social situations only, averaging about 2 drinks per month. Her review of systems is positive as previously noted, and is negative for low back pain, focal weakness, numbness, tingling, ataxia, fever, chills, or night sweats.

On examination, her height is 5 feet 9 inches and she weighs 245 lbs. She has normal bilateral hip range of motion and no pain during motion. She has normal bilateral knee range of motion, with bilateral knee crepitus. She has bilateral 10-degree varus alignment at the knee with bilateral normal pes cavus at the feet. She has right medial joint line tenderness and firm end point during both Lachman and anterior draw testing of the knee, but more anterior excursion of the right knee in comparison to the contralateral side. The right knee has a well-healed midline incision and a 2+ effusion with significant quadriceps atrophy measuring a 3 cm difference 10 cm superior to the medial tibial plateau. She has normal reflexes and normal strength on manual muscle testing. She has normal sensation for light touch, sharp/dull discrimination, and proprioception. She has a right antalgic gait pattern with a decreased time in stance phase on the right.

CASE STUDY DISCUSSION QUESTIONS

1. What is this patient's diagnosis, impairments, activity limitations, and participation restrictions?
2. Write a rehabilitation prescription for this patient.
3. What are her modifiable and nonmodifiable risk factors for her diagnosis?
4. Describe the components of a patient education plan for this patient's diagnosis and identify some patient education resources for her.
5. What are some strategies that you can use to check for patient understanding of your recommendations?
6. Describe the elements of professional behavior on the part of the physiatrist as it applies to this patient.
7. Identify the medical, surgical, and allied health team members that can be involved in the care of this patient and give examples of effective communication between them.
8. What are some potential patient safety concerns in the care of this patient? Identify some strategies to minimize them.

SELF-EXAMINATION QUESTIONS
(Answers begin on p. 367)

1. Which of the following best describes the correlation between obesity and osteoarthritis?
   A. Weight gain reduces both the development and progression of osteoarthritis
   B. Obesity is not a strong systemic risk factor for osteoarthritis development
   C. Prevention and education have the potential to impact this modifiable risk at the population level
   D. Weight reduction is associated with development and progression of knee osteoarthritis
   E. Weight gain is not associated with osteoarthritis of the knee

2. Which of the following imaging studies of the involved joint is indicated for the routine evaluation of patients suspected of having a diagnosis of osteoarthritis?
   A. Plain radiographs are often very helpful, especially in early osteoarthritis
   B. Musculoskeletal ultrasound of the medial meniscus
   C. MRI of the knee
   D. CT of the knee
   E. Osteoarthritis is a clinical diagnosis and imaging studies are often not necessary

3. Medications used in the management of osteoarthritis are often part of a comprehensive treatment plan. Which of the following statements is true when managing osteoarthritis?
   A. COX-2-selective NSAIDs have shown superior efficacy to nonselective NSAIDs
   B. There are no available agents to prevent the development or progression of osteoarthritis
   C. Opioids are first-line agents for use in osteoarthritis-related pain
   D. Use of intrathecal opioids is often used for the treatment of osteoarthritis
   E. There are several available agents that have been proven to prevent the development of osteoarthritis

4. Which of the following best describes the role of exercise in the treatment program for patients with osteoarthritis?
   A. It is not very helpful with weight management
   B. It has a limited role in improving muscle strength
   C. It has not been shown to be helpful against functional decline
   D. Exercise has been shown to reduce pain over time
   E. It does not have any benefit on protecting the articular cartilage from the effect of forces acting across the joint

5. Injury prevention programs to prevent ACL injuries use all of the following strategies *except*
   A. Concentric training programs
   B. Avoidance of high-risk behaviors
   C. Balance and proprioceptive training
   D. Training in sports-specific agility skills
   E. Standardized warm-ups and practices

REFERENCES

1. Powell RA, Downing J, Ddungu H, et al. Pain history and pain assessment. In: Kopf A, Patel NB, eds. *Guide to Pain Management in Low Resource Settings*. Seattle, WA: IASP; 2010:67–78.
2. Marx RG. Anterior cruciate ligament injuries and osteoarthritis. *Chronic OA Management*. 2012;1(3):1, 8–9.
3. Harold EJ. Managing osteoarthritis with comorbidities. *Chronic OA Management*. 2012;2(2):1, 4–6.
4. Suri P, Morgenroth DC, Hunter DJ. Epidemiology of osteoarthritis and associated comorbidities. *PM&R*. 2012;4(5S):S10–S19.
5. Neogi T, Zhang Y. Epidemiology of osteoarthritis. *Rheum Dis Clin North Am*. 2013;39(1):1–19.
6. Dodds JA, Gilli M, Hammerberg EM, et al. General orthopedics. In: Griffin LY, ed. *Essentials of Musculoskeletal Care*. 3rd ed. Rosemont, IL: AAOS; 2005:8–12.

7. Davies M, Donatelli R, Whiteside JA. Shoulder. In: Griffin LY, ed. *Essentials of Musculoskeletal Care.* 3rd ed. Rosemont, IL: AAOS; 2005:155–156.
8. Donatelli R, Hassinger DD, Lourie GM. Elbow and forearm. In: Griffin LY, ed. *Essentials of Musculoskeletal Care.* 3rd ed. Rosemont, IL: AAOS;2005:244.
9. Dalton JF, Donatelli R, Louthan A, et al. Hand and wrist. In: Griffin LY, ed. *Essentials of Musculoskeletal Care.* 3rd ed. Rosemont, IL: AAOS; 2005:299–300.
10. Della Valle CJ, Donatelli R, Klein GR. Hip and thigh. In: Griffin LY, ed. *Essentials of Musculoskeletal Care.* 3rd ed. Rosemont, IL: AAOS; 2005:412.
11. Donatelli R, Mauro CS. Knee and lower leg. In: Griffin LY, ed. *Essentials of Musculoskeletal Care.* 3rd ed. Rosemont, IL: AAOS; 2005:480–484.
12. Donatelli R. Foot and ankle. In: Griffin LY, ed. *Essentials of Musculoskeletal Care.* Rosemont, IL: AAOS; 2005:587.
13. Backman CL. Arthritis and pain. Psychosocial aspects in the management of arthritis pain. *Arthritis Res Ther.* 2006;8(221).
14. Lozada CJ. 100—treatment of osteoarthritis. In: Firestein GS, Budd RC, Gabriel SE, eds. *Kelley's Textbook of Rheumatology.* 9th ed. Philadelphia, PA: Saunders Elsevier; 2013: electronic version.
15. Hile ES, Studenski SA. Instability and falls. In: Duthie EH, Katz PR, Malone ML, eds. *Practice of Geriatrics.* 4th ed. Philadelphia, PA: Saunders Elsevier; 2007: electronic version.
16. Nelson AE. ACR guidelines update. *Chronic OA Management.* 2012;2(2):1, 7–9.
17. "Osteoarthritis." Centers for Disease Control and Prevention. July 28, 2013. http://www.cdc.gov/arthritis/basics/osteoarthritis.htm.
18. Brinker MR, O'Connor DP, Almekinders LC, et al. Physiology of injury to musculoskeletal structures: 3. articular cartilage injury. In: DeLee JC, Drez D, Miller MD, eds. *DeLee and Drez's Orthopedic Sports Medicine.* 3rd ed. Philadelphia, PA: Saunders Elsevier; 2010: electronic version.
19. Wilke WS, Carey J. Osteoarthritis. In: Carey WD, ed. *Cleveland Clinic: Current Clinical Medicine.* 2nd ed. Philadelphia, PA: Saunders Elsevier; 2009: electronic version.
20. Hunter DJ, Guermazi A. Imaging techniques in osteoarthritis. *PM&R.* 2012;4(5S):S68–S74.
21. McAlindon T. OA and obesity: more than mechanical. *Chronic OA Management.* 2011;1(2):1, 4–5.
22. Vincent HK, Heywood K, Connelly J, et al. Obesity and weight loss in the treatment and prevention of osteoarthritis. *PM&R.* 2012;4(5S):S59–S67.
23. De Luigi AJ. Complementary and alternative medicine in osteoarthritis. *PM&R.* 2012;4(5S):S122–S133.
24. Cheng DS, Visco CJ. Pharmaceutical therapy for osteoarthritis. *PM&R.* 2012;4(5S):S82–S88.
25. Hameed F, Ihm J. Injectable medications for osteoarthritis. *PM&R.* 2012;4(5S):S75–S81.
26. Grayson CW, Decker RC. Total joint arthroplasty for persons with osteoarthritis. *PM&R.* 2012;4(5S):S97–S103.
27. Silvers HJ, Bahr R, Giza E, et al. Principles of injury prevention. In: DeLee JC, Drez D, Miller MD, eds. *DeLee and Drez's Orthopedic Sports Medicine.* 3rd ed. Philadelphia, PA: Saunders Elsevier; 2010: electronic version.
28. Reid MC. Factors complicating management of osteoarthritis in later life. *Chronic OA Management.* 2012;1(4):1, 4–5, 8.
29. Lockyear PLB. Physician-patient communication: enhancing skills to improve patient satisfaction. Medscape. July 31, 2013. http://www.medscape.org/viewarticle/495199.
30. Holliman K. Integrated care of patients with osteoarthritis. *Chronic OA Management.* 2012;2(1):1, 7–10.
31. Allen KD. Osteoarthritis is underserved populations. *Chronic OA Management.* 2013;3(1):1, 4–6.

Basem Aziz
Neil Patel
Miksha Patel

21: Rehabilitation Following Total Knee Arthroplasty and Total Hip Arthroplasty

PATIENT CARE

GOALS

A physician trained in Physical Medicine and Rehabilitation (PM&R) should be able to competently evaluate, care for, educate, and advocate for individuals preparing for total knee arthroplasty (TKA) and total hip arthroplasty (THA) and the rehabilitation that occurs before and after these procedures. Patients should understand all of the risks, benefits, and course of rehabilitation before undergoing TKA and THA.

OBJECTIVES

1. Identify the key elements of the history and physical examination of the adult post hip and knee joint arthroplasty.
2. Discuss the impairments, activity limitations, and participation restrictions associated with hip and knee arthroplasty.
3. Describe the psychosocial aspects of hip and knee arthroplasty.
4. Identify the key elements in the rehabilitation of hip and knee arthroplasty.
5. Identify the injuries associated with hip and knee arthroplasty and the strategies to prevent them.

The key elements of making the diagnosis of a patient rely on a thorough history and physical examination.

HISTORY OF PRESENT ILLNESS

The history of present illness should include a description of the surgery performed and any immediate postoperative complications.

Past Medical History: With the increasing number of lower limb joint replacements, it is important to be aware of the comorbidities most common within the patient population undergoing these surgeries. A physiatrist needs to take into account the patient's lifestyle, age, and other risk factors for complications. For example, patients undergoing THA tend to be older with an average age of 66 years (1). It is estimated that 1% to 3% of those older than 65 years will undergo a THA at one point in their lifetime (1). Obesity is common in the United States and this contributes to the increasing need for total joint arthroplasties (2). Both groups require careful evaluation for other comorbid conditions, such as hypertension or diabetes. Other comorbidities to note are coronary artery disease, peripheral vascular disease, lumbar spinal stenosis, lumbosacral radiculopathy, and the presence of significant degenerative joint disease in other joints in the lower extremities (3).

Past Surgical History: The physiatrist should carefully record the patient's past surgical history, as the patient may have had previous postsurgical complications (such as poor wound healing, atelectasis, or deep venous thrombosis) associated with those procedures.

Allergies and Medications: It is important to record any history of allergies as well as a current list of medications.

Social and Functional History: Patient's type of work, hobbies, extent of family/friend support network, and level of function prior to the surgery should be recorded. A history of alcohol intake, smoking, or substance abuse should also be noted.

Review of Systems: The review of systems should include questions about cardiac, pulmonary, gastrointestinal, and genitourinary function. It is important to ask about pain in the operated joint (quality, intensity, aggravating, and alleviating factors) as well as in other parts of the musculoskeletal system (other joints, spine) since poorly controlled pain can have an adverse impact on the patient's rehabilitation and recovery.

PHYSICAL EXAMINATION

The physical examination of the post-joint arthroplasty patient should include elements to assess cardiovascular and pulmonary function. It is imperative that a thorough musculoskeletal assessment also be performed. This includes inspection, palpation, objective measurement of the active and passive range of motion of the major joints in the extremities, and muscle strength testing. The incision line should be inspected for signs of infection or dehiscence. The skin should also be inspected for pressure ulcers at the heels, sacrum, and ischium. Presence of edema in the lower extremities should also be recorded. Palpation can provide evidence of painful structures as well as subcutaneous fluid collections or adhesions. In performing range of motion testing, it is important to record the presence of any contractures. The measurements should be made using a goniometer. Strength testing should be performed in all of the key muscle groups in the lower extremities and upper extremities. Sensory testing should include light touch, pinprick, vibration, and proprioception. Muscle stretch reflexes for the upper and lower extremities should also be recorded. Proximal and distal pulses should be noted. A functional assessment should include bed mobility, transfers, and ability to ambulate using an appropriate assistive device.

Common impairments following lower extremity joint arthroplasty include weakness in the affected extremity, limited range of motion, reduced endurance, and impaired balance. Activity limitations include difficulty performing activities of daily living such as bathing, dressing, grooming, transfers from different surfaces, and ambulation on different terrains and stairs. Participation restrictions include inability to drive, return to work, and high-level recreational activities such as jogging and bicycle riding.

To ensure a complete recovery, it is important to understand the psychosocial impact on the physical recovery of the patient. The ability to function within the patient's social environment may become very difficult after surgery. The patient's role within his or her family prior to the surgery may need to be altered during the recovery period. The patient may experience a low level of self-esteem if he or she cannot return to his or her prior role (e.g., cooking and cleaning the home, primary financial provider for the family). It is important to identify for the patient a network of family and friends who can assist with the physical limitations and also have a positive impact on their mental health.

Some patients are highly motivated and push themselves in therapy so they can quickly resume their previous level of functioning; however, it is critical that this type of patient be educated about the disadvantages of pushing therapy too quickly. The other type of patient is one who is reluctant to participate in therapy and needs to be coaxed into undergoing the rehabilitative program. It is always important to remember that some patients may have a hard time adjusting to the physical limitations and dependency post surgery and can become clinically depressed. Patients will need to be counseled on lifestyle changes that will improve their overall health as well as the wear and tear on their joints. Connecting patients with a nutritionist or other weight loss programs will help them attain their appropriate weight for height goals and will ultimately help the patient get on the road to a healthier pain-free life. Along with a healthier lifestyle the benefits of exercise, stretching, and physical therapy go further into prevention of postoperative contractures.

Patients who have undergone total joint arthroplasty of the lower extremity will have limited ability to return to work for several weeks post surgery. Some will have to take an extended medical leave from work. Physical therapy, occupational therapy, and vocational therapy are all essential components for a quick recovery. Regaining the ability to walk without assistance on flat surfaces and stairs, increasing the range of motion in the affected joint, practicing household chores, and driving are all components of therapy to assist in the patient's return to previous functional status.

Ideally, the rehabilitation program for the lower extremity joint arthroplasty patient should begin prior to surgery. During this period the patient is educated about the surgery and postoperative rehabilitation and care. Exercise programs to improve overall endurance, range of motion, and strength in key muscle groups of the lower and upper extremities would be very beneficial.

Following surgery, the rehabilitation program begins on the first day post procedure. For hip arthroplasty patients, restrictions such as not crossing the legs or bending from the waist more than 90° are important to minimize the risk of hip dislocation (4). Therapies are guided by these restrictions. Physical therapists work with the patient on improving the range of motion of the lower extremities within restriction parameters and strength training of key muscle groups such as the hip flexors, abductors, and extensors; knee flexors and extensors; ankle dorsi and plantar flexors. Modalities such as cold therapy can be used to reduce pain. Functional activities such as bed mobility, transfers, and ambulation on different terrains and stairs are also performed. The patient is also provided with a home exercise program. Occupational therapists educate the patients on performing specific activities of daily living such as bathing, dressing, and toileting within the restrictions of their range of motion. In addition, they work with the patient on strengthening key muscle groups of the upper extremities and trunk that are essential for performing these types of activities and also provide the patient with appropriate assistive devices to assist them in these activities. In the inpatient rehabilitation setting, the patient may also require the services of other rehabilitation team members such as rehabilitation nurses, psychologists, social workers, and vocational counselors.

In order for the patient to fully benefit from the postoperative rehabilitation, he or she needs to have the pain well controlled. Joint arthroplasty can be a very painful procedure and post surgery it is important for patients to actively move painful joints. The pain can be controlled using modalities such as cold therapy and medications such as acetaminophen and opioid medications. The timing of medications is important so that the maximal analgesic benefit from the medications can coincide with the time the patient is actively getting rehabilitation.

Following the initial rehabilitation period, the patient post total joint arthroplasty typically continues with rehabilitation in an outpatient setting. Here the emphasis is on continuation of exercises to strengthen muscles in the affected extremity, improve flexibility, increase ambulation distance, and continue progress toward independence in activities of daily living. Most patients return to their normal activities within 3 to 6 months post surgery and are encouraged to maintain an active lifestyle thereafter (5). Issues such as return to work and resumption of driving are based on patient's level of function and remain barriers that would impede a safe return.

INJURIES FOLLOWING TOTAL JOINT ARTHROPLASTY IN THE LOWER EXTREMITIES

It is important to be aware of injuries that may occur after total joint arthroplasty. Complications and risks include but are not limited to venous thromboembolism in the lower extremities, dislocations, falls, fractures, infections, and pressure ulcers.

Venous Thromboembolism

When a patient undergoes a hip or knee arthroplasty, he or she is at an increased risk for the development of venous thromboembolism. Studies have shown rates of thrombosis after joint replacement have been as high as 31% even while on pharmacological anticoagulation. One study showed thrombosis in 16% of THA patients and 31% after TKA. It has been recommended to use a combination of pharmacological anticoagulation with mechanical anticoagulation, such as intermittent pneumatic compression (ICP) (6). It is important to educate the patient on the signs and symptoms of blood clots such as leg swelling, redness, and pain. It is essential to discuss all the medications with the patient and help him or her understand the importance of blood thinners.

There are many available options for doctors and patients to consider for venous thromboembolism prophylaxis such as warfarin, low-molecular-weight heparin, aspirin, rivaroxaban, fondaparinux, and compression devices for the lower extremities. It is important to not only understand the prophylaxis benefits of these drugs but also consider the bleeding risks that come with some of these therapies (7). Each drug has its negatives and positives that need to be considered and discussed with the patient. For example, warfarin is a low-cost anticoagulant that has shown efficacy in prevention of venous thromboembolisms and has lower rates of bleeding, but this benefit is only with compliance of the INR between 2 and 3 (7). Studies have shown that up to 83% of total hip and knee arthroplasty patients are nontherapeutic on postoperative day 4 (7). This shows that warfarin is an effective medication but is limited by the ability to control the medication within the therapeutic window. Before placing a patient on anticoagulants it is important to consider all of the risk factors and choose the medication that is best suited for the patient.

Hip Dislocation

Developing a hip dislocation is a potential complication following THA. Hip adduction or flexion greater than 90° can cause the newly implanted hip to dislocate. To prevent dislocations, hip precautions are prescribed: (a) no hip adduction across the midline, (b) no hip flexion greater than 90°. Placing an abduction pillow between the patient's legs can be of benefit. If a dislocation occurs, the patient may be fitted for a brace to maintain the correct position.

Hip Fracture

A fracture of the hip is another complication post surgery. Healthy areas of the hip may sustain small fractures, which can either heal on their own or require bone grafts to fix. To prevent fractures post THA, bisphosphonates can be used to decrease the risk through primary prevention and secondary prevention by 44% and 50% (8).

Infections

Infections are a complication of any surgery at the incision site. It is important to do proper wound care for the incision as well as be able to recognize whether the wound is infected early so antibiotics can be started appropriately. Removing a urinary catheter on postoperative day 1 can help reduce the predisposition for getting a urinary tract infection. By administering antibiotics before and after the surgery, infections can be prevented. Preoperative screening for nasal bacterial colonization several weeks prior to surgery can help detect potential sources that predispose prosthetics to infections (9).

Pressure Ulcers

Patients who are immobilized in a hospital bed have an increased likelihood of developing pressure ulcers. It is important to use devices that will alleviate pressure from dependent areas and rotate the patient when appropriate. It is also important to monitor any skin breakdown that will potentially lead to ulcer development. It is also important to monitor both the operated side and the nonoperated side. Areas such as the sacrum and heels are especially prone to developing pressure ulcers, so it is particularly important to monitor these areas for skin breakdown.

Falls

Injuries associated with falls can be avoided if the patient uses his or her walker or cane appropriately and waits until he or she has assistance. This is sometimes hard for a previously independent patient to understand. Along with the hip or knee being unstable to fully bear weight, the patient may also have postural hypotension from lying in bed for a long period of time. Educating the patient about the risk of falls and providing assistance can prevent these injuries from occurring in the inpatient setting. Environmental modifications such as lowering the patient's bed and ensuring that the brakes are on, eliminating clutter around the bedside, and educating the patient to use a call bell are all important to minimize risk of falls. Educating the patient on reoccurrence of falls if they do happen is just as important as preventing falls in the first place.

Contractures

Hip or knee flexion contractures can occur following lower joint arthroplasty. This is a significant complication since it can limit functional use of the limb post surgery. All efforts should be made to minimize contractures. This includes adequate pain control during rehabilitation so that the patient can perform range of motion and strengthening exercises and use of braces as necessary. Timely and effective communication with the orthopedist and treating therapists is essential.

Footdrop

Footdrop is a possible complication following joint arthroplasty of the hip or knee. Possible etiologies include injury to the sciatic or common peroneal nerve. The incidence of footdrop is fairly low with Weber et al. reporting a 0.07% incidence in 2,012 hip arthroplasties (10). Occasionally footdrop may occur secondary to acquired spinal stenosis after joint arthroplasty. Sometimes this can occur up to 9 months after surgery (11).

Physical examination can identify weakness in key muscle groups involved in knee flexion and foot dorsiflexion coupled with sensory loss depending on underlying location of injury. Nerve conduction studies and electromyography can help localize the site of nerve injury and determine severity. If the site is at the fibular neck, extra cushioning while sleeping and avoidance of crossing legs can help alleviate further compression at that site. Ankle-foot orthoses will help keep the foot dorsiflexed during the rehabilitation.

MEDICAL KNOWLEDGE

GOALS

Demonstrate knowledge of established and evolving biomedical, clinical epidemiological, and sociobehavioral sciences pertaining to hip and knee arthroplasty, as well as the application of this knowledge to guide holistic patient care.

OBJECTIVES

1. Discuss the following as they relate to hip and knee joint arthroplasty: (a) epidemiology, (b) indications and contraindications, (c) surgical procedure, and (d) rehabilitation.

EPIDEMIOLOGY

Knee and hip joint arthroplasty surgeries have increased over the past decade in North America (12). From 1991 to 2010 TKAs alone increased 162%, with an annual procedure rate of about 600,000 procedures (13). Kurtz et al. reported on the prevalence of primary and revision TKA and THA in the United States using data from the National Hospital Discharge Survey and U.S. Census from 1990 to 2002 and found 50% increase in the rate of primary THAs. Rates for primary TKAs almost tripled. Rates for revisions of TKAs and THAs also increased. The authors concluded that in the future the rates for these procedures will continue to increase (14). Mehrotra et al. reviewed the data from hospital discharges in Wisconsin from 1990 to 2000 and reported that the increase in the number of TKAs performed was greatest in the 40- to 49-year-old population. The cost associated with these procedures increased 109%, with Medicare receiving the highest proportion of charges (15). The finding that joint arthroplasty is being performed in younger populations has been reported elsewhere in the literature as well (16). Racial disparities between different groups have also been described, with fewer rates for TKAs being performed for African Americans, Hispanics, Chinese, and Filipino compared to Caucasians (12,17).

INDICATIONS AND CONTRAINDICATIONS

The primary indication for THA and TKA is to reduce pain and disability in the knee and hip, respectively, that have not responded well to conservative management. The cause of the pain and disability can be attributed to irreversible damage to the bone and cartilage in the joint. Some of the etiologies of joint disease requiring surgery include osteoarthritis, rheumatoid arthritis, avascular necrosis, trauma, and childhood joint disease (18).

Some relative contraindications to surgery include individuals who are (a) not good surgical candidates, (b) nonambulatory, and (c) have osteomyelitis (19). In the past older populations were not deemed good candidates for lower limb joint replacement surgery due to factors and comorbidities associated with advanced age; however, studies have shown that despite a long rehabilitation, this group of individuals can still have very good long-term outcomes (20).

SURGICAL TECHNIQUE

Total Hip Arthroplasty

This surgical procedure is performed in an operating room by an orthopedic surgeon and can take up to 3 hours. It can be performed with the patient under spinal/epidural or general anesthesia. The surgeons generally approach the surgery by making a single incision in either the posterior or lateral portion of the hip. A recent review of the literature did not find significant differences between these two approaches; however, it mentioned that there may be an increased risk of nerve injury utilizing a direct lateral approach (21). The procedure consists of removing the damaged femoral head and cartilage using a specialized tool called a reamer. The reamer scrapes away damaged tissue to prepare the socket for the new hip replacement. Once the socket is prepared, the acetabular component of the hip replacement (called the shell or cup) is placed into the acetabulum. This "cup" is fit to be slightly bigger than the cleared acetabular space to allow for a tight fit between the hardware and the pelvis. The femur is then prepared and a femoral stem is placed into the bone. The femoral stem can be held with or without the use of cement. Once the stem is in place, the metal ball is fit tightly into it. Once the ball is on the stem, the hip can be reduced and the hip joint is intact and in the proper location. The incision is closed and proper dressing placed.

Total Knee Arthroplasty Surgery

This surgical procedure is performed in an operating room by an orthopedic surgeon and can take up to 2 hours. In the initial step, the diseased distal end of the femur and proximal end of the tibia are removed to ensure a good surface for the new joint. In the second step, the metal implants used to recreate the joint are "press fit" or cemented into the bone for a secure placement (22). Once the implants have been placed, some surgeons resurface the underside of the patella with a plastic button. A spacer is then inserted between the two metal components to allow for a smooth articulating surface. A review of the literature reported a greater risk of future aseptic loosening for cemented fixation vs. cementless fixation (23).

REHABILITATION

Early rehabilitation after surgery can help improve outcomes such as achievement of functional milestones, fewer postoperative complications, and shorter hospital stay (24).

Cryotherapy has been used following TKA; however, a recent review of the literature found a low level of quality for the evidence of its effect on postoperative pain, range of motion, and length of stay (25).

There is evidence that the use of continuous passive motion (CPM) following TKA can improve active and passive range of motion of the joint a few degrees more than without the use of CPM; however, the total number of degrees is too small to be clinically relevant according to the authors (26). The use of neuromuscular electrical stimulation has been described for the purpose of improving quadriceps strength before and after TKA; however, its effectiveness and use is inconclusive at this time (27).

PRACTICE-BASED LEARNING AND IMPROVEMENT

GOALS

Demonstrate competence in continuously investigating and evaluating your own patient care practices for patients undergoing THA and TKA, appraising and assimilating scientific evidence, and continuously improving your patient care practices based on constant self-evaluation and lifelong learning.

OBJECTIVES

1. Describe learning opportunities for providers, patients, and caregivers with experience in THA and TKA.
2. Use methods for ongoing competency training in the rehabilitation and medical management of patients with a THA and TKA for physiatrists, including formative evaluation feedback in daily practice, evaluating current practice, and developing a systematic QI and practice improvement strategy.
3. Locate some resources including available websites for continuing medical education and continuing professional development.
4. Describe some areas paramount to self-assessment and lifelong learning such as review of current guidelines, including evidence-based, in treatment of patients with THA and TKA, and the role of the physiatrist as the educator of patients, families, residents, students, colleagues, and other health professionals.

As a physiatrist, it is essential to always self-evaluate and recognize one's own strengths and weaknesses. With respect to the care of the adult patient post lower extremity, hip, or knee arthroplasty, the physiatrist should keep up-to-date on the current surgical procedures, types of implants used, and complications associated with both of them. Examples of resources include Cochrane reviews, Knowledge NOW, orthopedic journals, and scientific meetings.

The physiatrist should also be familiar with advances in rehabilitative treatments as well as health insurance coverage issues as they pertain to rehabilitation following these surgeries.

Areas of quality and performance improvement activity in the care of adults post lower extremity joint arthroplasty may include (a) reduction of the incidence of flexion contractures of the hip and knee post joint arthroplasty, (b) reduction of the incidence of venous thromboembolism disease post surgery, (c) incidence of infections at surgical site as well as urinary tract infections, (d) length of stay on an inpatient rehabilitation facility, and (e) level of function at time of discharge from rehabilitation facility.

INTERPERSONAL AND COMMUNICATION SKILLS

GOALS

Demonstrate interpersonal and communication skills that result in the effective exchange of information and collaboration with patients, their families, and other health professionals.

OBJECTIVES

1. Discuss the key areas for physicians to counsel patients and families across socioeconomic and cultural backgrounds.
2. Identify key elements that need to be documented in the patient's medical record.
3. Demonstrate skills for effective communication and listening skills.
4. Demonstrate leadership skills and consultative role as it relates to hip and knee arthroplasty.

Communication and interpersonal skills are an integral part of the care of adults post lower extremity joint arthroplasty. In order to be effective, the physiatrist must be an excellent communicator with team members such as physical and occupational therapists, rehabilitation nurses, social workers, and consultants involved in the patient's care. Communication should be provided in a collaborative, collegial, and nonjudgmental manner. Opportunities for effective communication can be identified in formal (team conferences) and informal settings. An effective communication tool is the SBAR methodology (28) with read back. In this technique, the situation, background, assessment, and recommendations are communicated from one provider to another. To ensure that the message is clearly communicated, the recipient then repeats back the information provided. This approach can be used in person as well as on the phone.

Communication with the patient is equally important to ensure that the material provided is clearly understood by the patient. The patient should be provided with information on (a) what he or she needs to do, (b) why he or she needs to do it, and (c) the consequences if he or she doesn't follow the instructions. To ensure that the patient understands the information provided, he or she should be asked to repeat back the information to the clinician. This provides an opportunity for the clinician to correct any mistakes.

Documentation is an integral part of patient care. Maintaining good medical records is a skill that physiatrists learn in their residency training and continue learning throughout their career. The patient's chart is an important medium in which all members of the clinical team communicate with each other. The information provided can help inform other clinicians about pertinent information about the patient such as complications post surgery and relevant precautions to be carried out during rehabilitation.

Effective communication between patient and physician is one of the most important factors in developing trust and building a therapeutic relationship to ultimately improve the health of the patient. Starting from the initial appointment patients begin to form an opinion about how trustworthy, honest, intelligent, and reliable their physician is. It is important to understand how the relationship with the patient can either improve or deter from the ultimate treatment-based efforts. When gathering information about the patient, it is always important to ascertain his or her understanding of the joint arthroplasty procedure, its possible complications, and the rehabilitation process. The physiatrist should provide information at an appropriate level that takes into account the patient's prior educational level and then ask him or her to repeat back the information to ensure understanding. Personalized information can be especially effective in engaging the patient in his or her recovery.

In the field of physiatry, leadership skills are a very important "tool kit" that can greatly improve the physiatrist's ability to effectively manage his or her patients' care. During the course of their training, physiatrists have many opportunities to participate in and lead conferences, rounds, discharge planning, and other multidisciplinary meetings. The role of a physiatrist within team conferences is to monitor and guide the therapies and treatments. This open forum for all of the disciplines to participate can be quite daunting for physiatrists who are not used to facilitating a large group of professionals. As the leader, the physiatrist will need to make sure that the group is on task, that the best possible care is being provided to all patients, and that everyone has the opportunity to have input. It is also important to take the opportunity to review and reinforce specific precautions or medication alerts with the team that are relevant to the patient's care.

PROFESSIONALISM

GOALS

Reflect a commitment to carrying out professional responsibilities and an adherence to ethical principles in caring for joint arthroplasty patients.

OBJECTIVES

1. Demonstrate appropriate humanistic qualities.
2. Display sensitivity to a diverse patient population (culture, gender, age, race, religion, disabilities, sexual orientation).
3. Demonstrate respect for patient privacy and autonomy.
4. Demonstrate advocacy, responsibility, accountability, and commitment to excellence in quality care.
5. Demonstrate responsiveness to patient needs superseding self-interest as it relates to joint arthroplasty.

As with any patient, physiatrists should approach patient care with compassion and courtesy. Demonstrating respect to patients and their families is a cornerstone of developing an effective therapeutic alliance. Patients and their families should be treated in a courteous and kind manner by the health care team. Being diagnosed with osteoarthritis or undergoing a THA or TKA can be a very frightening proposition. Through a kind and compassionate bedside manner, physiatrists can help patients with the challenges faced during their rehabilitation.

It is important for the physiatrist to understand the impact of joint arthroplasty surgery in the context of the patient's cultural background, his or her religious beliefs, and role played in the family and community. When undergoing a large operation such as hip or knee surgery, a patient who was managing independently prior to the surgery has to become dependent on others for a period of time. This may be extremely difficult depending on the patient's role in his or her family and community. For example, in some cultures, the woman may be the only person in the home that cooks and cleans; however, once home following this major surgery she may not be able to completely fulfill this role until her recovery is complete.

Postoperative pain management is another area in which it is essential to have a good understanding of the cultural background of the patient. Cultural sensitivity is important when discussing treatment options for pain. In some cultures a homeopathic approach is preferred, whereas in other cultures a patient may prefer medications. Addressing the pain and being aware of the patient's wishes shows cultural sensitivity and respect for the patient and his or her family.

In this era of technology-based communication, it is important to maintain patient privacy and be vigilant for possible privacy violations. Discussing patient information in the hallways or elevators, checking laboratories or information on a computer in a common area, and leaving documents with patient information in conference rooms are all examples of violations of patient privacy.

Successfully advocating for the patient post THA or TKA when he or she is in a vulnerable state is a cornerstone of high-quality physiatric care. It requires carefully listening to the patient's needs and concerns and then acting on his or her behalf with his or her best interest in mind. Some examples include (a) coordinating medical care among the various medical and surgical consultants, (b) ensuring that clinical care is continued in a safe manner at transition points such as admission and discharge from an inpatient rehabilitation facility, and (c) case management with health insurance companies to ensure that the patient has adequate therapy services, medications, and adaptive equipment as he or she transitions to home or other rehabilitation settings (e.g., subacute rehabilitation).

SYSTEMS-BASED PRACTICE

GOALS

Awareness and responsiveness to systems of care delivery, and the ability to recruit and coordinate effectively resources in the system to provide optimal care in the rehabilitation continuum for patients that have undergone THA or TKA.

OBJECTIVES

1. Identify the components, systems of care delivery, services, referral patterns, and resources in the rehabilitation continuum for patients post THA or TKA.
2. Describe what constitutes effective patient safety following THA or TKA.
3. Discuss the importance of documentation throughout the care of the patient following THA or TKA.
4. Coordinate and recruit necessary resources in the system to provide optimal care for patients following THA or TKA, with attention to cost considerations, risk–benefit analysis, socioeconomics, and follow-up management.

5. Introduce quality improvement as a key factor in joint arthroplasty rehabilitation programs, including identification of systems errors.

Following a total joint arthroplasty of the lower extremities, rehabilitation is typically performed in a variety of settings such as (a) acute inpatient rehabilitation facilities, (b) subacute rehabilitation facilities, (c) outpatient rehabilitation facilities, and (d) patient's home. The decision on the most appropriate setting depends on a variety of factors such as his or her medical condition, ability to tolerate a rehabilitation program, health insurance coverage, and extent of family support upon discharge to home. The physiatrist is the ideal clinician to be involved in this type of decision making.

Once the patient is deemed to be medically stable to undergo intensive rehabilitation, he or she may be admitted to an acute inpatient rehabilitation facility where he or she will stay for approximately 5 to 7 days and receive approximately 3 hours of therapy per day. While in that facility, physical and occupational therapists will work with the patient on ambulation, transfers, and activities of daily living. Alternatively, the patient may be discharged to a subacute rehabilitation facility if he or she is older, frailer, has poor endurance to tolerate a rehabilitation program in an acute inpatient rehabilitation facility, or is deemed to require a longer and slower paced course of rehabilitation. This latter option is also available to patients who had a slower course of recovery in an inpatient rehabilitation facility and are not ready to return home.

Follow-up care of a patient who has had a total joint arthroplasty is important to achieve the maximal recovery. Once the surgery has been completed the process of continued rehabilitation is an essential component. Within 24 hours after surgery, rehabilitation will begin and daily physical therapy will continue through the course of the patient's stay at the hospital. Once the patient has been discharged, it is essential for him or her to understand the importance of attending therapy sessions as well as continuing the exercises at home. Outpatient therapy is a vital part of the rehabilitation process, and frequency of therapy sessions is variable among physiatrists but should initially be done at least weekly; in addition, a follow-up appointment with the physiatrist should be scheduled within a few weeks of discharge. It is also important for follow-up care to be provided by the surgeons to make sure that the incision is healing properly and that there are no surgical complications.

As previously mentioned, there are a number of complications that may occur following a THA or TKA. These include (a) dislocations of the hip, (b) hip or knee flexion contractures, (c) venous thromboembolism, (d) infections at the surgical site and of the urinary tract, (e) pressure ulcers, and (f) falls. It is important that the physiatrist use a proactive approach to minimize the risk of occurrence and actively address them once they have been identified. The patient should also be educated about these potential complications and be involved in efforts to minimize their occurrence.

To ensure that high-quality rehabilitative care is provided, there are a number of quality performance indicators that can be monitored and compared against appropriate benchmarks. If these benchmarks are not available, physiatrists should develop their own for their practices and institutions. Some benchmarks include (a) level of function at time of discharge from inpatient rehabilitation, (b) length of stay on an inpatient rehabilitation unit, (c) patient satisfaction with care rendered during period of rehabilitation, and (d) complication rate for the previously mentioned potential complications. Deviations from benchmarks can therefore trigger a quality improvement program.

The total joint arthroplasty patient moves through multiple transition points during his or her care. These are present in the acute hospital setting as the patient moves from the operating room to an intensive care unit or surgical ward. Once medically stable to undergo rehabilitation, the patient may be transferred to either a rehabilitation unit in the hospital or another institution that provides these services. During the rehabilitation stay, the patient may need to be transferred acutely if a complication develops. Once discharged from a rehabilitation facility, the patient will go to either his or her own home or an alternate facility. These transition points in care are especially vulnerable to communication errors between providers. Medication errors and errors regarding precautions following total joint arthroplasty are some examples.

To maximize patient safety during these transition points in care, it is important to ensure that the "hand-off" of patient care is done in an area free of distractions to allow proper communication between physicians. Important elements of a good hand-off include (a) updated medication list, (b) patient's medical and surgical history and pertinent complications, (c) weight-bearing status, and (d) pertinent precautions relevant to the rehabilitation program (e.g., THA precautions).

As mentioned earlier, the SBAR is a structured method of communicating patient information across the medical team that was described earlier (29). This method helps eliminate miscommunication between all of the members of the medical team during hand-offs at transition points in care. By using this mnemonic, physiatrists can help elucidate the information that is necessary for other team members to be well informed and make sure patient care is optimized.

There are many areas in the rehabilitation process that are very expensive and need to be evaluated for their cost-to-benefit ratio. It is important that all quality of care indices are evaluated and implemented to maximize patient outcomes while decreasing the cost of care. There are many costs associated with rehabilitation following THA or TKA starting with inpatient care. While the patient is admitted to the inpatient rehabilitation facility, there are many services that the patient will receive during his or her stay. These services typically include physical therapy, occupational therapy, imaging, and laboratory studies. Costs can be reduced through timely discharge planning, diligent management of medical comorbidities such as hypertension, and attentiveness to postsurgical complications. Being diligent in these areas helps the physiatrist decrease the length of stay and therefore decrease the health care expenditure for the patient.

CASE STUDY

A retired 61-year-old man with a past medical history significant for obesity, hypertension, diabetes mellitus, and myocardial infarction has been having increasing difficulty walking over the past 10 years. He was a police officer, who had played college football, before retiring 5 years ago due to difficulty performing his work-related duties.

Over the past 2 years, he has been suffering from chronic knee pain and has had difficulty performing activities of daily living. He suffers from decreased active range of motion in both knees, and bilateral pain in both knees, his right knee worse than his left knee. He describes pain that worsens with physical activity and is relieved by rest and over-the-counter pain medication. He had one fall at home 2 months ago, but did not suffer any negative sequela from it.

After conservative therapies failed to improve his function, he underwent a right TKA and is referred for physiatrist management of his rehabilitative care.

CASE STUDY DISCUSSION QUESTIONS

1. Identify the pertinent medical and rehabilitative issues for this patient during his postoperative care and rehabilitation and describe how you would manage them.
2. Write a rehabilitation treatment plan for this patient following the TKA.
3. Identify the patient safety concerns for this patient during his postoperative care and describe strategies to minimize their occurrence.
4. What important information needs to be communicated to the patient regarding the TKA, potential complications, and the rehabilitation program thereafter?
5. What are some key resources for furthering your education about total knee arthroplasty and the rehabilitation process thereafter using evidence-based resources?
6. Describe the key components of the rehabilitation continuum of care for this patient.

SELF-EXAMINATION QUESTIONS
(Answers begin on p. 367)

1. Which of the following is not a complication of THA or TKA?
   A. Deep vein thrombosis
   B. Paresthesia
   C. Increased muscle tone
   D. Infection
   E. Contractures

2. What is the average life span of a lower extremity joint arthroplasty?
   A. 1 to 4 years
   B. 5 to 9 years
   C. 10 to 20 years
   D. 20 to 30 years
   E. Forever

3. What complication of lower extremity joint arthroplasty can be directly avoided with postoperative antibiotics? (9)
   A. Bone fracture
   B. Joint dislocation
   C. Infection
   D. Contracture
   E. Joint pain

4. Which of the following could be a cause of adult hip pain?
   A. Rheumatoid arthritis
   B. Trauma
   C. Avascular necrosis
   D. Osteoarthritis
   E. All of the above

5. According to recent studies, what is the percent increase in the number of primary THAs?
   A. 5
   B. 15
   C. 25
   D. 50
   E. 75

REFERENCES

1. Passias P, Bono J. Total hip arthroplasty in the older population. *Geriatr Aging.* 2006;9(8):535–543.
2. Longo D, Fauci A, Kasper D, et al. *Harrison's Principles of Internal Medicine.* Vol. 2. 18th ed. New York, NY: McGraw Hill Companies Inc. 2012:2828–2836.
3. Bjorgul K, Novicoff WM, Saleh K. Evaluating co morbidities in total hip and knee arthroplasty: available instruments. *J Orthop Traumatol.* December 2010;11(4):203–209.
4. Rasul A, Wright J. Total joint replacement rehabilitation. http://emedicine.medscape.com/article/320061-overview#a30. Accessed January 9, 2013.
5. Up to Date. Total Hip Replacement (arthroplasty) (beyond the basics). http://www.uptodate.com/contents/total-hip-replacement-arthroplasty-beyond-the-basics?source=search_result&search=total+hip+arthroplasty&selectedTitle=3~88. Accessed January 10, 2013.
6. Silbersack Y. Prevention of deep-vein thrombosis after total hip and knee replacement. *J Bone Joint Surg.* 2004;86-B(6). http://www.bjj.boneandjoint.org.uk/content/86-B/6/809.full.pdf.
7. Knesek D, Peterson T, Merkell D. Review article thromboembolic prophylaxis in total joint arthroplasty. *Thrombosis.* 2012;2012:8. Article ID 837896.
8. Prieto-Alhambra D, Javaid MK, Judge A, et al. Fracture risk before and after total hip replacement in patients with osteoarthritis: potential benefits of bisphosphonate use. *Arthritis Rheumatol.* April 2011;63(4):992–1001.
9. "Joint Replacement Infection." American Academy of Orthopaedic Surgeons, October 2012. Web. February 2013. http://orthoinfo.aaos.org/topic.cfm?topic=A00629.
10. Weber ER, Daube JR, Coventry MB. Peripheral neuropathies associated with total hip arthroplasty. *J Bone Joint Surg.* 1976;58A:66. http://jbjs.org/pdfaccess.ashx?ResourceID=22491&PDFSource=
11. McNamara MJ, Barrett KG, Christie MJ, et al. Lumbar spinal stenosis and lower extremity arthroplasty. *J Arthroplasty* 1993;8(3):273–277. http://www.ncbi.nlm.nih.gov/pubmed/8326308.
12. Singh JA. Epidemiology of knee and hip arthroplasty: a systematic review. *Open Orthop J.* 2011;5:80–85. Published online March 16, 2011. doi:10.2174/1874325001105010080. PMCID: PMC3092498.
13. Ruiz D, Koenig L, Dall T, et al. The direct and indirect costs to society of treatment for end-stage knee osteoarthritis. *J Bone Joint Surg.* 2013;95(16):1473–1480.
14. Kurtz S, Mowat F, Ong K, et al. Prevalence of primary and revision total hip and knee arthroplasty in the United States from 1990 through 2002. *J Bone Joint Surg Am.* 2005;87(7):1487–1497.

15. Mehrotra C, Remington PL, Naimi TS, et al. Trends in total knee replacement surgeries and implications for public health, 1990–2000. *Public Health Rep.* 2005;120(3):278–282.
16. Ravi B, Croxford R, Reichmann WM, et al. The changing demographics of total joint arthroplasty recipients in the United States and Ontario from 2001 to 2007. *Best Pract Res Clin Rheumatol.* October 2012;26(5):637–647. doi:10.1016/j.berh.2012.07.014.
17. Centers for Disease Control and Prevention. Racial disparities in total knee replacement among Medicare enrollees—United States, 2000–2006. *MMWR Morb Mortal Wkly Rep.* 2009;58(6):133–138.
18. Total Hip Replacement. American Academy of Orthopaedic Surgeons, December 2011. http://orthoinfo.aaos.org/topic.cfm?topic=A00629. Accessed February 2, 2014.
19. Total Knee Replacement. OrthopaedicsOne review. In: *OrthopaedicsOne—The Orthopaedic Knowledge Network.* Created March 7, 2010 15:41. Last modified February 17, 2011 15:04 ver.13. http://www.orthopaedicsone.com/x/eQHYAQ. Accessed February 2, 2014.
20. Hamel MB, Toth M, Legedza A, et al. Joint replacement surgery in elderly patients with severe osteoarthritis of the hip or knee. *Arch Intern Med.* 2008;168:1430–1440. doi:10.1001/archinte.168.13.1430.
21. Jolles BM, Bogoch ER. Posterior versus lateral surgical approach for total hip arthroplasty in adults with osteoarthritis. *Cochrane Database Syst Rev.* 2006;(3). Article No.: CD003828. doi:10.1002/14651858.CD003828.
22. Total Knee Replacement. American Academy of Orthopaedic Surgeons. http://orthoinfo.aaos.org/topic.cfm?topic=a00389. Accessed January 10, 2013.
23. Hartl A, Schillinger M, Wanivenhaus A. Cemented versus cementless total hip arthroplasty for osteoarthrosis and other non-traumatic diseases. *Cochrane Database Syst Rev.* 2004;(3). Article No.: CD004850. doi:10.1002/14651858.CD004850 –.
24. Khan F, Ng L, Gonzalez S, et al. Multidisciplinary rehabilitation programmes following joint replacement at the hip and knee in chronic arthropathy. *Cochrane Collaboration.* January 2009;(1).
25. Adie S, Kwan A, Naylor JM, et al. Cryotherapy following total knee replacement. *Cochrane Database Syst Rev.* 2012;(9). Article No.: CD007911. doi:10.1002/14651858.CD007911.pub2.
26. Harvey LA, Brosseau L, Herbert RD. Continuous passive motion after knee replacement surgery. *Cochrane Summaries.* March 17, 2010.
27. Monaghan B, Caulfield B, O'Mathúna DP. Surface neuromuscular electrical stimulation for quadriceps strengthening pre and post total knee replacement. *Cochrane Database Syst Rev.* 2010;(1). Article No.: CD007177. doi:10.1002/14651858.CD007177.pub2.
28. SBAR: Situation-Background-Assessment-Recommendation. Institute for Healthcare Improvement. http://www.ihi.org/explore/sbarcommunicationtechnique/pages/default.aspx. Accessed February 14, 2013.
29. "Situation Background Assessment Recommendation—NHS Institute for Innovation and Improvement." Situation Background Assessment Recommendation—NHS Institute for Innovation and Improvement. NHS, n.d. Web. March 3, 2013. http://www.institute.nhs.uk/safer_care/safer_care/Situation_Background_Assessment_Recommendation.html.
30. Joint Revision Surgery—When Do I Need It? American Academy of Orthopaedic Surgeons. 2007. http://orthoinfo.aaos.org/topic.cfm?topic=A00510. Accessed February 1, 2014.

Navdeep Singh Jassal
Dayna McCarthy
Jennifer Schoenfeld
Matthew Shatzer

22: Spasticity

PATIENT CARE

GOALS

Provide competent patient care that is compassionate, appropriate, and effective for the evaluation, treatment, education, and advocacy for patients with spasticity-associated problems across the entire spectrum of care, and the promotion of health.

OBJECTIVES

1. Describe the key elements of the history and pertinent physical examination of the patient with spasticity.
2. Discuss the impairments, functional limitations, and activity limitations relevant to spasticity.
3. Describe the impact of spasticity on work, school, and community activity.
4. Propose the long-term consequences of spasticity (e.g., contractures, skin breakdown, etc.).
5. Identify potential injuries associated with spasticity (e.g., falls).
6. Identify the psychosocial and vocational implications of the patient with spasticity and strategies to address them.
7. Formulate the key components of a rehabilitation or treatment plan for the patient with spasticity (e.g., stretching program, modalities, etc.).

Clinical evaluation of the patient presenting with muscle overreactivity first and foremost requires an in-depth understanding of the patient's underlying condition (i.e., spinal cord injury [SCI], traumatic brain injury [TBI], cerebral palsy [CP], stroke) as this will help guide the physician's treatment plan. Long-term treatment goals and functional goals are heavily influenced by whether the underlying pathology is progressive versus static, whether the condition is acute or chronic, as well as past treatments utilized and their outcomes. Other etiologies of increased tone such as rigidity, catatonia, gegenhalten, or contractures (1) must also be ruled out. Identification of potential triggers such as pressure ulcers, ingrown toenails, catheter obstruction, kidney stones, urinary tract infection (UTI), deep venous thrombosis (DVT), heterotopic ossification, constipation/impaction, sepsis, and/or fractures commonly leads to increased tone and should be identified during initial evaluation. Improper body positioning can often contribute to worsening spasticity and contracture. Postures that have a negative impact include a scissoring posture (bilateral hip extension, adduction, internal rotation), windswept position (hip flexion, abduction, external rotation on one side and relative hip extension, adduction, and internal rotation on the other), and frog-leg position. Identification of a clinical pattern (e.g., location, duration, frequency), the presence of pain, the patient's ability to control involved muscle groups, and the functional impact are also included in comprehensive history pertaining to spasticity.

When approaching the physical examination, there are several key features that help the clinician identify spasticity. Velocity dependence is a requirement in the diagnosis of spasticity; this condition is defined as a velocity-dependent increase in tone. Currently, the Modified Ashworth Scale (MAS) that tests resistance to passive movement about a joint with varying degrees of velocity and is scaled from 0 to 4—with 0 indicating no tone and 4 indicating rigidity—is the most widely utilized scoring system to classify tone. In addition, there is the Tardieu scale, which quantifies muscle spasticity by assessing the response of the muscle to stretch applied at specified velocities. The MAS, in addition to motor strength testing and thorough ROM testing, comprises the most important clinical examination findings for spasticity. Special signs that may be present on examination are the "Clasp-knife" phenomenon as well as the "stroking effect," which are not pathognomonic but are commonly elicited. Spasticity more commonly affects antigravity muscles in the upper extremity. The most common patterns of upper motor neuron dysfunction include adducted/internally rotated shoulder, flexed elbow, pronated forearm, bent wrist, clenched fist, thumb in

257

palm, and an intrinsic plus hand. In the lower extremity most commonly seen patterns include flexed hip, scissoring thighs, stiff knee, flexed knee, equinovarus foot with curl or claw toes, valgus foot, and hyperextended first toe.

Limitations as a result of spasticity are dependent on severity and muscle involvement. At the very least it can cause discomfort and pain. Because it limits joint range of motion (ROM), it has the potential to limit mobility and produce deformities if left untreated. Most individuals will require orthosis for independent mobility. If the spasticity is severe enough, mobility may be limited to a wheelchair. Limited mobility may also result in pressure changes that can lead to skin breakdown. Spasticity can present challenges in respect to hygiene maintenance, bowel/bladder care, and sexual relationships, as the axilla, hands, and genitals can be difficult to access. It is important to understand that spasticity is not always detrimental. For instance, spasticity in trunk muscles may help with transfers; hip and knee extensor spasticity facilitates standing, transfers, and ambulation; soleus spasticity helps children with CP toe off; and finger flexor spasticity may allow people to manage utensils and self-care items.

Spasticity can substantially impact the quality of life in those affected. In surveys of patients' perceptions of problems, spasticity has been consistently identified in the top three to five life concerns (2). The Patient Reported Impact of Spasticity Measure (PRISM) was created to define and measure extents to which quality of life is affected in SCI patients with spasticity. The 7 factors assessed are social avoidance/anxiety, psychological agitation, daily activities, need for assistance/positioning, positive impact, need for intervention, and social embarrassment (3). Although this scale is used in a specific subset of patients with spasticity, it can be extrapolated for the spastic population and can offer insight into common difficulties that they face in interactive environments.

Left untreated, spasticity can lead to contractures that are difficult to correct and make self-care, hygiene, mobility, and transfers extremely difficult for both patient and caregiver. Over time asymmetric pull of overactive muscles can cause deformities and alter posture. Positioning and pressure relief are constant considerations as there is a high prevalence of skin breakdown in this patient population. Most common areas of skin breakdown include hands, axilla, elbows, genital area, sacrum, and ischium.

The most common injuries seen as a result of spasticity are those related to impaired mobility, such as falls, and pressure ulcers. When a patient is nonambulatory secondary to spasticity he or she has a higher propensity to sustain fractures especially in long bones. Hip dislocation may also occur in those that have hip joint involvement that is severe.

The severity of spasticity will guide the treatment plan, and rehabilitation must always be included. When constructing a therapy plan for spasticity, the goal is to reduce pain, regain function, and/or preserve function. This is accomplished by focusing on aggressive passive ROM, with a goal of 2 hours of stretching per day. In cases of focal spasticity, splinting/orthosis may also be indicated. There are several different approaches utilized by physical therapists to treat spasticity; most literature exists regarding techniques for stroke patients. The Bobath method aims to reduce spasticity through attention to trunk posture and controlled muscle stretch of the limbs. The Brunnstrom method advocates techniques to promote activity in weak agonists by facilitating contraction of either corresponding muscles in the unaffected limb or proximal muscles on the paretic side. No solid evidence exists for the use of modalities for spasticity; however, there is a small body of evidence that electrical stimulation techniques, although used for movement loss related to muscle paresis, may prove to be a useful adjunct to other treatments such as Botox (4).

MEDICAL KNOWLEDGE

GOALS

Demonstrate knowledge of established and evolving biomedical, clinical epidemiological, and sociobehavioral sciences pertaining to spasticity, as well as the application of this knowledge to guide holistic patient care.

OBJECTIVES

1. Describe the epidemiology of spasticity.
2. Describe the anatomy, physiology, and pathophysiology of spasticity.
3. Review the treatment options and rehabilitation components in spasticity.
4. Recognize the complications and red flags associated with spasticity.

Spasticity is a condition seen in upper motor neuron disorders (UMNDs). Conditions that include spasticity as a clinical feature include but are not limited to SCI, stroke, multiple sclerosis, amyotrophic lateral sclerosis, hereditary spastic paraparesis, and CP. It is rare for spasticity to occur on its own; rather, it occurs as one of the positive components of UMND, which also include exaggerated tendon reflex, clonus, spastic dystonia, increased tone, released reflexes, and Babinski sign. UMNDs also comprise negative components which include loss of motor control, loss of selective motor control and dexterity, slowed movements, and spastic cocontractions (1).

To understand the pathophysiology of spasticity, it is important to first understand normal anatomy and physiology of motor control. The motor system is a highly complex and integrated system that requires input and constant feedback. At the most distal aspect of the system there is the motor unit that comprises three main fibers, Type 1 (slow, aerobic), Type II (fast, anaerobic), and mixed (both Type I and Type II). When working properly, motor units fire with the coordination of an agonist and antagonist system, with normal patterns of recruitment (5). A feedback loop utilizes input regarding muscle length, muscle tension, joint position, and velocity. Muscle spindles are a major contributor to the feedback loop (Figure 22.1A, B). Attached to the muscle mass and containing both Ia and II fibers, the spindle is responsible for relaying information regarding position and rate of change of the muscle throughout ROM. The spindle also contains the gamma motor neuron, which is responsible for maintaining proper tension of the spindle. Within the muscle tendon exists the Golgi tendon organ. Comprised of Ib fibers, it is responsible for limiting muscle contraction to prevent musculotendinous

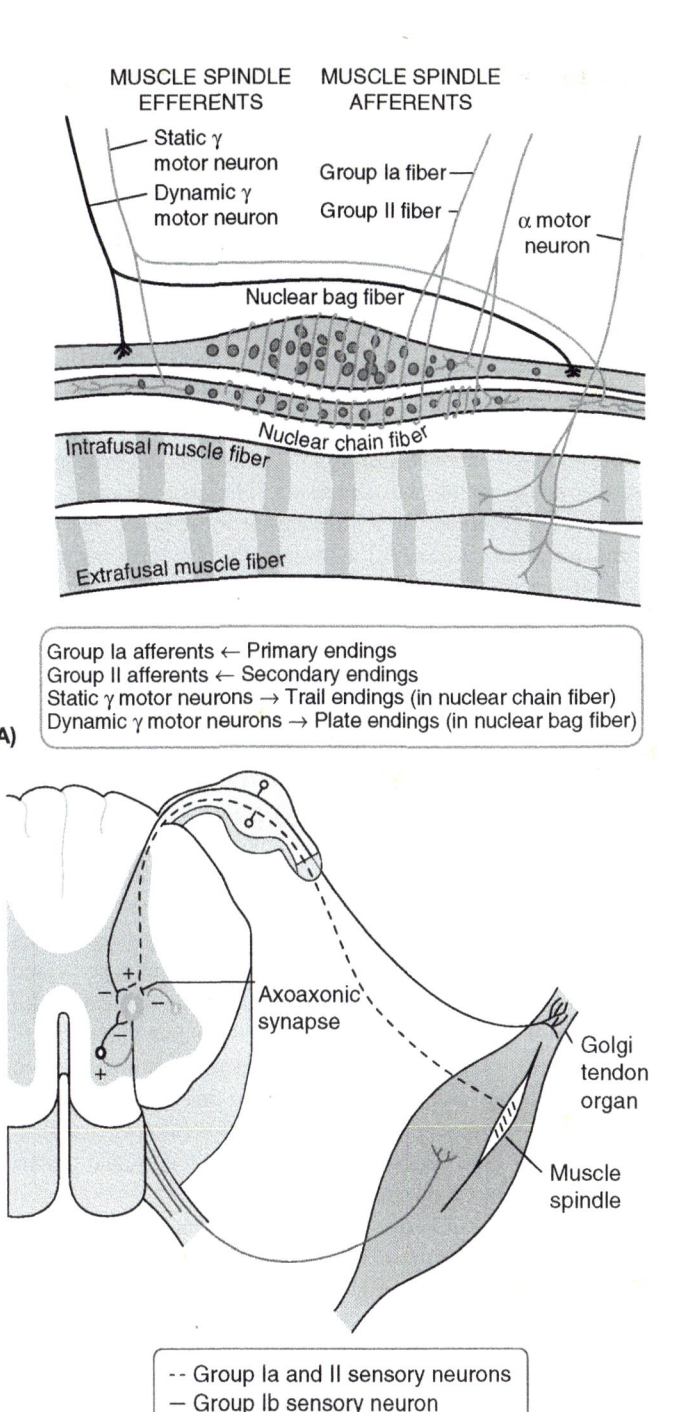

FIGURE 22.1 (A): Nuclear bag and nuclear chain fibers of the muscle spindle. **(B):** Influences on the stretch reflex. (Redrawn from Braddom, RL. *Physical Medicine & Rehabilitation*, 4th ed., Chapter 30, Philadelphia, PA: Elsevier; 2011.)

injury by initiating antagonist and inhibiting agonists. Moving proximally, spinal interneurons (Ia, Ib, Renshaw, propriospinal) play a large role in motor control. Ia and Ib interneurons work to facilitate both the muscle spindle and the Golgi tendon organs, respectively. Renshaw cells receive input directly from the alpha motor neuron allowing for direct cessation of agonist activity by directly engaging the alpha motor neuron. They also promote antagonist's function by way of the antagonist's Ia interneuron. Supraspinal stimuli are diverse and complex. The corticospinal tract is derived from extrapyramidal cells from the prefrontal region, the supplementary motor region, the cingulate gyrus, and the postcentral gyrus of the parietal lobe. Extensor pathways of the brain are the pontine medial reticulospinal and lateral vestibulospinal pathways. The pontine system facilitates the alpha and gamma motor neurons of the extensors of the limb muscles with some input into the system from the sensorimotor cortex. The lateral vestibular is found in the ventromedial portion of the cord and terminates at the spinal cord motor neurons. Stimulating this tract affects the motor neurons of the flexor muscles differently from the extensors, with the alpha and gamma motor neurons of the flexors inhibited and those of the extensors facilitated. The nucleus of the cerebellum also has an excitatory influence on extensor pathways (6). There are numerous pathways that facilitate flexion, whereas extensor inhibition occurs mainly in the medullary lateral reticular formation (MLRF). The cortex facilitates MLRF's action, and cortical injury can lead to net overactivity of the lower extremity extensor system. The MLRF demonstrates its effect through its connections to the motor neurons, type Ia interneurons, and type Ib system. In cats the corticospinal, corticoreticulospinal, and corticorubrospinal tracts all show significant flexor facilitation. Through interneurons, the corticorubrospinal tract excites flexor motor neurons and inhibits extensors. In addition, the medullary reticulospinal tract is a predominant part of a largely flexor-oriented system (7).

Spasticity is defined clinically as a motor disorder characterized by velocity-dependent increase in stretch reflexes with exaggerated tendon jerks, resulting from hyperexcitability of the stretch reflex. Although there is no definitive consensus on the pathophysiology of spasticity, the most commonly utilized theory is that a lower threshold exists for motor neuron response to stretch. This lower threshold is coupled with long discharges that result in an alteration of the balance between inhibitory and excitatory inputs to motor neurons, with the excitatory component being more frequently activated. Some have expressed the belief that the ionic properties of the membrane itself are changed as well. Other proposed theories involve central collateral sprouting, presynaptic disinhibition, and denervation hypersensitivity, as well as neurotransmitters serotonin and substance P malfunction (8).

There are a variety of treatment options available for spasticity. The clinician must be aware that increased tone is not always detrimental, in many cases the existence of tone allows for functional capacity that wouldn't be obtainable in its absence. As such, spasticity requires consistent monitoring and feedback by both the patient and the treatment team to maintain the appropriate balance for optimized function. Persistent neglect of this condition will lead to progression of spasticity and eventually rigidity and contractures. It is also a condition that fluctuates in severity based on nociceptive, visceral, or somatic stimuli. Depending on the primary pathology it may also worsen as the disease progresses. The goal of the provider when treating spasticity may include pain reduction, decreased spasms, facilitation of orthotic management, ease of care, changing positioning for pressure relief, release inhibition of antagonists, as well as improvement in hygiene, transfers, activities of daily living (ADLs), and mobility. As with most treatments it is always advisable to start conservatively, especially in the acute phase of the primary injury because more aggressive interventions may negatively impact recovery. As discussed previously, the mainstay of conservative management is constant stretching, minimum of 2 hours/day, to prevent progression of tone and to maintain ROM. In cases of focal spasticity, splinting/orthosis may also be indicated. There are several different approaches utilized by physical therapists to treat spasticity, and most literature exists regarding techniques for stroke patients. The Bobath method aims to reduce spasticity through attention to trunk posture and controlled muscle stretch of the limbs. The Brunnstrom method advocates techniques to promote activity in weak agonists by facilitating contraction of either corresponding muscles in the unaffected limb or proximal muscles on the paretic side. Other modalities that haven't been strongly studied but are still utilized by therapists include cryotherapy, electrical stimulation, splinting/casting, positioning, vibration therapy, and relaxation techniques.

If spasticity remains detrimental after conservative treatment and removal of inciting factors, then pharmacological management may be indicated. When considering oral medication for the treatment of spasticity the functional impairment and configuration of involved muscles must be factored into the choice of pharmacologic management. Generally speaking, individuals with processes that result in diffuse spasticity (i.e., SCI, MS) will respond to oral agents whereas those with focal spasticity will not. Current oral medications indicated for the treatment of spasticity focus on enhancement of segmental inhibition via GABA (baclofen), modulating the monoamines (tizanidine), alteration of ion channels (dantrolene, benzodiazepines, clonazepam, gabapentin, pregabalin, topiramate, vigabatrin, lamotrigine, riluzole, clonidine, cyproheptadine, and chlorpromazine), and inhibition of excitatory amino acids (orphenadrine, memantine, carisoprodol, and cannabinoids). Although the list of potentially beneficial oral agents is extensive, there are several that are more commonly used and therefore warrant more detailed descriptions. These include baclofen, diazepam, tizanidine, dantrolene, and clonidine.

Baclofen is a GABA agonist that is particularly useful for spasticity secondary to SCI and MS. Dosing is usually started at 5 mg twice daily and increased to three times daily with a maximum daily dose of 80 mg. The side-effect profile is somewhat extensive and includes but is not limited to a lower seizure threshold, sedation, weakness, GI symptoms, tremor, insomnia, and confusion. It is also important to note that baclofen should never be withdrawn suddenly and must be tapered off to prevent seizures.

Diazepam (Valium) has demonstrated benefits in those with SCI- and MS-related spasticity by facilitating GABA's effect on receptors. It is not indicated for those with TBI secondary to its negative effects on attention and memory. The starting dose is usually 4 mg at bedtime or 2 mg twice daily with a maximum dose of 60 mg/day. Side-effect profile most commonly includes sedation, memory impairment, and decreased REM sleep.

Tizanidine (Zanaflex) is a centrally acting alpha-2 adrenergic agonist with the typical side-effect profile of sedation, hypotension, dry mouth, bradycardia, dizziness, flushing, and liver toxicity. For the latter, baseline liver function tests (LFTs) are indicated before starting this medication as well as consistent LFT monitoring. Studies have shown tizanidine to be as effective as baclofen and diazepam in treating spasticity in SCI, MS, and TBI, as well as better overall tolerability. The starting dose is 2 to 4 mg at night, which may be increased to a maximum of 36 mg/day as tolerated.

Clonidine (Catapres) has the same mechanism of action as tizanidine with the same side-effect profile with a more profound effect on blood pressure leading to hypotension and syncope, as well as ankle edema and depression. This medication is most commonly prescribed in a transdermal form of 0.1 mg/week with a maximum dose of 0.3 mg/week. The oral form is dosed at 0.05 mg twice daily with a maximum dose of 0.4 mg/day.

Dantrolene, most commonly known for its treatment of malignant hyperthermia and neuroleptic malignant syndrome, has classically been used for spasticity of central origin based on its peripheral mechanism of action (blocks Ca++ release from sarcoplasmic reticulum of striated muscle). As with tizanidine this medication requires monitoring of LFTs as there is a high risk of liver toxicity. Other side effects include weakness, fatigue, paresthesias, diarrhea, nausea, and vomiting. The starting dose is 25 mg twice daily with maximum dose of 400 mg/day.

Individuals with more focal spasticity (i.e., stroke, TBI) respond favorably to injectables. Most commonly used particulates for chemodenervation are botulinum toxin type A and phenol. It should be noted that phenol is not recommended for treatment of upper limb spasticity (4). Phenol has the ability to block spasticity for months to years and is most commonly used in concentrations of 2% to 7%. Complications of phenol blocks include dysesthesias, muscle pain, muscle weakness, transient edema, DVT, skin sloughing if injected superficially, and serious systemic reactions if injected intravascularly.

The neurotoxin derived from *Clostridium botulinum* bacteria has seven serotypes of which only A (Botox, Dysport, Xeomin) and B (Myobloc) are available in the United States. When injected, the toxin is taken up by the nerve terminal where it prevents exocytosis of acetylcholine into the nerve terminal cleft. The effects of botulinum toxin last anywhere from 2 to 6 months with peak effect occurring around 4 to 6 weeks. Dosing is different depending on type. Type A dosing is 25 to 200 units per muscle, with a documented maximum dose of 400 units, although much higher doses have been administered without adverse effects. Type B starting dose is 10,000 units. The protocol for both forms is spacing of 3 months between injections and injections are most commonly administered using EMG guidance to ensure correct anatomical position of targeted muscle. Contraindications include known sensitivity, myasthenia gravis, Lambert-Eaton syndrome, motor neuron disease, and concomitant treatment with aminoglycoside or spectinomycin antibiotics. The side-effect profile includes weakness, ecchymosis, flu-like syndrome, dysphagia, nerve trauma, pain/soreness, antibody formation resulting in ineffectiveness of future botulinum toxin injections.

On the more invasive end of the treatment spectrum exists the intrathecal baclofen pump and surgical interventions. Intrathecal baclofen pumps (ITB) may be indicated in individuals with spasticity occurring diffusely in bilateral lower extremities, which has not responded well to therapeutic doses of oral baclofen. Surgical ablation of peripheral nerves is usually reserved for patients in whom conservative antispasticity treatments have failed. Surgical sectioning of tendon and muscle combined with postoperative serial splints can be used in patients with persistent deformity (e.g., Achilles tendon lengthening for equinus deformity at the ankle). In patients with potential for functional voluntary movement, fractional lengthening of forearm finger flexors, release of elbow flexors, and tenodesis may facilitate arm placement and grip (9).

There is an art to the treatment of spasticity and the approach to treatment should always be conservative. There exists the potential for serious adverse events with all of the treatment options discussed. It is imperative that the physician be thoroughly educated and understands the importance of introducing new treatments slowly, as well as closely weighing out the risks/benefits, including costs, before starting new treatments. For instance, it would be negligent for a physician to overdose a patient with Botox leading to weakness, a fall, and a hip fracture.

PRACTICE-BASED LEARNING AND IMPROVEMENT

GOALS

Demonstrate competence in continuously investigating and evaluating your spasticity patient care practices, appraising and assimilating scientific evidence, and continuously improving your patient care practices based on progressive self-evaluation and lifelong learning.

OBJECTIVES

1. Identify areas of self-assessment pertinent to the evaluation and management of spasticity.
2. Locate some resources including available websites for continuing medical education and continuing professional development.
3. Describe some areas paramount to self-assessment and lifelong learning such as quality improvement markers; review of current guidelines, including evidence-based, applicable in the treatment and management of patients with spasticity; and the role of the physiatrist as the educator of patients, families, residents, students, colleagues, and other health professionals.

Physiatrists providing care for patients with spasticity should have a working knowledge of the assessment of the patient with spasticity. The physiatrist should be cognizant of the impairments, activity limitations, and participation restrictions that are commonly seen in children and adults living with spasticity and use that knowledge to develop a comprehensive treatment plan to minimize complications associated with it.

Physiatrists should be up-to-date on the pathophysiology and treatment of spasticity, and have a working knowledge of side effects or adverse effects associated with the treatments. It is equally important that physiatrists have the necessary interpersonal and communication skills to effectively provide care and advocate for their patients with spasticity.

There are several strategies that physiatrists can use to identify gaps in their knowledge base about spasticity. Self-reflection on their clinical practice, self-assessment examinations, asking trusted colleagues to provide feedback to them on their practice, and asking patients under their care for their feedback on the care provided are just some examples.

Physicians should be current on published spasticity literature of major journals, be familiar with the teaching and learning resources produced by national and international professional organizations, attend local and national conferences on spasticity, and have a keen awareness of clinical practice guidelines (CPGs). The three major journals of Physical Medicine and Rehabilitation (PM&R) are *American Journal of PM&R*, *Archives of PM&R*, and *PM&R*. Two major SCI journals are the *Journal of Spinal Cord Medicine* and *Spinal Cord*. Two major PM&R professional organizations with a strong presence in the United States are Association of Academic Physiatrists (AAP) and American Academy of Physical Medicine and Rehabilitation (AAPM&R). American Spinal Injury Association (ASIA), the International Spinal Cord Society (ISCoS), and the Academy of Spinal Cord Injury Professionals (ASCIP) are three major SCI professional organizations. All of these organizations host annual educational and scientific conferences that may cover spasticity. Guidelines specifically regarding pharmacologic treatment of spasticity in both children and adolescents with CP and Botox neurotoxin for treatment of spasticity can be found published by the American Academy of Neurology (www.aan.com). The Paralyzed Veterans of America (www.pva.org) has produced CPGs specifically addressing spasticity management in multiple sclerosis that are available for free download.

Spasticity can be associated with or exacerbate conditions such as contractures, pressure ulcers, and predisposal to falls and joint subluxation. The incidence and prevalence of these potential spasticity-related complications can be tracked and benchmarks established as sources of comparison. The physiatrist can use this information to develop quality improvement projects that can minimize their occurrence.

INTERPERSONAL AND COMMUNICATION SKILLS

GOALS

Demonstrate interpersonal and communication skills that result in the effective exchange of information and build relationships and resolve conflicts with spasticity patients, their families, and other health professionals.

OBJECTIVES

1. Describe the importance of effective communication between physiatrists and rehabilitation teamwork, as applicable to patients with spasticity across socioeconomic and cultural backgrounds.
2. Identify key areas for physicians to educate patients and families specific to spasticity.

3. Identify key points to be documented in patient records to provide effective communication between team members with respect to spasticity.
4. Delineate the importance of the role of the physiatrist as the interdisciplinary team leader and consultant for the spasticity patient.

Effective communication and interpersonal skills between physicians and their patients and families are important in optimizing patient care. It is a central clinical function, and the resultant communication is the heart and art of medicine and a central component in the delivery of health care. Creating a good interpersonal relationship, facilitating exchange of information, and including patients in the decision-making process are the three main goals of doctor–patient communication. There are barriers that exist to proper communication: patient's anxiety and fear, doctor's burden of work, fear of litigation, and unrealistic patient expectations. It is important not only to recognize these barriers, but also to move past them, as the ultimate objective of any doctor–patient communication is to improve the patient's health and medical care. Effective communication between physicians and patients involves both style and content. Examples include allowing extra time for interactions, avoiding distractions, maintaining eye contact, listening, and frequently summarizing important points. Empathy and use of open-ended questions are other examples of integral communication skills (10).

These mentioned skills are of importance when caring for patients with spasticity and should be applied when counseling patients and families. Specifically, counseling should be on the causes of sudden increases in spasticity. This is clinically relevant, as spasticity can be caused by a worsening of a disease process, such as multiple sclerosis, or by irritants. It is important for patients, families, and caregivers to recognize potential irritants and seek appropriate medical attention in a timely manner. Of paramount importance in the spasticity management plan is maintaining ROM, either by the person with spasticity or passively by another person. Counseling individuals with spasticity and their caregivers of ROM is key to ensure that such a strategy is incorporated into normal daily life to maintain muscle length.

Spasticity and its associated symptoms can span the course of an individual's neurological condition and management may be necessary for a significant amount of their lifetime. Care is therefore often managed by many different disciplines across health and social care sectors. Teamwork is of importance, as all these disciplines offer their support to facilitate the patients to integrate management and treatment strategies into their daily life. It is fundamental to have input from several sources, as one service or provider in isolation is inadequate. Appropriate team members can assist in the management of spasticity and include a coordinated rehabilitation team consisting of a physiatrist, physical therapist (PT), occupational therapist (OT), speech and language pathologist (SLP), neurosurgery, and orthopedic surgery when appropriate (Table 22.1).

The physiatrist is in an excellent position to function as a team leader for the management of spasticity due to his or her

TABLE 22.1 The Spasticity Management Team

Physiatrist: May design the rehabilitation program, working with other team members to maximize the patient's function and minimize the disabling aspects of the neurologic injury. The physiatrist may also prescribe medications, identify key muscles for chemodenervation, and administer treatments. Also, he or she may assist with assessment of intrathecal baclofen pump trials and pump refills.

Physical Therapist (PT): May perform or direct another person to perform the exercises that are necessary to assist in maintaining the range of motion of limbs affected by spasticity. The PT may also apply and fit braces, splints, or casts that may be prescribed by the physiatrist. May direct training to improve the patient's gait and may instruct patients and caregivers on how to position affected arms and legs to help reduce spasticity. A PT often works closely with an occupational therapist to design changes in the home and equipment that might be necessary to accommodate the patient's needs.

Occupational Therapist (OT): May teach modifications for dressing, feeding, and grooming to both patient and caregiver. May also offer expertise on adaptive devices such as wheelchairs and bath equipment and may advise on home and workplace modifications to increase accessibility and ease of use. The OT is usually the medical professional that advises on issues such as seating, writing, and use of facilities.

Neurosurgeon (or certain pain physicians): May implant a baclofen delivery pump for patients with severe spasticity (Modified Ashworth Scale—grade 3 or greater), if the response is positive to a screening test. Neurosurgeons may also perform selective dorsal rhizotomy when other treatments are inadequate (11).

Orthopedic Surgeon: May perform procedure(s) to help reduce or correct contractures that lead to abnormal positioning of joints. Orthopedic operations often involve reconstruction or revision of tendons and bones.

clinical expertise in this area and the emphasis on teamwork that is part of his or her training.

Preventive stretching, applying modalities, educating caregivers about ROM, identifying muscles for chemodenervation, and assisting with assessment during ITB trials are all integral aspects of care that these team members can offer. The person with spasticity clearly needs to be central to the process, ensuring that the main goal of treatment is appropriate and beneficial to their desired outcome. This is the only way for spasticity management plans to truly be successful. Desired outcomes range from improved hygiene and decreased pain to more complex goals such as improved mobility.

PATIENT EDUCATION

Physicians should educate patients and families early about the sequelae of the upper motor neuron syndrome, positioning, and ROM activities. There are many options for spasticity treatment, including pharmacologic agents, chemical denervation, botulinum toxin therapy, intrathecal therapy, neurosurgical surgery such as dorsal rhizotomy, and even orthopedic procedures. Education should be provided in regard to the treatment options for diffuse areas versus focal or segmental areas with spasticity.

For example, chemodenervation may be more appropriate with affected discrete areas, and treatment that is more global should be applied if the condition is systemic. Other considerations when discussing treatment options are whether the spasticity affects upper or lower limbs. Patients with severe spasticity often receive multiple treatments in combination, as often is the case. When these spasticity treatments are offered, education about potential side effects is absolutely necessary, as well as the potential for reduced muscle strength or function. The overall medical condition of the patient is important. Patients dealing with hypotension, syncope, balance difficulty, and ataxia may not be able to tolerate the side effects of certain agents. These agents that can potentially cause somnolence and/or dizziness include baclofen, benzodiazepines, dantrolene, and gabapentin.

It is also critical to discuss costs when offering treatment options. When physicians, patients, and family deal with certain third-party payers or private health insurance companies, they may not cover the cost of intrathecal baclofen and botulinum toxins. These treatment options are expensive and paying out of pocket for certain modalities is not realistic. Financial issues should be addressed when dealing with the various treatment options. These are examples of topics that should be addressed and discussed in detail when educating patients and families with spasticity.

MEDICAL DOCUMENTATION

There are key points that should be documented in the patient record that provide effective communication between team members with spasticity. The MAS is used to score individual muscle movement as the limb is moved throughout the entire ROM. The amount of resistance (0–4) is recorded at each patient encounter and should be used to quantify the intensity of the spasticity. It is necessary to ensure ongoing documentation of compliance with therapeutic interventions and evaluation of orthotic or positioning devices. Functional changes (i.e., transfer difficulty) and limitations should be closely monitored and can be obtained from the patient or caregiver. Lastly, documenting skin integrity is essential because pressure ulcers may lead to devastating consequences if left unnoticed.

PROFESSIONALISM

GOALS

Reflect a commitment to carrying out professional responsibilities and an adherence to ethical principles in caring for patients with spasticity.

OBJECTIVES

1. Exemplify the importance of integrity, respect, compassion, ethics, and courtesy in the care of patients with spasticity.
2. Demonstrate the importance of patient-centered care, informed consent, and maintaining patient confidentiality in spasticity.
3. Respect the importance of patient's beliefs and goals, privacy, confidentiality, and autonomy as it applies to spasticity.
4. Demonstrate sensitivity to culture, diversity, gender, age, race, religion, disabilities, and sexual orientation as it may apply to patients with spasticity.
5. Exhibit responsibility and accountability of physiatry as it applies to spasticity.

The physiatrist should treat patients affected by spasticity in a respectful, compassionate, ethical, and courteous manner that is respectful of their cultural background, gender, race, religious beliefs, and sexual orientation. The physiatrist is responsible and accountable for the appropriate medical and rehabilitative care of the patient with spasticity and coordination of spasticity-related treatments in order to minimize complications.

Spasticity can present in varying degrees and in a plethora of diagnoses. A single generalized presentation of spasticity does not exist. Not fully recognizing its unique presentations and challenges would be a tremendous disservice to the patient. Often, this is not well understood even by health care professionals. The focus tends to be on the diagnosis and treatment plan, where the focus should be on the patient. Patients should not be defined by their diagnosis, but rather given the respect and courtesy to be seen as individuals dealing with something that has an impact on their daily lives. In physiatry, a field where the focus is on function and daily living, this needs to be paramount.

In conversing with and about patients with spasticity, great compassion must be implemented. The medical term *spastic* was first used to describe CP although this is not the only diagnosis that presents with spasticity. However, the word began to be used as an insult to imply stupidity, physical ineptness, or incompetence. Over time, it has lost its negative connotation and begun to be used to describe someone who is uncoordinated. However, use of any form of this word shows a lack of respect and understanding for those who are truly suffering with spasticity. These are individuals who are dealing with a true neurological condition. This is something to not only be careful of, but also something that should be taught to others who may not be as familiar with spasticity as physiatrists.

Each patient is affected by spasticity in a different way. For some, it may be hygiene that is their biggest concern; for others, it may be pain or function. It is important to listen carefully as to what the patient wishes to achieve with whatever intervention, if any, you choose to suggest based on his or her presentation. Although, as a physician, there may be goals one wishes to set for them and treatments one wishes to try to fulfill those goals, ultimately it is the patient's choice to choose what he or she believes is best for him or her. Patients should be active participants in the process with informed consent attained in each step. There should be clear understanding of what is going on by the patient or by the person assigned to make decisions, if the patient cannot do so himself or herself, so that he or she has all the information to make the best decision. For example, when prescribing medications or performing toxin injections, it is crucial that the physiatrist is very clear and specific as to possible side effects, duration of efficacy, follow-up requirements, and so on, to make sure patients have all the information to make an informed decision. It is also just as important to remember to guard a patient's privacy. This can often be forgotten, especially when there may be many people caring for the patient, or if the patient cannot communicate for himself or herself. But, it is a physician's duty to be mindful that the patient is at the center and that his or her privacy is guarded and wishes are respected at all times.

Often, patients suffering with spasticity need to rely on others for help. In severe cases, hygiene can be a problem for patients. The spasticity or even contractures can be so great, just to be able to clean private areas may present a challenge. In certain cultures and religions, this may present a real issue. Great respect and understanding must be taken with regard to a patient's age, sex, religion, cultural background, and sexual orientation. It is important to know the patients and not to offer treatments or interventions that may offend them in any way.

A physiatrist's goal is always for the patient to attain the greatest amount of functional independence with the least amount of burden or suffering. The physiatrist's responsibility is to present to the patient ways to attain the personal goals he or she set out, whether it be hygiene, pain control, or simply being able to shake someone's hand. The field of medicine is never stagnant. It is a physician's duty to be up-to-date on the latest research and treatment options available to patients. Although patients may decide not to pursue any of the avenues a physician suggests, it is nevertheless his or her responsibility to ensure that the patient has all the information necessary to make the best informed decision possible.

There are very few fields of medicine, let alone areas outside of medicine, that understand what spasticity is and how it can affect the day-to-day living of patients. Physiatrists must be their patients' best advocates. Sometimes, that includes the physician calling an insurance company to facilitate and expedite an approval of an oral medication, injection, or procedure that can benefit the patient. It is often an arduous process that can take hours, maybe days, to convince the insurance company of its benefits for a specific patient with spasticity. But, part of a physiatrist's role is to be that advocate. Physiatrists are uniquely qualified for that role because they can speak of specific functional goals/benefits in the spasticity population, where most other physicians cannot.

Another key component is knowledge. Arming people with knowledge of what spasticity is and why physiatrists do what they do can change how they view and interact with those who have spasticity. Often, patients or their families/caregivers, especially of the more disabled patients, find themselves frustrated, exhausted, and depressed. It takes time, energy, and patience to do or assist patients in their daily exercises, transfers, ambulation, medications, and so on. But physiatrists must advocate for their patients, especially those who cannot speak for themselves. They must ensure that the best is always being done for the patient. If there are concerns, a physiatrist should not to be afraid to broach a topic and provide support and compassion, sometimes just an ear, to make sure that with all the extraneous stuff, it is never forgotten that the patient is at the heart of it all.

SYSTEM-BASED PRACTICE

GOALS

Awareness and responsiveness to systems of care delivery, and the ability to recruit and coordinate effectively resources in the system to provide optimal continuum of care as it relates to spasticity.

OBJECTIVES

1. Identify the key components in the spectrum of rehabilitation continuum of care settings for patients with spasticity.
2. Coordinate and recruit necessary resources in the system to provide optimal and variety of care options available for the spasticity patient, with attention to safety, cost considerations, risk–benefit analysis, and management.
3. Identify the components, systems of care delivery, services, referral patterns, and resources.
4. Describe optimal long-term follow-up for spasticity patients, markers of quality of care, improvement metrics, and use of documentation in such rehabilitation programs.
5. Identify potential health care system errors in the care of spasticity.

The evaluation and treatment of spasticity commonly occurs in both inpatient and outpatient settings. Physiatrists can provide consultative services on spasticity-related matters, acute medical and surgical services, as well as in skilled nursing facilities. They can be actively involved in the treatment of adults and children admitted to inpatient rehabilitation facilities for acute rehabilitation services as well as rehabilitation in facilities providing subacute level rehabilitation services. Spasticity care can also occur in specialized multidisciplinary outpatient clinics or in the private offices of physiatrists. Ideally, spasticity care should occur in a coordinated manner across the rehabilitative health care continuum by a team of clinicians well versed in the practice of spasticity management providing specialized and individualized care for the patient.

Physiatrists, ideally, like to see patients from point A to point Z and follow with them in their journey providing support, advice, and interventions along the way. Spasticity is present in a multitude of diseases and conditions. They may evaluate patients in the early stages of their disease process with no spasticity, only to see them later with advanced spasticity. In theory, they would like to be able to intervene before their spasticity becomes advanced. Physiatrists turn to members of the rehabilitation team, including but not limited to the patient himself or herself, caregivers, and therapists for input on any issues that may be developing that they are unaware of. Once identified and evaluated, they can better serve their patients and their needs, whether it is offering a new therapy, medication, injection, and so on. They can then continually reassess and assure that no issue related to the patient's spasticity is left unaddressed.

Safety is a major concern in spasticity. Depending on the severity and location of the spasticity, safety concerns can range from gripping a hot cup of coffee to falls to developing skin breakdown and decubitus ulcers. Educating the patient and/or his or her caregivers as to what the patient's limitations are will help ensure their safety. Physiatrists always stress the importance of their patient's independence and autonomy, without sacrificing safety. It is not possible for physicians to be able to account for every situation that their patients might find themselves in. But, stressing what they can do while providing education as to what they may need assistance with can be effective as well. Physiatrists tend not to stress what a patient cannot do, but instead stress what they can do with whatever adaptations or devices are necessary. When it comes to their safety, it is crucial not to disillusion patients or their caregivers, as this can be potentially dangerous.

On first evaluation of a patient with spasticity, a full history and physical including a functional examination must be performed. Identifying the patient's goals and concerns should guide one as to what the next steps may be for each individual patient. If medication is prescribed, it is important to follow up closely with the patient to ensure there are no adverse side effects, verify he or she is tolerating the medications, or see if a dose increase or decrease is warranted. If physical or occupational therapies, or both, are prescribed, it is important to follow up with both the patient and therapist consistently to see what progress, if any, is being made, and especially to see if any issues are arising that the physiatrist is unaware of, but are being brought to the forefront in therapies.

If an orthotic is prescribed, close communication with the orthotist is important as well as follow-up with the patient once he or she receives the orthotic to assess both fit and function. If a patient is deemed a good candidate for an intervention such as with a botulinum toxin, close follow-up is important to know whether it is has helped, or in some cases made them worse. Some patients use their spasticity to function, like for standing or walking. Certain interventions may treat their spasticity but cause them to lose function. It is therefore very important to closely follow these patients to reassess and reevaluate on a consistent basis.

Caring for a person suffering with spasticity can be costly. Depending on what needs the patients have and the degree of assistance they require, costs can be quite high, placing a financial burden on both the patient and caregivers. When a physiatrist offers different treatments, device, or equipment options, it is important to be able to break down for the patient the cost, risks, and benefits of each. In an ideal world, everything would be covered by insurance and patients would not need to consider cost in their decision-making process, but this is a real concern for many. Another concern for patients is the risk–benefit analysis in varying treatment options for spasticity. There are few treatments that are risk free. Even seemingly benign interventions such as bracing can come with a risk of discomfort. For some patients, the benefits outweigh the discomfort, but others may prefer another modality, as the discomfort may be too great. As stated previously, education and information is key to allowing patients to make the most informed decision they can. For every option a physiatrist provides for a patient in regard to his or her spasticity, it is important to know the costs, risks, and benefits of each treatment, intervention, and/or modality.

There are few fields in medicine that have an intimate knowledge of spasticity. Few are experts in the recognition and grading of spasticity and even fewer are experts on how to approach/manage it. As previously stated, ideally physiatrists like to be able to start with patients from point A, the point where they are initially diagnosed, and be able to follow them through to point Z. Oftentimes, however, by the time they see a physiatrist, their spasticity has already begun to negatively impact their daily lives. Perhaps this is because physicians outside of physiatry are unaware that physiatrists are specifically trained in spasticity. A major source of error in our health care system is not knowing when to refer out, of not knowing when something is out of the realm of expertise, and where to then be able to refer a patient to receive the best care for his or her condition. This is especially true with spasticity as physicians, not necessarily trained in spasticity, try and manage it on their own. Only when it has progressed and is usually more severe do they start to seek out where to refer the patient. It is important for patients with spasticity to be followed by an expert in spasticity from as early on as possible because physiatrists can better identify barriers, safety concerns, and treatment pathways that are specific to this population.

CASE STUDY

JR is a 75-year-old African American man with a history of hypertension, diabetes type 2, hyperlipidemia, and left MCA CVA (diagnosed 2 years prior) that presents to your outpatient spasticity clinic because of difficulty walking. He also complains of pain in his right arm, most notably around his right elbow and right hand. He states that although he uses a rolling walker and right solid AFO in the community to ambulate, he still has difficulty advancing his right leg and has significantly worsened over the last year. JR denies any buckling of the knees or toe catching with use of his AFO. He denies any falls or near falls in the last year. His last therapy session was 4 years prior and he admits that he has not seen any physicians for follow-up since his stroke. He lives with his wife in a private home and has needed some more assistance from his wife with certain ADLs over the past year.

On motor examination the patient was noted to have the following findings on the right side: mild shoulder abduction, elbow flexion, and grip weakness of 4/5. Hip flexors were 4/5, hip extensors 4/5, hip abductors preserved 5/5, knee extensor strength preserved 4/5, knee flexors 4/5, ankle dorsiflexion was 0/5, planter flexion 1/5, and foot eversion 0/5. JR's left upper and lower extremity strength was grossly intact. His tone was found increased, most notably in right elbow flexor and right intrinsic hand muscles, MAS 3. On careful inspection of his hand, the patient was noted to have breakdown of his skin over the palmar aspect of his right hand. Tone in the right knee flexor was MAS 3. Sensory, DTRs, cranial nerves, and tone were all normal. Evaluation of gait revealed a slightly extended lordotic posture, short stance phase without push off on the right, diminished heel strike, and right steppage gait pattern. He was also noted to have difficulty advancing his right leg secondary to his increased knee flexion tone and his right elbow was flexed to 45° throughout ambulation. The patient's right solid AFO appeared to fit well and there was no apparent skin breakdown over his right lower extremity on careful inspection.

CASE STUDY DISCUSSION QUESTIONS

1. What are some of the key details of JR's history and physical that will contribute to his treatment plan and what further information might be warranted?
2. What is the indicated treatment cascade that should be utilized based on JR's findings?
3. As JR's physiatrist, what are some ways to strengthen future compliance in regard to spasticity follow-up visits?
4. What key points should you educate JR and his wife (caregiver) about with respect to his spasticity management?
5. As a physiatrist, what are some of your responsibilities as it pertains to professionalism in this case?
6. What is the optimal follow-up care for JR?

SELF-EXAMINATION QUESTIONS
(Answers begin on p. 367)

1. Which of the following is an example of effective communication between physicians and patients when dealing with spasticity?
   A. Not allowing extra time for interactions
   B. Minimal eye contact
   C. Being distracted during the patient encounter
   D. Using "open-ended" questions
   E. Infrequently summarizing points discussed with the patient during encounter

2. You are treating a 35-year-old male patient with a C5 ASIA. Which of the following antispasticity agents binds to GABA receptors in the spinal cord to inhibit reflexes that lead to increased tone?
   A. Tizanidine
   B. Clonidine
   C. Baclofen
   D. Dantrolene
   E. Botulinum toxin

3. In caring for a patient with spasticity, it is the responsibility of the physiatrist to
   A. Treat the patient based only on symptoms
   B. Be the patient's advocate
   C. Present treatment options only covered by insurance
   D. Set goals for the patient
   E. Exclude caregivers from the decision-making process

4. When considering a treatment option for a patient with spasticity, what is the most important factor to guide treatment?
   A. Cost
   B. Side effects
   C. Patient preference
   D. Insurance coverage
   E. Physician preference

5. A 15-year-old boy with spastic CP presents with worsening tone in his right elbow flexors. On examination the joint cannot be ranged due to the severity of his tone and is documented as a 4 on the MAS. Which term best defines this score?
   A. Flaccidity
   B. Contracture
   C. Rigidity
   D. Clonus
   E. Hypotonic

REFERENCES

1. Ammar Kheder & Krishnan Padmakumari Sivaraman Nair. Spasticity: pathophysiology, evaluation and management. *Pract Neurol* 2012;12:289–298.
2. Bhakta BB. Management of spasticity in stroke. Rheumatology and Rehabilitation Research Unit, University of Leeds, Leeds, UK. *Br Med Bull*. 2000;56(2):476–485.
3. Cook K, Teal C, Engebretson J, et al. Development and validation of Patient Reported Impact of Spasticity Measure (PRISM). *J Rehabil Res Dev*. 2007;44(3):363–371.
4. Skeil DA, Barnes MP. The local treatment of spasticity. *Clin Rehabil*. 1994;8: 240–246.
5. Brodal A. *Neurological Anatomy in Relationship to Clinical Medicine*. New York, NY: Oxford University Press; 1981.
6. Katz R, Pierrot-Deseilligny E. Recurrent inhibition of alpha-motor neurons in patients with upper motor neuron lesions. *Brain*. 1982;105(pt 1):103–124.
7. Magoun HW, Rhines R. An inhibitory mechanism in the bulbar reticular formation. *J Neurophysiol*. 1946;9:165–171.
8. Delisa JA. *Physical Medicine and Rehabilitation: Principles and Practice*. 5th ed. Chapter 50. Philadelphia, PA: Lippincott Williams & Wilkins; 2010.
9. Stevenson VL, Jarett L. *Spasticity Management: A Practical Multidisciplinary Guide*. London: Informa Healthcare; 2006.
10. Ha JF, Longnecker N. Doctor–patient communication: a review. *Oschner J*. 2010;1:38–48.
11. Shatzer M, Jassal NS. *Physical Medicine & Rehabilitation Pocketpedia*. 2nd ed. Chapter 26: Spasticity. Philadelphia, PA: Lippincott Williams & Wilkins; 2012.

Jonah Green
Monica Habib
Rachel Mallari
Tova Plaut

23: Musculoskeletal Disorders: Upper Extremity

PATIENT CARE

GOALS

Evaluate and develop a rehabilitation plan of care for patient with upper extremity musculoskeletal injuries (UEMIs) that is compassionate, appropriate, and effective for the treatment of neuromuscular problems across the entire continuum of care and the promotion of health.

OBJECTIVES

1. Perform a comprehensive evaluation of a patient with UEMI.
2. Formulate an optimal rehabilitation management plan for the patient with common acute, subacute, and chronic orthopedic and rheumatologic conditions including pain management and the role of medications and injections.

Disorders of the upper extremity comprise some of the most common reasons that a patient will seek the care of a physician. The most common presenting initial symptom is pain. Pain may be localized or may be referred to the neck or throughout the entire upper extremity; this is known as "referred pain." An appropriate medical history and physical examination should be performed to determine the location and etiology of any upper extremity disorder.

History should include when and where the pain originated, radiation of the pain, factors that worsen and improve the pain, associated neurologic symptoms, and maneuvers performed to alleviate or relieve the pain. History should also include recent traumatic events or sports or work-related maneuvers that may have induced the pain. Some good mnemonics to remember when taking a history for pain are "SOCRATES" or "PQRST" (see Table 23.1).

Physical examination, which includes many provocative tests, should begin with a basic examination of the entire cervical spine and upper extremity to determine the area with the most severe pain. Even after finding the location of the pain, care must be taken to examine the joint above and below that level of pain. Examination should include inspection, palpation, range of motion (ROM) measurement, and manual muscle testing. Sensory testing and the testing of reflexes are usually normal in musculoskeletal injuries but are also important to check in order to rule out other conditions. Table 23.2 provides the normal values for ROM of the upper extremity and Table 23.3 lists the grading system used for manual muscle testing. History and physical examination should not be overlooked as it is said that over 80% of diagnoses are made on history alone, a further 5% to 10% on examination, and the remainder on investigation (1).

This chapter focuses on a few of the most important upper extremity conditions divided by body location including rotator cuff (RTC) tears/syndromes, medial and lateral epicondylitis, and de Quervain tenosynovitis.

Shoulder disorders: The RTC is composed of four muscles: supraspinatus, infraspinatus, teres minor, and subscapularis. These muscles work cohesively to rotate the arm and stabilize the humeral head against the glenoid. RTC tears are frequently diagnosed, especially in those older than 60 years of age, and often occur from direct trauma, or the result of chronic impingement (2). Partial tears, however, are frequently idiopathic and incidentally diagnosed in the elderly. The partial RTC tear typically affects the supraspinatus tendon, which is often weakened from poor vascular supply, injury, and subacromial impingement. Pain often initially presents with repetitive overhead activities, and any action that involves flexion, abduction, and internal rotation. Patients may feel crepitus, clicking, or a catching sensation with overhead activities. Pain may be nocturnal and can be referred anywhere along the deltoid musculature. Tears of the RTC are the most common injury to any tendon in the body and can originate from an intrinsic or extrinsic cause. Extrinsic tears result from an attrition, which might have been caused by a subacromial bony prominence, while intrinsic tears can originate within the tendon body itself due to age-related degenerative changes, giving rise to partial and later complete rupture of the tendon body (3).

TABLE 23.1 Pain Mnemonics

SOCRATES	PQRST
S—Site	P—Provocation/palliation
O—Onset	Q—Quality of pain
C—Character	R—Region/radiation
R—Radiation	S—Severity
A—Alleviating factors	T—Timing
T—Timing	
E—Exacerbating factors	
S—Severity (scaled 1-10)	

TABLE 23.2 Upper Extremity Range of Motion

	MOVEMENT	DEGREES
Shoulder	Flexion	0-180
	Abduction	0-180
	Extension	0-45/60
	Internal rotation at 90° abduction	0-80/90
	External rotation at 90° abduction	0-90
	Internal rotation (walk finger up the back)	to T7
Elbow	Flexion	0-145/150
Forearm	Pronation/supination	0-80/90
Wrist	Flexion	0-80
	Extension	0-70
	Radial deviation	0-20
	Ulnar deviation	0-30/35
Thumb		
CMC	Abduction	0-70/80
	Flexion	0-15/45
	Extension	0-20
	Opposition	Tip of thumb to tip of fingers
MCP	Flexion	0-50/60
IP	Flexion	0-80
Digits (2-5)		
MCP	Flexion	0-90
	Hyperextension	0-45
PIP	Flexion	0-100
DIP	Flexion	0-90
	Hyperextension	0-10

TABLE 23.3 Grading for Manual Muscle Testing

5	Normal strength; ability to resist against maximal pressure throughout range of motion (ROM) against gravity
5−	Uncertain muscle weakness
4+	Inability to resist against maximal pressure throughout ROM
	Holds test position against moderate to strong pressure in antigravity position
4	Ability to resist against moderate pressure throughout ROM
4−	Ability to resist against minimal pressure throughout ROM
	Holds test position against slight to moderate pressure in antigravity position
3+	Ability to move through full ROM against gravity and to resist against minimal pressure through partial ROM, then contraction breaks abruptly
3	Ability to move through full ROM against gravity
3−	Ability to move through greater than one-half ROM against gravity
2+	Ability to move through less than one-half ROM against gravity
	Moves to completion of range against resistance with gravity eliminated
2	Ability to move through full ROM with gravity eliminated
2−	Ability to move through greater than one-half ROM with gravity eliminated
1+	Ability to move through less than one-half ROM with gravity eliminated
1	A flicker of movement is seen or felt in the muscle
	Tendon becomes prominent or feeble contraction felt in the muscle, but no visible movement of the part
0	No contraction palpable in the muscle

Physical examination should include strength, sensation, and ROM evaluation, as well as provocative testing including, but not limited to, the Neer and Hawkins tests for impingement, the supraspinatus test used to discover supraspinatus pathology, and the drop arm test to evaluate for a RTC tear. The Neer sign is performed with the examiner stabilizing the scapula and passively flexing the arm with the thumb pointing downward. Pain on forward flexion is an indication of a positive test for shoulder impingement. Hawkins test involves stabilizing the scapula, passively abducting the shoulder to 90°, flexing the shoulder to 30°, flexing the elbow to 90°, and internally rotating the shoulder. Again, pain is an indication of a positive test for impingement.

The supraspinatus test or "empty can" test involves patient testing at 90° elevation in the scapular plane and full internal rotation (empty can) with the patient resisting downward pressure exerted by the examiner at the patient's elbow or wrist. If weakness or pain occurs during the movement the supraspinatus tendon can be affected. In the drop arm test the examiner grasps the patient's wrist and passively abducts the patient's shoulder to 90°. The patient is then asked to hold the arm in that position. Inability to do so may be indicative of a severe or complete tear of the RTC. Sensory and reflex testing are usually found to be unaffected if the cause of the pain is a RTC tendinitis or tear. The differential diagnosis for a patient with a suspected RTC tendonitis or tear should include neurologic and nonneurologic conditions. Some nonneurologic conditions that should be considered are a glenolabral tear, acromioclavicular sprain, occult fracture, osteoarthritis, rheumatoid arthritis, adhesive capsulitis, myofascial pain syndrome, and myofascial thoracic outlet syndrome. The neurologic conditions that should be considered are cervical radiculopathy, brachial plexopathy, suprascapular neuropathy, or neurogenic (true) thoracic outlet syndrome.

Elbow and forearm disorders: Most common elbow disorders include medial epicondylitis, also known as golfer's elbow, and lateral epicondylitis, also known as tennis elbow. Medial epicondylitis is often caused by a repetitive valgus stress to the elbow. The repetitive throwing and swinging motions often lead to inflammation of the common flexor tendon at the elbow. Recurrent microtrauma can affect all medial elbow structures, which include the medial epicondyle, the medial condylar epiphysis, and the medial collateral ligament (MCL) of the elbow, which cause hypertrophy of the medial epicondyle (4). Patients usually report pain and sometimes swelling in the area just distal to the epicondyle, which may radiate proximally or distally. The patient may also provide a history of having difficulties with some wrist/hand movements like gripping a doorknob or carrying a shopping bag. On physical examination, the patient will illustrate tenderness distal to the medial epicondyle, reproducible with resisted wrist flexion. Sensation and deep tendon reflexes are usually normal except that ulnar neuropathy symptoms may occur in up to 20% of patients found to have a medial epicondylitis.

Lateral epicondylitis (aka tennis elbow) can occur insidiously from many different physical maneuvers, but is often attributed to poor technique during backhand swings or inappropriate grip strength or string tension, while playing racquet sports. These motions will cause microtearing of the extensor carpi radialis brevis. Patients will present with pain and weakness in grip strength and tenderness distal to the lateral epicondyle at the extensor muscle origin. Two tests that can be used to assess for lateral epicondylitis are Cozen test and the middle finger test. Cozen test is positive when resisted wrist extension triggers pain to the lateral aspect of the elbow, owing to stress placed upon the tendon of the extensor carpi radialis brevis tendon, with the elbow in extension. The middle finger test is positive for lateral epicondylitis when the proximal interphalangeal joint of the long finger is resisted in extension and pain is felt over the lateral epicondyle. The differential diagnosis for a patient with a suspected epicondylitis should include osteoarthritis, osteochondral loose body, triceps tendonitis, elbow synovitis, posterior interosseous nerve syndrome, median or ulnar neuropathy about the elbow, acute calcification about the lateral epicondyle, anconeus compartment syndrome, degenerative arthrosis, lateral ligament instability, bursitis, bone infection or tumor, radial head fracture, or collateral ligament tears.

Wrist and hand disorders: De Quervain tenosynovitis, a common disorder of the wrist/hand, most commonly occurs due to overexertion related to either household chores, one's occupation, or recreational activities causing a stenosing tenosynovitis of the synovial sheath of the tendons of the abductor pollicis longus (APL) and extensor pollicis brevis (EPB) in the first compartment of the wrist due to repetitive use. Patients will often report pain at the dorsolateral aspect of the wrist with referred pain toward the thumb and/or lateral forearm. Physical examination will reveal pain and tenderness on the radial side of the wrist associated with recurrent movements. Edema and crepitus may also be present. Physical examination should also include the Finkelstein test, which is positive when pain is elicited in the radial wrist while the wrist is forced into ulnar deviation with the thumb enclosed in a fist. Sensation and deep tendon reflexes will be normal. Symptoms of numbness should alert the clinician to consider an alternative diagnosis with a neurologic cause (i.e., carpal tunnel syndrome, cervical radiculopathy). In some cases, de Quervain disease is associated with rheumatoid arthritis, and thus a full examination of the hand should be performed bilaterally to evaluate for any swelling, malalignment, or deformities of any of the joints.

The differential diagnoses for de Quervain tenosynovitis are carpal joint arthritis, rheumatoid arthritis, radial nerve injury, cervical radiculopathy, carpal tunnel syndrome, Kienbock disease, triscaphoid arthritis, intersection syndrome, ganglion cyst, scaphoid fracture, and radioscaphoid arthritis.

The ailments discussed above are only a small list of the injuries that can occur to the upper extremity. Disorders of the shoulder, elbow, wrist, and hand can greatly impact a patient's activities of daily living (ADLs) and therefore are extremely important to diagnose and treat correctly in a timely manner, allowing the patient to return to his or her previous functional status.

Treatment of the above mentioned injuries should be individualized and take into account factors such as acuity and severity of the injury, first time occurrence vs. reoccurrence, complications associated with the injury, comorbid conditions that can have adverse impact on treatment plan, and age of the patient. Sample rehabilitation programs often consist of interventions such as modalities, strengthening and flexibility exercises, education on body mechanics with activities, and a home exercise program. Factors such as precautions while exercising, types of exercise equipment to be used, and rate of progression should also be considered.

MEDICAL KNOWLEDGE

GOALS

Demonstrate knowledge of established evidence-based evolving biomedical, clinical epidemiological, and sociobehavioral sciences pertaining to UEMI, as well as the application of this knowledge to guide holistic patient care.

OBJECTIVES

1. Describe the epidemiology, etiology, anatomy, physiology, and pathophysiology of UEMI.
2. Describe the role of imaging studies in the diagnosis of UEMI as well as their optimal timing and use.
3. Propose management approaches for UEMI.

Knowledge of anatomy and pathophysiology is the first step in developing a treatment plan for a patient with an upper extremity musculoskeletal disorder. This section focuses on the anatomy and pathophysiology of each disorder, the diagnostic testing used, and the available treatment options.

Shoulder disorders: RTC tears can either be traumatic or degenerative. Traumatic RTC tears are a common injury seen in the upper extremity in the younger population of athletes and laborers, whereas degenerative tears occur in older individuals. In a recent study by Mall et al., nine studies of traumatic RTC tears were analyzed, showing that the most common mechanism of injury was falling onto an outstretched arm, causing the supraspinatus muscle to be involved in 84% of tears, the infraspinatus torn in 39% of cases, and the subscapularis in 78% of injuries. Tear size was less than 3 cm in 22%, 3 to 5 cm in 36%, and greater than 5 cm in 42% of cases (5).

RTC tears can also occur in association with other shoulder injuries, such as a broken clavicle or dislocated shoulder. Chronic tears are indicative of extended use in conjunction with other factors such as poor biomechanics or muscular imbalance. Ultimately, most are the result of wear and tear that occurs slowly over time as a natural part of the aging process. They are more common in the dominant arm; however, a tear in one shoulder should raise suspicion for an increased risk of a tear in the opposing shoulder. Several factors contribute to degenerative or chronic RTC tears, of which repetitive stress is the most significant factor.

There are three types of tears that can occur to the RTC. A full-thickness tear can be massive and cause immediate functional impairments. A partial-thickness tear can be broken down into a tear on the superior surface into the subacromial space or inferior surface on the articular side. All these tears can be traumatic or degenerative (6).

As previously mentioned, history and physical examination are the most important elements in making any diagnosis; this includes diagnosing a RTC tear. There is no indication for any laboratory studies. Imaging studies can be helpful in confirming the diagnosis and eliminating other possibilities. MRI of the shoulder is the gold standard. A CT scan is a good study to see osseous structures but is not as effective in revealing soft-tissue injuries like a RTC tear. The initial imaging test usually performed is an x-ray to rule out any bony abnormalities. One might see a suggestion of a tear if there is upward migration of the humeral head or sclerotic changes at the greater tuberosity seen on x-ray. Over the past few years ultrasound is being used more frequently, as it is more cost effective and less invasive and has been proven comparable to MRI in efficacy in the diagnosis of supraspinatus tendon tears. It should be noted that a normal MRI cannot fully rule out a small tear (a false negative) and partial-thickness tears are also not as reliably detected (7).

Treatment of RTC disorders varies, and is dependent on its acute vs. chronic nature, the age and activity level of the patient, and how debilitating the tear is to the patient. Physical therapy is the mainstay of treatment and is successful in most patients. The basic phases of rehabilitation include (a) pain control and reduction of inflammation, (b) restoration of normal shoulder motion, (c) improved strength, (d) improved proprioception, and (e) return to task or sport-specific activities. Pain control and reduction of inflammation may be obtained by a combination of relative rest, icing, electrical stimulation, and acetaminophen or a nonsteroidal antiinflammatory medication. Subacromial injections of corticosteroid can also be therapeutic. If a patient's condition has not improved in 3 months then a surgical consultation should be considered. There is no evidence of better results from early rather than delayed surgery, and many with partial tears and some with complete tears will respond to nonoperative management. For this reason, many first recommend nonsurgical management of RTC tears. Early surgical treatment may be considered in acute tears that are significant (greater than 1 cm–1.5 cm) or in young patients with full-thickness tears who have a significant risk for the development of irreparable RTC changes (8).

Elbow and forearm disorders: Medial and lateral epicondylitis are the most common disorders of the elbow, with lateral epicondylitis accounting for the majority of cases. Medial epicondylitis, which accounts for 10% to 20% of epicondylitis in the elbow, is usually found in the dominant elbow of a golfer or pitcher due to the valgus stresses that are placed on the elbow by activities such as swinging the golf club or throwing a ball. The phase of throwing in which most stress is often placed on the medial elbow is during the late cocking and acceleration phases of a pitch. Medial epicondylitis in many cases is due to training errors (i.e., not warming up adequately), improper technique, or poor equipment. The muscles affected are of the flexor muscle group.

Lateral epicondylitis, on the other hand, also known as tennis elbow, is a term that can be misleading as most people who have it didn't get it from playing tennis. The mechanism of action for this type of injury is mostly due to overuse and poor mechanics that lead to an overload of the extensor and supinator tendons. Poor technique with racquet sports including improper backhand, inappropriate string tension, and inappropriate grip size are just some examples of how an athlete, especially an amateur athlete, can sustain this injury. The muscles mainly affected in a case of lateral epicondylitis are the extensor carpi radialis brevis, extensor carpi radialis longus, and the extensor digitorum communis.

The workup for diagnosing epicondylitis is often based on history and physical examination where laboratory studies are often of no value and imaging is rarely used. Plain radiographs of the elbow may show calcifications adjacent to the medial epicondyle in 20% to 30% of patients with medial epicondylitis but it has been shown that imaging is unnecessary in the workup of this condition (9). MRI is rarely used and only useful to rule out other causes of elbow pain like partial tendon tears, ligament injury, or in cases of recalcitrant epicondylitis.

Initial treatment of epicondylitis consists of relative rest, activity modification, thermal modalities, and anti-inflammatory medications. A forearm band (counterforce brace) worn distal to the flexor or extensor muscle group can dissipate forces over the forearm muscles and relieve stress from the tendon insertions. If the patient still has pain, a two-phase rehabilitation therapy program can be implemented. The first phase focuses on decreasing pain with different modalities (ultrasound, electrical stimulation) and education with biomechanical modifications. The second phase begins when the patient is pain free. This involves a strengthening program starting with static exercises and advancing to progressive resistive exercises. It also incorporates a stretching program. Injected corticosteroids have also been shown to be of benefit, but there are possible complications. The most feared complication postcorticosteroid injection use is tendon rupture, which can be minimized by ultrasound-guided techniques in which the tendon is visualized to avoid injecting directly into the tendon. No anatomic structure should be injected if unexpected resistance exists. The other dreaded complication from corticosteroid use is nerve damage (i.e., median nerve atrophy) following multiple attempted injections. Injection of botulinum toxin into the extensor digitorum communis muscles to the third and fourth digits has been reported to be beneficial in treating chronic treatment-resistant lateral epicondylitis (10). If conservative treatment fails (after 6–12 months), surgical treatment can be considered such as release of the origin of the extensor carpi radialis brevis and/or longus muscles and excision of excessive scar tissue.

Wrist and hand disorders: De Quervain tenosynovitis is defined as a stenosing tenosynovitis of the synovial sheath of tendons of the EPB and APL in the first dorsal compartment of the wrist due to repetitive use. Inflammation at this site is commonly seen in patients from cumulative microtrauma. Inflammation can also occur after a single episode of acute trauma to the site. Although this condition is seen in both males and females, it commonly has a predilection for females, especially during pregnancy and the postpartum period. No testing is available for de Quervain disease, other than serology testing for rheumatoid arthritis if clinical suspicion prevails. No imaging studies are needed and physical examination is often sufficient to make the diagnosis. However, in a setting of acute trauma, a radiograph can be performed, which may show a suggestion of fracture or osteonecrosis.

Initial treatment can start with rest, ice, splinting, and nonsteroidal anti-inflammatory medication, although there are some studies that show these treatments are ineffective (11). A rehabilitation therapy program can be implemented to reduce pain and improve function. In the acute phase, the therapist can use cryotherapy at the radial styloid to reduce inflammation and edema, followed by topical steroids that can be delivered into the subcutaneous tissue by phonophoresis and iontophoresis (12). The goals of therapy are to strengthen and regain ROM at the thumb, hand, and wrist. A thumb spica splint can be utilized to manage symptoms as it inhibits gliding of the tendon through the abnormal canal. Injection of anesthetic in combination with corticosteroid is currently the most frequently used treatment modality with an 83% cure rate (13). Surgery is considered a last resort reserved for those who fail injection therapy. Surgery involves incision of the skin, slitting or removal of a strip of the tendon sheath, closure of the skin, and application of a compression bandage that is removed in a week. The patient returns to normal activities after 2 to 3 weeks. On average, surgical success rates range from 83% to 92% (14).

In summary, for most upper extremity injuries a thorough history and physical examination are usually sufficient in obtaining the correct diagnosis. Laboratory studies and imaging should only be performed to accurately document the diagnosis and rule out other more serious conditions like tumors or rheumatologic disease. Radiologic examinations should start with an x-ray, and will range from CT, MRI, or ultrasound varying on the location and severity of the injury. Furthermore, blood work may be appropriate, such as uric acid levels, ESR, CRP, and rheumatoid factors, but only in cases where there is a high suspicion of underlying disease.

PRACTICE-BASED LEARNING AND IMPROVEMENT

GOALS

Demonstrate competence in continuously investigating and evaluating your own patient care practices in UEMI, appraising and assimilating scientific evidence, and continuously improving your patient care practices based on continuous self-evaluation and lifelong learning.

OBJECTIVES

1. Describe learning opportunities for providers, patients, and caregivers with experience in diagnostic and management decisions for patients with UEMIs.
2. Use methods for ongoing competency training in UEMI for physiatrists, including formative evaluation feedback in daily practice, evaluating current practice, and developing a QI and practice performance improvement activity strategy.
3. Locate resources including available websites and professional organizations for continuing medical education and professional development in UEMI.
4. Describe some areas paramount to self-assessment and lifelong learning in treatment and management of patients with UEMI.

The experienced physiatrist should have a myriad of tools at his or her disposal to improve decision making in clinical practice whether establishing a particular diagnosis, discussing treatment and prognosis, or matching patients to optimal interventions based on a parsimonious subset of predictor variables from the history and physical examination.

First and foremost, a physiatrist should evaluate his or her own breadth and scope of knowledge on the practice of upper extremity disorders and should be able to recognize any gaps in what he or she knows. For instance, practitioners should have history and physical examination abilities to determine the acuity and etiology of different disorders like RTC tears and de Quervain tenosynovitis. Only after a proper history and physical are obtained should imaging be utilized to further narrow the differential diagnoses made during the initial evaluation. Once a diagnosis is defined, the practitioner should reflect on the current level of success in his or her clinical practice regarding interventional vs. surgical vs. conservative treatments. Likely, the practitioner will need to facilitate a variety of treatment modalities to properly treat the patient's pain and disabilities.

A physiatrist should also undergo periodic reflection on outcomes in his or her clinical practice. For instance, patients should be instructed to fill out pain surveys on each office visit, which should be compared retrospectively and analyzed by the physiatrist. A physiatrist who performs interventional procedures can easily analyze improved pain scores, improved functionality, and the requirement for less oral or topical pain medications with each visit. If a patient requires more medication to treat his or her pain, then obviously the interventional techniques are inappropriate and perhaps the practicing physiatrist should change his or her treatment plan. In addition, one should utilize the practice of 360° analysis where patients, family members, therapists, nurses, and ancillary staff are all instructed to evaluate each other and comment on their communication and interpersonal skills, diagnosis, and therapeutic modalities. Physicians who are recent graduates from a residency program should seek the help of senior experienced physicians when making difficult clinical decisions, as they have a wealth of knowledge that they may offer to their junior colleagues.

There are also many resources currently available from which a physiatrist can obtain information and training to address his or her deficits and sharpen his or her skills. Knowledge NOW is a novel comprehensive online source for physiatrists organized by clinical topics (15). Knowledge NOW is still being developed and will be an important resource for physiatrists who wish to sharpen their knowledge base in an abbreviated manner. Another excellent web resource is PASSOR, which is the Physiatric Association for Spine, Sports, and Occupational Rehabilitation. This organization has published physical examination competency lists and guidelines for different interventional procedures. Another evidence-based website available to the practicing physiatrist is the Cochrane review, in which systematic reviews are performed and, in return, proper diagnostic evaluations and effects of interventions for prevention, treatment, and rehabilitation are discussed and analyzed (16). Full text and abbreviated articles are available for review in many languages and among multiple different disciplines. Other arenas that may provide innovative information on upper extremity disorders are literature reviews, white paper publications from organizations, and PubMed reviews.

Thus, there is no current shortage of resources for a physiatrist to become more knowledgeable in the diagnosis and treatment of upper extremity disorders. There are also an increasing number of procedure-based courses as technology continues to improve. The advent of the ultrasound has dramatically altered the field of physiatry and is becoming more of a daily tool that the physiatrist should utilize.

INTERPERSONAL AND COMMUNICATION SKILLS

GOALS

Demonstrate interpersonal and communication skills that result in the effective exchange of information and collaboration with UEMI patients, their families, and the rest of the rehabilitation team.

OBJECTIVES

1. Demonstrate skills used in effective verbal and nonverbal communication, listening, conflict resolution, and collaboration with UEMI patients and their caregivers, across socioeconomic and cultural backgrounds.
2. Delineate the importance of the role of the physiatrist as the interdisciplinary team leader and consultant pertinent to UEMI.
3. Demonstrate proper and timely medical record documentation and effective communication with consulting clinicians and referring physicians, and between health care professional team members in patient care as it applies to UEMI.
4. Identify key areas for physicians to counsel patients and families specific to UEMI.

As is the case for all conditions treated by a physiatrist, the care of patients with upper extremity musculoskeletal disorders also requires a multidisciplinary team approach. The first step in the care of a patient with an upper extremity disorder is not to perform a physical examination or order radiologic studies but to develop a strong doctor–patient relationship that involves mutual trust and respect. With the patient's permission, involving family, friends, or caregivers in the treatment plan can significantly speed up the patient's recovery time. These people can also assist the patient during healing when they are unable to perform many of their ADLs on their own due to their inability to use their upper extremity. The quality and safety of patient care can also improve when families play an active role. Family members can give unique information about the patient; interpret information from caregivers to the patient; and offer the patient touch and emotional comfort, personal hygiene, dressing changes, and coaching through painful procedures (17).

The importance of teamwork and communication skills among providers, patients, their families, and caregivers is of utmost importance in the care of patients with upper extremity musculoskeletal disorders, and a lot of what we know today is learned from programs developed by the U.S. military. From 1984 to 1989, research revealed that army aviation crew coordination failures contributed to 147 aviation fatalities and costs of more than $290 million, mostly attributed to issues with crew communication (18). This led the military to develop multiple training and evaluation systems to improve teamwork and communication, helping to develop a culture of safety in the military. One program developed by the Department of Defense Patient Safety Program in collaboration with the Department of Health and Human Services' Agency for Healthcare Research and Quality (AHRQ) is called Team STEPPS (Team strategies and tools to enhance performance and patient safety) (19). This is a teamwork system designed to improve the quality, safety, and efficiency of health care. The key components of the Team STEPPS program are leadership, situation monitoring, mutual support, and communication.

Leadership involves the ability to coordinate the activities of team members by ensuring team actions are understood, changes in information are shared, and that team members have the necessary resources to treat the patient properly. In the case of an upper extremity musculoskeletal disorder, the physiatrist needs to take on the role of team leader and treat the patient in a multidisciplinary team approach. He or she would be the one responsible for coordinating the patient's treatment plan and monitoring the patient's progress in the rehabilitation program. If there are any changes that need to be implemented—for example a change in weight-bearing status—it would be the physiatrist's responsibility to convey this information to the rest of the team.

In the case of a patient with a RTC tear, the patient will require a provider to take on a leadership role in making sure he or she gets the best treatment possible for a speedy recovery. This is an opportunity for a physiatrist with all the knowledge and skills learned during training to assume this leadership role. Once diagnosed with a RTC tear, the physiatrist can discuss with the patient, and his or her family if necessary, all available treatment options. If surgery is recommended, the physiatrist can coordinate the care between the orthopedist and himself or herself. Once surgery is completed, the physiatrist can develop a therapeutic rehabilitation program for improving the patient's strength, ROM, and ADLs while dealing with any pain issues due to the surgery. Whether working closely with the patient's insurance company to get approval for therapy visits or getting involved with the patient's employer to request modifications in work duties while the patient heals, good team leadership in the case of an upper extremity musculoskeletal disorder is of utmost importance.

Situation monitoring is another component of Team STEPPS, which is a process of actively scanning and assessing situational elements to gain information and understanding while maintaining awareness to support functioning of the team. The physiatrist is responsible for monitoring the actions of the other team members, ensuring that mistakes or oversights are caught quickly and easily so that the patient can progress toward the goals of healing.

Mutual support, another important concept of Team STEPPS, is crucial in dealing with upper extremity musculoskeletal disorders. It involves the ability to anticipate and support other team members' needs through accurate knowledge about their responsibilities and workload. In the case of an upper extremity musculoskeletal disorder, the physiatrist needs to work with many other physicians including orthopedics, radiologists, and primary care physicians. The physiatrist also works very closely with the therapists directly involved in the patient's care. Working in collaboration with all these members of the medical team helps achieve a mutually satisfying solution resulting in the best outcome for the patient.

Communication, the last and probably most important principle of Team STEPPS, is a process by which information is clearly and accurately exchanged among team members. Due to the fact there are many members of the health care team and many ongoing changing factors when dealing with a patient with an upper extremity musculoskeletal disorder, strategies and tools for effective communication are needed. One such structured communication method is known as "Brief, Huddle, Debrief." The Brief component involves a short session prior to the start of any treatment to discuss team formation, assign essential roles, establish expectations, and anticipate outcomes. The Huddle portion is an ad hoc planning to reestablish situation awareness, reinforce plans already in place, and assess the need to adjust the plan. Debrief is an informal information exchange session designed to improve team performance and effectiveness (20).

Documentation in the medical record has always been an important tool in the communication between providers; but in cases of patients with upper extremity musculoskeletal disorders medical documentation is used by nonclinicians too. Many upper extremity musculoskeletal issues are associated with lawsuits, whether due to an accident on the job or a motor vehicle accident. Precise documentation in the medical record by the physiatrist is extremely important, as it will most likely be used in a legal case. Lawyers, in many cases, will request copies of the medical record to use in their case and the physiatrist will be held responsible for anything written in the chart. In addition, anything they omit from the chart will be considered as if it did not occur.

Insurance companies are another nonphysician entity that will use the medical record; this is especially common in upper extremity musculoskeletal disorders. When requesting additional therapy visits for one's patient, insurance companies will request the medical record to evaluate if the patient is making progress in the therapy program prescribed. A well-documented medical record is needed to assist patients in getting the care they need.

In summary, patient care and medical knowledge are very important when treating patients with upper extremity musculoskeletal disorders, but if the physiatrist is lacking interpersonal and communication skills there is a higher chance for treatment failure. Demonstrating courtesy and respect for the patient, his or her families and caregivers, and all members of the health care team helps build relationships that lead to results with the best outcomes.

PROFESSIONALISM

GOALS

Reflect a commitment to carrying out professional responsibilities and an adherence to ethical principles in caring for patients with musculoskeletal injuries.

OBJECTIVES

1. Exemplify the humanistic qualities as a provider of care for patients with musculoskeletal injuries such as respect, promptness, efficiency, courtesy, kindness, altruism, integrity, honesty, compassion, and empathy.
2. Maintain professional behavior at all times including appropriate dress, language, and conduct.
3. Demonstrate ethical principles and responsiveness to patient needs superseding self and other interests.
4. Demonstrate sensitivity to patient population diversity including culture, gender, age, race, religion, disabilities, and sexual orientation.
5. Demonstrate and respect patient-centered care, confidentiality, patient privacy, autonomy, shared decision making, and informed consent as applicable to musculoskeletal injuries.
6. Recognize the importance of patient education in the treatment of and advocacy for patients with musculoskeletal injuries.

A physiatrist's job caring for patients with upper extremity musculoskeletal disorders from a diverse population can be rewarding and an eye-opening experience, while at the same time difficult due to obstacles that may arise from social, economic, and cultural differences. Ethical issues will also commonly arise during which time the physiatrist needs to maintain professional behavior without injecting his or her own personal judgment or beliefs that might interfere with medical decision making.

A social history is extremely important when developing a treatment plan for a patient with an upper extremity musculoskeletal disorder. Many upper extremity injuries require a certain amount of relative rest in order to heal properly (21). A patient who has young children and is their sole provider will be unable to comply with certain weight-bearing restrictions due to the need to lift the children. Upper extremity splints that are necessary for healing may not be practical for certain patients, again causing noncompliance. Knowledge of a patient's social situation can help the physiatrist provide the proper education necessary for a successful outcome.

Economic factors can also affect a patient's potential for a healthy recovery from an upper extremity musculoskeletal injury. Someone whose occupation requires a lot of upper extremity movement, like a housekeeper, will be unable to adhere to certain limitations due to the economic need to continue working. Also, physiatrists need to be aware that certain patients may not be able to afford to purchase equipment that may be recommended as part of their home exercise program to help speed their recovery. The high cost of medical equipment or the lack of insurance may also prevent patients from purchasing specific upper extremity braces or splints that are needed.

Culture affects all aspects of medical care and is something a physiatrist needs to be sensitive to and respect when caring for patients. Some cultures have modesty restrictions that, even though they might not prohibit them from participating in a therapy program, would hinder them from doing certain specific exercises in public areas. For example, a woman with strong religious beliefs with a shoulder injury may not be able to bare her shoulders in a public place for treatment. Professional sports players and extreme athletes also make up an interesting group of patients that follow a specific type of sports culture. Many athletes have been known to talk about the "play-through-it" culture of sports where if an athlete sustained an injury he or she would still continue to play (22). Also, during the rehabilitation process, the physiatrist needs to be wary of an athlete's desire to return to play before he or she is ready.

Ethical issues frequently arise when treating upper extremity musculoskeletal conditions. Based on reports from the CDC and the U.S. Census Bureau, the absolute number of disability claims has risen from during the time period between 1999 and 2005. The two most common complaints cited for disability are both musculoskeletal conditions, arthritis being the most common and back/spine problems a close second (23). Unfortunately some patients may experience negative reinforcement and not improve in function in order to be eligible for disability. The physiatrist's ethical principles are then called into play when he or she is required to fill out paperwork describing the patient's condition and functional status. Current evidence in work disability shows that advice to return to modified work and graded activity programs are most effective in reducing work absenteeism (24). Motor vehicle or work-related accidents are other examples of situations in which a patient may falsely exhibit an upper extremity injury in order to receive compensation from an insurance company or another individual. In all cases, the physiatrist should document all objective findings and maintain professional behavior and appropriate conduct at all times.

In addition to a physician being committed to performing professional responsibilities, going above and beyond to become a patient advocate separates good physicians from those known to be leaders in their field. In dealing with patients with upper extremity musculoskeletal disorders, a physiatrist needs to consider the patient as a whole by getting familiar with his or her work and social activities. For example, treating a patient with a repetitive stress injury in the upper extremity such as de Quervain tenosynovitis will be futile unless that patient modifies his or her daily routine. In the case of a stenographer who constantly uses his or her hands, the physiatrist will need to advocate for the patient to be placed on limited duty at his or her workplace until the condition heals. The physiatrist will also need to get familiar with the patient's work space in order to recommend changes in ergonomics. Another example where a physiatrist would need to advocate for his or her patient would be a case of lateral epicondylitis in an athlete who plays tennis for the school team. The physiatrist will need to play a key role in open discussions (with the patient's permission) with the coach of the team to allow the athlete some rest from sports until the epicondylitis heals. In addition, the physiatrist can assess the athlete's equipment and swing mechanics to prevent reoccurrence of the injury.

In summary, a physiatrist treating upper extremity musculoskeletal disorders needs to show commitment in performing his or her professional responsibilities and adhere to the ethical principles he or she undertook when reciting the Hippocratic Oath, attesting to practice medicine honestly. The physiatrist also needs to be sensitive to a patient's social, economic, and cultural beliefs and maintain professional behavior at all times.

SYSTEMS-BASED PRACTICE

GOALS

Awareness and responsiveness to systems of interdisciplinary care delivery, and the ability to access, evaluate, recruit, and coordinate effectively resources in the system to provide optimal continuum of care and outcomes as it relates to UEMI.

OBJECTIVES

1. Identify the key components, interprofessional team providers, systems of care delivery, services, referral patterns, coordination of care, and resources in the rehabilitation continuum of care.
2. Identify patient safety concerns and participate in patient safety activities, including identifying and avoiding potential systems-related and medical-related errors in the care of UEMI and strategies to minimize them.
3. Describe markers of quality in the care of the UEMI patient.

4. Describe cost/risk–benefit analysis, including ordering tests and discharge planning, utilization, and management of resources as they apply to UEMI.

Patients with UEMIs receive care in a variety of health care settings by a variety of health care providers. For example, occupational injuries involving the upper extremities can be treated in occupational medicine clinics or general physical medicine and rehabilitation clinics by physiatrists or occupational medicine physicians. Sports injuries of the upper extremities can be treated by orthopedists, physiatrists, family physicians, internists, and physical therapists in outpatient clinics.

UEMIs may also occur or be diagnosed in the inpatient setting in hospitals and skilled nursing facilities. Internists, physiatrists, orthopedists, physical therapists, and occupational therapists are some of the providers that can be involved in the care of patients with UEMIs.

Regardless of setting, coordination of care is essential among the providers to ensure that an appropriate treatment plan is carried out and monitored and that there is no duplication of services or diagnostic tests.

Close follow-up is important in the care of patients with UEMIs since impairments can quickly lead to significant activity limitations and participation restrictions. Painful RTC tears can lead to limited ROM of the shoulder, which can limit ADLs such as dressing as well as the ability to perform overhead activities in one's work setting. Painful inflammatory conditions of the elbows and wrists can lead to significant negative impact in ability to perform work in a work setting. The physiatrist should educate workers at risk for these types of injuries or injured athletes on strategies to minimize the risk of occurrence and recurrence. In addition, the physiatrist can educate employers about workplace modifications to minimize occupational injuries of the upper extremities and coaches of athletes on training techniques and equipment.

Quality of care in the treatment of UEMI should be timely, effective, and provided by competent, skilled, and compassionate providers so that secondary complications such as loss of function are minimized and the maximal level of function is achieved. The physiatrist should minimize the possibility of treatment-related complications from medications and injections.

Health care costs in the United States have continued to rise over the years. According to the World Health Organization (WHO), the United States spent more on health care per capita and more on health care as a percentage of its GDP (17.9%) than any other nation in 2011. The Commonwealth Fund ranked the United States last in the quality of health care among similar countries and notes U.S. care cost the most. In the 2013 Bloomberg ranking of nations with the most efficient health care systems, the United States ranks 46th among the 48 countries included in the study (25). The Institute for Health Improvement (IHI), an independent not-for-profit organization that is a leading innovator in health and health care improvement worldwide, then developed the Triple Aim as an approach to optimize the performance of the health system. The Triple Aim's goals are (a) improving the patient experience of care (including quality and satisfaction), (b) improving the health of populations, and (c) reducing the per capita cost of health care.

When a physiatrist is treating patients with upper extremity musculoskeletal disorders, he or she should always consider the Triple Aim when developing treatment plans. Cost efficiency in ordering tests, especially radiological studies, is a skill that can be difficult but one that every physiatrist should attempt to master. Preventive medicine also has been shown to be extremely important in reducing costs and improving the health of populations. Physiatrists dealing with patients with upper extremity musculoskeletal disorders will notice that many injuries, especially in their elderly population, occur due to falls. A plan to prevent falls in geriatric patients can decrease the high costs associated with the treatment of upper extremity injuries secondary to falls.

The ordering of radiologic imaging for patients with upper extremity musculoskeletal disorders continues to increase in the United States. Implementing guideline recommendations on when to order a certain radiologic study can not only decrease unnecessary ionizing radiation exposure but also decrease costs and improve accessibility (26). Imaging studies should only be considered if (a) they yield clinically important information beyond that obtained from the history and physical examination, (b) this information can potentially alter patient management, and (c) this altered management has a reasonable probability to improve patient outcomes. For example, patients with shoulder pain with no precipitating fall, no sudden onset of pain or swelling, no palpable mass or deformity, no pain at rest, and normal ROM are unlikely to require an initial radiographic examination (27). Radiographs are also not initially indicated for adult patients with nontraumatic elbow pain with full or limited movement of less than 4 weeks' duration. Following best practice models for ordering radiologic studies will not only reduce costs but will improve patient safety too.

In summary, the Triple Aim model of better health and better care at lower costs can only be successful if one understands and realizes how patient care and other professional practices impact on other health care professionals, health care organizations, and society. Practicing cost-effective evidence-based medicine, whether it be by being more efficient and diligent when ordering radiologic studies or by implementing preventive strategies to decrease falls, will be important for the survival of the health system in the United States and the continued success and development in the field of medicine.

CASE STUDY

A 15-year-old boy with no past medical history presents to your office with the chief complaint of pain in the lateral aspect of his right elbow over the past 3 weeks. He states that he has difficulty helping his mother carrying the groceries home from the supermarket and his mother, who accompanied him to his visit to your office, feels he is just being lazy and trying to make excuses in order not to help out. He denies any fever, nausea, vomiting, recent weight loss, or night sweats. He is an honor roll student and plays on his high school tennis team.

He currently lives with his mother and 7 siblings in a 2-bedroom apartment. He denies doing "anything out of the ordinary" over the past month. Physical examination of the right upper extremity is significant for some swelling over his lateral epicondyle. His muscle strength is 5/5 throughout the right upper extremity and he has full ROM. Cozen test is positive. He has no sensory deficits and his reflexes are normal.

CASE STUDY DISCUSSION QUESTIONS

1. What is your differential diagnosis for the patient's condition?
2. Discuss the anatomy involved and the mechanics of swinging a tennis racquet.
3. Utilize available medical resources to make appropriate treatment recommendations including side effects and efficacy of treatment for this patient's condition.
4. Discuss any social issues that might contribute to the patient's condition and any barriers to recovery.
5. Role-play a discussion between yourself, your patient, your patient's mother, and the coach of the team discussing your patient's condition, treatment options, and prevention from further injury.
6. What imaging studies and laboratory tests would you consider ordering for this patient? Discuss the cost efficiency.

SELF-EXAMINATION QUESTIONS
(Answers begin on p. 367)

1. Which of the following diagnostic tests will be most helpful in making the correct diagnosis for de Quervain tenosynovitis?
   A. Neer test
   B. Hawkins test
   C. Finkelstein test
   D. Green test
   E. Phalen test

2. Which of the following manual muscle testing grade would you expect if the patient is able to resist only against moderate pressure throughout ROM?
   A. 2 out of 5
   B. 3 out of 5
   C. 3+ out of 5
   D. 4 out of 5
   E. 5 out of 5

3. What is the normal ROM for elbow flexion?
   A. 0° to 90°
   B. 0° to 115°
   C. 5° to 115°
   D. 0° to 145°
   E. 0° to 180°

4. Which of the following is a feared complication of a cortisone injection for tendonitis?
   A. Pain
   B. Urinary retention
   C. Tendon rupture
   D. Risk of cancer
   E. Risk of bone fracture

5. Which muscle listed below is part of the RTC muscles?
   A. Teres major
   B. Teres minor
   C. Deltoid
   D. Rhomboid
   E. Triceps

REFERENCES

1. Epstein O, Perkin GD, Cookson J, et al. *Clinical Examination*. 4th ed. St. Louis, MO: Mosby Elsevier; 2008.
2. Braddom R, Chan L, Harrast, MA. *Physical Medicine and Rehabilitation*. 4th ed. Philadelphia, PA: Saunders/Elsevier; 2011.
3. http://www.ncbi.nlm.nih.gov/pubmed/17805510. Accessed January 27, 2014.
4. Cuccurullo S. *Physical Medicine and Rehabilitation Board Review*. New York, NY: Demos Medical Publishing; 2004.
5. Mall NA, Lee AS, Chahal J, et al. An evidenced-based examination of the epidemiology and outcomes of traumatic rotator cuff tears. *Arthroscopy*. February 2013;29(2):366–376. doi:10.1016/j.arthro.2012.06.024. Epub January 3, 2013.
6. Frontera W, Silver J. *Essentials of Physical Medicine and Rehabilitation*. Philadelphia, PA: Hanley & Belfus Inc.; 2002:90.
7. Stetson WB, Phillips T, Deutsch A. The use of magnetic resonance arthrography to detect partial-thickness rotator cuff tears. *J Bone Joint Surg Am*. 2005;87(suppl 2):81–88.
8. Tashjian RZ. Epidemiology, natural history, and indications for treatment of rotator cuff tears. *Clin Sports Med*. October 2012;31(4):589–604. doi:10.1016/j.csm.2012.07.001. PMID 23040548.
9. http://emedicine.medscape.com/article/97217-workup. Accessed January 27, 2014.
10. Wong SM, Jui AC, Tong PY, et al. Treatment of lateral epicondylitis with botulinum toxin: a randomized, double-blind, placebo-controlled trial. *Ann Intern Med*. 2005;143:793–797.
11. Moore JS. De Quervain's tenosynovitis: stenosing tenosynovitis of the first dorsal compartment. *J Occup Environ Med*. 1997;39:990–1002.
12. http://emedicine.medscape.com/article/327453-treatment. Accessed January 27, 2014.
13. Richie CA, Briner WW. Corticosteroid injection for treatment of de Quervain's tenosynovitis: a pooled quantitative literature evaluation. *J Am Board Fam Pract*. 2003;16:102–106.
14. Frontera W, Silver J. *Essentials of Physical Medicine and Rehabilitation*. Philadelphia, PA: Saunders/Elsevier; 2008:131.
15. http://www.aapmr.org/education/knowledge-now/Pages/default.aspx. Accessed January 27, 2014.
16. http://www.cochrane.org/cochrane-reviews. Accessed January 27, 2014.
17. Neal A, Twibell R, et al. Providing family-friendly care-even when stress is high and time is short: although liberal visiting policies can benefit patients and families, they pose challenges for nurses. *Am Nurs Today*. 2010;5(11):9–12.
18. www.drc.com/solutions/tps/high.htm. Accessed August 31, 2013.
19. Rivers R, Swain MD, Nixon B. Using aviation safety measures to enhance patient outcomes. *AORN J*. January 2003;77(1):158–162.
20. http://teamstepps.ahrq.gov. Accessed July 17, 2013.
21. Frontera W, Silver J. *Essentials of Physical Medicine and Rehabilitation*. Philadelphia, PA: Hanley & Belfus Inc.; 2002.
22. Fleming D. Not so crazy now, am I? *ESPN: The Magazine*. May 1, 2013.

23. CDC. Prevalence and most common causes of disability among adults—United States, 2005. *MMWR*. 2009;58(16):421–426.
24. Loisel P, Buchbinder R, et al. Prevention of work disability due to musculoskeletal disorders: the challenge of implementing evidence. *J Occup Rehabil*. December 2005;15(4):507–524.
25. Davidson KA. The most efficient health care systems in the world. *The Huffington Post*. August 29, 2013.
26. Bussieres AE, Peterson C, et al. Diagnostic imaging guideline for musculoskeletal Complaints in Adults-An evidence-based approach: Upper extremity disorders. *J Manipulative Physiol Ther*. January 2008;31(1):2–32.
27. Fraenkel L, et al. Improving the selective use of plain radiographs in the initial evaluation of shoulder pain. *J Rheumatol*. 2000;27:200.

Hamilton Chen
Danielle Perret Karimi

24: Lumbar Spine Disorders

PATIENT CARE

GOALS

Provide patient care that is compassionate, appropriate, and effective for the treatment of lumbar spine disorders and the promotion of good health.

OBJECTIVES

1. Perform a pertinent history and physical of the patient with low back pain.
2. Describe Waddell signs and its clinical use.
3. Identify "red flags" and key impairments, activity limitations, and participation restrictions for patients with lumbar pain.
4. Identify the psychosocial and vocational implications of low back pain and strategies to address them.
5. Discuss the implications for return to work for low back pain.
6. Describe a sample rehabilitation or treatment plan for low back pain.

PATIENT ASSESSMENT

The key elements of the history for lumbar spine pathology are obtained by eliciting the pain litany (1), a formulaic exploration of the patient's pain history. It includes the following:

1. Mode of onset (trauma, insidious, acute); note circumstances surrounding pain
2. Location and any radiation of pain (with consideration of dermatomes)
3. Chronicity (when did pain start?)
4. Tempo (constant or intermittent; if intermittent, duration and frequency of pain)
5. Character of pain (burning, aching, paroxysmal, shooting, etc.)
6. Severity/intensity of pain; note whether there is pain at night
7. Associated factors
   a. Precipitating factors (alleviating and exacerbating factors, including positions)
   b. Environmental factors (occupation, ergonomics)
   c. Family history
   d. Age at onset
   e. Pregnancy and menstruation
   f. Gender
   g. Past/current medical and surgical history
   h. Socioeconomic considerations
   i. Psychiatric history and current psychosocial considerations
   j. Medications, drug, and alcohol use
8. Treatments tried in the past and the level of effectiveness

Due to the high prevalence of lumbar spine pathology and the frequently benign course of the disease, there is an inherent necessity to tease out conditions that may pose significant threats to patients, such as fractures, tumors, and infections. The United States Agency for Health Care Policy and Research (AHCPR) published guidelines listing "red flags" in the clinical evaluation of the lumbar spine (Table 24.1) (2).

If any of these red flags are present, it is prudent for the physician to pursue further diagnostic testing.

In addition to the pain litany and evaluation for the red flags, another equally important aspect of the patient's history is the presence of any functional deficits resulting from the lumbar spine disease. The physiatrist should elicit the impairments in the patient's activities of daily living (ADLs) and functional mobility.

The key elements of the physical examination of the lumbar spine include a detailed neurologic and musculoskeletal examination. The neurologic component of the examination includes muscle strength testing, muscle stretch reflexes, and sensation testing. If there is suspicion for cauda equina or conus medullaris syndrome, examination maneuvers to determine upper motor neuron versus lower motor neuron pathology should be performed.

The musculoskeletal examination of the lumbar spine includes inspection, palpation, range of motion (ROM), and provocative tests for lumbar radicular pain (straight leg raise, crossed straight leg raise, slump tests), and for facet syndrome (Kemp test).

TABLE 24.1 Lumbar Spine "Red Flags"

POSSIBLE FRACTURE	POSSIBLE TUMOR OR INFECTION	POSSIBLE CAUDA EQUINA SYNDROME
From Medical History		
Major trauma, such as vehicle accident or fall from height	Age over 50 or under 20	Saddle anesthesia
Minor trauma or even strenuous lifting (in older or potentially osteoporotic patient)	History of cancer	Recent onset of bladder dysfunction, such as urinary retention, increased frequency, or overflow incontinence
	Constitutional symptoms, such as recent fever or chills or unexplained weight loss	Severe or progressive neurologic deficit in the lower extremity
	Risk factors for spinal infection: recent bacterial infection (e.g., urinary tract infection); recent spinal/epidural procedure; IV drug abuse; or immune suppression (from steroids, transplant, or HIV)	
	Pain that worsens when supine; severe nighttime pain	
From Physical Examination		
Examination limited by severe pain	Examination findings range from mild to severe, depending on progression; may also have positive tests for radicular pain	Unexpected laxity of the anal sphincter
Skin abrasions and contusions		Perianal/perineal sensory loss
Deviations from normal spine curves		Major motor weakness: quadriceps (knee extension weakness); ankle plantar flexors, evertors, and/or dorsiflexors (footdrop)

IMPAIRMENTS, ACTIVITY LIMITATIONS, AND PARTICIPATION RESTRICTIONS

The lumbar spine is associated with a wide range of clinical disorders. Although lumbar spine pathology may be a result of rheumatologic, hematologic, endocrinologic, and even neoplastic disorders, most impairments of the lumbar spine are the results of mechanical disorders.

Mechanical disorders refer to pain that results from overuse of a normal anatomic structure or pain that results from trauma or deformity of an anatomic structure (1). Common mechanical disorders from the lumbar spine include muscle strain, degenerative disc disease, osteoarthritis, lumbar stenosis, spondylolysis, and scoliosis. Discussion of the presentation of each differential diagnosis is beyond the scope of this text.

Disabilities that result from the lumbar spine may result in an inability to meet personal, social, and occupational demands. Patients with lumbar spine pathology often will have difficulty performing ADLs, functional mobility, and work duties.

General population studies have demonstrated that most low back pain episodes are mild and rarely disabling, with only a small proportion seeking care. Among patients who do present for care, 75% to 90% of those with "acute" low back pain recover in terms of pain and disability (3). This is in contrast to those with "chronic" low back pain, when pain is present greater than 3 months, and where prior studies have shown that two-thirds of patients still had not fully recovered 1 to 2 years after the initial onset of pain (3).

Biomechanical and anatomic factors often do not explain this variability in the clinical course of patients with lumbar spine pathology. There have been multiple psychosocial factors found to play a role in the prognosis for low back pain.

Prior literature reviews found that general psychological stress, negative cognitive characteristics, and depression are all associated with a poor prognosis for recovery (3). A study by Sullivan et al. found that depression is associated with increased pain intensity, disability, medication use, and unemployment among those with low back pain (4).

Prior literature reviews also reported that passive coping strategies, somatization symptoms, involvement of workers' compensation, involvement of legal representation, and fear avoidance were also associated with poor outcomes (3,5).

Other studied vocational psychosocial factors include job satisfaction, subjective appraisal of one's ability to work, significant prognostic factors in low back pain, and educational level (3,6).

When evaluating a patient with low back pain, it is important for the physician to consider these psychosocial variables for an estimation of prognosis. In addition, the physician should also consider Waddell signs (Table 24.2), which are signs/symptoms of low back pain that are nonorganic. It may suggest that there may be a psychological component to the patient's presentation.

The estimated annual cost for all occupational injuries and deaths in the United States is $128 billion to $155 billion, and the estimated annual cost for back pain is $20 billion to $50 billion (5). Maetzel et al. (7) estimated, in a review of studies published between 1996 and 2001, that lumbar spine injuries resulted in 149 million lost workdays per year. Bernacki et al. (8) found that patients covered by workers' compensation tended to have more office visits, hospital admissions, treating physicians, diagnostic referrals, and therapeutic procedures, and longer duration of care, compared with patients covered by other forms of insurance.

TABLE 24.2 Waddell Signs

- Tenderness tests: superficial and diffuse tenderness and/or nonanatomic tenderness
- Simulation tests: these are based on movements which produce pain, without actually causing that movement, such as axial loading and pain on simulated rotation
- Distraction tests: positive tests are rechecked when the patient's attention is distracted, such as a straight leg raise test
- Regional disturbances: regional weakness or sensory changes which deviate from accepted neuroanatomy
- Overreaction: subjective signs regarding the patient's demeanor and reaction to testing

Even though most patients with low back pain usually recover within a few weeks, work absenteeism can be a problem encountered by the physician. The biggest risk factors for delayed return to work and chronic disability are psychosocial variables, such as depression, level of education, excessive pain level, fear avoidance, job dissatisfaction, legal representation, somatization disorder, unemployment, and workers' compensation (5).

Recommendations for return to work should be highly individualized. In general, patients with nonspecific low back pain should continue to work, even when they continue to have low back pain symptoms during work. However, patients may require modified duty at work to prevent the aggravation of symptoms. A functional capacity evaluation (FCE) and vocational rehabilitation may assist in the preparation for return to work.

Associated conditions with mechanical low back pain include osteoarthritis of the peripheral joints. A prior epidemiologic study found a higher prevalence of hip and knee osteoarthritis in patients with spinal degenerative disorders (9).

In a patient presenting with acute low back pain, a comprehensive rehabilitation program begins with activity modification. Patients should avoid strenuous activity that may aggravate symptoms and nerve root irritation. Despite activity modification, the patient should be encouraged to ambulate and perform activities as tolerated. Strict bed rest is not recommended. Patients should be encouraged to return to work with modified duties.

Medication management includes nonsteroidal anti-inflammatory medications (NSAIDs), acetaminophen, muscle relaxants, and, in severe pain states, consideration for opioid analgesics (controversial). If there is a significant neuropathic component, membrane stabilizers, such as anticonvulsants and antidepressants, may be added as adjuvant treatment. There is no role for systemic glucocorticoids as an adjuvant treatment.

Formal physical therapy should include core strengthening, trunk coordination, and endurance exercises. If there is lower extremity pain, directional preference exercises may be helpful. Williams exercises (flexion-based exercises) may provide additional benefit in patients with neurogenic claudication symptoms from lumbar stenosis. McKenzie exercises (extension-based exercises) may provide additional benefit in patients with an acute disc herniation.

Additional forms of adjuvant treatment may include modalities, such as ice and/or heat, transcutaneous electrical nerve stimulation (TENS), and orthotics, such as lumbar corsets.

A comprehensive rehabilitation treatment may also include interventional procedures, depending on the presentation. Intraarticular facet injections and medial branch nerve blocks may be utilized as treatment for axial pain associated with facet disease. Epidural injections may be helpful for patients with lumbar radiculopathy/stenosis.

MEDICAL KNOWLEDGE

GOALS

Demonstrate knowledge of established and evolving biomedical, clinical epidemiological, and sociobehavioral sciences pertaining to lower back pain, as well as the application of this knowledge to guide holistic patient care.

OBJECTIVES

Discuss the following as they relate to lumbar spine/low back pain: (a) anatomy and clinical correlates; (b) epidemiology; (c) pathophysiology; (d) differential diagnosis; (e) diagnostic tests, common laboratories, and imaging; (f) treatment modalities; and (g) psychosocial and ethical issues.

The lumbar spine is comprised of 5 lumbar vertebrae, numbered L1 through L5. There is a small percentage of the population with 4 or 6 lumbar vertebrae. Directly beneath each lumbar vertebra, there is a pair of neural foramina with the same number designation. The neural foramina are bounded superiorly and inferiorly by pedicles, anteriorly by the intervertebral disc and vertebral body, and posteriorly by facet joints.

The spinal cord terminates at the conus medullaris, usually at the L1 or L2 level. Therefore, all lumbar and sacral spinal nerve roots originate from these levels. The dorsal root from the posterolateral aspect of the spinal cord and a ventral root from the anterolateral aspect of the cord join in the spinal canal to form the spinal nerve root. The spinal nerve roots then course down the intraspinal canal, forming the cauda equina until they exit at their respective foramina.

The primary function of the lumbar spine is for flexibility and protection of the spinal canal. The flexibility of the lumbar spine is accomplished through the functional units of the vertebral segments. Each vertebral segment is comprised of 3 functional units. One functional unit is formed between 2 vertebral bodies connected through an intervertebral disc. The 2 other functional units are the facet joints, formed from the articulation of the superior articular process of one vertebra with the inferior articular process of the vertebra above. The orientation of the lumbar facets is at a 90° angle to the transverse plane and at a 45° angle to the coronal plane. This makes the primary motion of the lumbar spine flexion and extension, with minimal side bending and rotation.

The intervertebral discs of the spine are composed of the annulus fibrosis, nucleus pulposus, and the vertebral end plates. The annulus fibrosis is composed of type I collagen that is arranged in organized, concentric lamellae, surrounding the nucleus pulposus. The nucleus pulposus is a gelatinous substance composed of water, proteoglycan, and type II collagen; it is largely an avascular structure. The annulus fibrosis has blood vessels in its superficial lamellae, while the nucleus has no direct blood supply. Nutrition is supplied by passive diffusion through the vertebral end plates and outer annulus fibrosis.

Any innervated structure in the lumbar spine can cause symptoms of low back and referred pain into the (usually proximal) extremity or extremities. Common pain generators in the lumbar spine include muscles, ligaments, dura mater, nerve roots, facet joints, annulus fibrosis of the disc, thoracolumbar fascia, and vertebrae.

Degeneration of the lumbar spine is postulated to be secondary to a degenerative cascade known as spondylosis (10). In phase I of this process (dysfunction phase), initial repetitive microtrauma leads to the development of circumferential tears of the annulus fibrosis and associated end-plate separation that may compromise disc nutrition supply. The circumferential annular tears will coalesce to form radial tears, resulting in loss of ability of the disc to retain water. This will lead to loss of disc height, disc desiccation, and disc bulging. In phase II (instability phase), there is loss of the mechanical integrity of the disc, with further loss of disc height. The loss of disc height increases the mechanical stress on the facet joints. This leads to facet degeneration, subluxation, and instability. In phase III (stabilization phase), continued disc space narrowing and fibrosis occur along with formation of osteophytes in the facet joints and vertebral bodies.

This cascade of degenerative anatomic changes in the lumbar spine may lead to lumbar stenosis, facet disease, and degenerative disc disease. Lumbar stenosis is the narrowing of the central lumbar spinal canal, lateral recess, or foramen from the process of spondylosis. If there is nerve root compression, the process is known as lumbar radiculopathy.

INCIDENCE AND PREVALENCE

A review by Hoy et al. (11) estimated the 1-year incidence of low back pain to range between 1.5% and 36%. The same review estimated the point prevalence to range from 1.0% to 58.1% (mean: 18.1%; median: 15.0%) and the 1-year prevalence to range from 0.8% to 82.5% (mean: 38.1%; median: 37.4%). The prevalence tended to be highest in the third decade, and increased with age until 60 to 65, then gradually declined (11). Women and individuals with lower educational status tended to have a higher prevalence of low back pain, while individuals in sedentary jobs had a lower prevalence of low back pain (12).

Low back pain has a significant psychosocial component. As mentioned previously, multiple psychosocial factors have been identified that are associated with low back pain. Therefore, psychological intervention may often play a role in the evaluation and treatment. One of the common psychosocial interventions for chronic pain is cognitive behavioral therapy (CBT) (13). CBT involves 3 basic components. The first component is a treatment rationale that helps patients understand that cognition and behavior may affect the pain experience and emphasizes the role that patients can play in controlling their own pain. The second component of CBT is coping skills training (relaxation techniques, distraction, etc.). The third component involves the application and maintenance of learned coping skills (13).

TREATMENT

Treatment of musculoskeletal disorders in the lumbar spine involves patient education, activity modification, lumbar support, therapy, medications, and injections.

Patient education topics include reassurance, methods of symptom control, and recognition of the red flags. Activity modification may include limiting prolonged sitting, heavy lifting, and excessive bending. Patients with radiculopathy, compression fracture, and disc disease should avoid flexion. Patients with stenosis and facet disease should avoid extension. Despite activity modification, patients should be encouraged to return to work as soon as possible.

Lumbar supports may prevent excessive spinal motion and/or reduce compressive loading of the spine by increasing intraabdominal pressure, but have limited evidence for efficacy. A thoracolumbar sacral orthosis (TLSO) is used in conditions requiring directional restriction, such as compression fractures and post laminectomy.

Therapy for the lumbar spine includes both physical therapy and exercise therapy. As mentioned previously, formal physical therapy may include core strengthening, trunk coordination, and endurance exercises. Directional preference exercises (Williams and McKenzie exercises) may be utilized in certain diagnoses. Patients may be candidates for aquatic therapy if land-based exercises are not tolerable. Modalities during therapy may include heat, ice, TENS, and traction.

Exercise therapy may include aerobic conditioning exercises, such as swimming, walking, and stationary biking. Home exercise programs may also be prescribed by the physician or therapist, where exercises will focus on correcting lumbar spine alignment, posture, and weakness.

Medications for treatment of musculoskeletal disorders in the lumbar spine include NSAIDs, acetaminophen, antidepressants, muscle relaxants, anticonvulsants, and opiates.

NSAIDs provide pain relief in both acute and chronic low back pain, but are associated with risks of gastrointestinal bleeding, renal dysfunction, exacerbation of hypertension, and cardiovascular risks. Antidepressants have been found to be more effective for chronic low back pain, but are also associated with many side effects.

Muscle relaxants are controversial due to the unclear role that muscle spasms play in low back pain. Opioids, like muscle relaxants, are also controversial. Opioids have potential for addiction, tolerance, and significant adverse effects.

Interventional treatments for musculoskeletal disorders of the lumbar spine include trigger point injections, epidural injections, facet injections, and medial branch nerve blocks.

Trigger point injections are indicated for myofascial pain, while epidural injections are indicated for lumbar radiculopathy, stenosis, and pain associated with discogenic disease. Facet injections and medial branch nerve blocks are indicated for axial pain associated with facet disease.

Surgical management of lumbar spine pain is often controversial, but the undisputed indications for surgical management are spinal instability, complicated infection, and progressive neurologic deficits.

One prior review (14) attempted to systematically assess the benefits and harms of surgery for nonradicular back pain with common degenerative changes, radiculopathy with herniated lumbar disc, and symptomatic spinal stenosis. The review found that surgery for radiculopathy with herniated lumbar disc and symptomatic spinal stenosis is associated with short-term benefits compared to nonsurgical therapy, though benefits diminish with long-term follow-up in some trials. Surgery for nonradicular back pain is no more effective than conservative management.

IMAGING, LABORATORY STUDIES, AND ELECTRODIAGNOSIS

Routine imaging of the lumbar spine should be discouraged due to the large number of "abnormal" imaging findings in asymptomatic individuals. One prior study found that one-third of asymptomatic subjects have a substantial abnormality on MRI (15).

An additional reason why routine imaging of the lumbar spine should be discouraged is because low back pain may often develop without radiologic change. Boos et al. (16) followed 46 asymptomatic patients with a herniated disc for an average of 5 years and found that MRI-identified disc abnormalities were poor predictors of the need for low back pain-related medical consultation when compared to the psychological aspects of work.

Current recommendations from the American College of Physicians (17) regarding imaging for low back pain are that (a) imaging is only indicated for severe progressive neurological deficits or when red flags are suspected and (b) routine imaging does not result in clinical benefit and may lead to harm.

When imaging is obtained, it is essential that radiologic findings be corroborated with patient presentation.

Common imaging modalities for the lumbar spine include plain films, CT, and MRI. Plain x-rays evaluate bony structural anatomy. Findings on lumbar spine plain films that may correlate with mechanical low back pain include fractures, transitional vertebra, spondylolisthesis, spondylolysis, excessive lordosis, scoliosis, disc space narrowing, osteophytes, facet disease, and neuroforaminal narrowing. Plain films are unable to evaluate soft-tissue structures. Flexion and extension x-rays may help determine if spinal instability is present, such as when spondylolisthesis is of concern.

CT scans are particularly useful for evaluating the details of bony structures. A CT scan may be indicated if there is suspicion of bony involvement with negative plain films. It may also be utilized in surgical planning. A CT may be combined with myelography, which significantly improves sensitivity. A CT myelogram may be indicated when the patient has a contraindication to MRI.

MRI is currently considered the "gold standard" in spinal imaging because of its ability to provide detailed imaging of the soft tissues, spinal canal, neuroforamen, ligaments, and disc. However, its high sensitivity may be detrimental to patient care because of its ability to mark "positive findings" in the asymptomatic patient.

Electrodiagnostic studies may play a pivotal role in the diagnosis of lumbar spine pathology. Nerve conduction studies and electromyography (EMG) assist in the physiologic (as opposed to anatomic in MRI) localization of a pathologic lesion. It is also useful in determining the type and severity of the neural injury, chronicity, as well as the prognosis for neural recovery. A nerve conduction study may be useful in ruling on peripheral nerve pathology, which may often present similar to lumbar spine radiculopathy or other pathology.

Laboratory studies are not typically useful in mechanical lumbar spine pathology, but may be useful for ruling out rheumatologic, hematologic, endocrinologic, and neoplastic disorders.

ETHICAL CONSIDERATIONS

Ethical issues in the management of low back pain involve both the physician and the patient. McGee et al. (18) held stakeholder meetings in 5 U.S. cities and found 6 main ethical issues relevant to chronic pain:

1. Reducing disparities in access to pain care among the young, elderly, and lower socioeconomic groups
2. Defining quality of care in pain management
3. The need to train qualified providers and the need for training programs in pain medicine
4. The need for evidence-based public policy regarding opioid use and diversion
5. The need to raise awareness about chronic pain as a disease to prevent stigmatization and discrimination
6. Promotion of multimodal therapies for pain as a way to prevent inappropriate opioid use as sole treatment

Other ethical issues involving the physician may include superfluous opioid prescription (pill mills), overutilization of interventional procedures, lack of evidence-based medicine to support treatment modalities, and physician relationships to industry (19).

PRACTICE-BASED LEARNING AND IMPROVEMENT

GOALS

Demonstrate competence in continuously investigating and evaluating your own lumbar spine pain patient care practices, appraising and assimilating scientific evidence, and continuously improving your patient care practices based on continuous self-assessment and lifelong learning.

OBJECTIVES

1. Conduct self-assessment and lifelong learning such as review of current guidelines, including evidence-based, in treatment of patients with low back pain and the role of the physiatrist as the educator of patients, families, residents, students, colleagues, and other health professionals.
2. Appraise the evidence-based guidelines and literature for treating lumbar spine pain.

3. Use methods for ongoing competency training in low back pain for physiatrists, including feedback from colleagues and patients in daily practice, evaluating current practice, and developing a systematic quality improvement (QI) and practice improvement strategy.
4. Locate some resources including available websites for continuing medical education and continuing professional development.

Key components of self-assessment and lifelong learning

- Appraise literature regarding the lumbar spine.
- Perform medical knowledge assessments to identify knowledge deficiencies and improvement plan.
- Utilize evidence-based treatments.
- Give and receive feedback from colleagues and patients.
- Discuss the basic sciences (anatomy, pathophysiology, etc.) and link with clinical practice.

PATIENT EDUCATION

Patients should be educated regarding the natural course of lumbar spine disease. Even though most low back pain is mild and rarely disabling, there are conditions that may pose significant threats. These conditions include fractures, tumors, infections, and cauda equina syndrome. Red flags suggestive of these conditions were discussed in a previous section. Patients should be educated about the presence of red flags and encouraged to seek immediate medical attention if these signs/symptoms are present.

Other key education points include pathophysiology; prognosis; impact on life/vocation, including impact on mood, sleep, and interpersonal relationships; and treatment risks and benefits.

PRACTICE-RELATED QUALITY IMPROVEMENT ACTIVITY

Key practice-related QI activities for low back pain might include frequent literature appraisal and application of evidence-based medicine, especially to the use of treatment modalities for this diagnosis. The consistent practice of evidence-based medicine will typically lead to the reduction of needless morbidity and mortality while improving patient outcomes. Outcome and morbidity tracking, with root cause analysis, and implementation of practice changes based on these data will also lead to quality and safety improvements. Another example of a practice performance activity might be a targeted process to improve the referral pattern for low back pain patients. One of the goals of this activity would focus on reversal of the referral cycle from primary care to surgery to PM&R/Pain changed to a primary care direct referral pattern to PM&R/Pain. Development of a process to reduce the use of diagnostic imaging in this population might be another performance improvement (PI) activity to consider.

The American College of Physicians and the American Pain Society have published evidence-based practice guidelines on the diagnosis and treatment of low back pain (20). The Orthopaedic Section of the American Physical Therapy Association has clinical practice guidelines for physical therapy treatments for low back pain (12). The North American Spine Society has also developed clinical practice guidelines for the diagnosis and treatment of specific lumbar spine diseases, such as lumbar stenosis and degenerative spondylolisthesis. Additional resources are also available from the AAPMR's online resources such as "Knowledge NOW" and Academe, PubMed searches, and the Cochrane Database. Physiatrists can also obtain education in pain medicine and interventional spine procedures through fellowship training.

INTERPERSONAL AND COMMUNICATION SKILLS

GOALS

Demonstrate interpersonal and communication skills that result in the effective exchange of information and collaboration with low back pain patients, their families, and other health professionals.

OBJECTIVES

1. Demonstrate skills used in effective communication, counseling, and collaboration with patients with chronic low back pain and their caregivers and families across socioeconomic and cultural backgrounds.
2. Discuss appropriate documentation strategies in a patient's medical records for low back pain.
3. Delineate the importance of the role of the physiatrist as the interdisciplinary team leader and consultant.

PATIENT COUNSELING

Key areas for physicians to counsel patients and families specific to the lumbar spine depend on the diagnosis. As mentioned previously, lumbar spine pathology may range from malignant disorders to musculoskeletal disorders. For all lumbar spine disorders, patients should be counseled regarding the lumbar spine anatomy, the overall favorable prognosis of low back pain (if from a musculoskeletal etiology), activity modification while resuming vocational activities, pain coping strategies, and treatment options.

MEDICAL DOCUMENTATION

For the initial consultation, adequate documentation includes all the components of a comprehensive history and physical examination: chief complaint, history of present illness, prior treatments, functional history, vocational history, disability history, medications, review of systems, red flags, physical examination, assessment, and plan.

Follow-up documentation should include the following: summary of prior visit, treatment response, pertinent review of systems (new or progressive weakness, sensory changes, bowel or bladder changes, and assessment for opioid-related side effects), physical examination, assessment, and multimodal treatment plan. Documentation of patient education is always warranted. If the practitioner is prescribing controlled substances, then medication name, dose, instruction, amount, refills, and reason for prescription are key points for documentation, as is assessment for patient aberrant behaviors.

EFFECTIVE COMMUNICATION AND LISTENING SKILLS

Suggestions for general communication and listening skills include maintaining proper eye contact, performing affirmative gestures/facial expressions, and appropriate use of other nonverbal communication skills, sitting down with the patient, giving appropriate feedback, and being clear, specific, and empathetic. The physician should assist the patient in providing and setting realistic expectations of care and realistic goals of treatment, which may include reductions in pain and improvements in mood, sleep, relations, and functionality. The physician should demonstrate empathy to the impact of chronic pain on one's life and approach treatment options as a patient-centered and team-based approach, where the physician articulates that the patient and physician will work through the elements of both the diagnosis and treatment of low back pain as a team. The physician is also encouraged to allow the use of patient pain logging (which may include pain intensity scores, diet/weight, activity logs), journaling, and other record keeping as a communication source.

To optimize outcomes, an interdisciplinary team approach is frequently needed for the treatment of patients with low back pain. Because of this, excellent communication is an essential skill for the physician. Tips for facilitating communication between treatment providers include the use of multidisciplinary conferences, frequent phone calls, and electronic communication. During the correspondence with the other treatment providers, physicians should always remember to respect others' views and have insight regarding one's own limitations.

PROFESSIONALISM

GOALS

Reflect a commitment to carrying out professional responsibilities and an adherence to ethical principles in lumbar spine physiatric management.

OBJECTIVES

1. Exemplify the humanistic qualities of a low back pain provider.
2. Demonstrate ethical principles and responsiveness to patient needs superseding self and other interests.
3. Demonstrate sensitivity to patient population diversity, including culture, gender, age, race, religion, disabilities, and sexual orientation.
4. Respect patient privacy and autonomy.
5. Recognize the socioeconomic factors and importance of patient education in the treatment of and advocacy for persons with chronic low back pain.
6. Describe the impact of demographics on the care of persons with lumbar spine pain.

To treat patients with low back pain, physicians should demonstrate humanistic qualities, such as compassion, empathy, altruism, integrity, and honesty. Humanism in medicine also includes use of therapeutic touch, especially in musculoskeletal medicine. Patients are frequently disrobed for the low back pain physical examination; sensitivity toward respecting patient privacy is applicable.

A prior study by Sanders et al. attempted to determine the cross-cultural differences in patients with low back pain (21). The study found that Mexican and New Zealander low back pain patients had significantly fewer physical findings than American, Japanese, Columbian, or Italian low back pain patients. The study also found that American, New Zealander, and Italian low back pain patients reported significantly more impairment in psychosocial, recreational, and/or work areas.

In addition, as mentioned previously, women as well as individuals with lower educational status tended to have a higher prevalence of low back pain, while individuals in sedentary jobs had a lower prevalence of low back pain.

Race and ethnicity have been previously identified as patient-related factors that influence whether an individual receives adequate pain management. Many prior studies have found that Hispanic and African American patients were less likely to receive adequate analgesia when compared to Caucasians (22).

In general, the physiatrist has the responsibility to provide education and allow the patient to have autonomy in the health care decision-making process. The risks and benefits of all treatment strategies, including the risks and benefits of conservative and no-treatment approaches, should be articulated to the patient. In this vein, patient autonomy also applies to the treatment of the lumbar spine and to low back pain. However, the prescription of opioid analgesics should be reserved for physician-determined appropriate patients. The physician must weigh the risks and benefits of opiate use for nonmalignant pain, especially since the use of opioid analgesics can be wrought with opioid misuse, addiction, opioid-related hyperalgesia, and other opioids-related adverse events, including overnarcotization and even death.

It is the responsibility of the physician to assess, manage, and follow up the patient's lumbar spine disorder. In addition, the physician should practice beneficence, nonmaleficence, social justice, and accountability as well as maintain competence with regard to the current evidence-based practices. The physician should also provide adequate patient education and communicate with other health care providers when appropriate.

For a review of the ethical issues in pain management, including social accountability for opioid prescribing, adherence to evidence-based medicine in the low back pain population, and professional responsibility, the reader is referred to the available ethics-based pain literature (19).

Patients with lumbar spine pathology may often present as challenging patients, with significant psychosocial overlay to the pain presentation, with comorbid medical conditions complicating treatment and with several pain generators or overlapping central pain syndromes, such as fibromyalgia. As a physician, it is essential to remain respectful, altruistic, and compassionate to patient needs. Physicians should be aware of the resources available in the medical system to provide assistance for challenging patients.

SYSTEMS-BASED PRACTICE

GOALS

Awareness and responsiveness to systems of care delivery, and the ability to recruit and coordinate effectively resources in the system to provide optimal continuum of care as it relates to low back pain.

OBJECTIVES

1. Identify the components, systems of care delivery, services, referral patterns, and resources in the low back pain rehabilitation continuum.
2. Coordinate and recruit necessary resources in the system to provide optimal care for the low back pain patient, with attention to safety, cost awareness, and risk–benefit analysis and management.
3. Introduce and define quality of care improvement markers for low back pain rehabilitation programs, including identification of systems errors.
4. Describe the role of the physiatrist in patient advocacy efforts.

The rehabilitation continuum of care of the lumbar spine involves both inpatient and outpatient environments. The inpatient rehabilitation environment involves admission to an acute rehabilitation unit for multidisciplinary care. Patients who typically require inpatient admission include those who had lumbar spine surgery or significant spinal cord injury (e.g., cauda equina syndrome). An inpatient rehabilitation admission will optimize patient function. Also, chronic back pain patients with multiple medications and poor physical condition may be considered for comprehensive multidisciplinary inpatient pain management programs.

Most patients with lumbar spine pathology will receive treatment in the outpatient setting. Outpatient rehabilitation treatment of the lumbar spine, like inpatient rehabilitation, may also involve multidisciplinary care. The treating physician must be aware of the resources available and when to utilize them to optimize patient outcomes. The outpatient physiatrist managing the patient with low back pain will work closely with other pain providers, including anesthesiology, neurology, and psychiatry team members, as well as pain psychologists, addiction specialists, and physical therapists. Providers of complementary and alternative medicine (CAM) therapies may also be members of this continuum of care, as may be orthotists.

PATIENT SAFETY

Patient safety components for the treating physician include effective triage of patients, awareness of red flags that may indicate a serious condition, adequate informed consent for procedures and for pharmacotherapy, opioid contracts, modified activity education, and principles of occupational health/safety and ergonomics. Urine toxicity screening to confirm opioid analgesic use and minimize diversion may also be required in some settings.

The optimal follow-up care is individualized for each patient, depending on the diagnosis and treatment. An individual with a serious diagnosis (e.g., lumbar spine malignancy) will require more frequent follow-up compared to an individual with a "benign" diagnosis (e.g., myofascial pain syndrome). Patients who have been treated with modalities that may have serious complications (opiates, injections, etc.) will also require more frequent follow-up.

MARKERS OF QUALITY

Important markers of the quality of care include the scales for measuring pain, such as the verbal numerical rating scale (NRS), verbal descriptor scale, visual analog scale (VAS), and brief pain inventory (BPI). Other markers may include common outcome measures used for clinical research, such as Short Form-36 (SF-36), Oswestry Disability Index (ODI), Roland Morris Disability Questionnaire, and Quebec Back Pain Disability Scale. In the pediatric population, the Faces Scale for pain intensity is typically used. Outcome assessments for low back pain frequently include reduction or change in pain intensity score, such as a 50% or greater subjective change in pain intensity reporting following a treatment modality. Changes in ambulatory function, independence in ADLs, strength, sensory gain, mood, appetite, sleep, and interpersonal relationships are also important markers of quality of care for assessing outcomes in this diagnosis.

COST-RELATED AND RETURN TO WORK CONSIDERATIONS

The total cost of low back pain in the United States is estimated to exceed $100 billion per year, with two-thirds from lost wages and reduced productivity (23). It is estimated that 5% of Americans miss at least 1 day of work annually due to low back pain. Of the patients who do miss work, more than 80% return to work within 1 month; more than 90% return by 3 months; and 5% never return (23). When a worker has been out of work for 6 months, the likelihood of returning to work is 50%; by the time a worker has been out for a year, the likelihood of returning to work is 25% (24).

Socioeconomic factors such as job dissatisfaction, physically strenuous work, psychologically stressful work, low education, and workers' compensation insurance are also important risk factors for the onset of back pain.

PATIENT ADVOCACY

Patient advocacy should extend beyond clinical care. Advocacy should also involve supporting patients in their psychosocial, employment, and interpersonal struggles. This may involve referral to appropriate consultants and use of multidisciplinary and interdisciplinary resources. Many physicians also play a role in political advocacy in terms of patient access to analgesics, including appropriate physician assessment and treatment of pain. Other potential roles include advocating for ergonomic modifications in various work settings.

SYSTEM-RELATED ERRORS

Examples of system-related errors in the management of low back pain might include inappropriate referral to a specialist consultant, inappropriate use of resources such as admission to acute rehabilitation for patients who do not require multidisciplinary care, use of diagnostic imaging such as MRI, and performance of an interventional procedure without insurance authorization. Strategies to minimize system-related errors include frequent evaluation of physician performance and patient outcomes, establishment of a quality improvement and patient safety dashboard for voluntary reporting of system-based errors, root cause analysis of errors, provider commitment to lifelong learning, and initiating change once a system-related error is found.

CASE STUDY

A 50-year-old man with no significant past medical history presents to your office with low back pain radiating to the right lower extremity. The pain is localized to the right buttock and radiates to the right great toe. The pain is described as a sharp, shooting pain and is associated with numbness and tingling. The pain worsens with lumbar flexion, and improves with bed rest.

On physical examination, the patient has decreased active ROM with flexion, but normal extension and lateral rotation. The patient has decreased strength in the right extensor hallucis longus and diminished sensation over the dorsum of the foot, including the great toe. Straight leg raise test is positive on the right side.

CASE STUDY DISCUSSION QUESTIONS

1. What is your differential diagnosis for this patient?
2. Would you order any imaging for this patient?
3. What would be your comprehensive rehabilitation treatment plan for this patient?
4. What are some key elements to patient education and counseling for this patient?
5. What are some patient safety concerns for the patient's condition?
6. You notice that a colleague of yours working in the same hospital has been ordering lumbar MRIs for every patient who presents with a similar presentation. What is a quality improvement project that may address the issue?
7. Identify lifelong learning, self-assessment, and professional development resources in caring for this type of patient.

SELF-EXAMINATION QUESTIONS
(Answers begin on p. 367)

1. Which of the following is not considered a red flag in the clinical evaluation of the lumbar spine?
   A. Major trauma
   B. IV drug abuse
   C. Severe nocturnal pain
   D. Numbness of bilateral feet
   E. Progressive motor weakness

2. The percentage of patients who recover from "acute" low back pain is
   A. 10% to 30%
   B. 30% to 50%
   C. 50% to 70%
   D. 70% to 90%
   E. 90% to 100%

3. A 45-year-old man presents with low back pain radiating down the right lower limb for 2 weeks. He has tried bed rest, as well as over-the-counter NSAIDs, with no benefit. He presents to your office for a consultation. On examination, you obtain a positive straight leg raise. There are no other red flags present. Of the following interventions, what is your next step?
   A. Initiate conservative treatment
   B. Order EMG
   C. Order MRI
   D. Order x-ray
   E. Order CT myelogram

4. A prior study attempted to characterize the ethical issues related to chronic pain. Which of these issues were identified as ethical issues?
   A. Reducing disparities in access to pain care among the young, elderly, and lower socioeconomic groups
   B. Defining quality of care in pain management
   C. The need to train qualified providers and the need for training programs in pain medicine
   D. The need for evidence-based public policy regarding opioid use and diversion
   E. All of the above

5. When a worker with low back pain has been out of work for 6 months, the likelihood of return to work is
   A. 20%
   B. 30%
   C. 40%
   D. 50%
   E. 60%

REFERENCES

1. Waldman S. *Pain Management.* 2nd ed. Philadelphia, PA: Elsevier; 2011.
2. Bigos S, Bowyer O, Braen G, et al. Acute low back problems in adults. Clinical Practice Guideline no. 14. In: *AHCPR Publication No. 95-0642.* Rockville, MD: Agency for Health Care Policy and Research, Public Health Service, U.S. Department of Health and Human Services; 1994.
3. Hayden JA, Dunn KM, van der Windt DA, et al. What is the prognosis of back pain? *Best Pract Res Clin Rheumatol.* 2010;24(2):167–179.
4. Sullivan MJ, Reesor K, Mikail S, et al. The treatment of depression in chronic low back pain: review and recommendations. *Pain.* 1992;50(1):5–13.
5. Nguyen TH. Nonspecific low back pain and return to work. *Am Fam Physician.* 2007;76(10):1497–1502.
6. Dionne CE, et al. A consensus approach toward the standardization of back pain definitions for use in prevalence studies. *Spine.* 2008;33(1):95–103.

7. Maetzel A, Li L. The economic burden of low back pain: a review of studies published between 1996 and 2001. *Best Pract Res Clin Rheumatol.* 2002;16(1):23–30.
8. Bernacki EJ. Factors influencing the costs of workers' compensation. *Clin Occup Environ Med.* 2004;4(2):v–vi, 249–257.
9. Horváth G, Koroknai G, Acs B, et al. Prevalence of low back pain and lumbar spine degenerative disorders. Questionnaire survey and clinical-radiological analysis of a representative Hungarian population. *Int Orthop.* 2010;34(8):1245–1249.
10. Middle K, Fish D. Lumbar spondylosis: clinical presentation and treatment approaches. *Curr Rev Musculoskelet Med.* 2009;2(2):94–104.
11. Hoy D, Brooks P, Blyth F, et al. The epidemiology of low back pain. *Best Pract Res Clin Rheumatol.* 2010;24(6):769–781.
12. Delitto A, et al. Low back pain: clinical practice guidelines linked to the international classification of functioning, disability, and health from the Orthopaedic Section of the American Physical Therapy Association. *J Orthop Sports Phys Ther.* 2012;42(4):A1–A57.
13. Keefe FJ. Cognitive behavioral therapy for managing pain. *Clin Psychol.* 1996;49(3):4–5.
14. Chou R, et al. Surgery for low back pain: a review of the evidence for an American Pain Society Clinical Practice Guideline. *Spine (Phila Pa 1976).* 2009;34(10):1094–1109.
15. Boden SD, Davis DO, Dina TS, et al. Abnormal magnetic-resonance scans of the lumbar spine in asymptomatic subjects. A prospective investigation. *J Bone Joint Surg Am.* 1990;72(3):403–408.
16. Boos N, Semmer N, Elfering A, et al. Natural history of individuals with asymptomatic disc abnormalities in magnetic resonance imaging: predictors of low back pain-related medical consultation and work incapacity. *Spine (Phila Pa 1976).* 2000;25(12):1484–1492.
17. Chou R, Qaseem A, Owens DK, et al. Diagnostic imaging for low back pain: advice for high-value health care from the American College of Physicians. *Ann Intern Med.* 2011;154(3):181–189.
18. McGee SJ, Kaylor BD, Emmott H, et al. Defining chronic pain ethics. *Pain Med.* 2011;12(9):1376–1384.
19. Perret D, Rosen C. A physician-driven solution–the Association for Medical Ethics, the Physician Payment Sunshine Act, and ethical challenges in pain medicine. *Pain Med.* 2011;12(9):1361–1375.
20. Chou R, et al. Diagnosis and treatment of low back pain: a joint clinical practice guideline from the American College of Physicians and the American Pain Society. *Ann Intern Med.* 2007;147(7):478–491.
21. Sanders SH, et al. Chronic low back pain patients around the world: cross-cultural similarities and differences. *Clin J Pain.* 1992;8(4):317–323.
22. Mossey JM. Defining racial and ethnic disparities in pain management. *Clin Orthop Relat Res.* 2011;469(7):1859–1870.
23. Katz JN. Lumbar disc disorders and low-back pain: socioeconomic factors and consequences. *J Bone Joint Surg Am.* 2006;88(suppl 2):21–24.
24. Benzon H. *Essentials of Pain Medicine*. 3rd ed. Philadelphia, PA: Elsevier; 2011.

Dallas Kingsbury
David Bressler

25: Rheumatoid Arthritis

PATIENT CARE

GOALS

Evaluate and develop a rehabilitative plan of care that is compassionate, effective, and targeted at the individual patient with rheumatoid arthritis (RA).

OBJECTIVES

1. Perform a detailed history and physical examination of a patient with RA.
2. Identify the key components of a rehabilitation program as they relate to the rheumatoid patient with RA.
3. Identify the psychosocial and vocational implications for the patient with RA and strategies to address them.
4. Formulate a sample rehabilitation treatment plan for the patient with RA.

HISTORY AND PHYSICAL

The history and physical examination in patients with either suspected or confirmed RA should reflect the understanding that it is an autoimmune disease primarily of the joints, with an array of possible comorbid systemic conditions. Areas of the patient history that are notably important for diagnosing and characterizing RA include the number and site of involved joints, as well as the duration of symptoms, as these questions are directly part of the diagnostic criteria. Especially at the onset, RA may be difficult to differentiate from other immune-mediated diseases. It may coexist with other rheumatologic diseases, such as mixed connective tissue disease and overlap syndrome, or the symptoms may be fleeting as in palindromic rheumatism. RA classically affects joints symmetrically, and more than other rheumatic disorders, it has a preference for small joints of the hands and feet. Protracted morning stiffness is a hallmark of the disease. Extraarticular manifestations of RA are common, with cardiac, pulmonary, integumentary, and hematologic systems being most affected (1).

Rheumatoid nodules are painless, firm areas of swelling of subcutaneous tissue, typically found on the extensor surfaces of the limbs (i.e., olecranon, dorsal hand at metacarpophalangeal [MCP] joints). Histologically, the nodules are comprised of a center of fibrinoid necrosis surrounded by a fibrous tissue shell, the larger of which can be multiloculated and contain synovial fluid. The appearance of rheumatoid nodules portends a poor prognosis and a sign of heightened disease activity.

The physical examination must be organized to include articular and extraarticular manifestations. As the patient transitions through the natural history of the disease, joint pathology will change over time. Fortunately, due to earlier diagnosis and earlier initiation of disease-modifying antirheumatic drug (DMARD) and biologic therapy, many of the debilitating, late-stage manifestations of RA are becoming less frequent. Initially, joint swelling and tenderness may appear similar to other forms of arthritis. Palpation can differentiate between the bogginess of synovial edema in RA from the bony osteophytes of osteoarthritis (OA). Periarticular edema is more common in gout, while the rheumatoid joint will have swelling confined to the capsule. As the disease progresses, abnormal synovium can proliferate and migrate across articular cartilage into the joint capsule or surrounding tendons. This boggy mass of synovium laden with inflammatory mediators is called a pannus.

The wrist is the most commonly affected joint in up to 75% of RA patients (2), with synovitis progressively weakening the ligaments between the radius, ulna, and carpal bones. One area to focus is the scapholunate ligament, assessing for laxity or subluxation, since compromise of this area leads to a cascade of events in which the radial support structures collapse, volar subluxation of the radius occurs, the metacarpals deviate radially, and the fingers deviate in an ulnar direction (3). Chronic synovitis of the MCP joints accentuates the ulnar drift of the fingers. Finger deformities are also very common in RA. One of the earliest physical findings is proximal interphalangeal joint edema, with tendon and ligament weakening or rupture occurring after many years of active disease. The two major late findings at the proximal interphalangeal (PIP) joint include the boutonnière deformity and swan-neck deformity. With a boutonnière deformity, the PIP is set into flexion, with reciprocal extension of the MCP and distal interphalangeal (DIP) joints. Synovial inflammation leads to a rupture of the extensor hood and causes the lateral bands to migrate downward, causing PIP flexion and DIP hyperextension. The swan-neck deformity is a hyperextension at the PIP joint, with MCP and DIP joint flexion. It can occur from multiple combinations of joint disruptions, which usually involve PIP volar support loss (e.g., volar plate rupture) and eventual contracture of the hand intrinsic muscles. In the upper extremity, elbow synovitis can lead to loss of extension and sometimes a compressive ulnar neuropathy. Shoulder and hip involvement is less common than the more distal joints, and typically occurs later in the disease process. Painful synovitis can lead to loss of range of motion (ROM) and joint contractures.

In the lower extremity, knee effusions are common and can sometimes lead to joint contracture. At the ankle, synovitis typically affects the tibiotalar joint. Synovial proliferation can extend to the tarsal tunnel or involve the posterior tibialis tendon resulting in a tenosynovitis and possible tendon rupture. Similar to the hand, chronic synovitis can cause weakening of the delicate ligamentous structures in the forefoot, at first leading to metatarsophalangeal (MTP) edema, tenderness, dorsal subluxation, and hallux valgus deformity. As noted, the painful metatarsal subluxation is caused by distention of the joint capsule, with the PIP joints moving superiorly, causing hammer toe deformities. The hip is one of the last joints to be involved in adult RA (but, paradoxically, is involved early in JRA). Remodeling of the acetabulum from chronic synovitis can result in "protrusio acetabuli," in which the femoral head migrates deeply into the acetabulum. The definitive treatment is total hip arthroplasty.

The spine is not frequently involved, with the notable exception of the atlantoaxial joint. Rupture of the transverse ligament between C1 and C2 can lead to myelopathy and possible death due to migration of the odontoid into the brainstem. It is important to obtain lateral, flexion/extension, and open mouth views, since an anterior subluxation of 9 mm or more between C1 and C2 increases the risk for cord compression (4). In advanced disease, atlantoaxial involvement becomes more of a concern, considering that up to 60% of RA patients who needed hip or knee arthroplasty were found to have cervical spine instability on radiographic screening (5) (Box 25.1).

FUNCTIONAL ASSESSMENT

A rehabilitation approach to RA should include an inventory of the patient's daily activities. This will allow the physiatrist to tailor a patient-specific rehabilitation program, as opposed to relying on a generic template. Two patients with similar severities of ulnar deviations and boutonnière deformities may compensate differently for manual tasks, and therefore may require separate rehabilitation approaches. Questions to ask include the following: Can you dress yourself? Get in/out of bed? Walk outdoors on flat ground? Wash/dry your entire body? Bend down to pick up clothing from the floor? Turn faucets on/off? Get in/out of the car?

Based on American College of Rheumatology (ACR) guidelines (6), patients can be given a functional classification, from I to IV increasing in severity of disability (Boxes 25.2, 25.3).

Box 25.1 Pearl: Atlantoaxial Instability

- Cervical spine disease (C1–C2) parallels peripheral joint disease

---

Box 25.2 Functional Classification

- Class I: no functional limitations
- Class II: joint discomfort or limitations in ROM, but activities of daily living (ADLs) not significantly compromised
- Class III: ADLs significantly compromised
- Class IV: incapacitated, and unable to perform ADLs

Box 25.3 Pearl: Disease Activity Index

- Functional status is most traditionally assessed by the health assessment questionnaire (HAQ)

REHABILITATION PROGRAM

Historically, any exercise for RA was controversial, but now therapeutic exercise is considered a basic component of any comprehensive rehabilitation program. Areas that have shown notable success include aerobic exercise, strengthening exercises, cognitive behavioral therapy, and self-efficacy training. Joint and energy conservation, adaptive equipment, and orthotic support are the basic tenets of a comprehensive occupational therapy program (7).

In RA patients, short-term (less than 3 months) land- or water-based dynamic exercise programs have a positive effect on aerobic capacity, muscle strength, and functional ability (8). Low-impact activities, such as swimming and biking, are preferred. One study directly compared land-based aerobic capacity training (walking) with water-based aerobic capacity training, and found no differences with regard to safety (9). Overall, studies have shown decreased inflammation, joint pain, and joint tenderness (10). Specifically for aerobic exercises (at 50%–90% maximum heart rate [HR]), a meta-analysis of 14 randomized controlled trials (RCTs) showed small, beneficial effects on cardiorespiratory function, functional ability, and disease activity (11).

For ROM therapy and stretching, it is recommended that each joint is moved through its complete ROM at least once daily. Joint movement is gently encouraged despite pain, and it needs to be emphasized that *ROM therapy is not done to relieve pain*, but to prevent contractures. All types of strengthening exercises may be employed, as long as they do not result in muscle soreness greater than 2 hours post exercise, or fatigue lasting more than 1 hour after exercise, or increased joint pain noted during exercise. Initially isometrics can be employed due to decreased dynamic/sheer forces on the joints compared to isotonic and isokinetic training.

Modalities can also assist in physical and occupational therapy programs. Cold therapy is ideal for acute flares, especially in joints with effusions. Deep heat is indicated for patients with chronic inflammation and contractures (Box 25.4).

HOW SHOULD THE REHABILITATION PROGRAM BE MODIFIED DURING A FLARE?

In a word, *rest!* Reevaluate and reduce all resistive exercises, especially those that stress the small joints of the hands and feet. In this case, splinting is helpful to ensure that joint stress is minimized. Limited passive ROM is performed to prevent contracture. Medically, flares often require steroid supplementation, in addition to considering a change in DMARD therapy (Box 25.5).

PAIN MANAGEMENT

Patients often come to the physiatrist, either directly or from another consulting physician, with the expectation of complete pain relief. The first step is explaining that complete pain relief is often unachievable. A reasonable goal is pain reduction sufficient enough to allow greater participation in activities of daily living (ADLs) (Box 25.6).

Box 25.4 *Pearl*: Exercise Precautions

- Caution when ordering isometric exercise (especially in the upper extremity)
- Sustained isometric contractions increase intrathoracic pressure and decrease cardiac output (Valsalva effect). To compensate, heart rate and vasoconstriction occur to maintain blood pressure and cardiac output
- Rheumatoid arthritis patients frequently have hypertension and/or cardiovascular disease, and patients with impaired hemodynamics may respond to isometric exercises with exaggerated or dangerous increases in blood pressure
- High-risk cardiac patients should be monitored closely for chest pain, abnormal BP elevations, and arrhythmias (12)

Box 25.5 *Pearl*: Exercise Prescription Modification Should Be Considered in Rheumatoid Arthritis Patients With:

- Fatigue lasting greater than 1 hour post exercise
- Muscle soreness lasting greater than 2 hours post exercise
- Increased joint pain during exercise

Box 25.6 Sample Rehabilitation Prescription

- Diagnosis: Rheumatoid arthritis
- ICD-9 Code: 714.0
- Impairment: decreased ROM right MCP and PIP joints; right knee 20° flexion contracture, decreased muscle strength in all 4 extremities
- Disability: decreased ambulation, decreased ADLs
- Precautions: avoid Valsalva maneuver, do not overfatigue, postexercise pain not greater than 2 hours, contact MD if acute flare
- Goals: pain relief, inflammation reduction, joint preservation, functional restoration
- Modalities: cryotherapy for acute flares, paraffin/fluidotherapy for the hands, orthotic splinting as needed, deep heating for joint contracture and stiffness
- PT/OT: ROM, mobilization to affected joints, stretching (after preheating, if contractures), strengthening exercises (especially closed-chain), light isotonics, isometrics (only for acute flare), general conditioning exercises (aerobics), cross training using low-impact exercise (cycling, swimming), gait training with appropriate assistive device, ADL evaluation and training, adaptive equipment and training, joint protection, and energy-conservation techniques, home exercise program

---

MEDICAL KNOWLEDGE

GOALS

Demonstrate knowledge of established evidence-based and evolving biomedical, clinical epidemiological, and sociobehavioral sciences pertaining to RA, as well as the application of this knowledge to guide holistic patient care.

OBJECTIVES

1. Define RA, and describe the epidemiology, natural history, and pathophysiology of the disease.
2. Describe how RA is diagnosed and what treatment options are available.
3. Review the range of prognoses associated with RA depending on severity and risk factors.
4. Educate patients on making patient-centered decisions regarding their plans of care.

EPIDEMIOLOGY AND PATHOPHYSIOLOGY

RA is a symmetric, systemic, autoimmune, polyarthritis caused by abnormal growth of inflammatory synovial tissue, resulting in cartilage destruction and surrounding bone erosion. The worldwide prevalence is approximately 1%, annual incidence is about 3/10,000 adults, and it is two to three times more common in women (13). This incidence has remained stable over many years. New criteria for diagnosing early RA were published in 2010, and follow-up studies estimating incidence rates using the new criteria have yielded similar results (14). The etiology of RA remains unknown, but is considered to be multifactorial, resulting from an interaction between a genetic predisposition and environmental exposure, the exact contributions of which are still being elucidated. The important genetic contributors are major histocompatibility genes (mostly HLA-DRB1), in addition to minor immunomodulation genes. Environmental associations include alcohol, tobacco (increases susceptibility up to 20- to 40-fold), and even oral cavity flora (15).

The latest theories cite that preclinical RA likely develops via an immunologic conflict, unintuitively outside the joints or synovial membrane, in the mucous membranes of the upper gastrointestinal (GI) tract or airways. Subsequently, upon exposure to a second event, the autoimmune process spreads to the synovium, with eventual systemic involvement, giving rise to typical RA symptoms and signs. The "second event" is still being investigated (16). The hallmark of this disease is "synovitis," that is, a joint synovium laden with autoantibodies, several classes of leukocytes, and inflammatory cytokines that initially cause joint pain and stiffness. Over time, this synovitis causes diffuse systemic manifestations, in addition to the hallmarks of joint and bone destruction.

NATURAL HISTORY

Stage 1 is characterized by morning fatigue and joint stiffness, and lasts for several weeks to 2 months. Joint pain is primarily localized to the hands and wrists, which may begin to show signs of edema. At this point, no deformities or rheumatoid nodules are present, serological rheumatoid factor (RF) titers are usually negative, and there is no synovial proliferation on pathological or physical examination.

By the time a patient enters stage 2, the diagnosis of RA has been established, and 70% have a detectible RF titer. An experienced clinician may be able to appreciate palpable proliferative synovium surrounding affected joints. Radiographically, x-rays will show early diffuse juxtaarticular osteopenia but there is not yet evidence of erosions.

If treatment is not initiated, patients may enter stage 3, where they will begin to experience tangible losses in function secondary to joint damage. Common examples include soft-tissue contractures and tendon ruptures of the hand (the extensor tendon being a common site of rupture). The appearance of rheumatoid nodules on examination and x-ray evidence of erosions are hallmarks of stage 3. Also, systemic manifestations begin to develop in this stage, the most common of which include anemia of chronic disease, pericarditis, weight loss, and various vasculitides.

Stage 4 is considered the "end stage" of RA. By this time, joints have undergone so much degeneration, there is little synovium left to serve as a site for inflammation (i.e., the so called burned out phase). Of note, patients with disease activity greater than 15 years may develop amyloidosis. The mortality rates of patients in this late stage rival that of cancer, stage 4 Hodgkin lymphoma, and three-vessel coronary disease (17).

RA affects a broad population ranging from children to the elderly and has a spectrum of presentation from transient episodes of monoarthritis to the more common active systemic disease. In children, it is classified as juvenile rheumatoid arthritis (JRA), for which there is a separate set of diagnostic criteria and treatment protocols, the specifics of which are beyond the scope of this chapter. The onset and pattern of RA typically follow the natural history as described above (i.e., an insidious onset of a symmetric polyarthritis), but occasionally some patients present with a series of transient, self-limited episodes of monoarthritis or polyarthritis that subsides completely in days to weeks. This presentation is called *palindromic rheumatism*. Fifty percent of these patients will eventually progress to full RA (1).

DIAGNOSIS

In 1987, the ACR developed a set of criteria that could distinguish patients with established RA from those with other rheumatic diseases. In 2010, the ACR and European League Against Rheumatism (EULAR) revised those criteria to identify patients at an earlier stage of the disease, highlighting symptoms associated with persistent and/or erosive disease. Research has shown that earlier diagnosis that led to earlier treatment resulted in improved outcomes and minimized irreversible sequelae, because the majority of joint destruction with fixed deformities occurs within 2 years of onset (18).

The 2010 criteria screen patients with confirmed presence of synovitis in at least one joint and the absence of an alternative diagnosis that better explains the synovitis. The criteria focus on scoring four different domains of disease, with a higher score indicating more severe disease: number and site of involved joints (range 0–5), serologic abnormality (range 0–3), elevated acute-phase response (range 0–1), and symptom duration (range 0–1). A total score of 6 or greater, within a 6-month time frame, in properly screened individuals indicates "definite RA" (19,20).

Physical examination findings are described in the Patient Care section, but regarding the 2010 ACR criteria, it is important to note that the presence of small joint involvement (MCP, PIP, 2–5 MTP, thumb IP joints, and wrists) is a more powerful predictor of RA.

LABORATORY TESTS

RF *with titer* is a serologic marker commonly used to assess for RA, and at a cellular level is defined by autoantibodies (mostly IgM) with a specificity for the Fc portion of the IgG molecule. The importance of RF lies in the positivity of the test (i.e., a higher titer portends a worse prognosis). Extraarticular findings are almost exclusively confined to RF-positive patients. Negative RF results are less helpful, highlighting the utility value of anti-citrullinated peptide antibodies (ACPAs) in making an earlier diagnosis. Of patients with confirmed RA, 35% with an initial negative RF titer will test positive for ACPAs. The mean ACPA titers increase markedly 2 to 4 years before symptom onset.

Four laboratory tests are incorporated into the 2010 ACR criteria. RF with titer and ACPAs contribute to the "serological abnormality" section. For either RF or ACPA, a "low positive" (above the upper limit of normal [ULN]) is worth 2 points, whereas a "high positive" (greater than three times the ULN) contributes three points. Either erythrocyte sedimentation rate (ESR) or C-reactive protein (CRP) levels above the ULN contribute 1 point to the "elevated acute phase" section of the criteria.

Other laboratory tests that do not directly contribute to the diagnosis are often ordered for the purposes of ruling out other diseases or in preparation for starting pharmacologic therapy. For example, a negative ANA helps exclude systemic lupus erythematosus (SLE). Arthrocentesis is helpful for ruling out crystal arthropathies and pyogenic infection. A complete blood count and liver function tests are required prior to treatment with methotrexate. A purified protein derivative (PPD) test is required prior to initiation of biologic agents due to the risk of reactivation of tuberculosis (Box 25.7).

RADIOLOGY

During the initial evaluation, plain radiographs of affected joints should be obtained. It is important to note that small joints in the hand may have commensurate changes in the foot and ankle. As previously described, osteopenia is seen in stage 2 and bony erosions in stage 3. Pathologically, erosions on x-ray represent sections of joint margins where the outer cortex has been destroyed by synovial proliferation. Erosions are seen in affected joints in up to 90% of patients not responding to treatment (21). MRI is more sensitive than plain radiography in early detection of erosions (22), but hasn't yet been incorporated into any official clinical decision-making criteria. A normal chest x-ray is important prior to initiation of methotrexate due to hepatotoxic side effects and interstitial pulmonary fibrosis (Box 25.8).

DIFFERENCE BETWEEN RHEUMATOID ARTHRITIS AND OSTEOARTHRITIS

Many patients do not understand the difference between RA and osteoarthritis (OA). Of paramount importance is an understanding that RA is a systemic disease with potential multiorgan involvement. Radiological differences between RA and OA are described below.

Overall, joints affected by RA are warm and tender, reflecting an inflamed synovium. Areas of synovial proliferation may be palpably soft, whereas joints in OA are hard and bony due to osteophyte formation. RA predominates in joints with robust synovium, which in the hand include the MCP and PIP joints. In contrast, OA affects the distal interphalangeal joints and carpometacarpal joint of the thumb. Typically, patients with RA will notice the worst joint stiffness in the morning for a prolonged period of time, as compared to the brief stiffness or "gelling" which is typical for the OA patient. As opposed to RA, there are no specific serologic markers for OA (Table 25.1).

MEDICAL TREATMENT

Pharmacologic therapy for RA has changed drastically since the early 20th century, starting with aspirin and gold salts through the 1940s.

The discovery of steroids in the 1950s was initially greeted with great fanfare by the medical community; however, over time further use revealed their limitations and shortcomings. Nonetheless, they remain an important part of medical management of RA. Further advances were seen with the discovery of DMARDs in the 1970s, but significant systemic side effects also frequently interfered with long-term use. The turn of the 21st century brought advancements with the advent of the "biologic" class of medications, which targets specific immunologic cytokines or receptor sites.

In 2012, the ACR revised their 2008 guidelines for the use of DMARD and biologic agents for RA (24). Examples of currently utilized DMARDs include hydroxychloroquine, leflunomide, and methotrexate. Biologic agents include the nontumor necrosis factor (TNF) abatacept, rituximab, and tocilizumab; and the anti-TNF: adalimumab, etanercept, and infliximab. New biologic agents are constantly being introduced in the market (Figure 25.1).

Prior to initiation of pharmacologic therapy patients should meet the proper diagnostic criteria (see above). ACR recommendations diverge between patients with early and established RA.

Box 25.7 *Pearl*: Synovial Fluid Analysis Findings In Rheumatoid Arthritis

- Cloudy & yellow
- Won't pass "newspaper test" (i.e., newsprint print cannot be read through the vial of inflammatory fluid)
- 5,000 to 50,000 leukocytes
- >50% PMNs

Box 25.8 *Pearl*: Advanced Imaging

- When clinical status is worsening (i.e., increasing joint pain) and x-rays remain normal, consider musculoskeletal sonography or MRI, which can detect erosions up to 2 years earlier than conventional roentography (23).

TABLE 25.1 Radiological Differences (24)

	RHEUMATOID ARTHRITIS	OSTEOARTHRITIS
Sclerosis	±	++++
Osteophytes	±	++++
Osteopenia	+++	0
Symmetry	+++	+
Erosions	+++	0
Cysts	++	++
Joint space narrowing	+++ (symmetric)	+++ (asymmetric)

Source: From West et al (23).

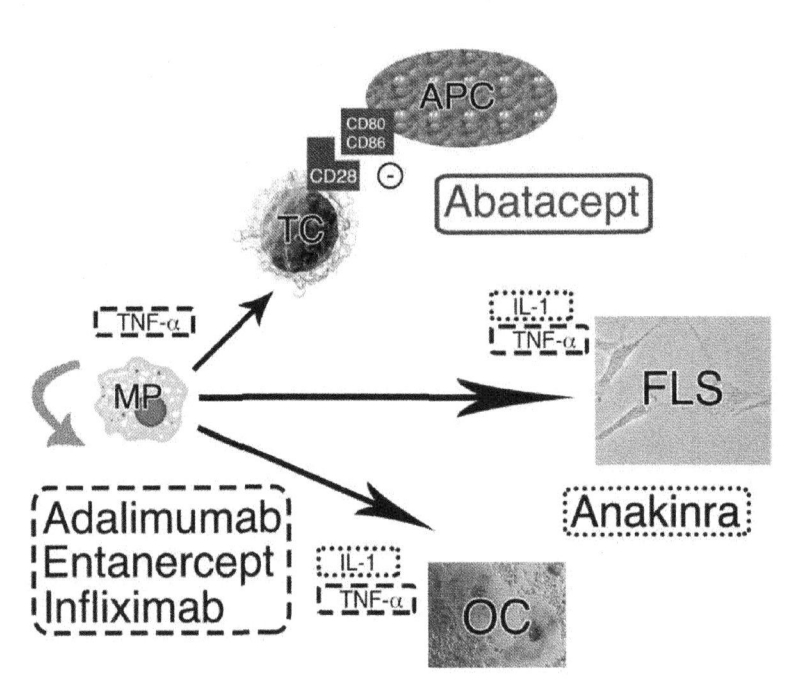

FIGURE 25.1 Cytokine networks are displayed, along with accompanying sites of action of several popular biologic agents. Macrophages (MP[i]), fibroblast-like synovioctyes (FLS[ii]), and T cells (TC[iii]) are depicted with selected cytokines and their targets. Several cytokines activate osteoclasts (OC[iv]), the primary cell identified in the bony erosions seen in rheumatoid arthritis. IL-1 and TNF-alpha are integral parts of the cascade of cellular autoimmunity. Adalimumab (Humira®), entanercept (Enbrel®), and infliximab (Remicade®) are examples of TNF-alpha blockers [dashed outline]. Anakinra (Kineret®) is an antagonist of the interleukin-1 (IL-1) receptor [dotted outline]. Abatacept (Orencia) is a selective costimulation modulator [solid outline], as it inhibits T-cell activation by binding to CD80 and CD86 on antigen presenting cells (APC), thus blocking the required CD28 interaction shared between APCs and T cells.

In early RA, suggestions for therapy depend on disease activity (scored as low, moderate, or high) and on presence or absence of "features of a poor prognosis." For early RA, low disease activity, and no poor prognostic factors, the recommendation is to start with DMARD monotherapy (which is most often methotrexate). In early RA, as disease activity and prognostic factors worsen, the ACR recommends adding an additional DMARD. Anti-TNF agents for early RA are reserved for patients with both high disease activity and poor prognostic factors.

For patients with established RA, making modifications to pharmacologic therapy becomes a complex process that not only depends on disease activity and prognostic factors, but also takes into consideration failed therapies and adverse reactions.

EULAR has a similar, but separate set of recommendations regarding medical therapy (29).

Glucocorticoids

Glucocorticoids are being used as a bridging medication (i.e., in the interim between the initiation of DMARD therapy and the time that it has a clinical effect, often measured in months from treatment initiation), for combination strategies along with DMARDs (due to delayed onset of action), for flares, and for treatment of vasculitis.

Several studies evaluated groups of patients, all of whom were starting a DMARD, and compared those who were also started with a glucocorticoid (usually prednisone) versus those whose initial therapy only added a nonsteroidal anti-inflammatory drug (NSAID) or placebo. Better clinical outcomes, including pain and joint tenderness, were reported in the glucocorticoid groups (30). When glucocorticoids are added to an already existing DMARD monotherapy regimen, studies have shown improvements in signs, symptoms, and function, especially radiographic progression (31). Difficulties still remain regarding the optimal duration and dosage of glucocorticoid treatment, and in addition, when to consider discontinuation.

REMISSION

While the goal of rehabilitation is preservation of function, the goal of medical therapy ultimately is remission. The original ACR criteria for clinical remission, published in 1981 (32), depended on the presence of five of the following six factors for 2 months (assuming a lack of systemic symptoms, i.e., vasculitis, pericarditis, myositis, pleuritis, weight loss, fever): no fatigue, morning stiffness for 15 minutes or less, no joint pain, no joint tenderness to palpation or ROM testing, no soft tissue or tendon sheath swelling, ESR less than 30 (women) or 20 (men). ACR/EULAR redefined remission in 2011 (33) as the fulfillment of all of the following: tender joint count less than or equal to 1, swollen joint count less than or equal to 1, CRP less than or equal to 1 mg/dL, patient global assessment less than or equal to 1 (on a 0–10 scale). These criteria have been effective in identifying patients who have long-term courses that were better than those who did not meet the definition of remission. The 2011 guidelines set the new standard for remission for future clinical research trials.

FLARES

A flare is described as "a worsening of disease activity of sufficient intensity and duration to consider a change in therapy," (34) but there is no current consensus for objectively diagnosing a flare period. Physiologically, flare represents an activation of inflammatory mediators in the synovium. The EULAR recommends that rapid remission is the primary goal of treatment in every patient, and strict monitoring should dictate the adjustment of medication as frequently as every 1 to 3 months (31).

PROGNOSIS

Predictors of a poor prognosis include functional limitation (e.g., Health Assessment Questionnaire [HAQ] score or similar valid tools), extraarticular disease (e.g., presence of rheumatoid nodules, RA vasculitis, Felty syndrome), positive RF or anticyclic citrullinated peptide antibodies, and bony erosions by radiograph (25). Other poor prognostic factors include persistent swelling of the PIP joints, flexor tenosynovitis of the hands, a large number of swollen joints, and impaired functional status at time of diagnosis. A good prognosis has already been outlined in the section on remission.

PRACTICE-BASED LEARNING AND IMPROVEMENT

GOALS

Demonstrate competence in continuously investigating and evaluating your RA patient care practices, appraising and assimilating scientific evidence, and continuously improving your patient care practices based on progressive self-evaluation and lifelong learning.

OBJECTIVES

1. Identify learning opportunities for providers, patients, and caregivers with experience in RA, including professional RA organizations.
2. Appraise the evidence-based practice guidelines, benchmarks, and literature in the specific rehabilitation management of RA patients.
3. Use methods for ongoing competency training in RA for physiatrists, including feedback from colleagues and patients in daily practice, evaluating current practice, and developing a quality improvement (QI) and practice performance improvement (PI) RA project activity.
4. Locate some resources including available websites for continuing medical education and professional development.
5. Conduct self-assessment and lifelong learning such as review of current quality of care markers, including evidence-based, in treatment of patients with RA and the role of the physiatrist as the educator of patients, families, residents, students, colleagues, and other health professionals.

Physiatrists providing care for patients with RA should have a working knowledge of the key elements of the medical history and physical examination of the patient with RA. They should be able to identify impairments, activity limitations, participation restrictions, and then, in conjunction with clinicians involved in the care of the RA patient, develop rehabilitation programs to address them.

They should be able to recognize patient safety concerns in this population and implement strategies to minimize them from occurring. Physiatrists should be up-to-date on advances in the understanding of the pathophysiology of RA and its medical, surgical, and rehabilitative treatment. Given the complexity of the medical treatments for RA, the physiatrist should have a working knowledge of side effects or adverse events associated with commonly used medications.

Physiatrists should also be aware of community resources available for patients with RA in their communities. Lastly, it is equally important that physiatrists have the necessary interpersonal and communication skills to effectively provide care for their patients with RA in the medical, community, school, and work settings as applicable.

There are several strategies that physiatrists can use to identify gaps in their knowledge base about RA and the medical and rehabilitative care of the patient with RA. Self-reflection on their clinical practice, self-assessment examinations sponsored by the AAPMR, asking trusted colleagues to provide feedback to them on their practice, and asking patients with RA under their care for feedback on the care provided by the physiatrist are some examples.

MAJOR RHEUMATOID ARTHRITIS ORGANIZATIONS

The ACR is the primary group in the United States responsible for setting new standards for diagnosis and treatment of RA. Seminal publications include comparisons of disease activity measurement tools (35), guidelines for choosing medications (25), and QI assessment (36). The EULAR (37) plays a role similar to that of the ACR, but among countries in Europe, and occasionally the two organizations jointly publish practice guidelines, such as the updated 2011 remission criteria (35).

There are many organizations that can be useful resources for patients and their families. Some of the major nonprofits include the *Arthritis Foundation* (38), the *Arthritis National Research Foundation* (39), and the *Rheumatoid Patient Foundation* (40). It is important to be aware of the official organizations involved in RA for patients and families seeking more information. Just having inquisitive patients "refer to the Internet" isn't enough, since pharmaceutical companies often sponsor websites that appear to be unbiased informational resources, but eventually link directly to the pharmaceutical corporate website (41).

EVIDENCE-BASED PRACTICE BENCHMARKS FOR REHABILITATION-CENTERED TREATMENT OF RHEUMATOID ARTHRITIS

Table 25.2 highlights some of the best evidence for rehabilitation, as well as other nonpharmacologic treatments and modalities for RA.

QUALITY IMPROVEMENT/PERFORMANCE IMPROVEMENT (41)

New approaches to QI and PI advocate for a Plan-Do-Study-Act (PDSA) framework over the standard model of running clinical trials because it places responsibility on the author and reader to implement the report's results. An example of

TABLE 25.2 Summary of Available Cochrane Reviews Related to Treatments for Rheumatoid Arthritis

TREATMENT/NO OF STUDIES	SUMMARY
Dynamic exercise/8	■ Land-based dynamic exercise moderately improved aerobic capacity and strength, and was safe both in the short and long term (8) ■ Aquatic-based exercise did not provide any additional benefit versus land-based exercise ■ In a different meta-analysis of 14 randomized controlled trials (RCTs), aerobic exercises (at 50%–90% maximum heart rate [HR]) showed small, beneficial effects on cardiorespiratory function, functional ability, and disease activity (11)
Occupational therapy/38	■ Strong evidence for the efficacy of "instruction on joint protection" ■ High-quality evidence that OT can help patients perform ADLs with less pain ■ Limited evidence in improving functional ability ■ Splints can decrease pain, but may decrease range of motion (ROM) (42)
Balneotherapy (spa)/6	■ Evidence is insufficient to support the claims of positive findings in most of the studies due to poor methodologic quality, the absence of an adequate statistical analysis, and the absence of essential outcome measures (i.e., pain & quality of life) (43)
Thermotherapy (heat and cold)/7	■ No significant effects for hot and ice pack applications and faradic baths on objective measures of disease activity ■ However, there were positive results for paraffin wax baths alone for arthritic hands on objective measures of ROM, pinch function, grip strength, pain, and stiffness after 4 weeks of treatment ■ Adding therapeutic ultrasound did not improve positive effects (44)
TENS/3	■ Conflicting results between different subsets of TENS therapy ■ AL-TENS (acupuncture-like TENS) reduced pain and improved strength when compared to placebo ■ C-TENS (conventional TENS) showed no objective benefit versus placebo; however, patients rated C-TENS better than AL-TENS on subjective scores of disease activity
Tai chi/4	■ Tai Chi-based exercise programs had no clinically important or statistically significant effect on most outcomes (i.e., ADLs, swollen/tender joints, global overall rating) ■ Significantly improved ankle ROM ■ Does not exacerbate rheumatoid arthritis symptoms
Herbal/22	■ Patients who took evening primrose oil, primrose oil, borage seed oil, or black current seed oil (with the active ingredient gamma-linolenic acid [GLA]) rated their pain to be 33 points lower (9–56 points lower) on a scale of 0 to 100 after 6 months of treatment versus placebo, which rated 19 points lower ■ Patients who took GLA rated their disability 16% better versus placebo which rated 5% better ■ None of the above caused significant unwanted side effects (45)
Diet/15	■ The effects of dietary modification, including vegetarian, Mediterranean, elemental, and elimination diets, on rheumatoid arthritis are still uncertain. Some small, single trials showed a reduction of pain, but not physical function or morning stiffness. Dietary modification groups had higher drop-out rates and weight loss (46)
Splinting/10	■ Resting hand and wrist splints do not significantly affect ROM or pain, although participants preferred wearing a resting splint to not wearing one ■ Extra-depth shoes and molded insoles decrease pain during weight-bearing activities (i.e., standing, walking, and stair climbing) (47)
Acupuncture and electro-acupuncture/2	■ In one study, pain, number of swollen and tender joints, disease activity, overall well-being, laboratory results, and amount of pain medication needed were about the same whether they had acupuncture or sham ■ Another study, comparing electroacupuncture to sham, showed that knee pain significantly improved with true acupuncture at both 24 hours and at 4 months. However, reviewers concluded that the poor quality of the trial, including the small sample size, preclude its recommendation (48)
Neuromodulators/4	■ Weak evidence that oral nefopam, topical capsaicin, and oromucosal cannabis are all superior to placebo in reducing pain in patients with rheumatoid arthritis ■ Capsaicin can be considered as an add-on therapy for patients with persistent local pain and inadequate response or intolerance to other treatments ■ Oral nefopam and oromucosal cannabis have more significant side effects, and potential harms may outweigh modest benefits (49)

(continued)

TABLE 25.2 Summary of available Cochrane reviews related to treatments for Rheumatoid Arthritis (*continued*)

Opioid therapy/11	■ Weak oral opioids (codeine, tramadol) can provide effective analgesia for some patients with rheumatoid arthritis (18% absolute improvement over placebo) ■ However, adverse effects (e.g., nausea, vomiting, dizziness, and constipation) are common and may offset the benefits (30% absolute difference compared to placebo) ■ There is insufficient evidence regarding the use of weak opioids for longer than 6 weeks, or the role of strong opioids (oxycodone, morphine, fentanyl) (50)
Muscle relaxants (benzodiazepines)/6	■ Failed to find evidence of a beneficial effect of muscle relaxants (diazepam and triazolam) over placebo, alone (at 24 hours, 1 or 2 weeks) or in addition to NSAIDs (at 24 hours), on pain intensity, function, or quality of life ■ Short-term muscle relaxant use (24 hours–2 weeks) is associated with significant adverse events (e.g., drowsiness and dizziness) (absolute difference of 49% when compared to placebo) (51)
Laser therapy/6	■ Given mostly on the hands and generally for two to three times a week for 4 weeks ■ Decreased pain and morning stiffness more than "placebo" laser therapy; also increased hand flexibility more than placebo therapy ■ Pain decreased by 1.10 points on a scale of 1–10. The length of time for morning stiffness decreased by 28 minutes ■ Effects lasted for up to 4 weeks, but not longer ■ Some evidence indicates that longer administration times and shorter wavelengths produced better effects (52)
Patient education/31	■ Significantly improved first follow-up (i.e., short-term) scores on disability, joint counts, patient global assessment, psychological status, and depression, but no significant effects were found in the long-term after final follow-up (3–14 months) (53)

an effective PDSA addressed the original 68-joint count survey, the original time-intensive intake for rheumatologists, and whether fewer joints could be assessed, while still providing adequate information for clinical decision making (54).

Plan: Use an available pool of RA patients to analyze the standard 68-joint count compared to other counts of 42, 36, or 28 joints and how this related to other measures of clinical status, such as patient questionnaires, radiographs, and laboratory tests.

Do: 210 patients in the clinical cross-sectional RA database were assessed with different joint counts and analyses of clinical trials to compare the results of the 28-joint count versus the standard 68-joint count.

Study: The analysis revealed that the 28-joint count was as informative as the standard 68-joint count with respect to both clinical care decisions (55) and for use in clinical trials (56).

Act: Since the reduced number was found to be equal to the higher joint count, it established an easier and more efficient intake survey. Future areas of study include developing earlier therapeutic interventions to reduce pain and improve functional status, and developing protocols that help patients exercise more frequently and have better access to physicians when their disease activity limits their ability to exercise.

INTERPERSONAL AND COMMUNICATION SKILLS

GOALS

Demonstrate interpersonal and communication skills that result in optimizing the effective exchange of information and collaboration with patients with RA, their families, and the rest of the rehabilitation team.

OBJECTIVES

1. Describe the importance of effective communication between physiatrists, rehabilitation team providers, and patients with RA across socioeconomic and cultural backgrounds.
2. Identify key areas for physicians to educate patients and families specific to RA.
3. Identify key points to be documented in patient records to provide effective communication between team members with respect to RA.
4. Delineate the importance of the role of the physiatrist as the interdisciplinary team leader and consultant for the patient with RA.

PATIENT-CENTERED COMMUNICATION

Building a positive relationship is especially important when caring for patients with RA, as they require ongoing pain management and functional reassessments as their disease activity waxes and wanes. It is important to develop a strong patient-centered interaction style in these long-term patients, as increased trust was significantly correlated with fewer side effects and better global health. In a study of systemic lupus and RA patients, physician interview style was assessed based on factors such as sensitivity, informativeness, reassurance, and patient-centeredness. Patient-centered interviewing was assessed by asking patients to rate whether the following was true: "My doctors always ask me what I need." The only clinical interaction variable studied that was significantly and independently associated with patient disclosure of information was patient-centeredness (57).

Part of optimal patient communication is addressing common misconceptions about RA and its treatment. A recent Medscape symposium revealed that 43% of patients with RA did not think that their doctor truly understood their condition (58). This article highlights the differences in perception between physician and patient with statements such as "You don't look swollen enough"; "it shouldn't hurt that bad"; "your 'inflammation markers' look good, so what's the problem?"

Many patients will have guilt of causation (i.e., a feeling that some lifestyle choice led to the disease), and it is important to stress that they are not responsible for their condition. Patients often seek complementary therapies, especially if pain control is inadequate or they experience side effects from medications, so it is important to address which alternative treatments are effective (see Table 25.1). It should also be discussed that the choice of DMARD or biologic therapy is individualized to each patient, and the efficacy of a particular medication is not impacted by its novelty, popularity, or cost (59).

Flares represent another area of impaired patient/physician communication. The Outcome Measures in Rheumatology (OMERACT) RA Flare Group sought to identify domains to define flares based on questionnaire data collected from international groups of patients and health care professionals (HCPs). There was close agreement among all participants in the domains of pain, physical function, stiffness, and tender joint count. However, there was a discrepancy between patients and physicians in several areas. Patients rated "participation" and "self-management" as important domains to consider when evaluating for a flare, whereas health care providers rated "swollen joint count" and "global assessment scores." These differences underscore the reality that many HCPs still perceive RA through the limited set of criteria defined by the ACR, which clearly misses several domains that patients find significant. Clearly, physicians should seek to take inventory of a patient's own rating of his or her participation in life events, and ability to manage daily activities, in order to broaden and improve communication.

MORTALITY

RA is a disease that not only affects small joints, but also has widespread systemic ramifications, which can significantly contribute to morbidity and mortality. The leading cause of mortality in RA is cardiovascular disease. The overall mortality in patients with RA is reported as 2.5 times higher than the general, age-matched population (60). For patients with severe articular and extraarticular disease, the mortality approaches that among patients with three-vessel coronary disease or stage 4 Hodgkin disease (20) (Box 25.9).

MEDICAL RECORD

The medical record must accurately reflect the current functional status of the patient. It must contain all the medications, including holistic and nutraceuticals, to monitor for side effects and potentially dangerous interactions.

An index of joint surgeries and deformities will determine joint protection measures and weight-bearing precautions. Nurses, physicians' assistants, and occupational and physical therapists may all be involved in managing patient care, and will look to the medical record for guidance on how certain joints

---

Box 25.9 Key Counseling Points

- What have I done to get rheumatoid arthritis?
- Will my children get it?
- Are the drugs safe to take?
- Is there a diet that will help?
- Are there dangers if I become pregnant?
- Are alternative therapies effective?
- Will exercise help or make me worse?
- Can I take birth control?
- Can I drive a car?
- Should I move to a different climate?

---

can be mobilized. Just as in the Barthel Index (an ADL-focused scale to evaluate function in the stroke patient), RA requires a similar evaluation by the rehabilitation team to assess ADL skills and physical limitations. Functional status updates to the medical record should include items such as ambulation (number of blocks walked), stair negotiation, and difficulty with bathing, toileting, and dressing.

PATIENT EDUCATION

RA is typically a chronic, slowly progressive inflammatory disease that includes not only synovial structures, but also extraarticular systems. Limited mobility due to pain and stiffness are associated with depression and fatigue. The effects of RA on an individual's occupation can cause emotional stress, which compounds the negative impact on personal well-being and interpersonal relationships. Patient education should target a wide variety of both medical and nonmedical issues faced by patients such as flares, physical activity, intimacy (sexuality), mental health/depression, stress management, osteoporosis, home care services, nutrition, and joint replacement (61). Sexual dysfunction is common in approximately 50% of patients with RA. In men, sexual dysfunction correlated significantly to pain score, cardiovascular disease, age, and disease activity (61). Many studies have shown significant beneficial effects on functional status, when comparing the effects of group-based education and information on exercises by a physical therapist compared with information by a physical therapist only (62).

Self-efficacy, defined as "the belief in one's ability to carry out a task with a desired outcome," has been a popular area of investigation in RA research. Scores attained by the Arthritis Self-Efficacy Scale (ASES) are associated with physical disease-related variables such as pain, fatigue, disease activity, and disability (63).

PROFESSIONALISM

GOALS

Reflect a commitment to carrying out professional responsibilities and an adherence to ethical principles in caring for patients with RA.

OBJECTIVES

1. Exemplify the humanistic qualities in patient-centered care.
2. Demonstrate ethical principles, responsibilities, and responsiveness to patient needs superseding self and other interests.
3. Demonstrate sensitivity to patient population diversity, cultural competence, gender, age, race, religion, disabilities, and sexual orientation.
4. Respect patient privacy, confidentiality, autonomy, and shared decision making.
5. Recognize the socioeconomic factors and importance of patient education in the treatment of and advocacy for persons with RA.

SOCIOCULTURAL FACTORS

As with all rheumatic disease, RA can be a chronic, lifelong struggle complicated by flares, functional loss, and medication side effects. Close doctor–patient relationships must be cultivated to properly address ongoing issues. In a study of 102 patients with rheumatic disease, patients completed a self-response survey aimed at characterizing their perceptions of medical encounters and subsequent trust in their care providers (57). The results showed that nonwhite males trusted physicians less than nonwhite females. Furthermore, the diminished trust by Latino and African American patients persisted after controlling for features of patient–doctor communication (i.e., patient-centeredness, sensitivity). This indicates that there is a gap in the current understanding of how to optimize clinical interactions across a variety of cultural settings.

PRIVACY ISSUES

Patients with RA may be reluctant to discuss depression, sexual dysfunction, and fear of incapacitation or death. It becomes the responsibility of the physician to address these issues with sensitivity and respect.

ADVOCACY

It is important to be aware of shortcomings in the current health care system approach to RA, and strongly support patients who are not receiving equality of care. A 2003 study (64) assessed whether patients receiving the standard of care for RA meet the inclusion criteria for clinical trials of biological agents, with the results showing that most patients do not meet those criteria. The authors advocated for less stringent inclusion criteria for clinical trials to better represent the population of patients who may benefit from that research. Other areas include advocating for the patients with RA in their workplace, school, and community for wheelchair-accessible ramps and doors. Adaptations may be required to accommodate for handicaps imposed by environmental constraints. The physiatrist should be prepared to educate the patient, public, and other HCPs about the wide scope of benefits of rehabilitative medicine outlined in this chapter.

ETHICAL ISSUES

Some authors have suggested that a detailed discussion of the full scope of RA, including its multisystemic effects and numerous treatment options, can overwhelm patients with unwanted information, exacerbate patient anxiety, and increase reported side effects via a negative placebo mechanism. This raises the ongoing bioethical issue of balancing beneficence (i.e., keeping the welfare of the patient in mind) with autonomy (respecting the capacity of the patient to make an informed decision). Considering the previous example in which physicians were concerned with giving patients too much information, a study of 100 patients with RA found that nearly 90% agreed with statements suggesting that they preferred full disclosure (i.e., "Even if the news is bad, I should be well informed" versus "I should be given information only when I ask for it"). Current employment and female gender were correlated with stronger preferences for being informed (65).

When considering the four bioethical principles of autonomy, beneficence, nonmaleficence, and justice, there are potential ethical conflicts that can arise during the course of patient care. For example, the patient's wishes with respect to certain medical treatments may go against the recommended treatment from the medical establishment (autonomy versus beneficence). Another example is related to limited access to rehabilitative care, adaptive equipment, and specialty care due to factors such as limited health insurance coverage, finances, and inaccessibility to treatment (principle of justice). For example, the economically advantaged patient may be able to afford new DMARDs or anti-TNF agents, or afford lighter and more customizable assistive devices (66).

SYSTEMS-BASED PRACTICE

GOALS

Awareness and responsiveness to systems of care delivery, and the ability to recruit and coordinate resources to provide optimal continuity of care options relating to RA.

OBJECTIVES

1. Identify the key components in the rehabilitation continuum of care from the inpatient to community setting for patients with RA.
2. Coordinate and recruit necessary resources in the system to provide optimal and variety of care options available for the patient with RA, with attention to safety, cost considerations, and risk–benefit analysis and management. Identify the components, systems of care delivery, services, referral patterns, and resources.
3. Describe optimal follow-up, markers of quality of care, improvement markers, and use of documentation in RA rehabilitation programs.

CONTINUUM OF CARE

RA patients receive care from a wide variety of health care providers, ranging from visiting nurse services and physical therapists, to rheumatologists, physiatrists, and orthopedists. Rehabilitative services for patients with RA can be provided in a variety of settings. For the vast majority of patients, RA can be managed in a home environment, which has the advantages of patient independence, family support, and familiar and comfortable environment. In the community setting, the patient with RA has access to multispecialty care, and these visits typically focus on nonemergent pain or functional limitations.

The inpatient setting is usually reserved for significant changes in the patient's medical status that require close monitoring and coordinated medical care; for example, a systemic exacerbation of the disease (i.e., vasculitis, pericarditis, myelosuppression) or the result of the side effect of medication (i.e., infection, sepsis, interstitial fibrosis). One risk imposed by hospitalization is exposing an already immunocompromised patient to an environment that leaves him or her susceptible to infections and other medical complications (Box 25.10).

MARKERS OF QUALITY OF CARE

Quality of care can be measured by the degree to which health services increase the likelihood of desired health outcomes and are consistent with current professional knowledge (41,67). Many advances have been made in the therapeutic approach to RA, but there is concern that not all physicians treating RA reliably incorporate new research into their daily clinical care. The ACR has endorsed quality measures for treating RA and monitoring patient care. Some fall into safety categories, such as documenting a tuberculosis screen within 6 months before receiving a first course of therapy with a biologic agent. Others focus on monitoring, such as assessing and classifying disease activity and functional status at least once every 12 months. Quality of care is also measured by adherence to ACR treatment guidelines, such as ensuring that all patients with an established diagnosis of RA are treated with a DMARD unless there is a contraindication to the medication, there is inactive disease, or the patient refuses treatment.

Also, if there are signs of increased disease activity, or evidence of bone erosion progression over any 6-month period, a DMARD or glucocorticoid must be added, or a DMARD must be changed to assure adherence to quality of care guidelines (68). Although there are no specific quality of care markers from the ACR regarding rehabilitation medicine, the physiatrist may assist in the noted yearly assessment. Patients with RA may interact with the physiatrist and rehabilitation team more frequently than other specialists. This close interaction allows for building rapport between the patient and the rehabilitation team, with the physiatrist being the primary patient advocate within the multidisciplinary specialties.

PATIENT SAFETY ISSUES

While earlier diagnosis and prompt initiation of DMARD and biologic therapies has become the new standard for RA treatment, it creates a group of medications unfamiliar to many providers.

It is important to be able to know and recognize the side effects of the newer medications in order to ensure ongoing patient safety. Although most of the DMARDs can cause systemic symptoms such as nausea, abdominal discomfort, rashes, and diarrhea, methotrexate in particular can cause myelosuppression, interstitial pulmonary fibrosis, and hepatotoxicity. It is also teratogenic, so premenopausal patients should be adequately screened. It should be noted that patients might not always recognize signs and symptoms of these systemic effects. This is highlighted by evidence from one study showing that, despite a nurse-led education program for methotrexate, less than 15% of patients with RA recognized the lethal interaction with trimethoprim/co-trimoxazole), and less than 60% recognized major adverse effects related to methotrexate, such as liver toxicity and increased risk of infection (69).

With respect to rehabilitation medicine, high-intensity exercise and strength training have been found to be safe (8,41), although the risk for joint flare-up exists. Postoperatively, patients with RA may be at a higher risk for hip dislocation due to pannus formation and the presence of joint erosions (66,70). For patients with atlantoaxial instability, cervical spine manipulation or traction should be strictly avoided, as several cases of severe neurological complications have been described (71).

Additional patient safety concerns can arise at transition points in the patient's care from acute hospital admission to the rehabilitation unit or home setting. Effective communication between clinicians at these transition points is essential to minimize risk of adverse events by making sure that all treatment providers are "on the same page." For example, the physiatrist should communicate specific precautions with respect to the use of modalities, forms of resistive exercise, spinal manipulation techniques, and the degree of exercise tolerance.

COST CONSIDERATIONS

As the interplay evolves between the advancement of medical technology with rising health care costs, there is a consistent effort to establish a cost–benefit analysis relative to current clinical recommendations. One study presented an economic evaluation of the Rheumatoid Arthritis Patients In Training (RAPIT) study (10) that compared a long-term, high-intensity exercise program with

---

Box 25.10 Rehabilitation Goals

The physiatrist and physical/occupational therapy team typically spend more time with patients than other specialties, placing them at the center of a systems-based practice. This gives the rehabilitation team an opportunity to monitor changes closely and intervene when problems develop.

- Reduce pain
- Limit deformity
- Increase muscle strength
- Reduce fatigue
- Teach coping skills to deal with preexisting limitations
    - Joint conservation
    - Adaptive equipment
- Manage therapy prescriptions and home exercise programs/modalities during flares
- Recognize depression and provide access to treatment

"usual care" (72). In both groups, patients could receive individual physical therapy. Over the 2-year period, there was a cost reduction of 62% in the high-intensity exercise group compared to the "usual care group"; however, this was not able to offset the overall cost of implementing the RAPIT program (cost of two physical therapists teaching 94 classes/year at 75 minutes/class).

Another area of potential cost savings lies in the prescription of devices meant to improve quality of life. There are many orthotic devices designed to augment function of impaired limb kinematics ("*function over form*"). However, some devices can be expensive, with lack of supporting evidence for their efficacy at improving "core measures" of RA disability or discomfort. A Cochrane review identified studies that evaluated working wrist splints, resting hand and wrist splints, and special shoes or insoles in patients with RA. The authors were unable to show that wrist splints statistically improved function or decreased pain. However, patients stated that they preferred wearing them, and evidence showed that wearing resting hand or wrist splints does not limit long-term ROM or cause additional pain. Another study showed that patients who wore extra-depth shoes with semirigid insoles had significantly less pain on walking and stair climbing (55). Several other orthotics did not improve pain or function in these trials. When deciding what assistive devices to prescribe, consideration should be given to those devices that have demonstrated proven effectiveness.

CONCLUSION

RA has been, and remains, the prototypical autoimmune disease. Despite the fact that the etiology of RA remains unknown, the pathway leading to joint destruction has been more clearly elucidated with a wellspring of new biologic agents targeted at specific sites of the inflammatory pathway. The rehabilitation team remains an integral part of the multidisciplinary approach to the management of RA.

CASE STUDY

A 21-year-old Spanish-speaking woman presents with a 2-month history of symmetrical wrist, hand, and knee pain and limitation of motion, pain, swelling, and stiffness in both wrists, knees, and feet. She was seen by a community primary care physician and was presumptively diagnosed with RA.

She is being referred to you for "physical therapy." She has a past medical history of childhood tuberculosis, diagnosed and treated in Mexico. The patient reports no known history of rheumatologic disease.

She has been taking naproxen twice a day but has experienced minimal pain relief. The patient is employed as an off-the-books housekeeper, but has been unable to work due to the multiple joint pains as described. She has no insurance, and lives alone in a second-floor walk-up.

On questioning, it is clear that she has no understanding of RA. She is reluctant to engage in any exercise program because of pain.

CASE STUDY DISCUSSION QUESTIONS

1. Formulate a rehabilitation program to address the patient's current pain, swelling, and joint limitation of motion.
2. What is the current understanding of the pathophysiology of RA and the role of biologic agents in the treatment of this disease?
3. What is the current understanding of the role and limitations of exercise, modalities, and orthotic devices in the treatment of RA?
4. What are the socioeconomic obstacles that impact this patient's care and how can you best advocate for this patient?
5. Identify the various clinical specialties that are involved in the patient's care, describe their role, and provide examples of effective communications between team members.
6. What are some examples of patient safety risks for this patient?

SELF-EXAMINATION QUESTIONS
(Answers begin on p. 367)

1. Which of the following is the earliest symptom of atlantoaxial (C1–C2) instability?
   A. Gait imbalance
   B. Diffuse symmetric upper extremity weakness and paresthesias
   C. Cervical pain radiating to the occiput
   D. Bowel and bladder incontinence
   E. Skin rash over the cervical spine

2. The best established environmental risk factor for RA is
   A. Viral infection
   B. Family member with a history of RA
   C. Alcohol consumption
   D. Smoking
   E. Silica exposure

3. Which of the following are predictors of a good prognosis for the patient with RA?
   A. Extraarticular disease
   B. Erosions within 2 years of disease onset
   C. Education level less than 11th grade
   D. Persistently elevated CRP
   E. Morning stiffness for 15 minutes or less

4. Which of the following modifications would be made to a rehabilitation prescription in the setting of a flare?
   A. Progress isometrics to isotonics
   B. Reduce exercise intensity, splinting, and limited ROM to affected joints
   C. Add ultrasound to treatment regimen
   D. Eliminate all ROM exercises
   E. Exercise is not a part of the rehabilitation prescription in RA

5. Which of the following is an IL-1 inhibitor?
   A. Etanercept (Enbrel®)
   B. Anakinra (Kineret®)
   C. Infliximab (Remicade®)
   D. Adalimumab (Humira®)
   E. Gabapentin (Neurontin®)

REFERENCES

1. Tehlirian CV, Bathon JM. Chapter 6: rheumatoid arthritis—Figure 6B-2. In: Klippel JH, ed. *Primer on the Rheumatic Diseases*. 13th ed. New York: Springer; 2008.
2. Ono S, et al. Reconstruction of the rheumatoid hand. *Clin Plast Surg*. 2011;38:713–727.
3. Chung KC, Pushman AG. Current concepts in the management of the rheumatoid hand. *J Hand Surg Am*. April 2011;36(4):736–747.
4. Weissman BN, Aliabadi P, et al. Prognostic features of atlantoaxial subluxation in rheumatoid arthritis patients. *J Radiol*. 1982;144(4):745.
5. Collins DN, Barnes CL, Fitzrandolph RL. Cervical spine instability in rheumatoid patients having total hip or knee arthroplasty. *Clin Orthop Relat Res*. 1991;(272):127–135.
6. Hochberg MC, Chang RW, Dwosh I, et al. The American College of Rheumatology 1991 revised criteria for the classification of global functional status in rheumatoid arthritis. *Arthritis Rheum*. 1992;35:498–502.
7. Theodora PM, et al. Nonpharmacological treatment of rheumatoid arthritis. *Curr Opin Rheumatol*. 2011;23:259–264.
8. Hurkmans E, et al. Dynamic exercise programs (aerobic capacity and/or muscle strength training) in patients with rheumatoid arthritis. *Cochrane Database Syst Rev*. 2009;(4):CD006853.
9. Minor MA, Hewett JE, Webel RR, et al. Efficacy of physical conditioning exercise in patients with rheumatoid arthritis and osteoarthritis. *Arthritis Rheum*. 1989;32(11):1396–1405.
10. De Jong Z, Munneke M, Zwinderman AH, et al. Is a long-term high-intensity exercise program effective and safe in patients with rheumatoid arthritis? Results of a randomized controlled trial. *Arthritis Rheum*. 2003;48(9):2415–2424.
11. Baillet A, et al. Efficacy of cardiorespiratory aerobic exercise in rheumatoid arthritis: meta-analysis of randomized controlled trials. *Arthritis Care Res*. 2010;62:984–992.
12. Meka N, et al. Endurance exercise and resistance training in cardiovascular disease. *Ther Adv Cardiovasc Dis*. 2008;2(2):115–121.
13. Spector TD. Rheumatoid arthritis. *Rheum Dis Clin North Am*. August 1990;16(3):513–537.
14. Humphreys JH, Verstappen SM, Hyrich KL, Chipping JR, Marshall T, Symmons DP. The incidence of rheumatoid arthritis in the UK: comparisons using the 2010 ACR/EULAR classification criteria and the 1987 ACR classification criteria. Results from the Norfolk Arthritis Register. *Ann Rheum Dis*. 2013;72(8):1315–1320.
15. Cooles FA, Isaacs JD. Pathophysiology of rheumatoid arthritis. *Curr Opin Rheumatol*. May 2011;23(3):233–240.
16. Schaeverbeke T, et al. When and where does rheumatoid arthritis begin? *Joint Bone Spine*. December 2012;79(6):550–554.
17. Harris ED, Genovese MC. *Primary Care Rheumatology*. Philadelphia, PA: W.B. Saunders; 2000:256–257.
18. Quinn MA, Emery P. Window of opportunity in early arthritis: possibility of altering the disease process with early intervention. *Clin Exp Rheumatol*. 2003;21(suppl 31):S154–S157.
19. http://www.rheumatology.org/practice/clinical/classification/ra/ra_2010.asp.
20. Aletaha D, et al. 2010 rheumatoid arthritis classification criteria: an American College of Rheumatology/European League Against Rheumatism collaborative initiative. *Ann Rheum Dis*. 2010;69(9):1580.
21. Fuchs HA, et al. Evidence of significant radiographic damage in rheumatoid arthritis within the first 2 years of disease. *J Rheumatol*. 1989;16(5):585.
22. Klarlund M, Ostergaard M, Jensen KE, et al. Magnetic resonance imaging, radiography, and scintigraphy of the finger joints: one year follow up of patients with early arthritis. The TIRA Group. *Ann Rheum Dis*. 2000;59(7):521.
23. West SG. Rheumatology Secrets. 2nd edition. Elsevier Health Sciences; 2002: 121.
24. Singh JA, et al. 2012 update of the 2008 American College of Rheumatology recommendations for the use of disease-modifying antirheumatic drugs and biologic agents in the treatment of rheumatoid arthritis. *Arthritis Care Res (Hoboken)*. May 2012;64(5):625–639. doi:10.1002/acr.21641.
25. Image used under Creative Commons/GNU Free Documentation License: http://en.wikipedia.org/wiki/Image:Hematopoiesis_%28human%29_diagram.png.
26. Image used under Creative Commons/GNU Free Documentation License (Attribution: SubtleGuest at English Wikipedia) http://en.wikipedia.org/wiki/File:NIH_3T3.jpg.
27. Image used under Creative Commons/GNU Free Documentation License (Attribution: BruceBlaus at English Wikipedia) http://en.wikipedia.org/wiki/File:Blausen_0625_Lymphocyte_T_cell.png.
28. Image used under Creative Commons/GNU Free Documentation License: http://en.wikipedia.org/wiki/File:TRAPosteoclastculture.jpg.
29. Smolen JS, et al. EULAR recommendations for the management of rheumatoid arthritis with synthetic and biological disease-modifying antirheumatic drugs. *Ann Rheum Dis*. May 5, 2010. doi:10.1136/ard.2009.126532. Published Online First.
30. Gotzsche PC, Johansen, HK. Short-term low dose corticosteroids vs placebo and nonsteroidal antiinflammatory drugs in rheumatoid arthritis. *Cochrane Database Syst Rev*. 2005;1:CD000189.
31. Gorter SL, Bijlsma JW, Cutolo M, et al. Current evidence for the management of rheumatoid arthritis with glucocorticoids: a systematic literature review informing the EULAR recommendations for the management of rheumatoid arthritis. *Ann Rheum Dis*. 2010;69(6):1010–1014.
32. Pinals RS, Masi AT, Larsen RA. Preliminary criteria for clinical remission in rheumatoid arthritis. *Arthritis Rheum*. 1981;24:1308–1315.
33. Felson DT, et al. American College of Rheumatology/European League Against Rheumatism Provisional Definition of Remission in Rheumatoid Arthritis for Clinical Trials. *Ann Rheum Dis*. 2011;70:404–413. doi:10.1136/ard.2011.149765.
34. Bartlett SJ, Hewlett S, et al. Identifying core domains to assess flare in rheumatoid arthritis: an OMERACT international patient and provider combined Delphi consensus. *Ann Rheum Dis*. 2012;71:1855–1860.
35. Anderson J, et al. Rheumatoid arthritis disease activity measures: American College of Rheumatology Recommendations for Use in Clinical Practice. *Arthritis Care Res*. May 2012;64(5):640–647.
36. Saag KG, et al. Defining quality of care in rheumatology: the American College of Rheumatology White Paper on Quality Measurement. *Arthritis Care Res*. January 2011;63(1):2–9. doi:10.1002/acr.20369.
37. http://www.eular.org
38. http://www.arthritis.org/conditions-treatments/disease-center/rheumatoid-arthritis/

39. http://www.curearthritis.org/rheumatoid-arthritis/
40. http://rheum4us.org/
41. http://www.ra.com/
42. Seultjens EEMJ, Dekker JJ, Bouter LM, et al. Occupational therapy for rheumatoid arthritis. *Cochrane Database Syst Rev.* 2004;(1). Art. No.: CD003114.
43. Verhagen AP, Bierma-Zeinstra SMA, Boers M, et al. Balneotherapy for rheumatoid arthritis. *Cochrane Database Syst Rev.* 2004;(1). Art. No.: CD000518
44. Welch V, Brosseau L, Casimiro L, et al. Thermotherapy for treating rheumatoid arthritis. *Cochrane Database Syst Rev.* 2002;(2). Art. No.: CD002826.
45. Cameron M, Gagnier JJ, Chrubasik S. Herbal therapy for treating rheumatoid arthritis. *Cochrane Database Syst Rev.* 2011;(2):CD002948.
46. Hagen KB, Byfuglien MG, Falzon L, et al. Dietary interventions for rheumatoid arthritis. *Cochrane Database Syst Rev.* 2009;(1). Art. No.: CD006400.
47. Egan M, Brosseau L, Farmer M, et al. Splints and orthosis for treating rheumatoid arthritis. *Cochrane Database Syst Rev.* 2001;(4). Art. No.: CD004018.
48. Casimiro L, Barnsley L, Brosseau L, et al. Acupuncture and electroacupuncture for the treatment of rheumatoid arthritis. *Cochrane Database Syst Rev.* 2005;(4). Art. No.: CD00378.
49. Richards BL, Whittle SL, Buchbinder R. Neuromodulators for pain management in rheumatoid arthritis. *Cochrane Database Syst Rev.* 2012;(1). Art. No.: CD008921.
50. Whittle SL, Richards BL, Husni E, et al. Opioid therapy for treating rheumatoid arthritis pain. *Cochrane Database Syst Rev.* 2011;(11). Art. No.: CD003113.
51. Richards BL, Whittle SL, Buchbinder R. Muscle relaxants for pain management in rheumatoid arthritis. *Cochrane Database Syst Rev.* 2012;(1). Art. No.: CD008922.
52. Brosseau L, Welch V, Wells GA, et al. Low level laser therapy (Classes I, II and III) for treating rheumatoid arthritis. *Cochrane Database Syst. Rev.* 2005;(4). Art. No.: CD002049.
53. Riemsma RP, Kirwan JR, Taal E, et al. Patient education for adults with rheumatoid arthritis. *Cochrane Database Syst Rev.* 2003(2). Art. No.: CD003688.
54. Pincus T, et al. Quantitative measurement of patient status in the regular care of patients with rheumatic diseases over 25 years as a continuous quality improvement activity, rather than traditional research. *Clin Exp Rheumatol.* November–December 2007;25 (6 suppl, 47):69–81.
55. Fuchs HA, et al. A simplified twenty-eight joint quantitative articular index in rheumatoid arthritis. *Arthritis Rheum.* 1989;32: 531–537.
56. Fuchs HA, Pincus T. Reduced joint counts in controlled clinical trials in rheumatoid arthritis. *Arthritis Rheum.* 1994;37:470–475.
57. Berrios-Rivera JP, et al. Trust in physicians and elements of the medical interaction in patients with rheumatoid arthritis and systemic lupus erythematosus. *Arthritis Rheum (Arthritis Care Res).* June 15, 2006;55(3):385–393.
58. Young K. Rheumatoid arthritis warrior. n.p. web. January 26, 2014. http://rawarrior.com/medscape-symposium-reveals-attitudes-rheum-patients-encounter/.
59. http://emedicine.medscape.com/article/331715.
60. Lemon J, Marichal-Williams B, Blum E, Bracero M. Rheumatoid arthritis educational series: a nurse-led project. *Orthop Nurs.* 2012;31(4):205–209.
61. Palmer D, El Miedany Y. Sexual dysfunction in rheumatoid arthritis: a hot but sensitive issue. *Br J Nurs.* 2011;20(17):1134–1137.
62. Taal et al. (1993). Group education for patients with rheumatoid arthritis. *Patient Educ Couns.* 1993;20:177–187.
63. Primdahl J, et al. Self-efficacy as an outcome measure and its association with physical disease-related variables in persons with rheumatoid arthritis: a literature review. *Musculoskelet Care.* 2011;9:125–140.
64. Sokka T, Pincus T. Most patients receiving routine care for rheumatoid arthritis in 2001 did not meet inclusion criteria for most recent clinical trials or American College of Rheumatology criteria for remission. *J Rheumatol.* 2003;30:1138–1146.
65. Fraenkel L, Bogardus S, Concato J, Felson D. Preference for disclosure of information among patients with rheumatoid arthritis. *Arthritis Rheum.* 2001;45(2):136–139.
66. Hunt PC, et al. Demographic and socioeconomic factors associated with disparity in wheelchair customizability among people with traumatic spinal cord injury. *Arch Phys Med Rehabil.* November 2004;85(11):1859–1864.
67. Committee on Quality of Health Care in America. Institute of Medicine. *Crossing the Quality Chasm: A New Health System for the 21st Century.* Washington, DC: National Academy Press; 2001.
68. Bombardier C, Mian S. Quality indicators in rheumatoid arthritis care: using measurement to promote quality improvement. *Ann Rheum Dis.* 2013;72 Suppl 2:ii128-31.
69. Sowden E, et al. Limited end-user knowledge of methotrexate despite patient education. An assessment of rheumatologic preventive practice and effectiveness. *J Clin Rheumatol.* 2012;18:130–133.
70. Kohan KJ, Thomas MA. Acute atraumatic hip dislocation in an adult with rheumatoid arthritis. *Am J Phys Med Rehabil.* April 2012;91(4):346–348.
71. La Francis ME. A chiropractic perspective on atlantoaxial instability in Down's syndrome. *J Manipulative Physiol Ther.* March–April 1990;13(3):157–160.
72. Van den Hout WB, de Jong Z, Munneke M, et al. Cost-utility and cost-effectiveness analyses of a long-term, high-intensity exercise program compared with conventional physical therapy in patients with rheumatoid arthritis. *Arthritis Rheum.* 2005;53(1):39–47.

Lauren R. Eichenbaum
Geet Paul
Stephen Nickl
David Bressler

26: Fibromyalgia

PATIENT CARE

GOALS

Provide competent patient care that is team based, patient centered, compassionate, appropriate, and effective for the evaluation, treatment, education, and advocacy of fibromyalgia (FM) patients across the continuum of care and the promotion of health.

OBJECTIVES

1. Describe the key components of fibromyalgia and the assessment of FM, including history and physical examination.
2. Define the impairments, activity limitations, and participation restrictions of the patient with FM.
3. Identify the psychosocial and vocational implications of the patient with FM and strategies to address them.
4. Formulate an optimal rehabilitation program for the treatment and management of FM.

WHAT IS FIBROMYALGIA SYNDROME?

The etiology of the fibromyalgia syndrome (FMS) is not well understood. FMS is a common medical condition, which causes intermittent, chronic, widespread pain. It is more prevalent in women 20 to 60 years of age, affecting 0.5% to 5.0% of the population (1). It is exacerbated by poor sleep, activity, inactivity, and emotional stress (2). FMS continues to be a process in evolution, with symptoms being recognized since the 1700s. It was initially termed *fibrositis*, which was discarded when no inflammatory marker(s) could be identified. To date there are no specific tests for the diagnosis of FMS. In the 1990s the American College of Rheumatology (ACR) adapted diagnostic criteria that relied on the identification of "classical" tender points. In 2010, although still part of the physical examination, the identification of tender points was deemed no longer mandatory for a diagnosis of FMS. Instead, FMS is now considered a syndrome characterized by widespread pain due to the sensitization of the central nervous system. The cause(s) of this central maladaptation is multifactorial and has not been fully elucidated.

WHAT IS THE CURRENT PROPOSED CRITERIA FOR THE DIAGNOSIS OF FIBROMYALGIA?

As previously noted, the ACR first developed the main diagnostic criteria for fibromyalgia in 1990. At that time, patients included in the diagnosis presented with widespread pain for a minimum of 3 months and reported pain in at least 11 of 18 defined tender points. At that time, the exclusion of concomitant disease was not necessary.

In 2010, the ACR developed new guidelines for the diagnosis of FM. These guidelines no longer exclusively relied on the identification of select tender points (which were frequently performed incorrectly or not at all), but instead focused on a presentation of widespread pain with associated somatic and cognitive complaints (2,3,4). Three criteria were developed relating to the severity, the duration, and the exclusion of other diseases (Table 26.1).

WHAT IS CHRONIC WIDESPREAD PAIN?

Chronic widespread pain is characterized by pain for a minimum duration of 3 months in all four quadrants of the body, including the axial skeleton. The pain must be present on both sides of the body, both above and below the waistline (5). In addition, all other possible diseases must be ruled out (4).

WHAT IS THE WIDESPREAD PAIN INDEX?

The widespread pain index (WPI) broadens the tender point criteria to general areas of pain. It measures the presence of pain over the last week in 19 areas of the body thereby being scored from 0 to 19. The WPI includes the locations given in Table 26.2.

WHAT IS THE SYMPTOM SEVERITY SCALE?

The symptom severity (SS) scale score is a composite scale based on the severity of four specific symptoms (4). The first

TABLE 26.1 2010 ACR Diagnostic Criteria for Fibromyalgia

1. Widespread Pain Index (WPI) and Symptom Severity (SS)

    a. WPI ≥ 7 and SS ≥ 5

    or

    b. WPI 3–6 and SS ≥ 9

2. Symptoms present for at least 3 months
3. Other possible disorders ruled out

TABLE 26.2 WPI Tender Point Location

MIDLINE	RIGHT	LEFT
Neck	Jaw	Jaw
Chest	Shoulder girdle	Shoulder girdle
Abdomen	Upper arm	Upper arm
Upper back	Lower arm	Lower arm
Lower back	Hip (buttock, trochanter)	Hip (buttock, trochanter)
	Upper leg	Upper leg
	Lower leg	Lower leg

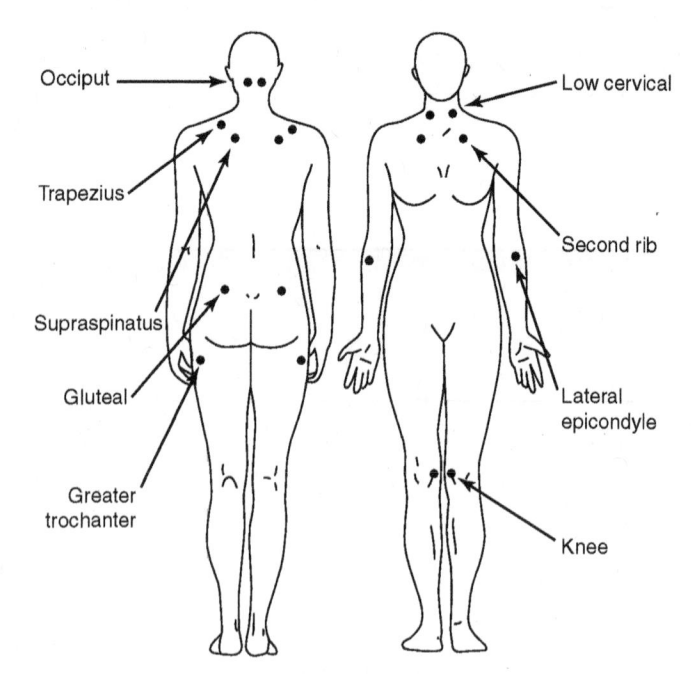

FIGURE 26.1 Tender point locations according to 1990 ACR guidelines.

3 symptoms are fatigue, waking unrefreshed, and cognitive symptoms. These symptoms are rated from 0 to 3 based on severity over the last week. The final category is the severity of somatic symptoms which include muscle pain, diarrhea, constipation, headache, dry mouth, insomnia, and depression. Somatic symptoms are rated from 0 to 3 (no symptoms, few, moderate, and a great deal of symptoms). The cumulative score for SS is between 0 and 12 (Table 26.3).

WHAT ARE TENDER POINTS?

A tender point (Figure 26.1) is the presence of pain upon digital palpation of a muscle or tendon. The force with palpation should not exceed 4 kg/cm^2 (approximately the amount of force that it takes to whiten your nail bed) (6). For a tender point to be positive, the patient must state that the palpation was painful. Note that a complaint of "tenderness" is not considered painful (5).

TABLE 26.3 Somatic Symptom Score

SYMPTOMS	GRADING	SOMATIC SYMPTOMS
Fatigue	0 — Denies	0 — Denies
Waking unrefreshed	1 — Mild	1 — Few
Cognitive symptoms	2 — Moderate	2 — Moderate
	3 — Severe	3 — Great deal of symptoms

WHAT ARE THE PRIMARY SOMATIC AND COGNITIVE SYMPTOMS ASSOCIATED WITH FMS?

SOMATIC	COGNITIVE
IBS - Irritable Bowel Syndrome	Chronic fatigue
Palpitations	Memory impairment ("fibrofog")
Subjective sensory deficits	Depression
Headache	

WHAT ARE THE KEY PSYCHOSOCIAL ASPECTS ASSOCIATED WITH FIBROMYALGIA SYNDROME?

According to Winfield, the population suffering from FM is likely to have had traumatic experiences in their childhood or other emotional stressors throughout their life (7). It is known that depression and emotional stress are strongly associated with FM (8). It is highly important that all patients diagnosed with FM be evaluated for depression or other psychiatric disorders. The disability and pain experienced in FM patients are associated with a poor quality of life (7). FM and depression have overlapping symptoms; therefore, the diagnosis and treatment of depression can often improve the somatic symptoms and quality of life of the patient with FM.

SAMPLE REHABILITATION PROGRAM

Goals: An education for the patient and family, modalities, aerobic exercise (AE), stretching, strengthening, and cognitive behavioral therapy (CBT). The program should be tailored to the needs of each individual. Warm water pool exercises have been shown to produce significant improvement (9). Aerobic training improves fatigue and depression, and participants were found to tolerate increased levels of pressure over their tender points (10). Aerobic training has also been shown to reduce muscle and cognitive fatigue, and to decrease symptoms of depression (11). A sample physical therapy (PT) prescription is presented in Table 26.4.

Alternative Treatment

There are many alternative treatments such as yoga, acupuncture, and meditation; however, Tai Chi is one of the most researched alternative exercise programs. Tai Chi is a low-intensity exercise, which utilizes a slow and constant shifting of body weight for balance training. This exercise has low impact on the spine and is void of abrupt movements, which can be a source of pain. It also incorporates deep breathing exercises for relaxation, making it a multidisciplinary treatment (12).

TABLE 26.4 Sample Physical Therapy Prescription

Diagnosis: Fibromyalgia
Impairment: Symmetrical above and below waist tender points (11/18)
Disability: Compromised activities of daily living
Precautions: Standard
Short-term goals: Reduction of tender point tenderness by 40%; increase of aerobic exercise tolerance to 10 minutes/session
Long-term goals: Reduction of tender point tenderness by 75% to 80%; increase of aerobic exercise tolerance to 20 to 30 minutes/session
Treatment: Tetanizing electrical stimulation + moist hot pack to area (s) of maximum tenderness for 20 minutes or massage for 20 minutes; progressive stretching/flexibility training to upper/lower extremities
Cardiovascular conditioning with progressive aerobic training: Treadmill, bicycle, or recumbent bike (resistance free) as tolerated for 5 to 10 minutes at 50% to 60% of maximal heart rate (HR); increase as tolerated to progress to 20 to 30 minutes at 70% to 80% maximal HR
Strength training: Isometric, isotonic, or isokinetics as tolerated
Stretching and relaxation exercises
Home exercise program (HEP) reflecting exercise protocol outlined earlier (HEP should be advanced to 20–30 minutes aerobic and flexibility training 5 to 6 times/week)
Frequency: 2 to 3 times/week for 6 to 8 weeks
At 6 to 8 weeks patient should be reevaluated and program adjusted to reflect progress to date

COGNITIVE BEHAVIORAL THERAPY

CBT is the integration of cognitive and behavioral therapies. Cognitive and behavioral factors play a large role in the symptomatic manifestations of FM. CBT provides psychological treatment that leads to modifications of dysfunctional thoughts and behavioral modifications. CBT was found to have efficacy in reducing depressed mood and in improving pain (13). The American Pain Society (APS) gave CBT a strong recommendation while the European League Against Rheumatism (EULAR) only gave CBT a weak recommendation.

MEDICAL KNOWLEDGE

GOALS

Demonstrate knowledge of established and evolving biomedical, clinical, epidemiological, and sociobehavioral sciences pertaining to FM, as well as the application of this knowledge to guide holistic patient care treatment.

OBJECTIVES

1. Describe the epidemiology, anatomy, physiology, pathophysiology, and pharmacology of FM.
2. Discuss the central sensitization theory.
3. Describe the role of neuroimaging in FMS.
3. Describe the neurotransmitters in pain signaling.
4. Evaluate both pharmacological and nonpharmacological treatment of FMS.

According to the National Institutes of Health, FM has been diagnosed in over 5 million Americans who are over 18 years of age, the large majority of whom are women (14). Goldenberg and coauthors report that the disease is stratified in a ratio of 3.4% for women and 0.5% for men (15).

Studies have shown that there is a genetic predisposition toward the development of FMS (16). After osteoarthritis, FM is the second most common disorder seen by rheumatologists (15). Of interest, only 20% of the diagnosed population in the United States receives treatment (15). The medical costs of treating individuals suffering from FM increase with the severity of the disease, and can be an economic burden with annual expenditure ranging from $6,951 to $9,869 per patient (17).

Yunus (2001) introduced the term *central sensitivity syndromes* (CSS) to describe the group of syndromes that have significant overlap of symptoms with FM. These include chronic fatigue syndrome, irritable bowel syndrome, tension-type headache, migraine, temporomandibular disorder, myofascial pain syndrome, restless legs syndrome, interstitial cystitis, and more (18).

Yunus states that "Central sensitivity syndromes (CSS) comprise an overlapping and similar group of syndromes without structural pathology and are bound by the common mechanism of central sensitization (CS) that involves hyper excitement of the central neurons through various synaptic and neurotransmitter/neurochemical activities" (19).

While there are no specific diagnostic tests for FMS, an interesting electromyography (EMG)-based procedure has been proposed to establish the presence of "central sensitization" (20). An electrical correlate, which reflects central sensitization can be objectively demonstrated by using the nociceptive flexion reflex (NFR). The test is performed as follows: the sural nerve that is purely sensory is slowly (start at 1 mA) stimulated over the lateral malleolus until a spinal flexion reflex contraction is recorded at the ipsilateral biceps femoris muscle tendon. The current threshold required to produce the initial contraction, has been shown to be consistently reduced, reflecting the hypersensitivity and central sensitization in FMS patient (20).

In FMS patients, the pain pathway is altered due to imbalance of several neurotransmitters resulting in centrally mediated augmentation of pain and sensory processes. Neurotransmitters that act to facilitate nociceptive processing are upregulated. This includes substance P, nerve growth factor, and brain-derived neurotrophic factor. Glutamate levels are also increased in the cerebrospinal fluid (CSF) and the brain. Glutamate is a key player responsible for the pain "wind-up" phenomenon, which results in greater hyperalgesia and allodynia. Pain wind-up phenomenon is the perceived increase in pain intensity over time after repeated painful stimulation. Along with the upregulation of the ascending pathway there is decreased activity in the descending, antinociceptive pathway. There is a significant reduction in the CSF levels of metabolites of neurotransmitters that typically inhibit pain transmission, such as serotonin, norepinephrine, and dopamine. Opioid levels are also altered in FM patients. Opioid levels are found to be increased with decreased μ-opioid receptor availability. This can explain why opioid therapy may be ineffective in treatment of FM (21).

Neuroimaging studies have substantiated the growing body of evidence that FM is characterized by cortical or subcortical augmentation of pain processing. Functional MRI studies demonstrated, in FM patients, increased neuronal activation and cerebral blood flow at the pain processing centers of the brain at lower pain producing pressures compared to healthy individuals (22). Other neuroimaging studies have showed hypoperfusion of the striatum and thalamus, decreased dopamine binding in the striatum, and changes in the brain structures in the cingulated cortex, insular cortex, striatum, and thalamus. Results of these studies show that there are functional and morphological changes that occur in CNS structures involved in the pain pathway in patients with FM (23).

PHARMACOLOGICAL TREATMENT OF FIBROMYALGIA

Historically, the most common agents used to treat FM were Tylenol, opioids, nonsteroidal anti-inflammatory drugs (NSAIDs), tricyclic antidepressants (TCAs), and cyclobenzaprine. But none of these medications or group of medications have been approved by the FDA to treat FM, and the studies that support their use are poorly designed. Currently there are only 3 drugs approved by the FDA for treatment of FM: pregabalin (Lyrica), duloxetine (Cymbalta), and milnacipran (Savella). These medications all serve as neuromodulating agents that alter the abnormal signaling in the spinal cord and brain of patients with FM.

The APS gave the highest level of recommendation to AE, CBT, amitriptyline, and multicomponent therapy (24). EULAR gave the highest level of recommendations to the pharmacologic treatments (tramadol, amitriptyline, fluoxetine, duloxetine, milnacipran, pregabalin, and more) (25). Note the APS recommendations are old, predating the FDA approval of pregabalin, duloxetine, and milnacipran (Table 26.5).

Tricyclic Antidepressants

TCAs, such as amitriptyline and cyclobenzaprine, have been shown to be beneficial in the treatment of pain as well as treating fatigue and poor sleep that is commonly associated with FM. TCAs increase the synaptic concentration of serotonin and norepinephrine by inhibiting the reuptake of these neuropeptides. However, due to their side-effect profile, including sedation, dry mouth, constipation, and cardiovascular issues, many patients are unable to tolerate these medications (26).

Selective Serotonin Reuptake Inhibitors

Selective serotonin reuptake inhibitors (SSRIs) that have been studied include fluoxetine, citalopram, and paroxetine. Controlled studies have shown mixed results. Mease (26) states that SSRIs are generally not as effective as TCAs and serotonin–norepinephrine reuptake inhibitors (SNRIs), though they aid in the treatment of depression. APS gave SSRIs a moderate level of evidence, while EULAR gave it the highest level of evidence.

Serotonin–Norepinephrine Reuptake Inhibitors

SNRIs have been found to be most effective in treating FM and include venlafaxine (Effexor), duloxetine (Cymbalta), and milnacipran (Savella). Venlafaxine was the first of the SNRIs to be studied but the results were mixed (26). Duloxetine is the first of the SNRIs to be approved by the FDA for treatment of FM. In two separate double-blind randomized controlled trial (RCT) studies, duloxetine was found not only to decrease widespread pain but also to improve overall function, quality of life, and fatigue (27,28). Both studies demonstrated that the decrease in pain was direct, and not indirect through treatment of depression. The other SNRI to be approved by the FDA for FM is milnacipran (Savella). It has a higher ratio of norepinephrine to serotonin than the other SNRIs mentioned. Two separate but similarly designed double-blind RCT studies revealed that milnacipran significantly reduced pain and fatigue, and improved cognition (29,30). APS gave SNRIs a moderate level of evidence, while EULAR gave it the highest level of evidence.

Anticonvulsants

Gabapentin and pregabalin are both widely used for treating neuropathic pain. They bind to the alpha-2-delta protein associated with voltage-gated calcium channels and modulate calcium influx, resulting in the decreased release of Substance P and glutamate (26). Pregabalin was the first drug to be approved by the FDA for the treatment of FM. It was shown to be efficacious in the reduction of pain, disturbed sleep, and fatigue compared with placebo (32).

TABLE 26.5 Comparison of Evidence-Based Recommendations by APS and EULAR

	AMERICAN PAIN SOCIETY		EULAR	
	LEVEL OF EVIDENCE	STRENGTH OF RECOMMENDATION	LEVEL OF EVIDENCE	STRENGTH OF RECOMMENDATION
Aerobic exercise	I	A	IIb	C
CBT	I	A	IV	D
Amitriptyline	I	A	Ib	A
Cyclobenzaprine	I	A	—	
Multicomponent therapy	I	A	—	
Tramadol	II	B	Ib	A
Balneotherapy	II	B	IIa	B
Education alone	II	B	—	
Hypnotherapy	II	B	—	
Biofeedback	II	B	—	
Massage therapy	II	B	—	
Anticonvulsants	II	B	Ib	A
SSRI	II	B	Ib	A
SNRI	II	B	Ib	A
Opioids	III	C	IV	Not D
Acupuncture	II	C	—	
Trigger point injections	III	C	—	

Source: Derived from Hauser et al 2010.

Tramadol

Tramadol is a weak opioid with mild SSRI properties. Both APS and EULAR gave it a high level of recommendation. Bennett et al. in 2003 in a double-blind RCT demonstrated that tramadol combined with acetaminophen was effective in reducing pain in patients with FM (33).

NONPHARMACOLOGICAL TREATMENT OF FIBROMYALGIA

Exercise Program

Evidence supports the efficacy of AE for patients with FM. In a Cochrane review from 2008 (34), the authors concluded that moderate evidence supports AE having a positive effect on global well-being and physical function. In another meta-analysis, the Ottawa Panel (2008) found Grade A evidence that AE reduced pain and improved endurance and quality of life. AE should be performed at low intensity (50%–60% of maximal HR) to moderate (60%–80%) intensity, two to three times a week, and for at least 4 to 6 weeks in order to see a reduction of symptoms (35). It is important to remember that patients with FM are often overweight and with reduced cardiovascular fitness level. Overexertion can worsen pain. Start with low-intensity exercise, such as walking in place and aquatic therapy, and increase the intensity as tolerated (14). For a sedentary person who has moderate to severe FM, Jones and Liptan recommend the following progression: (a) breath, posture, and relaxation training; (b) flexibility; (c) strength and balance; and (d) aerobics (36). According to Busch et al. in a Cochrane review, strength-only and flexibility-only training remain incompletely evaluated as the studies are of either poor quality or completely lacking (34).

PRACTICE-BASED LEARNING AND IMPROVEMENT

GOALS

Demonstrate competence in continuously investigating and evaluating your FM patient care practices, appraising and assimilating scientific evidence, and continuously improving your patient care practices based on constant self-evaluation and lifelong learning.

OBJECTIVES

1. Describe learning opportunities for providers, patients, and caregivers with experience in FM.
2. Use methods for ongoing competency training in FMS for physiatrists, including formative evaluation feedback in daily

practice, evaluating current practice, and developing a systematic QI and practice performance improvement strategy to improve patient care.
3. Locate national organizations and resources including available websites for continuing medical education and continuing professional development.
4. Describe some areas paramount to self-assessment and lifelong learning such as review of current guidelines, including evidence-based guidelines, in treatment and management of patients with FMS and the role of the physiatrist as the educator of patients, families, residents, students, colleagues, and other health professionals.

Physiatrists providing care for patients with FMS should have a working knowledge of the key elements of the medical history and physical examination of the patients with FMS. They should be able to identify impairments, activity limitations, and participation restrictions and then, in conjunction with members of the rehabilitation team, develop rehabilitation programs to address them. Physiatrists should be up-to-date on advances in the understanding of the pathophysiology of FMS and its pharmacological and nonpharmacological treatment and have a working knowledge of side effects or potential adverse events associated with treatments. It is equally important that physiatrists have the necessary interpersonal and communication skills to effectively provide care for their patients with FMS.

There are several strategies that physiatrists can use to identify gaps in their knowledge base about FMS and the medical and rehabilitative care of the patient with FMS. Self-reflection on their clinical practice, self-assessment examinations, asking trusted colleagues to provide feedback to them on their practice, and asking patients with FMS under their care for their feedback on the care provided by the physiatrist are just some examples.

As the understanding of FM continues to grow, the approach to diagnosis and treatment should be evidence based. Diagnosis should be based on the criteria put forward by ACR. Physicians should keep up-to-date on current breakthroughs in research by reading literature published by ACR. *Arthritis & Rheumatism* is the official monthly journal published by ACR. This journal includes peer-reviewed articles on diagnosis, treatment, laboratory research, and socioeconomic issues related to rheumatic disease. ACR also has annual meetings where leaders in the field will provide lectures and overview of current research in the field. The National Fibromyalgia Association has been involved in increasing awareness of FM by providing important media campaigns, implementing continuing medical education programs, and providing assistance for scientific research. The treatment plan should follow recommendations set forth by APS and EULAR. Both EULAR and APS recommend a multidisciplinary approach emphasizing both pharmacological and nonpharmacological treatment modalities. Treatment should be tailored individually based on presenting symptoms and comorbid conditions. Other resources available to the physiatrist include AAPMR Knowledge NOW and Cochrane reviews.

Quality and practice performance improvement should be based on relief of the patient's symptoms. Unfortunately, FM symptoms are multifaceted. Management of patient's symptoms requires a holistic team approach, including physicians, physical and occupational therapists, and a psychologist. Each visit should include an accurate assessment and modification of the treatment plan based on the patient's self-reported pain, sleep, fatigue, and overall well-being. Two well-known validated scales used to assess pain intensity are the Visual Analog Scale (VAS) and Verbal Rating Scale (VRS). Pain location can be documented using body maps or pain diagrams. The Revised Fibromyalgia Impact Questionnaire (FIQ-R) is widely used to assess changes in overall functional ability with treatment (Figure 26.2). Other common assessment tools include the Health Assessment Questionnaire, Arthritis Impact Measurement Scale, the Symptom Interpretation Questionnaire, and The Patient Global Impression of Change (PGIC)Scale (38). These outcome measurement tools should be used to track the effectiveness of the current treatment. If the patient is no longer improving, these assessment tools can identify specific hurdles, and appropriate alterations can be made in the management regimen. Data can be compared with national results and appropriate improvement strategies should be implemented.

INTERPERSONAL AND COMMUNICATION SKILLS

GOALS

Demonstrate interpersonal and communication skills that result in the effective exchange of information and collaboration with FM patients, their families, and the rest of the rehabilitation team.

OBJECTIVES

1. Demonstrate skills used in effective verbal and nonverbal communication, listening skills, and collaboration with FMS patients and their caregivers across socioeconomic and cultural backgrounds.
2. Delineate the importance of the role of the physiatrist as the interdisciplinary team leader and consultant pertinent to FMS.
3. Identify key areas for physicians to counsel patients and families specific to FMS.
4. Demonstrate proper documentation and effective communication between health care professional team members in patient care as it applies to FMS.

When it comes to fibromyalgia, perhaps no other disease entity requires more comprehensive patient communication in combination with best diagnostic practices. The initial and most important step in effective patient communication is an acknowledgment that FMS is real and has a medical explanation. The physician should assure the patient that the condition is not life-threatening, and that while no cure currently exists, treatment strategies are available to lessen pain and improve function.

Physiatrists are well suited to lead a team of clinicians involved in the care of the patient with FMS due to their training on the clinical presentation and treatment of patients with this diagnosis as well as experience in leading multidisciplinary

Domain 1: Functional Domain

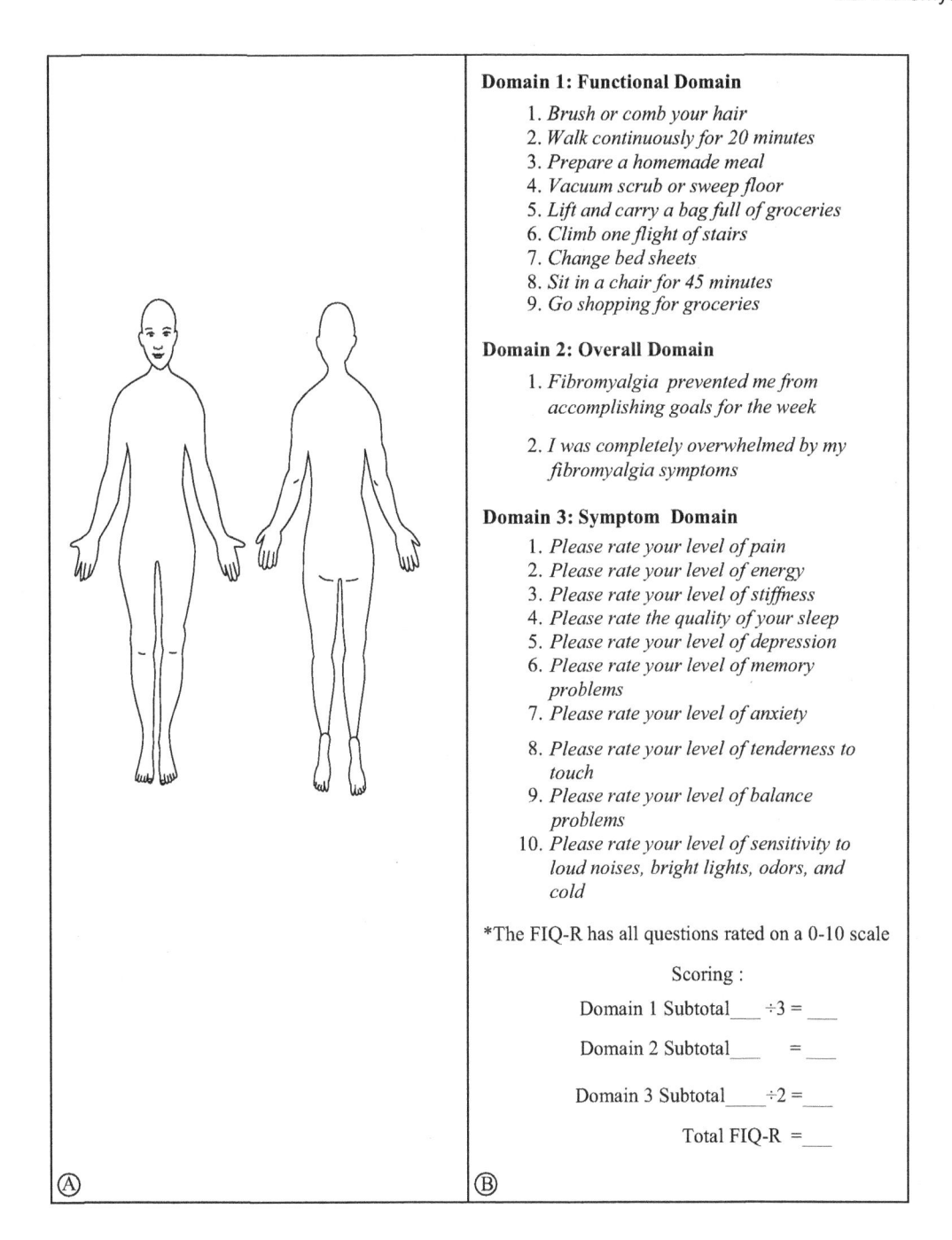

1. *Brush or comb your hair*
2. *Walk continuously for 20 minutes*
3. *Prepare a homemade meal*
4. *Vacuum scrub or sweep floor*
5. *Lift and carry a bag full of groceries*
6. *Climb one flight of stairs*
7. *Change bed sheets*
8. *Sit in a chair for 45 minutes*
9. *Go shopping for groceries*

Domain 2: Overall Domain

1. *Fibromyalgia prevented me from accomplishing goals for the week*
2. *I was completely overwhelmed by my fibromyalgia symptoms*

Domain 3: Symptom Domain

1. *Please rate your level of pain*
2. *Please rate your level of energy*
3. *Please rate your level of stiffness*
4. *Please rate the quality of your sleep*
5. *Please rate your level of depression*
6. *Please rate your level of memory problems*
7. *Please rate your level of anxiety*
8. *Please rate your level of tenderness to touch*
9. *Please rate your level of balance problems*
10. *Please rate your level of sensitivity to loud noises, bright lights, odors, and cold*

*The FIQ-R has all questions rated on a 0-10 scale

Scoring :

Domain 1 Subtotal____ ÷3 = ____

Domain 2 Subtotal____ = ____

Domain 3 Subtotal____ ÷2 = ____

Total FIQ-R = ____

FIGURE 26.2 (A) Pain Diagram and (B) Revised Fibromyalgia Questionnaire

teams. The physiatrist develops a treatment plan for the patient. This plan should establish treatment goals that are (a) specific, (b) realistic, (c) measurable, and (d) have a targeted date of completion. Adhering to this plan establishes a format for follow-up visits where progress and/or impediments can be reviewed and new treatment goals established.

Patient education plays an important role in the management of FM. A study done in 2002 showed that providing a patient with a proper diagnosis of FM significantly increased health satisfaction as well as led to fewer symptoms reported in 3 years post labeling (39). The diagnosis of FM should be made by an experienced doctor using guidelines provided by the ACR.

Once patients are properly diagnosed with FM, they should be thoroughly educated about the disease and its manifestations. A well-educated patient will have better coping techniques and make proper adjustments to his or her treatment regimen based on symptom changes. Education should focus on how FM is diagnosed, signs and symptoms, current understanding of the etiology, and treatment options. Education should also be provided on exercise, diet, sleep hygiene, relaxation techniques, stress management, socialization, pain behaviors, planning for a difficult day, communication styles, and goal setting. Therapists should provide education on energy conservation, techniques for moderation, ergonomics, and a proper home exercise program (40). Multiple studies have shown that physical therapy supplemented with education can significantly improve quality of life and self-efficacy (41,42).

Documentation is an important communication tool between clinicians involved in the care of the patient with FMS. The documentation should provide key elements of the patient's medical history and physical examination that are consistent with the diagnosis of FMS as well as pharmacological and nonpharmacological treatments rendered and their level of effectiveness. Side effects and/or adverse events secondary to medications used to treat FMS should also be clearly documented. The names and contact information of clinicians involved in the care of the patient should be readily available. The physiatrist should also be available to discuss the patient's diagnosis and recommended treatments with therapists providing rehabilitative care.

PROFESSIONALISM

GOALS

Reflect a commitment to carrying out professional responsibilities and an adherence to ethical principles in caring for patients with FM.

OBJECTIVES

1. Exemplify the humanistic qualities as a provider of care for patients with FM.
2. Demonstrate ethical principles and responsiveness to patient needs superseding self and other interests.
3. Demonstrate sensitivity to patient population diversity, including culture, gender, age, race, religion, disabilities, and sexual orientation.
4. Respect patient privacy and autonomy.

Professionalism is a core principle for practitioners in the medical profession. While the principle extends back to the Hippocratic Oath (43), professionalism in the modern day has been formally studied by a number of the major governing bodies. The American College of Physicians, in conjunction with the American Board and the European Federation of Internal Medicine, developed a Physician Charter for Professionalism. This charter holds that professionalism, buttressed by public trust, forms the foundation for medicine's social contract. Within this contract, interests of the patient take primacy over those of the physician, and threshold levels of integrity and competence are requisite to satisfy the standards that should be clearly evident to both the practitioner and society (44).

Patients with FM should be treated with respect and compassion, particularly given that they are often misdiagnosed with rheumatologic conditions or psychiatric disorders prior to the arrival at a diagnosis of FM. Patients suffering from FMS have seen on average four physicians and waited 2.3 years prior to receiving their correct diagnosis. Furthermore, 59% of patients found it difficult to communicate with their physician (45). From the patient's perspective, it is concerning when there are no discrete findings to substantiate his or her complaints. As a physician, arriving at the diagnosis is difficult and often involves excluding other diseases. This is particularly true when the patient presents with many somatic complaints.

Rehabilitative care should be delivered in a manner that is sensitive to the person's cultural, ethnic, and religious beliefs. The treating clinicians should be sensitive to issues such as gender, age, race, religion, and sexual orientation whenever they may arise in the treatment of FMS. In keeping with the bioethical principle of autonomy, the patient's wishes regarding his or her care should be respected.

In the context of treating a patient with FM, it can be difficult for both the patient and the physician to achieve complete satisfaction with management of the complexity of the symptoms and the lack of definitive treatment. Managing this process involves having the patient and the physician build a foundation of confidentiality and trust. Caregivers must take the responsibility to correctly diagnose and manage this patient population and help the patient achieve appropriate expectations.

SYSTEMS-BASED PRACTICE

GOALS

Awareness and responsiveness to systems of care delivery, and the ability to access, evaluate, recruit, and coordinate effectively resources in the system to provide optimal continuum of care and outcomes as it relates to FM.

OBJECTIVES

1. Identify the key components, providers, and systems of care delivery and services in the rehabilitation continuum of care for the patient with FMS.
2. Identify patient safety concerns as they apply to FMS and strategies to minimize their occurrence.
3. Describe cost/risk–benefit analysis, utilization, and management of resources as they apply to FMS.

The management of FMS naturally lends itself to a system-based practice of medicine, where the health care provider sees himself or herself as part of a larger integrated system of patient care (Figure 26.3). In doing so, the risk of care being performed in a vacuum is avoided. A multidisciplinary team approach provides the best pathway toward comprehensive, cost-effective patient care. Members of this team can include a physiatrist, physical therapist, occupational therapist, and rheumatologist depending on the setting where the treatments are rendered.

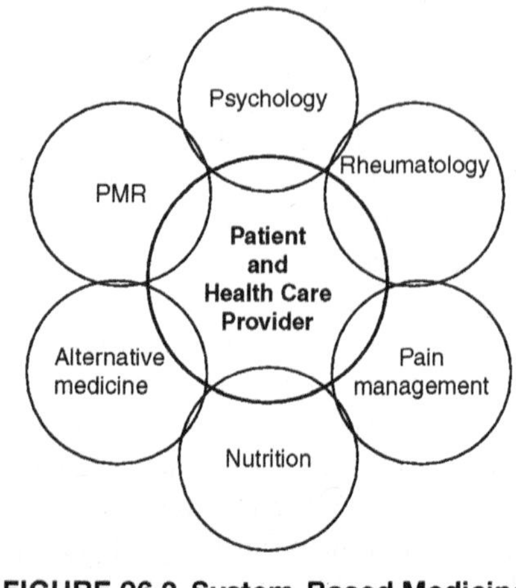

FIGURE 26.3 System-Based Medicine

Minimizing the risk of harm begins with an early accurate diagnosis of FMS in order to reduce the risk of injury associated with unnecessary or invasive diagnostic tests. Once the diagnosis is made, it is important to minimize the risk of side effects or adverse events associated with medications commonly used to treat FMS. Under ideal circumstances, the FMS patient is properly managed by caregivers who are competent and experienced in providing comprehensive care for individuals living with this diagnosis. This implies that the patient is able to function at the highest level possible in activities that are important to him or her with minimal adverse impact from pharmacological and nonpharmacological interventions.

FM has been associated with substantial health care cost; therefore, appropriate cost consideration and risk–benefit analysis are necessary in order to decrease spending. The annual direct costs for FM in the United States were found to be $7,973 per subject. Costs were mostly due to medication and physician visits. The majority of patients with FM in the United States (73%) take two or more prescription medications. This number is higher than that of France (70%) and Germany (56%). In the United States, prescriptions included antidepressants (56%), analgesics other than anti-inflammatories (51%), and antiepileptics (36%). Despite the liberal use of these medications, only 14% of U.S. subjects reported being extremely satisfied with their prescription medications (46). Another area of cost saving includes limiting unnecessary tests and radiology examinations. Given the many presenting symptoms of FM, physicians may be tempted to order multiple laboratory and radiology tests. Providers should exercise prudence in ordering tests and decisions should be based on the current standard of care.

CASE STUDY

A 42-year-old right-handed woman without any significant past medical history presents to clinic with a chief complaint of global body pain for 8 months. There was no inciting event, although patient notes that the onset of symptoms appeared to coincide with the death of her mother. Patient describes pain as achy in character and waxes and wanes over time. Patient also reports occasional numbness in all digits of the hand bilaterally. She denies any cervical or radicular symptoms. Patient describes awaking from sleep unrefreshed in the morning and feeling extremely tired throughout the day. Patient also reports difficulty in concentrating and occasional forgetfulness. She has taken Tylenol and several NSAIDs with little pain relief. Patient is divorced and currently living in a third-floor walk-up apartment. Patient works in a garment factory; however, she was recently laid off due to downsizing and has been unable to find new employment.

Patient has visited several physicians and has had an extensive workup; however, she has not yet received a diagnosis to explain her symptoms. She is frustrated because physicians seem to dismiss her complaints and tell her "it is in her head." The following laboratory work has all come back within normal limits: thyroid function panel, C-reactive protein, erythrocyte sedimentation rate, rheumatoid factor, cyclic citrullinated peptide, antinuclear antibody, liver function tests, and CBC. She also had a normal EMG. She is scheduled for a sleep study in the future. A cervical spine x-ray showed mild to moderate degenerative changes.

On physical examination, the patient appeared to be an obese woman in mild distress. She had full range of motion in all of her extremities and her cervical thoracolumbar spine. She had full strength in all of her extremities, but had some giveaway weakness with resistance. Her sensation was intact to light touch and pinprick and her deep tendon reflexes were 1+ throughout. She was diffusely tender to palpation throughout her upper and lower extremities and entire dorsal spine. She had myalgic pain to digital compression of major muscle groups in the upper and lower extremities.

CASE STUDY DISCUSSION QUESTIONS

MEDICAL KNOWLEDGE: What are the classic features of FM described in this patient? What is "fibrofog"? Does the diffuse pain outside of the classical tender points rule out the diagnosis of FM? What is the relevance of the pending sleep study? What will be the next step in her management?

PATIENT CARE: What are the key psychosocial features that are associated with FM? Is there another specialty that you should consult for the management of this patient? What will be the next step in her management? Formulate a sample therapy prescription for this patient. What facilities, organizations, and support groups are available to assist in the management of this patient?

PRACTICE-BASED LEARNING AND IMPROVEMENT: Describe national organizations or Internet resources that serve as tools for patient education. What are some key tools or surveys that can be used for quality improvement projects for the management of FM? Where can providers find the most up-to-date, evidence-based guidelines for the management of FM?

INTERPERSONAL AND COMMUNICATION SKILLS: What are the key issues the provider must discuss in this initial encounter? What were the possible shortcomings of previous providers that led to increased frustration in this patient?

PROFESSIONALISM: What role does confidentiality and trust play in achieving success in the management of patients with FM? Describe the barriers that providers face in maintaining professionalism when treating patients with FM.

SYSTEM-BASED PRACTICES: Describe an effective comprehensive, cost-effective team-approached treatment plan for this patient.

SELF-EXAMINATION QUESTIONS
(Answers begin on p. 367)

1. What is chronic widespread pain?
   A. Pain for a minimum of 2 months, including all 4 musculoskeletal body regions and the axial skeleton above or below the waistline

B. Pain for a minimum of 3 months, including the four musculoskeletal body regions, excluding the head but including the axial skeleton
C. Pain for a minimum of 6 months, including the four musculoskeletal body regions, excluding the head but including the axial skeleton
D. Pain for a minimum of 3 months in all four quadrants of the body, including the axial skeleton both above and below the waistline
E. Pain for a minimum of 9 months in three musculoskeletal body regions, excluding the head but including the axial skeleton

2. Which of the following exercise regimens has the ACR recommended for the treatment of FM?
    A. Aerobic training with low-intensity exercise
    B. Aerobic training with low- and high-intensity exercise
    C. Limit aerobic training until the symptoms resolve
    D. Limited to only range of motion and stretching
    E. Limited to high-intensity exercises

3. According to the ACR and EULAR recommendation, which of the following approaches optimizes treatment of FMS?
    A. A generic multidisciplinary approach with an emphasis on low-intensity aerobic activity
    B. A multidisciplinary approach emphasizing nonpharmacological treatment modalities
    C. A multidisciplinary approach emphasizing pharmacological treatment modalities
    D. A multidisciplinary approach emphasizing both pharmacological and nonpharmacological treatment modalities
    E. An approach that emphasizes high-intensity exercises and opioid medications

4. When counseling patients with FMS, the initial and most important step in effective patient communication is explaining that FMS is
    A. Real and has a medical explanation
    B. A condition for which no cure exists
    C. Not life-threatening
    D. A condition with temporary symptoms
    E. Not a real disease that requires treatment

5. Persons suffering from FMS have seen an average of ___ physicians and have waited ___ years prior to receiving their correct diagnosis.
    A. Two physicians, 2.5 years
    B. Four physicians, 2.3 years
    C. Five physicians, 4 years
    D. Ten physicians, 5 years
    E. Seven physicians, 5 years

REFERENCES

1. White KP, Harth M. Classification, epidemiology, and natural history of fibromyalgia. *Curr Pain Headache Rep.* 2001;5(4):320–329. doi:10.1007/s11916-001-0021-2.
2. Bennett RM. National Fibromyalgia Association: Science of Fibromyalgia. *National Fibromyalgia Association: Science of Fibromyalgia.* n.p., n.d. Web. March 30, 2013.
3. Wolfe F. The fibromyalgia syndrome: a consensus report on fibromyalgia and disability. *J Rheumatol.* 1996;23:534–539.
4. Wolfe F, Clauw DJ, Fitzcharles M-A, et al. The American College of Rheumatology Preliminary Diagnostic Criteria for Fibromyalgia and Measurement of Symptom Severity. *Arthritis Care Res.* 2010;62.5;600–610.
5. "American College of Rheumatology (ACR) 1990 Diagnostic Criteria for Fibromyalgia Syndrome." *American College of Rheumatology (ACR) 1990 Diagnostic Criteria for Fibromyalgia Syndrome.* n.p., February 26, 2013. Web. March 30, 2013.
6. Harden RN, Revivo G, Song S, et al. A critical analysis of the tender points in fibromyalgia. *Pain Med.* March 2007;8(2):147–156. doi:10.1111/j.1526-4637.2006.00203.x.
7. Winfield JB. Psychological determinants of fibromyalgia and related syndromes. *Curr Rev Pain.* 2000;4:276–286.
8. Yunus MB. Psychological aspects of fibromyalgia syndrome: a component of the dysfunctional spectrum syndrome. *Baillieres Clin Rheumatol.* 1994;8:811–837.
9. Gowans SE, DeHueck A. Pool exercise for individuals with fibromyalgia. *Curr Opin Rheumatol.* 2007;19.2:168–173.
10. Busch AJ, Barber KA, Overend TJ, et al. Exercise for fibromyalgia. *Cochrane Summaries.* n.p., October 8, 2008. Web. April 20, 2013.
11. Häuser W. Efficacy of multicomponent treatment in fibromyalgia syndrome; a meta-analysis of randomized clinical trials. *Arthritis Rheum.* February 15, 2009;61(2):216–224.
12. Peng PW. Tai Chi and chronic pain. *Reg Anesth Pain Med.* July–August, 2012;37(4):372–382.
13. Bernardy K, Füber N, Köllner V, et al. Efficacy of cognitive-behavioral therapies in fibromyalgia syndrome—a systematic review and metaanalysis of randomized controlled trials. *J Rheumatol.* October 2010;37(10):1991–2005.
14. National Institute of Arthritis and Musculoskeletal and Skin Diseases (NIAMS) Information Clearinghouse. Fibromyalgia. *What Is Fibromyalgia.* National Institutes of Health, July 2011. Web. Accessed November 16, 2013.
15. Goldenberg DL, Burckhardt C, Crofford L. Management of fibromyalgia syndrome. *JAMA.* November 17, 2004;292(19):2388–2395.
16. Arnold LM, Hudson JI, Hess EV, Ware AE, Fritz DA, Auchenbach MB, Stark LO, Keck PE Jr. Family study of fibromyalgia. *Arthritis Rheum.* 2004 March; 50 (3):944–952.
17. McNett M, Goldenberg D, Schaefer C, et al. Treatment patterns among physician specialties in the management of fibromyalgia: results of a cross-sectional study in the United States. *Curr Med Res Opin.* March 2011;27(3):673–683.
18. Yunus MB: Central sensitivity syndromes. *JIRA.* 2001;8:27–33.
19. Yunus MB. Central sensitivity syndromes: a new paradigm and group nosology for fibromyalgia and overlapping conditions, and the related issue of disease versus illness. *Semin Arthritis Rheum.* 2008;37:339–352.
20. Desmeules JA, Cedraschi C, Rapiti E, Baumgartner E, Finckh A, Cohen P, Dayer P, Vischer TL. Neurophysiologic evidence for a central sensitization in patients with fibromyalgia. *Arthritis Rheum.* 2003 May; 48 (5):1420–1429.
21. Clauw DJ, Arnold LM, McCarberg BH; FibroCollaborative. The science of fibromyalgia. *Mayo Clin Proc.* September 2011;86(9):907–911.
22. Gracely RH, Petzke F, Wolf JM, et al. Functional magnetic resonance imaging evidence of augmented pain processing in fibromyalgia. *Arthritis Rheum.* May 2002;46(5):1333–1343.

23. Schmidt-Wilcke T, Clauw DJ. Fibromyalgia: from pathophysiology to therapy. *Nat Rev Rheumatol*. July 19, 2011;7(9):518–527.
24. Burckhardt CS, Goldenberg D, Crofford L, et al. *Guideline for the Management of Fibromyalgia Syndrome. Pain in Adults and Children*. APS Clinical Practice Guideline Series No. 4. Glenview, IL: American Pain Society; 2005.
25. Carville SF, Arendt-Nielsen S, Bliddal H, et al. EULAR evidence-based recommendations for the management of fibromyalgia syndrome. *Ann Rheum Dis*. 2008;67:536–541.
26. Mease PJ, Dundon K, Sarzi-Puttini P. Pharmacotherapy of fibromyalgia. *Best Pract Res Clin Rehumatol*. April 2011;25(2):285–297.
27. Arnold LM, Rosen A, Pritchett YL, et al. A randomized, double-blind, placebo-controlled trial of duloxetine in the treatment of women with fibromyalgia with or without major depressive disorder. *Pain*. December 15, 2005;119(1–3):5–15.
28. Russell IJ, Mease PJ, Smith TR, et al. Efficacy and safety of duloxetine for treatment of fibromyalgia in patients with or without major depressive disorder: results from a 6-month, randomized, double-blind, placebo-controlled, fixed-dose trial. *Pain*. June 2008;136(3):432–444.
29. Mease PJ, Clauw DJ, Gendreau RM, et al. The efficacy and safety of milnacipran for treatment of fibromyalgia. A randomized, double-blind, placebo-controlled trial. *J Rheumatol*. February 2009;36(2):398–409.
30. Clauw DJ, Mease P, Palmer RH, et al. Milnacipran for the treatment of fibromyalgia in adults: a 15-week, multicenter, randomized, double-blind, placebo-controlled, multiple-dose clinical trial. *Clin Ther*. November 2008;30(911):1988–2004.
31. Mease PJ, Dundon K, Sarzi-Puttini P. Pharmacotherapy of fibromyalgia. *Best Pract Res Clin Rehumatol*. April 2011;25(2):285–297.
32. Crofford LJ, Rowbotham MC, Mease PJ, et al. Pregabalin for the treatment of fibromyalgia syndrome: results of a randomized, double-blind, placebo-controlled trial. *Arthritis Rheum*. April 2005;52(4):1264–1273.
33. Bennett RM, Kamin M, Karim R, et al. Tramadol and acetaminophen combination tablets in the treatment of fibromyalgia pain: a double-blind, randomized, placebo-controlled study. *Am J Med*. May 2003;114(7):537–545.
34. Busch AJ, Schachter CL, Overend TJ, et al. Exercise for fibromyalgia: a systematic review. *J Rheumatol*. June 2008;35(6):1130–1144.
35. Häuser W, Klose P, Langhorst J, et al. Efficacy of different types of aerobic exercise in fibromyalgia syndrome: a systematic review and meta-analysis of randomized controlled trials. *Arthritis Res Ther*. 2010;12(3):R79.
36. Jones KD, Liptan GL. Exercise interventions in fibromyalgia: clinical applications from the evidence. *Rheum Dis Clin N Am*. 2009;35:373–391.
37. Brosseau L, Wells GA, Tugwell P, et al. Ottawa Panel evidence-based clinical practice guidelines for aerobic fitness exercises in the management of fibromyalgia: part 1. *Phys Ther*. July 2008;68(7):857–871.
38. Perrot S, Dickenson AH, Bennet RM. Fibromyalgia: harmonizing science with clinical practice considerations. *Pain Pract*. May–June 2008;8(3):177–189.
39. White KP, Nielson WR, Harth M, et al. Does the label "fibromyalgia" alter health status, function, and health service utilization? *Arthritis Rheum*. 2002;47:260–265.
40. Pfeiffer A, Thompson JM, Nelson A, et al. Effects of a 1.5-day multidisciplinary outpatient treatment program for fibromyalgia: a pilot study. *Am J Phys Med Rehabil*. March 2003;82(3):186–191.
41. Burckhardt CS, Mannerkorpi K, Hedenberg L, et al. Randomized, controlled clinical trial of education and physical training for women with fibromyalgia. *J Rheumatol*. 1994;21:714–720.
42. Rooks DS, Gautam S, Romeling M, et al. Group exercise, education, and combination self-management in women with fibromyalgia: a randomized trial. *Arch Intern Med*. November 12, 2007;167(20):2192–2200.
43. Oath of Hippocrates. In: *Harvard Classics*. Vol. 38. Boston, MA: P.F. Collier and Son; 1910.
44. Project of the ABIM Foundation, ACP–ASIM Foundation, and European Federation of Internal Medicine*; Medical Professionalism in the New Millennium: a physician charter. *Ann Intern Med*. February 2002;136(3):243–246.
45. Choy E, Perrot S, Leon T, et al. A survey of the impact of fibromyalgia and the journey to diagnosis. *BMC Health Serv Res*. 2010;10:102.
46. Knight T, Schaefer C, Chandran A, et al. Health-resource use and costs associated with fibromyalgia in France, Germany, and the United States. *Clinicoecon Outcomes Res*. April 23, 2013; 5:171–180.

Samuel P. Thampi
Travis R. von Tobel
Monica Habib

27: Cervical Radiculopathy

PATIENT CARE

GOALS

Evaluate and develop a rehabilitative plan of care for the patient with a cervical radiculopathy that is compassionate, appropriate, and effective.

OBJECTIVES

1. Perform a detailed history and physical examination of the adult with a cervical radiculopathy.
2. Identify the psychosocial and vocational implications of cervical radiculopathy.
3. Identify the key components of a rehabilitation program for the patient with cervical radiculopathy and formulate a sample rehabilitation treatment plan.

Comprehensive assessment of the adult with cervical radiculopathy involves close attention to the following:

- The duration of the pain (years/months/weeks)
- The mode of onset (motor vehicle accident/job-related accident/insidious): In case of a motor vehicle accident, obtain history of specifics of the accident such as date of accident, restraint used if any, driver versus passenger, front-end collision/rear-end collision/side-impact collision
- The location of pain: It is important to note if the pain is located on the right side, left side, or both, as you need to correlate the symptoms with the physical examination signs and radiological findings
- Radiation of pain: Radicular pain is a common presentation in cervical radiculopathy. This is in contrast to axial pain as seen in facet and/or myofascial pain syndrome
- Neurologic symptoms: Evaluate of symptoms of tingling, numbness, weakness or bowel/bladder symptoms
- Quality of pain
- Intensity of pain
- Aggravating factors
- Alleviating factors
- Neck trauma associated with neck pain
- Ask if this is the first time that the pain has occurred or if this is an exacerbation of an ongoing neck pain
- Functional impact of the neck pain on activities such as driving, work, reading, sexual activity
- Diagnostic tests and treatments prior to current visit to physiatrist

In reviewing the past medical history, it is important to ask about unplanned weight loss, fever, chills, and night sweats as malignancies and infections can present with neck pain. It is also important to ask about kidney disease, stomach ulcers, liver disease, and bleeding diathesis as these can be important considerations in planning treatment. For example, epidural injections can cause epidural hematomas in patients with platelet deficiency.

In past surgical history ask about prior spine surgeries, including the level of surgery and type of surgical instrumentation. Spinal fusion can lead to early degeneration in the levels above and below the level of fusion.

In family history, it is important to ask about history of malignancies.

When taking a social, vocational history, it is useful to inquire about the type of work the patient does, if working, and hobbies that have been limited because of the neck pain.

A listing of current drug allergies and medications should be made.

Physical examination consists of inspection, palpation, range of motion assessment, motor strength testing of key muscle groups, sensory examination, and special tests.

On inspection, the physiatrist should evaluate the cervical spine and upper extremities for any abnormal skin markings, scars, masses, alignment and bony deformities, erythema, and atrophy. Superficial and deep palpation should be performed with focus on tenderness of muscles, tendons, and bony structures

TABLE 27.1 Range of Motion Cervical Spine (Measured by Goniometer)

	NORMAL (°)
Flexion	60
Extension	50
Side bending, right	45
Side bending, left	45
Lateral rotation, right	80
Lateral rotation, left	80

of the spine and upper extremities. Active and passive range of motion values for the cervical spine and upper extremities should be recorded and compared against normal values. Table 27.1 provides some normative data for movement of the cervical spine.

Relevant neurological examination consists of (a) sensory examination of the upper and lower extremities in key dermatomes using light touch and pinprick, (b) manual muscle testing of key muscle groups of the upper and lower extremities, and (c) muscle stretch reflexes in both upper and lower extremities (Table 27.2). It is important to check for evidence of upper motor neuron pathology as manifested by brisk reflexes, clonus, Hoffman sign in the upper extremity, and Babinski sign in the lower extremity.

Spurling test is used to assess root compression. The test involves turning the head to the affected side and applying downward pressure. The test is positive if the patient experiences increased pain into the shoulder and into the hand in a radicular pattern. The sensitivity of the Spurling test to nerve root pathology on CT scan was 95% and specificity was 94% (1). One has to observe for facet joint line tenderness and myofascial trigger points.

IMPAIRMENTS, ACTIVITY LIMITATIONS, AND PARTICIPATION RESTRICTIONS ASSOCIATED WITH CERVICAL RADICULOPATHY

Impairments associated with cervical radiculopathy include decreased range of motion of the neck, weakness, and decreased sensation in the neck and upper extremities. These impairments

TABLE 27.2 Neurologic Deficits in Radiculopathies

LEVEL	SENSORY LOSS	MUSCLE WEAKNESS	REFLEX CHANGE
C5	Outer arm	Shoulder abduction	Biceps
C6	Thumb	Wrist extension	Brachioradialis
C7	Middle finger	Wrist flexion	Triceps
C8	Little finger	Finger flexion	
T1	Inner arm	Interossei	

can limit activities such as driving, overhead movements, and lifting, which can in turn restrict ability to work and engage in avocational activities. Neck pain at night can impair sleep, leading to daytime drowsiness.

Psychosocial implications due to cervical radiculopathy can include anxiety and depression due to the limitations in social activities and hobbies with friends and family. Work restrictions can lead to loss of/decreased productivity, reduction in wages, and even potential loss of employment. Prescription drug overdose and prescription drug diversion can also be potential problems.

TREATMENT PLAN FOR THE PATIENT WITH NECK PAIN

The treatment plan for neck pain is developed once an accurate diagnosis has been made. The differential diagnosis of neck pain is quite broad; however, some examples include the following: (a) myofascial pain syndrome, (b) cervical radiculopathy, (c) facet joint pathology, (d) cervical spinal stenosis, (e) cancer (primary vs. metastatic disease), (f) infectious, and (h) systemic (e.g., rheumatoid arthritis). Diagnosis is based on a combination of factors that include the history and physical examination as well as appropriate imaging and electrodiagnostic studies as needed. It is not uncommon to have one or more concurrent diagnoses such as cervical radiculopathy, myofascial pain, and degenerative disease of the spine.

The treatment plan for nociceptive and/or neuropathic pain originating in the neck that is noninfectious or nonmalignant in nature often includes a combination of interventions such as (a) medications (e.g., steroids, nonsteroidal anti-inflammatory drugs, muscle relaxants, antiepileptics, opioids), (b) injections (e.g., trigger point injections, spinal injections—epidural, transforaminal, medial branch blocks), (c) physical therapy, (d) chiropractic care, and (e) acupuncture.

MEDICAL KNOWLEDGE

GOALS

Demonstrate knowledge of established and evolving biomedical, clinical, and epidemiological sciences pertaining to cervical radiculopathy, as well as the application of this knowledge to guide holistic patient care.

OBJECTIVES

1. Describe the anatomy, physiology, and pathophysiology of cervical radiculopathy.
2. Identify the pertinent laboratory and diagnostic studies important in the evaluation of cervical radiculopathy.
3. Review the treatment of cervical radiculopathy.

Cervical radiculopathy is a disorder in which conduction along the nerve root is blocked, resulting in objective neurologic signs such as numbness or weakness, and/or a condition in which the blood supply to a nerve root is compromised, resulting in paresthesias (2).

Cervical radiculopathy is a very common cause of neck pain in the United States, and is one of the most common reasons for a patient to seek physician care. The most frequently presenting symptom is pain, although not all patients with cervical radiculopathy will have pain, especially in medial disc protrusion (3). There are many potential pain generators in the cervical spine. They include the intervertebral disc, the facet joint, the atlanto-occipital joint, the ligaments of the muscles, and the bone of the cervical spine region. The intracanalicular structures include the meninges, blood vessels, and the neural tissue of the spinal cord. There are 7 cervical vertebrae and 8 cervical nerve roots. The intervertebral discs are located between the vertebral bodies of C2 to C7. Each intervertebral disc is composed of an outer annulus fibrosis and an inner gelatinous nucleus pulposus, providing transmission of axial loads to dissipate forces throughout various ranges of motion. Apart from the nerve roots, structures such as the intervertebral discs, zygapophyseal joint, posterior longitudinal ligament, and the muscles can also serve as pain generators and produce somatic referral of pain into the upper limb. Biomechanical and/or biochemical insults to nonneural structures can trigger nociceptive nerve fibers via stretching, compression, or inflammation, causing pain referral. Mechanical stimulation of the cervical zygapophyseal joints or their innervating nerves is well documented in studies to produce head and neck pain with upper limb referral patterns.

After a thorough history and physical is obtained, imaging studies should be performed to diagnose the etiology of the cervical radiculopathy. Imaging should begin with basic anteroposterior (AP) and lateral x-rays to evaluate vertebral body alignment and disc space height, evaluate facet joints for arthritis, and exclude bony lesions (lytic and blastic), and then progress to a CT or MRI if appropriate diagnosis is still unclear.

Plain radiographs have limited value in diagnosing etiology of cervical radiculopathy, as these studies focus primarily on the bony structures. Thus, MRI remains the gold standard in imaging for cervical radiculopathy, as it can accurately visualize all soft-tissue structures within the cervical spine.

The author follows a simple "ABC" approach to reviewing an MRI of the cervical spine looking for

A = Alignment: Evaluate for spondylolisthesis.
B = Bone: Evaluate for bony infiltrates due to metastasis, infections, or fractures.
C = Canal/Cord: Evaluate for central canal stenosis and spinal cord myelomalacia.

Then at each level, look for disc pathology, epidural lesions, facet hypertrophy, and foraminal stenosis.

Electrodiagnosis has a role in evaluating radiculopathy. It can help localize a nerve injury (e.g., cervical root), determine its severity, determine if it is acute or chronic, and provide some information regarding prognosis for recovery. Laboratory studies such as uric acid or rheumatoid factor, erythrocyte sedimentation rate (ESR), and C-reactive protein can evaluate for inflammatory arthropathy.

Once the diagnosis is made, various treatment options can be considered. Initial care should focus on controlling pain and inflammation to curb the injury response and ensure participation in a functional restoration program. Nonsteroidal anti-inflammatory drugs (NSAIDs) should be initiated early to reduce the inflammatory response and the release of thromboxane and prostaglandins. Muscle relaxants, antineuropathic agents, and antidepressants can be used as adjuvants for pain control. Opiates can be used as a modality; however, they carry the risk of opiate-induced morbidity and mortality. Initially, the patient should be advised to avoid any actions that aggravate the symptoms. Physical therapy should be initiated soon after the pain symptoms begin to diminish and should include modalities such as massage, superficial and deep heat, and electrical stimulation. Use of a soft cervical collar remains controversial and may be beneficial for short periods of time, but may cause atrophy-related immobilization if used excessively. Transcutaneous electrical nerve stimulation (TENS) may also be used to modulate musculoskeletal pain. Once the acute pain symptoms have resolved, proper spinal biomechanics should be emphasized, and therapy should focus on proper movement patterns. Proprioceptive training, balance, and postural conditioning should be incorporated into the patient's therapy regimen. Once the patient is entirely pain free and able to perform a full cervical range of motion, then dynamic exercises can be initiated.

Unfortunately, a subset of patients with cervical radiculopathy will not improve with general physical therapy and modalities, and interventional spine techniques will need to be considered. Cervical steroid injections can be considered in the treatment of radicular pain. Cervical epidural steroid injections (i.e., interlaminar and transforaminal epidurals) can be performed under radiographic guidance. Transforaminal epidural steroid injections can be utilized to both diagnose and treat the radiculopathy. Cervical transforaminal epidural steroid injections carry a high risk for spinal cord and brain infarction. Particulate steroid can act as an embolus. Inadvertent intravascular injection of the blood vessels in the vicinity of the transforaminal can compromise the blood supply to the spinal cord and the brain. Approximately one-third of patients with cervical radiculopathy who are treated nonoperatively have persistent symptoms, and should be referred to a surgical spine specialist for consideration of surgical intervention (4).

PRACTICE-BASED LEARNING AND IMPROVEMENT

GOALS

Demonstrate competence in continuously investigating and evaluating patient care practices for cervical radiculopathy, appraising and assimilating scientific evidence, and continuously improving patient care practices based on constant self-evaluation and lifelong learning.

OBJECTIVES

1. Describe key components of self-assessment and lifelong learning for the physiatrist with respect to continuing professional development as related to cervical radiculopathy.
2. Describe the importance of clinical reflection in the professional growth of the physiatrist taking care of a patient with cervical radiculopathy.
3. Identify resources, including websites and professional organizations, for clinical guidelines, evidence-based practice,

and continuing medical education and professional development as it pertains to cervical radiculopathy.
4. Describe the key elements of effective patient education methodology as it applies to the care of the patient with cervical radiculopathy, as well as educating families, residents, and the interdisciplinary team.

The experienced physiatrist should have a myriad of tools at his or her disposal to improve decision making in clinical practice in making a particular diagnosis, establishing a prognosis, or matching patients to optimal interventions based on a frugal subset of predictor variables from the history and physical examination.

First and foremost, a physiatrist should evaluate his or her own knowledge on the diagnosis of cervical radiculopathy. The field of pain medicine has grown and advanced greatly in the past 10 years, and it is of importance that every physiatrist should sharpen his or her diagnostic and therapeutic skills on a periodic basis. For instance, practitioners should have good history and physical examination techniques to determine the location and the etiology of cervical radiculopathy. After a proper history and physical are obtained, imaging should be obtained to further narrow the differential diagnoses made during the history and physical examination. Once a diagnosis is defined, the practitioner should plan the appropriate treatment.

The physiatrist who follows patients should analyze improved pain scores, improved functionality, and requirement for pain medications with each visit. Interventional procedures can reduce the need for opiates. In addition, one should utilize the practice of 360° multisource analysis, in which patients, family members, therapists, nurses, and ancillary staff are instructed to provide feedback to the physiatrist and comment on communication and interpersonal skills, diagnosis, and therapeutic modalities. There are many resources currently available from which a physiatrist can obtain information and training to address his or her deficits and sharpen his or her skills. There are many Accreditation Council of Graduate Medical Education (ACGME)-accredited fellowship programs as well as non-ACGME accredited programs which a physiatrist might want to consider. Knowledge NOW is a novel comprehensive online source for physiatrists organized by clinical topics (5). Knowledge NOW is still being developed and will be a resource for physiatrists who wish to sharpen their knowledge base in an abbreviated manner. Physiatric Association for Spine, Sports, and Occupational Rehabilitation (PASSOR) has published guidelines for interventional procedures. Cochrane review is another source in which systematic reviews and meta-analyses examine treatments for a variety of neuromusculoskeletal disorders (6). Full-text and abbreviated articles are available for review in multiple languages and among multiple different disciplines.

Other arenas that may provide innovative information on cervical radiculopathy are literature reviews, white paper publications from organizations, and PubMed reviews. The International Spine Intervention Society (ISIS) is a multifaceted organization that is committed to "the development, evaluation, validation, education, and advocacy of percutaneous techniques used in the diagnosis and treatment of spine disorders" (7).

Additionally, the physiatrists must sharpen not only their intellectual skills, but also their communication skills with patients, their families, and other professional colleagues. Effective communication is of the utmost importance. A holistic approach is often required to treat the many different causes of cervical radiculopathy, which may include medications, procedures, and a specialized rehabilitation program. Each of these techniques should be discussed with the patient and his or her family, including the potential risks, benefits, and limitations of these treatment modalities. Furthermore, if possible, a timeline should be given to the patient, as most types of cervical radiculopathy take weeks or even months to improve, and the patient may not understand the chronicity of the disease process.

According to the National Network of Libraries of Medicine (NNLM), health literacy is defined as "the degree to which individuals have the capacity to obtain, process, and understand basic health information and services needed to make appropriate health decisions." It is important to acknowledge that more than half of the patients read at less than a sixth-grade level. Thus, it is vital that physiatrists use a variety of techniques in communicating with patients. Some techniques advertised by the NNLM are allowing patients to take an active role in health-related decisions and develop strong health information skills, utilizing the need for written and printed information using simple nonmedical language, and the technique referred to as "teach-back" in which patients are asked to reiterate the information just given to them in their own terms, allowing them to ask questions and clarify difficult terminology.

The National Patient Safety Foundation is currently utilizing a novel technique being used by health care professionals across the United States, called "Ask Me-3" (8). This technique encourages patients to seek answers to three major questions: What is my main problem? What do I need to do? Why is it important for me to do this? If this technique is utilized properly, studies have shown that patients tend to make fewer mistakes, compliance is increased, and patients are better able to manage chronic health conditions, thus ensuring an improved quality of life.

Many other resources exist that discuss quality of care issues and training in quality improvement methodology. One such course is the Institute for Healthcare Improvement (IHI). This organization serves to provide professional development programs, such as conferences, seminars, and audio- and web-based programs, that seek to raise the quality of health and health care for all (9).

INTERPERSONAL AND COMMUNICATION SKILLS

GOALS

Demonstrate interpersonal and communication skills that result in the effective exchange of information and collaboration with patients with cervical radiculopathy, their families, and other health professionals.

OBJECTIVES

1. Demonstrate skills used in effective communication and collaboration with patients with cervical radiculopathy and their caregivers, across socioeconomic and cultural backgrounds.
2. Demonstrate proper documentation and effective communication between health care professional team members in patient care as it applies to cervical radiculopathy.

Effective communication in medicine is a team effort made up of two parts: the patient and his or her expectations and beliefs, and the medical provider with his or her clinical expertise and experience. Maintaining effective medical records is a documentation of this communication. The goal is to unite the team, getting all the parts working together for the common good of the patient while not violating the patient's culture, beliefs, and wishes. The informed patient should be allowed to have control of his or her care, complying with patient-centered care, by providing all the information to make an informed decision.

According to Bartlett et al., compliance may be hindered by physician failure. It was found that quality of interpersonal skills influenced patient outcomes more than quantity of teaching and instruction. Secondary analyses found that all the effects of physician communication skills on patient adherence are mediated by patient satisfaction and recall. These findings indicate that the physician might pay particular attention to these 2 variables in trying to improve patient adherence, and that enhancing patient satisfaction may be pivotal to the care of patients with chronic illness (10).

Physicians sometimes fail to communicate effectively to their patients. Patient adherence is mediated by patient satisfaction and recall. The physician has to take the time to sit and speak with the patient, explain the medical issues, and ensure the patient comprehends the information. The patient must then repeat the plan, and show an understanding of the treatment and rationale for care. If on each and every encounter the physician does not use this methodology, patient adherence is hindered. Interpersonal skills of physicians are crucial to patient satisfaction and compliance, more than the quantity of teaching (10). Empowering the patient enhances patient satisfaction, thus improving the quality of care.

Effective communication among the interventional pain specialist, the patient, family members, and professional colleagues is one of the cornerstones of good patient care and is essential for quality care and patient satisfaction (10). The key components of effective communication and conflict resolution are (a) relationship building: (b) the ability to listen, reflect, redirect, and validate; (c) shared understanding and common ground; (d) framing and reframing the issues; (e) collaborative brainstorming and shared decision making; and (f) aligned expectations.

Relationship building with the patient is an important way to establish trust and good rapport. It is important to get to know the patient and find out what is truly meaningful and important to him or her; it is also useful to determine the patient's values, preferred style of communication, role in the family and community, job, hobbies, and interests. It is equally important to recognize the emotional impact of the cervical neck pain and review and summarize, often using the patient's own words, to describe his or her challenges. The physician must be the leader but should demonstrate leading through suggestion.

To be an effective communicator requires active listening skills on the part of the interventional pain specialist. Ask open-ended questions initially, followed by more focused questions. Reflect back what the patient says, using his or her own words whenever possible. If the patient goes off on a tangent, redirect him or her.

A shared understanding of the issues involved in the care of cervical neck pain requires an understanding of the problem from several different perspectives: the interventional pain specialist, the primary care provider, the patient, the family, at times the institution or setting where the patient is receiving rehabilitative care, and the communication through use of electronic medical records (EMRs). Once these have been defined, a shared understanding of the problem that combines the perspectives of all the stakeholders can be developed. Based on this shared understanding, the issues can be framed in a mutually acceptable way and common ground achieved. Better communication between all the parties involved leads to improved patient outcomes (11,12). A helpful perspective is to have the interventional pain specialist and the patient working on the same side against the challenges faced by the patient.

In our current era with EMR, are we making positive gains in communication? Patients' and clinicians' level of satisfaction with interpersonal communication has declined (13,14). According to O'Malley et al., commercial EMRs both help and hinder physician interpersonal communication—real-time, face-to-face, or phone conversations—with patients and other clinicians, based on in-depth interviews with clinicians in 26 physician practices. EMRs assist real-time communication with patients during office visits, primarily through immediate access to patient information, allowing clinicians to talk with patients rather than search for information from paper records. For some clinicians, however, aspects of EMRs pose a distraction during visits. Moreover, some indicated they rely on EMRs for information gathering and transfer at the expense of real-time communication with patients and other clinicians. Given time pressures already present in many physician practices, EMRs and office workflow modifications could help ensure that EMRs advance care without compromising interpersonal communication. In particular, policies promoting EMR adoption should consider incorporating communication skills training for medical trainees and clinicians using EMRs (15).

EMRs and the implementation pushed by the federal government is a work in progress. The benefits of EMRs are clear, legible, and transportable documentation, but errors are most apparent during times of transition and implementation. Immediate access to EMR data enables the physician to focus on the patient rather than gathering information from a variety of paper sources. But the physician may be distracted by the technology and presume that he or she has so much more information about the patient that communication is reduced with the patient and colleagues. As a result, a physician sitting in front of a computer screen may fail to make proper eye contact with the patient or fail to double check the EMR reports with the patient, a practice that was widely conducted with paper records. During this transition to EMRs, physicians should take the time to review each patient's problem list and medication list with the patient to fill the gaps that are plausible with EMRs (15).

Once a shared understanding has been developed, shared goals can be developed that are based on the goals of the interventional pain specialist, patient, family, and often the interdisciplinary team caring for the patient. Based on these shared goals, collective brainstorming occurs in which all the treatment options and potential consequences of options are discussed and the patient is assisted in his or her risk–benefit analysis and decision making, giving the patient the control.

In providing feedback, the clinician should use objective markers of success that are mutually agreed upon with the patient, use positive statements as often as possible, and emphasize the positive things that the patient is doing in his or her care plan. The progress and issues should be presented in a nonjudgmental and nonemotional way. The clinician should check for understanding. In giving negative feedback, it is important to be tough on the behavior and easy on the person. Ask for reasons why the behavior is occurring (the why, how, what, who, when of the problem) and focus on key discrepancies. Describe the expected behavior and the discrepancy. It can be very helpful to enlist support from family members whenever possible.

When communicating with the patient, the clinician should speak at a moderate pace, varying the tone of speech, and pausing effectively for emphasis or when making a point. It is also important to draw the patient into conversation and take frequent turns while speaking and avoiding dual monologues.

Nonverbal communication is equally important. The clinician should (a) maintain good eye contact; (b) sit at eye level with the patient; (c) remove barriers between the physiatrist and patient (i.e., computer, furniture, telephone, cellular phones); (d) keep an open posture; (e) face the patient; (f) sit next to the patient, rather than across from him or her; and (g) resist folding arms across the chest or crossing legs.

A good medical record is an essential tool of communication between clinicians caring for cervical neck pain, but EMRs are even better. The documentation should be provided on a timely basis and reflect the patient's medical, rehabilitative, psychosocial, and emotional barriers, as well as treatment plan to address the barriers. In an age of EMRs, it is essential that the physiatrist refrain from the "cut, copy, paste" of medical record material from one note to another.

PROFESSIONALISM

GOALS

Reflect a commitment to carrying out professional responsibilities and an adherence to ethical principles in caring for patients with cervical radiculopathy.

OBJECTIVE

1. Demonstrate importance of integrity, respect, compassion, ethics, and courtesy in the care of patients with cervical radiculopathy.
2. Exhibit the importance of patient-centered care, informed consent, and maintaining patient confidentiality in cervical radiculopathy.
3. Discuss the importance of patient's beliefs and goals, privacy, and autonomy as it applies to cervical radiculopathy.
4. Demonstrate sensitivity to culture, diversity, gender, age, race, religion, disabilities, and sexual orientation as it may apply to cervical radiculopathy.
5. Describe responsibility and accountability of physiatry as it applies to cervical radiculopathy.
6. Discuss the role of the physiatrist as an advocate for the patient with cervical radiculopathy.

Chronic cervical neck pain is debilitating for an individual. It can have a profound impact on the person's ability to work, drive, care for himself or herself (and other family members), and engage in activities that were once meaningful. It is very important to show respect, compassion, and empathy for the patient and to provide the best possible care in an honest and respectful manner.

According to Murinson et al., the overarching goal of medical training is to nurture the growth of knowledgeable, caring, and insightful clinicians guided by the ideals of medical professionalism. Recent definitions of professional competence identify essential clinical skills, including cognitive expertise, emotional competence, and reflective capacity. This modern framework reflects the increasingly complex nature of the patient–clinician interaction, in which the clinician must exchange diagnostic information while supportively engaging the patient on a deeper, affective level. The affective dimension can be particularly potent when pain is the primary symptom, as it is for the majority of medical visits. Unfortunately, however, current models of professionalism, used as an early guide for medical trainees to develop an understanding of the clinical exchange, largely focus on interactions in the cognitive domain. To emphasize the importance of emotions in professional development, we propose the Cognitive and Emotional Preparedness Model, which describes the clinical encounter occurring on 2 channels, one cognitive and the other emotional, and stresses the importance of multidimensional development in preparing the clinician to (a) communicate clinical information, (b) provide emotional support, and (c) actively reflect on experiences for continued improvement. Together, acquisition of knowledge, emotional development, and reflective skill will improve the clinical interaction. We know that the proficiency of medical trainees in developing clinical skills profoundly shapes patient satisfaction and treatment outcomes. This article reviews the cognitive, emotional, and reflective development of medical trainees and presents a model illustrating how clinical development impacts pain care. For improved efficacy, pain education should be calibrated to students' developmental needs (11).

It is important that all attempts be made to have the patient and his or her needs at the center of the care plan of the interdisciplinary team. Systems and processes should support this fundamental tenet of patient care. The interventional pain specialist and interdisciplinary team members should work together with the patient in a collaborative manner in making clinical care decisions that are consistent with the patient's wishes and values. An example of shared decision making can come in determining the treatment for the patient. The physiatrist has the clinical expertise to guide the patient in the most appropriate treatment, but the fears of a patient can hinder the process. Together, they share in the decision-making process.

The patient's age and cultural beliefs can also have an impact on the care of the cervical neck pain. For example, an individual's phobia of needles can severely hinder the interventional pain specialist's ability to alleviate pain. The physiatrist's role is to educate the patient, directly address the patient's phobia, and delve into his or her fears and concerns about needles. By taking the time to communicate effectively, the root and source of the fear can be alleviated, while developing trust in the doctor–patient relationship. In the end, a strong relationship can help the patient overcome a phobia of needles and alleviate the cervical neck pain.

Ethical issues can come up in the care of cervical neck pain. There are times when a patient's health care insurance denies the procedure based on peer reviews of clinical documents. In all these instances it is important to define and understand the ethical issues in question and review existing laws, policies, and guidelines for guidance. The physiatrist sometimes has to take a stand against denials for treatment by referring to the guidelines through an appeal process.

SYSTEM-BASED PRACTICE

GOALS

Awareness and responsiveness to systems of care delivery, and the ability to recruit and coordinate effectively resources in the system to provide optimal care as it relates to cervical radiculopathy.

OBJECTIVES

1. Describe key components and available services in the rehabilitation continuum of care and community rehabilitation facilities as it applies to cervical radiculopathy.
2. Discuss how to work effectively in various systems of care as it applies to cervical radiculopathy.
3. Discuss patient safety, cost-effectiveness, utilization, and management of resources as it applies to cervical radiculopathy.
4. Participate in identifying and avoiding potential systems- and medical-related errors for cervical radiculopathy and strategies to minimize them.

Physiatrists are often asked to evaluate and provide treatment for cervical radiculopathy in a variety of settings. These include (a) medical/surgical unit of an acute care medical center, (b) acute inpatient rehabilitation facility, (c) subacute rehabilitation unit in a skilled nursing facility, (d) visiting therapy services in a patient's home, and (e) outpatient pain management centers.

In a medical/surgical unit of an acute medical center, a patient with acute cervical radiculopathy typically receives physical and occupational therapy at the bedside or in the facility's rehabilitation gym. Pain management and physiatrist consultations services should be available. If the patient's symptoms are severe and have failed to respond to conservative treatment, cervical epidural steroid injection can be performed as an inpatient procedure. The decision on which of these options is selected is often dependent on the patient's medical stability and comorbidities, the patient's current level of function, and the number of hours per day that the patient can participate in a rehabilitation program. Additional factors include the level of support at home and the patient's health care insurance program.

Cost considerations and risk–benefit analysis are an important part of the decision-making process in the care of cervical neck pain. This is especially evident in the selection of procedures as insurance carriers can deny procedures.

The interdisciplinary team that is involved in the care of cervical neck pain typically includes an interventional pain specialist, a physiatrist, a physical therapist, an occupational therapist, a chiropractor, a massage therapist, an acupuncturist, a rehabilitation nurse, a social worker, and a psychologist. This team is usually seen in rehabilitation wards/hospitals, skilled nursing facilities, outpatient offices, and in interventional pain specialist offices. An interventional pain specialist generally meets a patient on a monthly basis to discuss the patient's progress and management of pain. Based on the patient's feedback, appropriate services are identified, and a treatment plan is developed and carried out within an agreed-upon time frame.

The patient with cervical neck pain encounters several potential safety risks during treatment, across the continuum of care described above. These include but are not limited to (a) adverse effects and side effects associated with medications commonly prescribed for cervical radiculopathy, and (b) direct nerve injury secondary to cervical epidural steroid procedure.

Interpreting and understanding evidence synthesis, systematic reviews, and other analytic literature is an arduous task. As a pain physician, it is crucial to understand the goals, principles, and processes of evidence-based medicine to meaningfully improve its applications. This knowledge not only affords better insight into the analytic reviews in interventional pain management, but also ultimately allows future information to be selected, evaluated, and used with prudence in a technically competent, ethically sound interventional pain management practice in order to better care for the individual.

Good communication among rehabilitation team members, the patient, and family is an essential factor in minimizing these risks. This communication is especially important at transition points as the patient moves through the continuum of care. At these points, clinicians should review medications, educate the patient and the professional to whom transfer of care is relegated about the risk of each medication prescribed, and provide strategies to minimize them.

CASE STUDY

A 40-year-old woman presents with neck pain radiating to the right upper extremity following a motor vehicle accident.

CASE STUDY DISCUSSION QUESTIONS

1. What are the questions you would ask the patient during her assessment?
2. Discuss a plan for conservative treatment.
3. Discuss a plan for interventional treatment after failed conservative treatment.
4. Discuss the resources available for updates in cervical radiculopathy.
5. How would you communicate treatment options with the patient?

SELF-EXAMINATION QUESTIONS
(Answers begin on p. 367)

1. A patient presents with neck pain and upon examination is found to have a positive Hoffman sign. Which of the following is the most likely diagnosis?
   A. Peripheral neuropathy
   B. Cervical radiculopathy
   C. Cervical myelopathy
   D. Brachial plexopathy
   E. Cervical dystonia

2. You examine a 32-year-old man with cervical radiculopathy. You find that he has weakness of the wrist extension. Which of the following is the most likely explanation for this finding?
   A. C4 root involvement
   B. C5 root involvement
   C. C6 root involvement
   D. C7 root involvement
   E. C8 root involvement

3. A patient whom you examine presents with C5 root involvement. You would expect sensory loss in which of the following areas?
   A. Shoulder region
   B. Thumb
   C. Little finger
   D. Middle finger
   E. Inner arm

4. A 50-year-old woman sees you with a diagnosis of cervical radiculopathy. Upon physical examination she has a diminished brachioradialis reflex. This finding suggests that the most likely root involved is
   A. C4 root
   B. C5 root
   C. C6 root
   D. C7 root
   E. C8 root

5. Which of the following interventional procedures carries the highest risk of cerebrovascular accident (CVA)?
   A. Interlaminar epidural steroid injection
   B. Transforaminal epidural steroid injection
   C. Facet blocks
   D. Medical branch blocks
   E. Trigger point injections

REFERENCES

1. Shabat S, Leitner Y, David R, Folman Y. The correlation between Spurling test and imaging studies in detecting cervical radiculopathy. *J Neuroimag.* October 2012;22(4):375–378.
2. Merskey H, Bogduk N. *Classification of Chronic Pain. Description of Chronic Pain Syndromes and Definition of Pain Terms.* IASP Press; 1994.
3. Bogduk N. *Medical Management of Acute Cervical Radicular Pain Evidence Based Approach.* New Castle Bone and Joint Institute, Cambridge Press; 1999.
4. Eubanks JD. Cervical radiculopathy: nonoperative management of neck pain and radicular symptoms. *Am Fam Physician.* January 1, 2010;81(1):33–40.
5. The AAPM&R Knowledge Now website. http://www.aapmr.org/education/knowledge-now/Pages/default.aspx.
6. The Cochrane Collaboration website. http://www.cochrane.org/cochrane-reviews.
7. The International Spine Intervention Society website. http://www.spinalinjection.org/.
8. The National Patient Safety Education website. http://www.npsf.org/for-healthcare-professionals/programs/ask-me-3/.
9. The Institute for Healthcare Improvement website. http://www.ihi.org/about/pages/default.aspx.
10. Bartlett EE, Grayson M, Barker R, et al. The effects of physician communications skills on patient satisfaction; recall, and adherence. *J Chronic Dis.* 1984;37(9–10):755–764.
11. Murinson BB, Agarwal AK, Haythornthwaite JA. Cognitive expertise, emotional development, and reflective capacity: clinical skills for improved pain care. *J Pain.* November 2008;9(11):975–983.
12. Manchikanti L, Boswell MV, Giordano J. Evidence-based interventional pain management: principles, problems, potential and applications. *Pain Physician.* 2007;10:329–356.
13. Stille CJ, Jerant A, Bell D, et al. Coordinating care across diseases, settings and clinicians: a key role for generalist in practice. *Ann Intern Med.* April 19, 2005;142(8):700–708.
14. Montgomery JE, et al. Primary care experiences of Medicare beneficiaries, 1998 to 2000. *J Gen Intern Med.* October 2004;19(10):991–998.
15. O'Malley AS, Cohen GR, Grossman JM. *Electronic Medical Records and Communication With Patients and Other Clinicians: Are We Talking Less?* Center for Studying Health System Change Issues Brief, NO. 131. Washington, DC: Center for Studying Health System Change; April 2010.

Kiran Vadada
Mahmud Ibrahim
Joseph Herrera

28: Sports Medicine: Preparticipation Evaluation

PATIENT CARE

GOALS

Evaluate and develop a plan of care for athletes prior to sports participation and the promotion of health.

OBJECTIVES

1. Describe the purpose of preparticipation evaluations.
2. Outline the responsibilities of the physician prior to deciding on clearance for participation.
3. Identify the key elements of the screening history and physical examinations.
4. Support the rationale for giving clearance to participate in sports.
5. Identify factors specific to athletes with disability.
6. Identify factors specific to female athletes.

The fundamental purpose of the preparticipation evaluation (PPE) is to ensure that a given athlete can safely perform the functions required of a given sport. The evaluation should be detailed and thorough, yet focused and efficient. It is important to differentiate this from the role of a primary care physician performing a routine wellness evaluation. The PPE is intended for diagnosis and management of all medical conditions that are present in the athlete. Its purpose is to identify life-threatening conditions that may preclude participation, as well as conditions that may require appropriate treatment and conditioning prior to participation. Many young athletes have had minimal interactions with physicians prior to this evaluation; therefore, any cause for concern should be referred for further investigation prior to clearance.

The history is usually performed using a questionnaire that is filled out by the athlete in advance for the sake of time efficiency. During the visit it is reviewed, and pertinent positives are explored further. Items of particular concern are history of organ loss, concussion, seizure, syncope, palpitations, dyspnea, paresthesias, and family history of early cardiac events.

KEY ELEMENTS OF HISTORY

Current Condition
- Injuries or illnesses since last checkup
- Active acute or chronic illness
- Recent viral illness—mononucleosis
- Medications, allergies, and supplements
- Adequate caloric intake
- Stress
- Menstrual abnormalities (as applicable)
- Sleep
- Pain
- Paresthesias
- Weakness

Past Medical/Surgical History
- Hospitalizations
- Surgeries
- Loss of consciousness/syncopal episodes (particularly during exercise)
- Cardiac conditions (prompt about pain, palpitations, and murmurs)
- Diabetes
- Seizures
- Heat exhaustion/stroke
- Asthma (prompt for exercise-induced symptoms)
- Vision problems (ask about glasses/contacts)
- Musculoskeletal injuries
- Prior restriction from sports

Family History
- Cardiac disease (myocardial infarction [MI] before age 50, sudden death)

Social History
- Alcohol/tobacco/substance abuse
- Family support
- Behavioral problems

The physical examination pays more attention to functional capacity than subtle examination findings. While it is acceptable to describe routine findings as "normal" without further elaboration, gross abnormalities must be described in detail.

KEY ELEMENTS OF PHYSICAL EXAMINATION

Vitals:	Blood pressure, pulse, height, weight
General:	Body habitus, posturing
Skin:	Rashes or lesions
Head:	Pupillary reflex, extraocular muscles, tympanic membrane, sinuses, nares, oropharyngeal mucosa, vision screen (Snellen eye chart)
Lymph:	Cervical, axillary, inguinal
Cardiovascular:	Radial and femoral pulses, rate and rhythm, murmurs
Pulmonary:	Symmetrical expansion, wheezing, rales
Abdomen:	Splenomegaly, hernia
Spine:	Cervical and lumbar range of motion (ROM), kyphosis, scoliosis
Extremities:	ROM and strength, look for major side-to-side discrepancy
Genitalia:	Presence of both testicles, whether nontender, check for hernia (males only)

Marfanoid features are particularly important to catch due to the cardiac implications of the syndrome. It is also important to be aware of normal variants seen in certain sports: for example, baseball pitchers routinely have increased external rotation in their throwing arm compared to the contralateral side. This should not be mistaken for instability or acute ligamentous injury, and need not be documented or worked up further. Pain is a fairly reliable indicator for pathology in athletes, who generally tend to minimize their symptoms. If any examination maneuver produces pain or visible discomfort, more focused examination for the affected part should be performed and documented. If there is any uncertainty, referral to the appropriate provider should be done with a specific request for clearance to participate.

Granting clearance for participation assumes responsibility for the athlete's well-being to a certain degree. Participation in sports involves a certain level of risk that is unavoidable, and it is understood that all adverse events cannot be predicted or prevented. By systematically ruling out any contraindications and identifying factors that need further attention, the physician is attempting to protect the participant as much as can be reasonably expected. An athlete may be granted full clearance without restrictions, conditional clearance pending further evaluation, or not cleared for participation. Conditional clearance requires referral and follow-through with the appropriate health care provider, depending on the medical concern.

Impairment in sports is addressed in a very delicate fashion, as there are many psychosocial factors involved. Physiatrists are attuned to the needs of patients who have suffered loss of function, and are well suited to addressing these issues in athletes. When dealing with single conditions, such as paraplegia or amputation, adjustments are relatively straightforward. Wheelchair sports, for instance, have a systematic method of accounting for various levels of functionality in order to evenly balance opposing teams. Significant challenges arise when dealing with the integration of disabled athletes with their able-bodied counterparts. In 2012, paralympian Oscar Pistorius was the first amputee to participate in the Olympics, raising much controversy about the potential advantage of his bilateral carbon composite flex-foot sprinting prostheses. There are many cases of amputees in wrestling who compete with the same rules as their able-bodied opponents. It is impossible to objectively quantify the mismatch that may be occurring, due to the complexity of both physical and mental interactions between competitors. While the able-bodied athletes have the seemingly obvious advantage, it is reasonable to suggest that there are sport-specific advantages in certain conditions. The low center of mass in a double amputee may serve to his advantage in the wrestling ring. On a separate note, it is theorized that an able-bodied participant may unknowingly attenuate his or her performance out of sympathy for the disabled opponent.

Female athletes must be screened with particular emphasis on three factors affecting their well-being. The "female athlete triad" consists of menstrual disturbances, disordered eating, and impaired bone mineralization, and is found more in participants of sports that favor lower body weight such as gymnastics.

MEDICAL KNOWLEDGE

GOALS

Demonstrate knowledge of established and evolving biomedical, clinical epidemiological, and sociobehavioral sciences pertaining to sports medicine, as well as the application of this knowledge to screening and guiding evaluation of athletes.

OBJECTIVES

1. List key elements for proficiency prior to conducting PPEs.
2. Identify areas likely to be injured in common high-school and collegiate sports.
3. Support the rationale for the use of diagnostic and imaging testing during the screening process.
4. Identify ethical considerations that should be taken during the screening process and prior to giving clearance.
5. Educate athletes on making patient-centered decisions regarding their sports participation.

In order to safely clear athletes for sports participation, one must possess a strong understanding of common musculoskeletal ailments as well as the functional demands of the given sport of interest. While general anatomy and biomechanics of the spine, shoulder, and hip girdles, as well as the rest of the upper and lower extremities, should be studied, sport-specific knowledge must also be obtained. For example, the rotator cuff is well known for its importance in throwing athletes, particularly baseball pitchers. What might not be as obvious is its critical function in boxing. Without a strong rotator cuff, a boxer cannot adequately defend the head and neck by blocking punches with his or her upper extremities. Furthermore, punch force is also dependent on active shoulder stabilization at the moment of impact. This highlights the importance of understanding sport-specific functionality when evaluating athletes for clearance.

In 2007, an extensive review of 16 years' of injury surveillance data over 15 different National Collegiate Athletic Association sports was done. Sports included baseball, softball, basketball, football, hockey, soccer, lacrosse, and gymnastics in a variety of combinations of men's and women's divisions. More than 50% of overall injuries involved the lower extremity, with the ankle ligament sprain being the single most common injury. Football had the highest rate of injury of all sports (1).

While the routine musculoskeletal examination is more or less identical for all sports, certain sport-specific emphasis should be maintained. A commonly overlooked area in football players is the wrist. They are prone to carpal bone fractures and dislocations due to the repetitive falling as well as the grabbing and pulling motions required during play. Boxers are prone to nasal, orbital, and hand fractures to a greater degree than most other sportsmen. Basketball players are at increased risk for eye injuries, in addition to the general ailments involved with running and throwing athletes. All contact sports require deeper inquiry about prior contusions and concussions compared to noncontact sports. These examples only touch the surface of the extensive body of evidence regarding injury mechanisms based on sport type. Prior to evaluating athletes of a particular sport, physicians must do adequate groundwork to familiarize themselves with their particular athletic population.

Evaluating athletes is often very rewarding because one can appreciate the determination and focus that they dedicate to their sport. This, however, can become challenging when an athlete minimizes symptoms in order to achieve clearance to play. Although the physician may sympathize with such concerns, it is unethical to deviate from protocol due to a persuasive athlete. Any findings on evaluation that may impair his or her ability to safely perform his or her functions must be further evaluated without question.

Besides checking routine vital signs, there is no mandatory laboratory work or diagnostic testing required in preparticipation screening. However, when pertinent positives are found on history and physical examination, further evaluation is warranted. Any history of syncope, palpitations, chest pain, or an early cardiac event in the family requires an EKG. It is controversial whether routine screening EKGs should be done even in the absence of risk factors due to the relatively low incidence of cardiac events in athletes. Females showing signs of any of the 3 conditions seen in the female athlete triad should be screened with electrolyte panels, caloric intake assessments, and bone mineral density testing.

PRACTICE-BASED LEARNING AND IMPROVEMENT

GOALS

Demonstrate competence in appraising and assimilating scientific evidence into your team physician and sports medicine care practices, and making improvements based on progressive self-evaluation and lifelong learning.

OBJECTIVES

1. Describe learning opportunities for providers, patients, and caregivers as applicable to PPEs of athletes.
2. Locate resources including available websites and professional organizations for continuing medical education and professional development in sports medicine.

Physiatrists performing PPEs should have a working knowledge of musculoskeletal anatomy, sports-specific injuries, and medical conditions commonly seen in athletes. They should be able to perform an appropriate assessment of the athlete prior to participation in sports and be able to recognize the potential safety risks to the athlete associated with the sports. Physiatrists involved in the care of athletes should have excellent interpersonal and communication skills in order to effectively communicate with the athletes, coaches, and athletic trainers.

There are several strategies that physiatrists can use to identify gaps in their knowledge base about sports medicine and the PPE. Self-reflection on their clinical practice, self-assessment examinations, asking trusted colleagues to provide feedback to them on their practice, and asking athletes under their care for their feedback on the care provided by them are just some examples.

There are several organizations that provide resources related to the treatment of athletes involved in organized sports. A brief list includes the American Academy of Family Physicians, American Academy of Pediatrics, American College of Sports Medicine, American Medical Society for Sports Medicine, American Orthopaedic Society for Sports Medicine, and American Osteopathic Academy of Sports Medicine. In 2010, these organizations collectively released the fourth edition of their joint consensus statement about PPEs. The publication extensively covers various aspects of the process and serves as a comprehensive tool for involved providers.

Maintaining a successful relationship with an athletic department requires routine reevaluation of protocol as well as review of emerging evidence relevant to the sport. For instance, the management of concussion has evolved significantly in the past few years based on new understanding of brain injury and recovery. The concept of second impact syndrome is relatively new and highlights the devastating effects of compounded, seemingly minor events involving brain trauma. This has in turn tightened up the requirements for clearance to participate in the setting of prior concussions.

INTERPERSONAL AND COMMUNICATION SKILLS

GOALS

Demonstrate interpersonal and communication skills that result in optimizing the effective exchange of information and collaboration with athletes, their families, and the rest of the sports medicine team.

OBJECTIVES

1. Describe the importance of effective communication between the sports medicine professional and other team members, as applicable to athletes across socioeconomic and cultural backgrounds.
2. Discuss the perspective of the athlete in the process of obtaining clearance for participation.
3. Provide an example of an injury that warrants counseling and education for the athletes as well as the family and coaching staff.
4. Identify key points to be documented in patient records to provide effective communication between team members with respect to athletic participation.
5. Delineate the importance of the role of the sports medicine specialist as the interdisciplinary team leader and consultant for the athlete.

It is important to keep the perspective of the athletes in mind in order to facilitate a meaningful encounter. Oftentimes, particularly in younger populations, the PPE is viewed as an unnecessary formality. Rather than approach them as patients with underlying conditions to be diagnosed, they should be seen as healthy individuals with potential conditions that may warrant further attention. Many of these athletes have had minimal interaction with physicians and may therefore be hesitant and guarded during the encounter. Some may view the physician as the person who might prevent them from playing sports, and not understand the importance of the screening. Continually providing reassurance that there is a common goal in mind can put some of these fears to rest. Athletes should also have the chance to speak to the physician in private without any scrutiny from his or her peers.

Maintaining good rapport with the coaching and administrative staff can also make a drastic difference in the efficiency of the process. They know the athletes well and can provide valuable insight on potential problems. They should be given an opportunity to voice any concern they may have. For example, when dealing with an athlete with a history of concussion, it is important that the coaches, coaching staff, athletic trainers, and the athlete's family members all learn to recognize the symptoms of a concussion. It is important to emphasize that a loss of consciousness is not necessary for a concussion to occur and that athletes younger than 18 years of age take longer to recover from a concussion than older athletes. It is also important to reiterate that decisions regarding return to play should be individualized (2). Education and counseling of the coaches and staff while maintaining open communication results in a team effort in the continued monitoring of the athlete's condition.

Documentation in PPE is extremely important. Many times, the physician performing the physical examination will not be the same physician who is covering the sporting event. Physicians need to be able to communicate with one another when an athlete is at risk for an injury or has a prior injury. Some key points that need to be documented include the following:

- Personal or family history of any sudden death, cardiac abnormalities, or lightheadedness when exercising
- History of concussion
- Medications, prior medical conditions, and details of limited clearance
- Loss of any paired organs (eyes, kidneys, testicles, ovaries), which may disqualify an athlete from competing in many contact sports
- History of seizures

With regard to athletes with disability, it is important to document any prosthetics or orthotics the athlete may be using, skin breakdown, hearing and vision impairment, muscle spasticity, and bowel or bladder issues.

The medical history is the most sensitive and specific component of the PPE. More than 75% of important medical and orthopedic conditions affecting the athletes can be identified by asking the right historical questions. In the fourth edition of the PPE monograph, the authors have rewritten and expanded the questionnaire to now include more than 50 questions (2). Parents can help fill out the questionnaire in order to ensure accuracy. It is important to emphasize the importance of answering the questions truthfully.

Teamwork is essential in the successful completion of a round of PPEs. It is important to have the medical stations set up in such a way as to allow efficient flow of the athletes from one station to another. Some argue that one physician should perform the complete physical examination on an athlete, rather than split up the stations by body system (3). Others feel that this sacrifices efficiency and is not useful, especially during mass participation events. Regardless of the setup of the evaluations, the physician must take a leadership role in organizing an efficient team during these examinations.

The actual encounters can take place at any available space that can facilitate a waiting area and an evaluation area. Depending on the number of physicians present, the tasks can be divided into stations, with the athletes circling around the stations before arriving at the final stop where their paperwork is reviewed once more. This type of setup is usually a dynamic process, with adjustments being made based on the flow of the athletes. If a particular station is backed up, the entire operation suffers; therefore, appropriate adjustments need to be made. When fewer hands are available it may be more efficient to have each physician do the entire history and physical examination from start to finish. At the end of every session, it would benefit all who were involved to briefly discuss strategies of making the encounters more efficient. Every session is a learning experience, and over time, optimal protocols can be determined for every scenario based on available manpower, tools, and rooms.

PROFESSIONALISM

GOALS

Reflect a commitment to carrying out professional responsibilities and an adherence to ethical principles in the screening approach for athletes.

OBJECTIVES

1. Exemplify the humanistic qualities as a provider of care for the athlete.
2. Demonstrate ethical principles and responsiveness to needs of the athlete superseding self and other interests.
3. Demonstrate sensitivity to athlete population diversity, including culture, gender, age, race, religion, disabilities, and sexual orientation.
4. Respect patient privacy, confidentiality, and autonomy.
5. Demonstrate the process of referring for further workup when a concern is found during screening.

Although maintaining a good rapport with the coaching and administrative staff as well as the athletes is vital, one must also maintain professional boundaries. There must be a mutual respect for the process by all parties involved. When the physician decides that further investigation is needed for any reason it should be clear that these are mandatory requirements, not just recommendations.

When performing the evaluation, it is important to respect the athlete's privacy. Oftentimes, mass preparticipation physicals are set up in large venues and offer little to no privacy. Although this can usually increase efficiency, there are advantages to the office setting. This setting offers privacy to discuss other issues, such as smoking, alcohol, drug use, and sexual activity. Risk-taking behaviors, such as use of helmets and seat belts, can also be addressed. Many adolescents do not have a primary care physician, and thus, the evaluation may be the only contact the athlete has with a medical provider the entire year (2).

One particular area of the evaluation in which sensitive issues may arise is with female athletes suspected of having the female triad of disordered eating, menstrual abnormalities, and poor bone mineralization. Eating disorders are actually quite common among female athletes (4). Oftentimes, this nutritional deficiency is what leads to the other two components of the triad, via vitamin D deficiency and inadequate production of sex hormones. Without extensive patient counseling and education, correction of these deficiencies is nearly impossible. Such issues are better addressed in the privacy of the physician's office.

Other issues that may arise during the PPE are other medical conditions that may not disqualify an athlete from competing, but should be addressed, such as skin disorders, sickle cell trait, and sexually transmitted diseases. It is important to respect the athlete's privacy when handling sensitive issues.

It is also essential to ensure that appropriate follow-up care is sought. When an area of concern is found, the athlete and coaching staff must be provided with the referring physician's contact information, and instructed to make an appointment in a timely fashion. Thoroughly documenting the abnormal findings with the reasons for consultation as well as contacting the consultant will help ensure that the patient receives appropriate follow-up. For example, if a cardiac murmur is found, it should be described with various different positions including standing, supine, and squatting. The referral to cardiology should include the physical examination findings as well as the intended sports participation so that a recommendation can be made based on the level of exertion required.

SYSTEMS-BASED PRACTICE

GOALS

Awareness and responsiveness to systems of athletic care delivery, and the ability to recruit and coordinate effectively resources in the system to provide optimal continuum of care as it relates to sports medicine and the athlete.

OBJECTIVES

1. Identify the key components in the spectrum of athlete continuum of care settings.
2. Discuss some limitations of the PPE.
3. Coordinate and recruit necessary resources in the system to provide optimal and variety of care options available for the athlete, with attention to safety and cost–benefit considerations.
4. Identify the components, systems of care delivery, services, referral patterns, and resources available to the athlete.
5. Describe optimal long-term follow-up for athletes, markers of quality of care and improvement metrics, and use of documentation in such sports medicine programs.

The PPE is a screening tool to detect any potentially life-threatening or disabling medical conditions or musculoskeletal conditions and to screen for such conditions that may predispose the athlete to injury. Secondary goals include determining the overall health of the athlete, to serve as an entry point into the health care system for adolescents, and to initiate a discussion on health-related topics (2). For a screening tool to be effective, it must be able to identify medical issues that can be positively impacted upon, affordable, practical, and sensitive. Controversy exists regarding the effectiveness of the PPE as a screening tool. Research has failed to demonstrate that the PPE is effective in reducing morbidity or mortality of athletes (3). However, when thoroughly and consistently performed by qualified licensed physicians, the PPE may be an effective tool to identify medical and musculoskeletal conditions that affect an athlete's ability to perform in a sport.

There is no standardization of the PPE in the United States. The requirements are determined by each state. In addition, the type of provider who is licensed to perform the PPE also varies by state. Thus, the PPE process varies from state to state. This has been a significant barrier to determining the effectiveness of the PPE. There is a need for a national standardized PPE. This would allow for meaningful data collection and outcome measures (2).

The current recommendation in the United States in regard to the cardiovascular screen is a detailed past medical and family history, as well as a focused physical examination (2). The European Society of Cardiology and the International Olympic Committee have both endorsed the routine use of electrocardiogram (ECG) in the PPE. These recommendations are based on an Italian study that showed an 89% reduction in the incidence of sudden cardiac death in athletes over a 25-year period (5). However, the American Heart Association recommended against the routine use of ECG in screening athletes. It was determined that use of ECG was not a feasible option in the

United States due to low prevalence of disease, poor sensitivity, high false-positive results, poor cost effectiveness, and lack of properly trained physicians to interpret the results (6). Any athlete with symptoms of exertional syncope, near syncope, chest pain, palpations, or excessive exertional dyspnea will require a thorough cardiovascular evaluation to exclude underlying heart disease (2).

The use of an electronic medical record (EMR) can be useful not only for documenting the PPE, but also when covering events. There is often a lack of continuity of care, where the physician who covers the sporting event is not the same one who cleared the athletes for participation. Using an EMR will allow instant access to all prior documented issues, which can be very useful while evaluating an athlete on the field. Although this may not be critical for musculoskeletal injuries, it can be life-saving in a collapsed athlete with a documented history of seizure disorder, hyponatremia, heat stroke, or anaphylaxis.

CASE STUDY

A 17-year-old high-school senior is seen as part of her routine preparticipation screening for the girls' volleyball program. Prior to this, she has not been involved with any organized sports. She does not have a primary care physician and has had minimal interactions with health care providers.

Detailed history reveals no active medical issues and no past medical history. Her family history is noncontributory. She exercises 6 days a week, running 5 miles every morning and doing 1 hour of weight training every evening. She performs well in her classes and has a good relationship with her teachers and fellow students.

Physical examination reveals normal vital signs with a height of 5 feet 8 inches and a weight of 97 lbs. The rest of her physical examination is normal.

CASE STUDY DISCUSSION QUESTIONS

1. What are some key points in the history that need further elaboration?
2. On further history, she admits that she has had pain in her right foot for the past several months. She has tried changing her footwear with no improvement. What are some diagnostic tests that may be useful in addition to the routine evaluation?
3. Describe the issues that may arise in this athlete if suspected of having the female triad, and strategies that the physiatrist may use to address these issues in a professional manner.
4. Describe the pros and cons of the effectiveness of the PPE as a screening tool in this athlete.
5. Describe effective interpersonal and communication skills between the physiatrist, the athlete, and her coaches if the athlete was to develop an acute shoulder injury that could affect her ability to play on the team.
6. Discuss possible ethical conflicts that may arise for the physiatrist performing the PPE.

SELF-EXAMINATION QUESTIONS
(Answers begin on p. 367)

1. The designation of "conditional clearance" for sports participation indicates which of the following?
   A. The athlete is cleared for participation as long as a referred clinician also agrees
   B. The athlete can participate as long as a waiver is signed
   C. The athlete can only participate under certain weather conditions
   D. The athlete can participate if his or her parents agree
   E. The athlete can participate if his or her siblings agree

2. Which of the following collegiate sports has the highest injury rate?
   A. Volleyball
   B. Soccer
   C. Football
   D. Gymnastics
   E. Badminton

3. What is a major difference between screening for contact sports versus that for noncontact sports?
   A. Contact sports require greater emphasis on aerobic endurance
   B. Noncontact sport screenings are less thorough
   C. Noncontact sport screenings do not require the routine laboratory work that is required in contact sport screenings
   D. A history of concussion is a greater concern in contact sports
   E. A history of concussion is a greater concern in noncontact sports

4. Which of the following is the most sensitive component of the routine PPE?
   A. History
   B. Physical
   C. Laboratory work
   D. EKG
   E. X-rays

5. When an abnormal finding requires further evaluation, whose responsibility is it to ensure that appropriate follow-up care is sought prior to clearance?
   A. The athlete
   B. The physician performing the screening
   C. The coaching staff
   D. The athlete's parents
   E. The athletic trainer

REFERENCES

1. Hootman JM, Dick R, Agel J. Epidemiology of collegiate injuries for 15 sports: summary and recommendations for injury prevention initiatives. *J Athl Train*. April–June 2007;42(2):311–319. Review. PubMed PMID: 17710181; PubMed Central PMCID: PMC1941297.

2. American Academy of Family Physicians, American Academy of Pediatrics, American College of Sports Medicine, et al. In: Roberts W, Bernhardt D, eds. *Preparticipation Physical Evaluation.* Systems-Based Examination 4th ed. Elk Grove, IL: American Academy of Pediatrics; 2010.
3. Seto C. The preparticipation physical examination: an update. *Clin Sports Med.* 2011;30:491–501.
4. Sundgot-Borgen J. Prevalence of eating disorders in elite female athletes. *Int J Sport Nutr.* 1993;3(1):29–40.
5. Corrado D, Basso C, Pavei A, et al. Trends in sudden cardiovascular death in young competitive athletes after implementation of a preparticipation screening program. *JAMA.* 2006;296:1593–601.
6. Maron BJ, Thompson PD, Ackerman MJ, et al. Recommendations and considerations related to preparticipation screening for cardiovascular abnormalities in competitive athletes: 2007 update: a scientific statement from the American Heart Association Council on Nutrition, Physical Activity, and Metabolism. *Circulation.* 2007;115:1643–1655.

Todd R. Lefkowitz

29: Entrapment Neuropathies

PATIENT CARE

GOALS

Provide patient care that is compassionate, appropriate, and effective for the treatment of the adult with an entrapment neuropathy.

OBJECTIVES

1. Describe the key components of the assessment of the adult with an entrapment neuropathy.
2. Discuss the long-term implications of entrapment neuropathies.
3. Assess the impairments, activity limitations, and participation restrictions associated with entrapment neuropathies.
4. Describe potential injuries associated with entrapment neuropathies.
5. Formulate the key components of a rehabilitation treatment plan for the adult with an entrapment neuropathy.

Examination of a patient with a peripheral entrapment neuropathy begins with a thorough history. The physician should inquire about dysesthesias or weakness in the distribution of the peripheral nerve involved, as well as any symptoms outside of the peripheral nerve's distribution if a more proximal lesion (e.g., radiculopathy or plexopathy) is suspected. It is helpful to ascertain if a patient's symptoms radiate distally from the neck or shoulder or proximally from the wrist or elbow, although pain patterns often overlap, making it difficult for patients and physicians alike to discriminate between two sites of compression. Concomitant shoulder pain should raise suspicion for a shoulder impingement syndrome.

In the upper limb, hand diagrams are useful screening tools for evaluating patients with suspected entrapment neuropathies at the wrist (e.g., carpal tunnel syndrome [CTS]) and elbow (cubital tunnel syndrome [CuTS]) (1,2). The Katz hand diagram (Figure 29.1) is a self-administered inventory where patients' depiction of pain, numbness, tingling, and decreased sensation can be compared against a symptom classification system of classic, probable, possible, or unlikely CTS.

A sensitivity of 80% and a specificity of 90% were reported in one cohort study (3).

The presence of more generalized symptoms in the limbs may suggest an underlying systemic process such as a peripheral polyneuropathy.

A history of recent abdominal, pelvic, gynecologic, or orthopedic surgery should be ascertained in patients with suspected peripheral entrapment neuropathies of the lower limb. Extended lithotomy positions and anterior approaches to hip replacement have been associated with femoral neuropathies at the inguinal ligament (4,5). The obturator nerve and, less commonly, the common peroneal nerve can be injured in the lithotomy position (6). Workers who habitually squat or kneel (e.g., carpenters or farm workers) may preferentially injure the peroneal nerve at the fibular head.

Physical examination of persons with distal entrapment neuropathies of the upper limb should incorporate sensory testing of dually innervated digits (e.g., ring finger and thumb) to help discriminate median from ulnar nerve and median from radial nerve involvement. Two-point discrimination and monofilament testing are commonly used modalities to assess for sensory loss. Atrophy of the thenar eminence, hypothenar eminence, or intrinsic hand muscle weakness should be documented if present. Muscle stretch reflexes should remain unaffected in the absence of a cervical radiculopathy or brachial plexopathy. The Tinel test has historically been used to elicit paresthesias with varying degrees of sensitivity and specificity (7). Other provocative tests such as Phalen's and the elbow hyperflexion tests have been used to reproduce symptoms suggestive of CTS and ulnar neuropathy at the elbow, respectively.

Sensory testing of patients with suspected distal entrapment neuropathies of the lower limb may be confounded by the presence of a peripheral polyneuropathy, especially in those individuals with a history of diabetes mellitus, chemotherapy (e.g., vincristine, cisplatin), or other toxin exposure (e.g., EtOH). Clinical documentation of muscle weakness is paramount in preparing for the electrodiagnostic (EDX) evaluation. Examination of muscles that have the same spinal nerve root innervation but different peripheral nerve innervation may help distinguish a peripheral entrapment neuropathy from a lumbosacral radiculopathy or plexopathy.

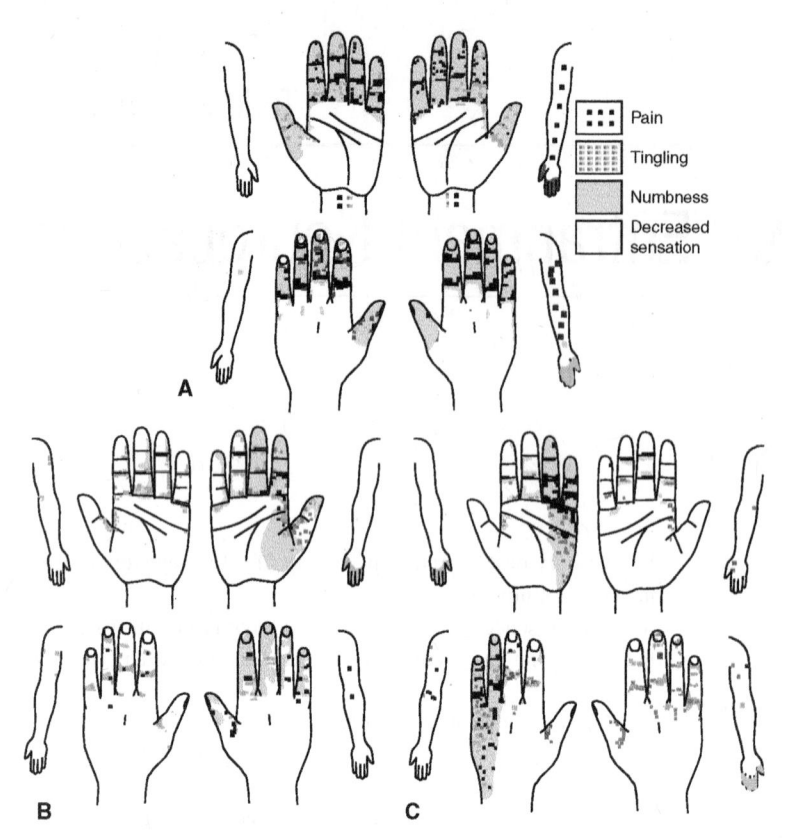

FIGURE 29.1 The Katz Hand Diagram
Source: Adapted from Katz and Stirrat (1990). Copyright 1990, with permission from Elsevier.

Patients with CTS or ulnar neuropathy in their dominant hand may complain of bothersome paresthesias which impair certain work activities requiring fine motor skills (e.g., typing, driving, and electrical work). Ulnar neuropathy, in particular, may be associated with decreased grip strength as the ulnar part of the hand provides a powerful grip. These patients may require written work restrictions from the physician if symptoms are thought to endanger the safety of the patient or those under his or her care. The physician is well advised to image the cervical spine in patients whose hand symptoms are accompanied by new-onset gait disturbance or urinary incontinence to rule out symptomatic cervical stenosis with spinal cord compression.

The physician should counsel patients on how best to modify their work activities such that vibratory and mechanical forces are reduced; however, patients are ultimately responsible for communicating these recommendations directly to their employers (8). This may prove impractical, however, as employers may not allow certain workers with hand-intensive jobs to return to the workplace with restrictions in place in the absence of available light-duty positions.

A trial of non-operative therapy may be attempted in patients with mild-to-moderate symptoms prior to surgical consideration. A referral to an occupational therapist or a certified hand therapist for neurodynamic mobilization exercises or carpal bone mobilization exercises is often prescribed, although the evidence supporting its use is very limited (9). Static splinting of the wrist in persons with CTS may provide relief of symptoms, but evidence is lacking regarding design, wearing regimen, and efficacy compared to other non-surgical treatments (10). Dynamic splinting of the elbow in persons with CuTS may be excessive as a padded elbow sleeve is often sufficient to protect the ulnar nerve at the medial elbow.

There is poor quality evidence from very limited data which suggests that therapeutic ultrasound is more effective than placebo for short- or long-term symptom relief in persons with CTS (11). Likewise, the evidence supporting low-level laser therapy in CTS is also limited (12). Pooled data from four trials found significant short-term benefit from a 2-week course of oral steroids in patients with CTS (13). Compared to placebo, however, patients prescribed diuretics or nonsteroidal anti-inflammatory drugs (NSAIDs) did not demonstrate significant improvement (13).

Roughly 50% of patients with mild CTS may experience pain relief for up to 15 months after a single corticosteroid injection into the carpal tunnel despite earlier reports of no increased benefit after 1 month (14,15). The safest approach for a carpal tunnel injection remains controversial. Historically, physicians used the palmaris longus (PL) tendon as an anatomical landmark to guide their injections. This approach, however, risks injury to the median nerve and inadvertent injection of the nearby ulnar artery. The median nerve was found to extend ulnarly beyond the PL tendon in 88% of hands with CTS in one series (16). As such, some authors advocate injecting through the flexor carpi radialis tendon as the safest route of administration despite the theoretical risk of tendon rupture (17). Ultrasound-guided injections have since been recommended to avoid nerve, tendon, and arterial injuries (17).

Optimal timing of surgical decompression in CTS or CuTS has not been established in the medical literature. Ideally, patients should be referred for decompression after an adequate trial of nonoperative therapy has been attempted, but prior to the development of thenar muscle atrophy or intrinsic muscle weakness. It is certainly reasonable to stop or defer nonoperative therapies in those patients presenting with moderate-to-severe findings on EDX studies or those patients with progressive motor deficits in their hands.

Follow-up care of patients with peripheral entrapment neuropathies is necessary, especially after decompression surgery. The recurrence rate of CTS ranges from 3% to 25% with persistent symptoms seen in up to 95% of patients (18–20). Factors associated with poorer outcomes following a carpal tunnel decompression include early symptomatic recurrence, diabetes mellitus, obesity, cervical spine pathology, involvement of the non-dominant hand, and intraoperative scar tissue or fibrosis (21). Recurrence rates of 10% to 13% have been reported following open cubital tunnel release surgery (22,23).

Patients presenting with symptomatic recurrences of a peripheral entrapment neuropathy should be counseled on adopting healthy lifestyle modifications to reduce the burden of systemic disease (e.g., diabetes, thyroid, EtOH consumption) that may be stressing their peripheral nervous system. Consideration should be given to a trial of a nerve membrane stabilizing agent (e.g., gabapentin, pregabalin), although the available literature on these medications primarily reflects experience with patients who have painful diabetic peripheral neuropathy or postherpetic neuralgia and not necessarily peripheral entrapment neuropathies (24).

MEDICAL KNOWLEDGE

GOALS

Demonstrate knowledge of established and evolving biomedical, clinical, and epidemiological sciences pertaining to entrapment neuropathies, as well as the application of this knowledge to guide holistic patient care.

OBJECTIVES

1. Describe the epidemiology, anatomy, physiology, and pathophysiology of entrapment neuropathies.
2. Discuss the common types of entrapment neuropathies and their characteristics.
3. Identify the pertinent laboratory and diagnostic studies important in the evaluation of entrapment neuropathies.
4. Review the treatment of common entrapment neuropathies.

CTS is the most commonly reported nerve compression syndrome followed by ulnar neuropathy at the elbow; however, ulnar neuropathy is only 1/13 as common as CTS (25). CTS affects 3 out of every 10,000 full-time workers according to 2004 National Institute of Occupational Safety and Health data, with a higher prevalence among electrical assembly, food packing/processing, and poultry workers (8). The loss of future earnings of workers

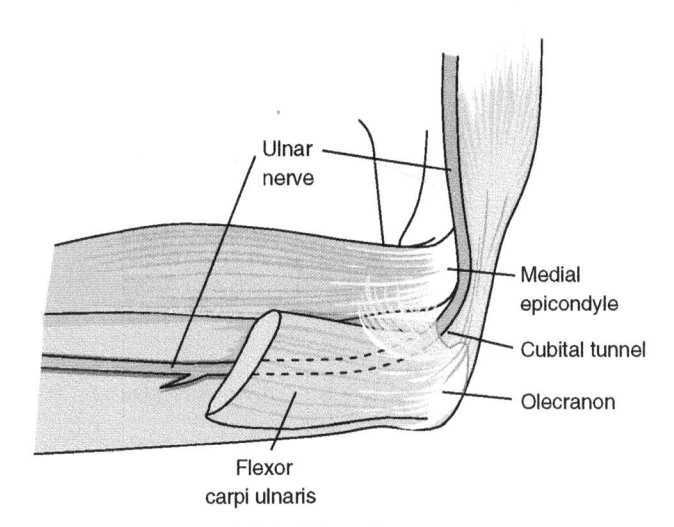

FIGURE 29.2 The Cubital Tunnel
Source: Adapted from Cuccurullo SJ. In: *Physical Medicine & Rehabilitation Board Review*, 2nd ed. Demos Medical Publishing; 2010.

with CTS has been estimated to range from $45,000 to $89,000 in one study of workers in Washington State (26).

Compression of the median nerve may result in focal demyelination with or without ischemic changes (27). The ulnar nerve is vulnerable to mechanical compression as it passes between the medial epicondyle of the humerus and olecranon process of the ulna. Repetitive flexion and extension of the elbow can predispose to a traction injury of the nerve as it traverses beneath the proximal edge of the flexor carpi ulnaris (FCU) (Figure 29.2) aponeurosis and the arcuate ligament (e.g., humeroulnar arcade), causing CuTS.

Injuries to the ulnar nerve in the vicinity of the Guyon's canal are exceedingly rare but may be seen in cyclers (e.g. cycler's palsy) or those with space-occupying lesions (e.g., ganglion cysts) of the wrist (Figure 29.3).

Distal ulnar nerve entrapments have been previously described by Shea (28).

The existence of a distal entrapment neuropathy with a concomitant cervical radiculopathy (e.g., double crush syndrome) remains controversial. Proponents of this theory argue that a proximal nerve lesion increases the likelihood of a distal entrapment neuropathy by decreasing net axoplasmic flow to an already compromised distal nerve segment, resulting in further axonal damage (29). The median nerve's extensive root innervation from C6 through T1 may be responsible for the proximal radiation of pain into the upper limb often reported by patients with CTS. Whether this phenomenon represents retrograde degeneration of distal median nerve axons from an initial compressive lesion at the wrist or concomitant compression and sensitization of the dorsal root ganglion in the cervical neural foramen is still unclear.

Peroneal neuropathy at the fibular head is the most common entrapment neuropathy in the lower extremity. The peroneal and tibial divisions of the sciatic nerve run as distinct nerve bundles that do not exchange branches in the posterior thigh. After innervating the short head of the biceps femoris (SHBF) muscle, the peroneal nerve wraps around the fibular head and neck where it

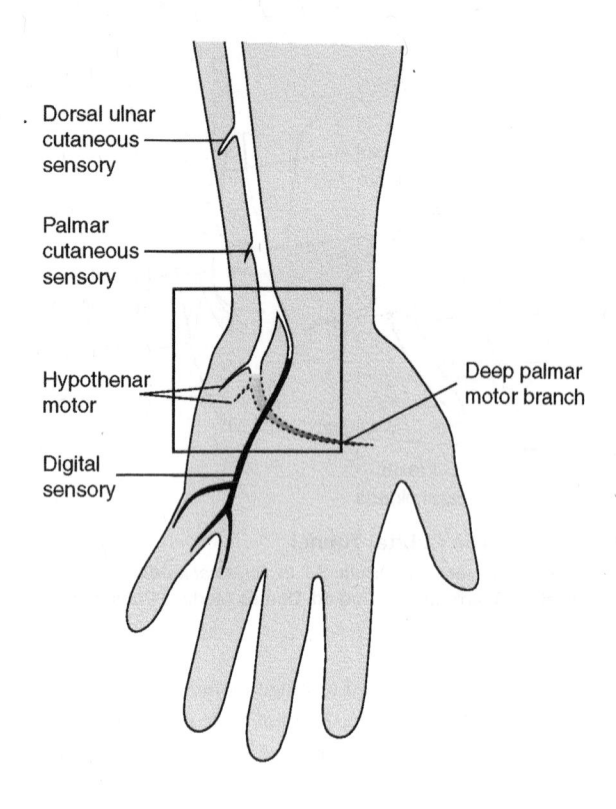

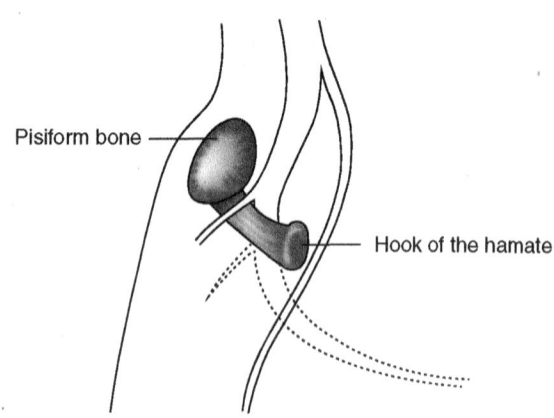

FIGURE 29.3 Anatomy of the Ulnar Nerve at the Wrist
Source: Adapted from Cuccurullo SJ. *Physical Medicine & Rehabilitation Board Review*, 2nd ed. Demos Medical Publishing; 2010.

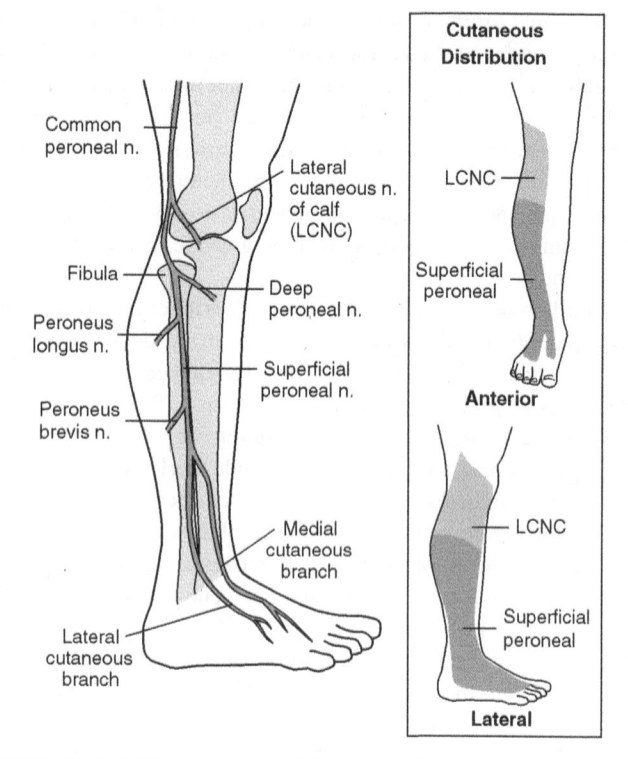

FIGURE 29.4 The Superficial Perineal Nerve
Source: Adapted from Cuccurullo SJ. *Physical Medicine & Rehabilitation Board Review*, 2nd ed. Demos Medical Publishing; 2010.

widespread use in clinical practice for diagnosing patients with buttock and proximal posterior thigh pain (Figure 29.5). The mean diameter of the piriformis muscle as measured in one cadaveric study was approximately 6.3 mm as compared to 19 mm (~¾ inch) of the sciatic nerve, making true entrapment unlikely in the absence of anatomic variants (34). Most commonly, the sciatic nerve passes undivided below the piriformis closely adheres to the periosteum, making it vulnerable to compression and trauma (Figure 29.4).

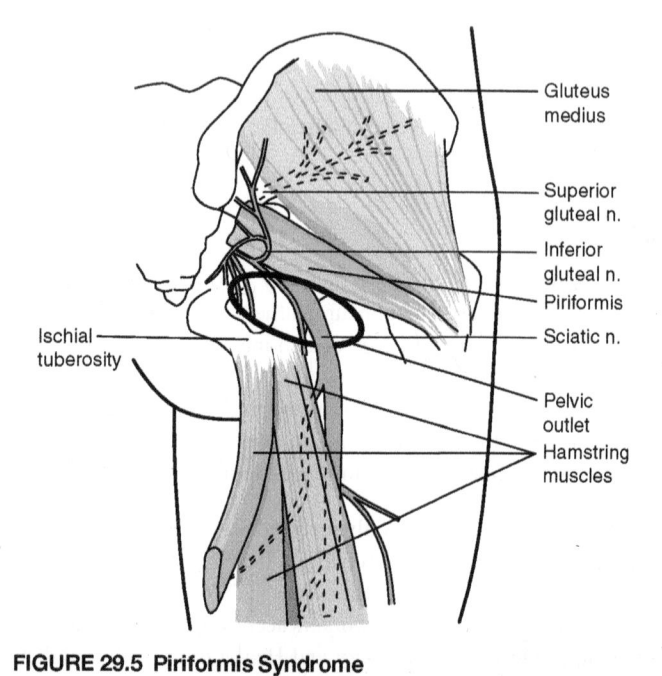

The larger fascicles of the peroneal nerve are surrounded by less supportive epineural tissue rendering them relatively intolerant to mechanical compression compared to the tibial division of the sciatic nerve (30). In addition to the more common causes of peroneal neuropathy, severe flexion and inversion ankle sprains can cause traction injuries to the nerve from tearing of the vasa nervosum (31).

The incidence of sciatic neuropathy has been reported to range from 0.05% to 1.9% (32). In patients undergoing traditional hip replacements (via a posterolateral approach), the incidence may be higher with electromyographic evidence of neurologic injury reported to be as high as 70% (33).

Entrapment of the sciatic nerve by the piriformis muscle (e.g., piriformis syndrome) is relatively uncommon despite its

FIGURE 29.5 Piriformis Syndrome
Source: Adapted from Cuccurullo SJ. *Physical Medicine & Rehabilitation Board Review*, 2nd ed. Demos Medical Publishing; 2010.

muscle, but divisions of the nerve may pass between and below the muscle or between and above the muscle (35,36).

EDX studies can help confirm the physician's clinical suspicion of a peripheral entrapment neuropathy. Practice parameters have previously been set forth by the American Association of Neuromuscular and Electrodiagnostic Medicine (AANEM) for CTS and ulnar neuropathy at the elbow (37,38). In addition to standard median and ulnar sensory nerve conduction studies (NCS) across the wrist, the median-ulnar sensory latency difference to digit 4 and the median-radial sensory latency difference to digit 1 can be helpful in cases where the diagnosis of CTS is equivocal. A mixed sensorimotor mid-palm stimulation study comparing the latencies of the median and ulnar nerves can also be performed to supplement the standard EDX workup. Robinson et al. proposed a combined sensory index (CSI) using the previous three comparative studies to improve the reliability, sensitivity, and specificity of NCS in diagnosing CTS (39). A summated latency difference greater than or equal to 0.9 ms is considered abnormal with a sensitivity of 83% and a specificity of 95%. If one comparison study is abnormal, then there is a 98% likelihood that the CSI will be abnormal (40).

The performance of needle electromyography (EMG) in patients with suspected CTS remains at the discretion of the examining physician. It can be used to document axonal loss in those patients with thenar muscle atrophy and decrements in the median compound muscle action potential (CMAP) amplitude in the palm. An abnormal median sensory or motor latency or amplitude, however, does not predict abnormal needle EMG findings (41). Needle EMG should be included as part of the EDX evaluation of patients whose differential diagnosis includes cervical radiculopathy and brachial plexopathy.

In patients with CuTS, there is a 25% chance of finding an abnormality on EMG in the ulnar-innervated forearm muscles compared with a 70% chance of finding an abnormality in the ulnar-innervated intrinsic hand muscles due to the topography of the nerve fascicles traversing the retrocondylar groove (42). Sampling the medial half of the flexor digitorum profundus (FDP) muscle may be of higher diagnostic yield than sampling the FCU muscle, as the branch of the ulnar nerve to the FCU traverses the cubital tunnel in only 50% of individuals (42). A dorsal ulnar cutaneous (DUC) NCS can also help localize a lesion to the cubital tunnel as this nerve does not pass through the Guyon's canal.

A sciatic neuropathy is a relatively uncommon diagnosis in the EMG laboratory. An absent sural sensory nerve action potential (SNAP) and normal needle examination of the lumbar paraspinal muscles places the suspected lesion distal to the dorsal root ganglion, effectively ruling out a lumbosacral radiculopathy. If the gluteus medius and vastus muscles are normal and the saphenous SNAP is intact, then the lumbar plexus can be considered intact. If there are neuropathic motor units in the external hamstrings and absence of neuropathic motor units in the SHBF muscle, then the most affected portion of the sciatic nerve is proximal to the SHBF.

The EDX evaluation of patients with a suspected entrapment neuropathy of the peroneal nerve is helpful in localizing the lesion above or below the knee. Motor conduction studies to the extensor digitorum brevis (EDB) muscle should be performed. If the EDB muscle is atrophied or a response is difficult to obtain, then recording from the tibialis anterior muscle may be used instead. An accessory peroneal nerve should be suspected if, during routine peroneal NCS to the EDB, the CMAP amplitudes obtained at the fibular head and popliteal fossa are greater than the CMAP amplitude obtained at the ankle. A response obtained by stimulating posterior to the lateral malleolus confirms the diagnosis. Needle EMG of the SHBF can further localize the lesion as the SHBF is the only peroneal-innervated muscle above the knee. Denervation potentials in the SHBF muscle may suggest a sciatic neuropathy if needle EMG of the lumbar paraspinals and gluteal muscles is normal.

An ultrasound examination of the median nerve can complement the EDX survey in cases where the diagnosis of CTS is equivocal. Approximately 10% to 15% of patients with a clinical diagnosis of CTS will have normal NCS, reflecting a sensitivity of 85% to 90% (42). In the early stages of the disease, morphologic changes of the median nerve do not occur; however, a normal ultrasound examination in a patient with clinical symptoms suggestive of CTS does not preclude the diagnosis. As the disease progresses, flattening of the median nerve may be seen at the distal part of the carpal tunnel with enlargement of the nerve at the proximal portion of the tunnel at the level of the scaphoid-pisiform (43).

An 8-point ultrasonographic "inching test" measuring the cross-sectional area (CSA) of the median nerve across the wrist has been shown to positively correlate with NCS severity and duration of CTS symptoms (44) (Figure 29.6).

The area 2 cm distal to the distal wrist crease (location *i*2) had the smallest measured median nerve CSA and is thought to be the most likely site of entrapment in cases of idiopathic CTS (44) (Figure 29.7).

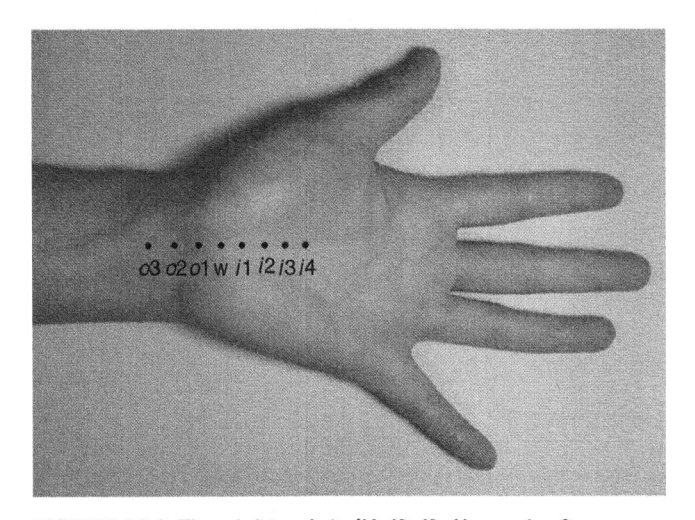

FIGURE 29.6 The eight points (*i*4, *i*3, *i*2, *i*1, w, *o*1, *o*2, and *o*3) for recording in both the "inching test" and ultrasonography; *i*4, *i*3, *i*2, *i*1 represent levels at 4, 3, 2, and 1 cm distal to the wrist crease in the inlet of the carpal tunnel; w is at the level of the wrist crease; and *o*1, *o*2, and *o*3 levels at 1, 2, and 3 cm are proximal to the wrist crease in the outlet of the carpal tunnel.

Source: Copyright ©2012 Chen et al.; BioMed Central Ltd.

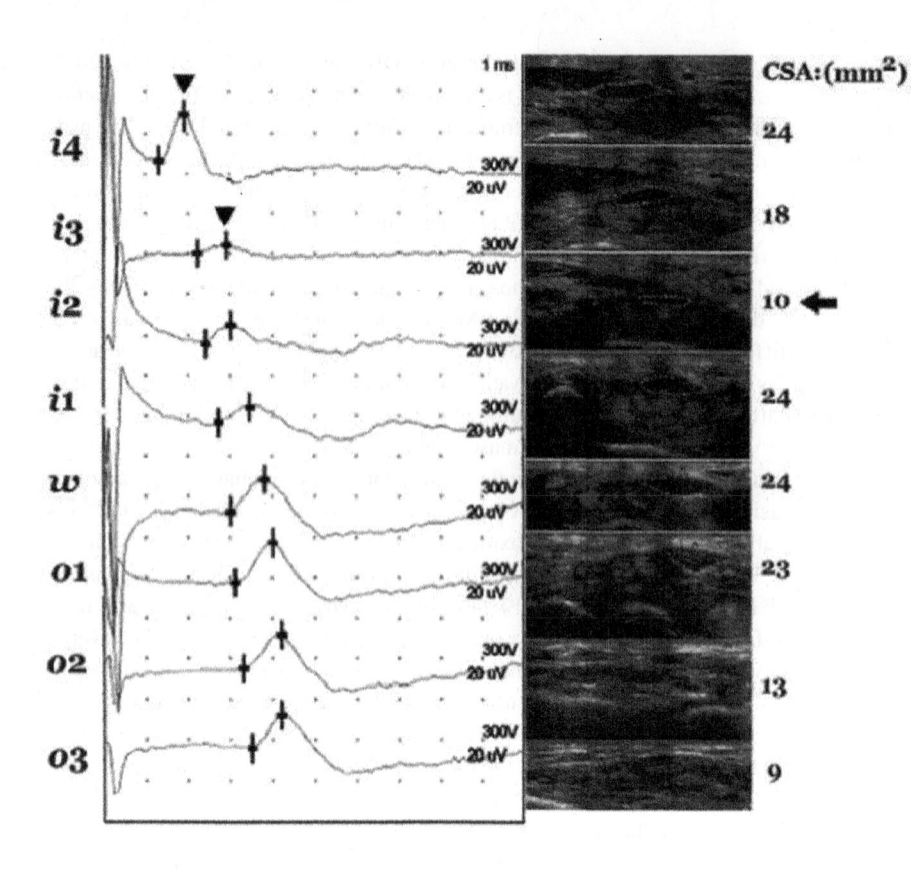

FIGURE 29.7 An example of "positive-site" between i4 and i3 corresponding to the relatively smaller cross-section area (CSA) at i2. The peak latencies (arrowhead) at i4 and i3 are 1.9 ms and 2.9 ms, respectively, and the difference between them is 1.0 ms, i.e. >0.4 ms. The CSA measured at i2 (arrow) is smaller than those measured at nearby levels. Markers of the 8-point: i4, i3, i2, i1, w, o1, o2, and o3.

Interestingly, longer duration of CTS symptoms correlated with a larger measured median nerve CSA, a finding that has not been previously reported. Diabetic patients with CTS also have larger measured median nerve CSA (45).

Ultrasonographic examination of patients with CuTS may also be performed to complement the EDX survey. Cut-off values for the CSA of the ulnar nerve at the level of the medial epicondyle vary from greater than or equal to 7.5 to 7.9 mm^2 (43).

PRACTICE-BASED LEARNING AND IMPROVEMENT

GOALS

Demonstrate competence in continuously investigating and evaluating your own entrapment neuropathy patient care practices, appraising and assimilating scientific evidence, and continuously improving your patient care practices based on constant self-evaluation and lifelong learning.

OBJECTIVES

1. Describe learning opportunities for providers, patients, and caregivers with experience in entrapment neuropathies.
2. Use methods for ongoing competency training in entrapment neuropathies for physiatrists, including formative evaluation feedback in daily practice, evaluating current practice, and developing a systematic quality improvement (QI) and practice improvement (PI) strategy.
3. Locate some resources including available websites for continuing medical education and continuing professional development.
4. Describe some areas paramount to self-assessment and lifelong learning such as review of current guidelines, including evidence-based, in treatment of patients with entrapment neuropathies and the role of the physiatrist as the educator of patients, families, residents, students, colleagues, and other health professionals.

In addition to the evidence-based EDX practice parameters set forth by the AANEM for evaluating patients with suspected peripheral entrapment neuropathies, there are other resources available for physiatrists to assess and improve their knowledge needs. The American Academy of Physical Medicine and Rehabilitation has compiled an extensive listing of EDX didactic case studies, as well as concise synopses of related clinical topics in the PM&R Knowledge NOW database for online learning. Systematic quality reviews and PI strategies for physiatrists caring for patients with peripheral entrapment neuropathies can be found in the May 2013 Supplement to the PM&R journal titled *Electrodiagnostics and Clinical Correlates*. Furthermore, a comprehensive series of live lectures, workshops, and courses dedicated to the advancement of neuromusculoskeletal ultrasound has been established to meet the growing need for continued medical education in this field. Resources for patients and their caregivers are available at the National Institute of Neurological Disorders and Stroke website: www.ninds.nih.gov.

How physicians apply this newly acquired knowledge and skill set to patient care in the clinic or office setting is essential. For example, the medical literature suggests that using normative data for diagnosing CTS in patients with diabetes or in workers with hand-intensive jobs is problematic as the rate of false-positive diagnoses increases (42). QI measures have since been developed using comparison EDX techniques with higher cutoff values (e.g., ≥1.0 ms for sensory latencies and ≥2.0 ms for motor latencies) to avoid this potential problem (42).

The learning curve for neuromusculoskeletal ultrasound is steep as it requires the physician to familiarize himself or herself with normal and pathological sonographic anatomy which can take time to learn. However, the appearance of certain structures under sonographic imaging can be readily appreciated in both their normal and diseased states and, thus, be quickly applied to patient care. Using the median nerve as another example, cut-off values of the median nerve CSA have been proposed to confirm cases of idiopathic CTS. Values of 12.5 mm^2 at the carpal tunnel inlet, 11.5 mm^2 at the distal wrist crease, and 10.1 mm^2 at the carpal tunnel outlet have been used and are easily reproducible on most commercially available ultrasound machines (44); 15 mm^2 has been proposed as the cut-off value for surgical decompression of the median nerve (46).

INTERPERSONAL AND COMMUNICATION SKILLS

GOALS

Demonstrate interpersonal and communication skills that result in the effective exchange of information and collaboration with entrapment neuropathy patients, their families, and other health professionals.

OBJECTIVES

1. Demonstrate skills used in effective communication and collaboration with patients with entrapment neuropathies and their caregivers across socioeconomic and cultural backgrounds.
2. Identify strategies to use in the prevention of reinjury after entrapment neuropathies.
3. Delineate the importance of the role of the physiatrist as the team leader and consultant.
4. Demonstrate proper documentation and effective communication between health care professionals in patient care.

If the physician believes that a patient's symptoms are work related, then this should be documented in the medical record and the patient should be informed of his or her right to file a Workers' Compensation claim. Failure of the physician to document causation or to provide a rationale supporting his or her judgment will delay timely treatment of the patient's condition and prolong symptoms. It is also essential for the physician to document whether or not patients are working, especially during the first 3 months after a diagnosis of CTS is made, as this is the time period where disability and functional status have been shown to undergo the greatest change (8).

Effective communication of a patient's clinical, EDX, and/or sonographic findings to the referring surgeon is an integral part of pre-operative planning for peripheral nerve decompression surgery in patients who have failed non-operative management. More important is the confirmation or elimination of confounding neurological conditions (e.g., cervical/lumbar radiculopathy, brachial/lumbosacral plexopathy) from the differential diagnosis. A careful EDX examination that excludes the presence of a radiculopathy or plexopathy and confirms the presence of a peripheral entrapment neuropathy refutes a more proximal etiology of a patient's painful symptoms. This may help avoid unnecessary spinal surgery and prevent further morbidity, as seen when patients presenting with lower back pain are mandated to have a physiatric consultation prior to surgical referral (47).

High rates of false-positive findings have recently been associated with MRI scans of the lumbar spine, with 27% of normal subjects found to have a disc protrusion in one study (48). The presence of degenerative disease on MRI can offer an attractive explanation for a patient's presumed radicular pain and paresthesias. The physiatrist should be mindful to interpret these imaging studies cautiously in the absence of frank central or foraminal stenosis on the patient's symptomatic side.

The EDX and sonographic impression is also highly valuable to the treating physical or occupational therapist when the etiology of a patient's symptoms is unclear. For example, differentiating an ulnar entrapment neuropathy at the elbow from a C8 radiculopathy may change the patient's treatment plan from manual decompression of the symptomatic cervical neural foramen to neurodynamic mobilization exercises directed at releasing myofascial restrictions that may be entrapping the ulnar nerve at the elbow. This information should also be provided to the patient's primary care physician in an attempt to maintain continuity of care. Prevention of re-injury after successful treatment of a peripheral entrapment neuropathy is challenging, especially in those patients with highly repetitive, hand-intensive jobs. Physician communication with a patient's employer or human resources representative is often necessary to ensure that proper ergonomic modifications are made and work restrictions are adhered to once the patient returns to work.

PROFESSIONALISM

GOAL

Reflect a commitment to carrying out professional responsibilities and an adherence to ethical principles in entrapment neuropathies.

OBJECTIVES

1. Exemplify the humanistic qualities as a provider of care for patients with entrapment neuropathies.
2. Demonstrate ethical principles and responsiveness to patient needs superseding self and other interests.
3. Demonstrate sensitivity to patient population diversity, including culture, gender, age, race, religion, disabilities, and sexual orientation.
4. Respect patient privacy and autonomy.
5. Recognize the importance of patient education in the treatment of and advocacy for persons with entrapment neuropathies.
6. Describe the impact of demographics on the care of persons with entrapment neuropathies.

Physiatrists may likely be the first physicians consulted to make the diagnosis of a peripheral entrapment neuropathy. They are therefore uniquely positioned to help patients navigate the various non-operative and operative treatments available to them. To be an effective patient advocate often requires restraint from recommending overaggressive therapies. This is especially true when counseling older patients who present with long-standing disease who are unlikely to benefit from injections or surgery given their pre-morbid medical history or lower level of functioning.

Helping patients maintain their current level of functioning by recommending the use of adaptive equipment (e.g., button threaders, jar openers) while palliating painful symptoms may help preserve older patients' dignity and foster independence. Older patients with more advanced disease may require static splinting of their hand or foot in a functional position that prevents contracture formation.

Physicians should be sensitive to the fact that the loss of fine motor skills associated with CTS or CuTS may render certain patients unemployable, especially those with hand-intensive jobs. These patients may not have the option of working light duty or retraining for an alternative career. The loss of professional identity may foster the development of a reactive depression that the astute clinician should inquire about and, if present, make the appropriate referral for supportive psychotherapy.

SYSTEMS-BASED PRACTICE

GOALS

Awareness and responsiveness to systems of care delivery, and the ability to recruit and coordinate effectively resources in the system to provide optimal care as it relates to entrapment neuropathies.

OBJECTIVES

1. Identify the components, systems of care delivery, services, referral patterns, and resources in the entrapment neuropathy rehabilitation continuum.
2. Coordinate and recruit necessary resources in the system to provide optimal care for the patient with entrapment neuropathies, with attention to safety, cost awareness, and risk–benefit analysis and management.
3. Introduce QI as a key factor in entrapment neuropathy rehabilitation programs, including identification of systems errors.

The rehabilitation continuum of care for patients with peripheral entrapment neuropathies spans multiple clinical disciplines. Rehabilitation and occupational medicine physicians, orthopedic surgeons and neurosurgeons, physical and occupational therapists, and vocational counselors all may be involved in the health care delivery system for these patients. Although a majority of patient care is delivered in outpatient settings by individual providers, a coordinated multidisciplinary rehabilitation program is often necessary in certain subgroups of patients such as those with orthopedic trauma, polyarticular arthritis, traumatic brain injury, and burn injuries where superimposed peripheral entrapment neuropathies are more common. This system of care, with the physiatrist serving as team leader, is employed primarily in acute rehabilitation settings once the patient is medically stabilized, to expedite functional recovery and promote community reintegration.

For example, an orthopedic trauma patient whose injuries include a proximal tibia–fibula fracture is admitted to the rehabilitation unit of the hospital. The patient underwent a successful open reduction and internal fixation surgery. He is noted to have ankle dorsiflexion weakness as his physical therapist attempts to advance his weight-bearing status. This information is conveyed back to the attending physiatrist who orders EDX testing, which is consistent with a partial lesion of the common peroneal nerve at the level of the fibula head. The patient is placed in a dynamic ankle foot orthosis to assist his dorsiflexion while ambulating. Upon discharge from the rehabilitation unit, an appointment is made for outpatient follow-up in 6 weeks with a repeat EMG planned for 6 months post-discharge to document further neurological recovery.

Safety concerns for patients with peripheral entrapment neuropathies should be discussed at each follow-up visit. If a patient or employer is unable to modify the work activities that were thought to have brought about symptoms, then a referral to a vocational counselor should be made. Braces or splints should be regularly checked to ensure adequate fit without compromising peripheral circulation or causing paresthesias. Close communication with the patient's treating physical or occupational therapist will ensure that these issues do not become problematic. The risks associated with injection therapy and peripheral nerve decompression surgery have previously been discussed.

CASE STUDY

A 45-year-old female assembly line worker presents to clinic with complaints of right wrist pain with numbness and tingling in the first three digits of her right hand. Her symptoms started insidiously over the course of 3 months without antecedent trauma or injury. Physical examination is significant for a positive Tinel's test over the volar aspect of the right wrist, a positive Phalen's test, and slight weakness of thumb abduction. The patient is noted to have decreased pinprick sensation over the median half of her right ring finger compared to the ulnar half consistent with "splitting."

A presumptive diagnosis of CTS was made, and the patient was appropriately counseled. She was placed in a static wrist splint. An EDX study was performed, which was consistent with moderate CTS. An ultrasound examination of the median nerve showed a CSA of approximately 10 mm^2 at the carpal tunnel outlet.

CASE STUDY DISCUSSION QUESTIONS

1. The patient returns to clinic 6 months later complaining of worsening symptoms in her right hand despite brace treatment and work modifications. Discuss the relative risks and benefits of a corticosteroid injection into the carpal tunnel.

2. You are considering repeating the patient's EDX examination. Discuss the utility of including needle EMG as part of the EDX work-up for patients with CTS.
3. Describe the problems using normative data for defining CTS in special populations (i.e., diabetics, workers with hand-intensive jobs) and offer a solution.
4. Describe the most important part of communicating the EDX and/or ultrasonographic findings in patients being considered for surgical intervention.
5. Describe the factors associated with a poor outcome in patients undergoing carpal tunnel decompression surgery.

SELF-EXAMINATION QUESTIONS
(Answers begin on p. 367)

1. Anterior approaches to total hip replacements are best associated with which of the following peripheral entrapment neuropathies?
   A. Pudendal neuropathy
   B. Femoral neuropathy
   C. Sciatic neuropathy
   D. Tibial neuropathy
   E. Peroneal neuropathy

2. Which of the following is the only peroneal-innervated muscle above the knee?
   A. Adductor magnus
   B. Rectus femoris
   C. Short-head biceps femoris
   D. Long-head biceps femoris
   E. Semimembranosus

3. Robinson's CSI has a sensitivity of 83% and a specificity of 95% for diagnosing CTS when the summated latency difference is greater than
   A. 0.3 ms
   B. 0.6 ms
   C. 0.9 ms
   D. 1.2 ms
   E. 1.5 ms

4. Which of the following ulnar-innervated forearm muscles has the highest yield on needle EMG in patients with CuTS?
   A. Medial half FDP
   B. FCU
   C. First dorsal interosseous muscle
   D. Superficial head flexor pollicis brevis
   E. Pronator teres

5. In patients undergoing ultrasonographic evaluation for idiopathic CTS, where is the most likely site of entrapment?
   A. 2 cm proximal to distal wrist crease
   B. 4 cm proximal to distal wrist crease
   C. At the distal wrist crease
   D. 2 cm distal to distal wrist crease
   E. 4 cm distal to distal wrist crease

REFERENCES

1. Katz JN, Stirrat CR. A self-administered hand diagram for the diagnosis of carpal tunnel syndrome. *J Hand Surg.* 1990;15A:360–363.
2. Werner RA, Chiodo A, Spiegelberg T, et al. Use of hand diagrams for screening for ulnar neuropathy: comparison with electrodiagnostic studies. *Muscle Nerve.* 2012;46:891–894.
3. Katz JN, Stirrat CR, Larson MG, et al. A self-administered hand symptom diagram for the diagnosis and epidemiologic study of carpal tunnel syndrome. *J Rheumatol.* 1990;17(11):1495–1498.
4. Moore A, Stringer M. Iatrogenic femoral nerve injury: a systematic review. *Surg Radiol Anat.* 2011;33:649–658.
5. Bohrer JC, Walter MD, Park A, et al. Pelvic nerve injury following gynecologic surgery: a prospective cohort study. *Am J Obstet Gynocol.* 2009;201:531–537.
6. Sorenson EJ, Chen JJ, Daube JR. Obturator neuropathy: causes and outcome. *Muscle Nerve.* 2002;25:605–607.
7. Lifchez SD, Means KR Jr, Dunn RE, et al. Intra- and inter-examiner variability in performing the Tinel's test. *J Hand Surg Am.* 2010;35(2):212–216.
8. Nuckols T, Harber P, Sandin K, et al. Quality measures for the diagnosis and non-operative management of carpal tunnel syndrome in occupational settings. *J Occup Rehabil.* 2011;21:100–119.
9. Page MJ, O'Connor D, Pitt V, et al. Exercise and mobilization interventions for carpal tunnel syndrome. *Cochrane Database Syst Rev.* 2012, Jun 13;6.
10. Page MJ, Massy-Westropp N, O'Connor D, et al. Splinting for carpal tunnel syndrome. *Cochrane Database Syst Rev.* 2012, July 11;(7).
11. Page MJ, O'Connor D, Pitt V, et al. Therapeutic ultrasound for carpal tunnel syndrome. *Cochrane Database Syst Rev.* 2012, Jan 18;(1).
12. Barbosa RI, da Silva Rodrigues EK, Tamanini G, et al. Effectiveness of low-level laser therapy for patients with carpal tunnel syndrome: design of a randomized single-blinded controlled trial. *BMC Musculoskelet Disord.* 2012;13:248.
13. O'Connor D, Marshall S, Massy-Westropp N. Non-surgical treatment (other than steroid injection) for carpal tunnel syndrome. *Cochrane Database Syst Rev.* 2003, Art. No.: CD003219;(1).
14. Visser LH, Ngo Q, Groenwewq SJ, et al. Long term effect of local corticosteroid injection for carpal tunnel syndrome: a relation with electrodiagnostic severity. *Clin Neurophysiol.* 2012;123(4):838–841.
15. Marshall S, Tardif G, Ashworth N. Local corticosteroid injection for carpal tunnel syndrome. *Cochrane Database Syst Rev.* 2007, CD001554;(2).
16. Racasan O, Dubert T. The safest location for steroid injection in treatment of carpal tunnel syndrome. *J Hand Surg Br.* 2005;30(4):412–414.
17. Kim DH, Jang JE, Park BK. Anatomical basis of ulnar approach in carpal tunnel injection. *Pain Physician* 2013;16:E191–E198.
18. Botte MJ, von Schroeder HP, Abrams RA, et al. Recurrent carpal tunnel syndrome. *Hand Clin.* 1996;12:731–743.
19. Fusetti C, Garavaglia G, Mathoulin C, et al. A reliable and simple solution for recalcitrant carpal tunnel syndrome: the hypothenar fat pad flap. *Am J Orthop.* 2009;38:181–186.
20. Strasberg SR, Novak CB, Mackinnon SE, et al. Subjective and employment outcome following secondary carpal tunnel surgery. *Ann Plast Surg.* 1994;32:485–489.
21. Karthik K, Nanda R, Stothard J. Recurrent carpal tunnel syndrome: analysis of the impact of patient personality in altering functional outcome following a vascularized hypothenar fat pad flap surgery. *J Hand Microsurg.* 2012;4(1):1–6.
22. Seradge H, Owens W. Cubital tunnel release with medial epicondylectomy: factors influencing the outcome. *J Hand Surg.* 1998;23A:483–491.

23. Lankester B, Giddins G. Ulnar nerve decompression in the cubital tunnel using local anaesthesia. *J Hand Surg.* 2001;26B:65–66.
24. Athanasakis K, Petrakis I, Karampli E, et al. Pregabalin versus gabapentin in the management of peripheral neuropathic pain associated with post-herpetic neuralgia and diabetic neuropathy: a cost effectiveness analysis for the Greek healthcare setting. *BMC Neurol.* 2013;13:56.
25. Schappert SM, Rechtsteiner EA. *Ambulatory Medical Care Utilization Estimates for 2006.* National Health Statistics Reports, No. 8. Hyattsville, MD: National Center for Health Statistics; 2008:1–29. p. 19.
26. Foley M, Silverstein B, Polissar N. The economic burden of carpal tunnel syndrome: long-term earnings of CTS claimants in Washington State. *Am J Ind Med.* 2007;50(3):155–172.
27. Sunderland S. *Nerves and Nerve Injuries.* New York, NY: Churchill Livingstone; 1978:15.
28. Shea JD, McClain EJ. Ulnar nerve compression syndromes at and below the wrist. *J Bone J Surg.* 1969;51A:1095–1103.
29. Upton A, McComas A. The double crush in nerve entrapment syndromes. *Lancet.* 1973;2:329–362.
30. Sunderland S. The relative susceptibility to injury of the medial and lateral popliteal division of the sciatic nerve. *Br J Surg.* 1953;411:300–302.
31. Stewart JD. Foot drop: where, why and what to do? *Pract Neurol.* 2008;8:158–169.
32. Brown GD, Swanson EA, Nercessian OA. Neurologic injuries after total hip arthroplasty. *Am J Orthop.* 2008;37:191–197.
33. Weber ER, Daube JR, Convenry MB. Peripheral neuropathies associated with total hip arthroplasty. *J Bone Joint Surg Am.* 1976;58:66–69.
34. Windisch G, Braun EM, Anderhuber F. Piriformis muscle: clinical anatomy and consideration of the piriformis syndrome. *Surg Radiol Anat.* 2007;29(1):37–45.
35. Beason LE, Anson BJ. The relation of the sciatic nerve and its subdivisions to the piriformis muscle. *Anat Rec.* 1937;70:1–5.
36. Benzon HT, Katz JA, Benzon HA, et al. Piriformis syndrome: anatomic considerations, a new injection technique, and a review of the literature. *Anesthesiology.* 2003;98:1442–1448.
37. American Academy of Neurology, American Association of Electrodiagnostic Medicine, American Academy of Physical Medicine and Rehabilitation. Practice parameter for electrodiagnostic evaluation of carpal tunnel syndrome: summary statement. *Muscle Nerve.* 2002;25:918–922.
38. American Academy of Neurology, American Association of Electrodiagnostic Medicine, American Academy of Physical Medicine and Rehabilitation. Practice parameter for electrodiagnostic studies in ulnar neuropathy at the elbow: summary statement. *Muscle Nerve.* 1999;22:408–411.
39. Robinson LR, Micklesen P, Wang L. Strategies for analyzing nerve conduction data: superiority of a summary index over single tests. *Muscle Nerve.* 1998;21:1166–1171.
40. Robinson LR, Micklesen PJ, Wang L. Optimizing the number of tests for carpal tunnel syndrome. *Muscle Nerve.* 2000;23:1880–1882.
41. Werner RA, Albers JW. Relation between needle electromyography and nerve conduction studies in patients with carpal tunnel syndrome. *Arch Phys Med Rehabil.* 1995;76:246–249.
42. Werner RA. Electrodiagnostic evaluation of carpal tunnel syndrome and ulnar neuropathies. *PM&R.* 2013;5(5S):18.
43. Kara M, Özçakar L, De Muynck M, et al. Musculoskeletal ultrasound of peripheral nerve lesions. *Eur J Phys Rehabil Med.* 2012;48:665–674.
44. Chen SF, Lu CH, Huang CR, et al. Ultrasonographic median nerve cross-section areas measured by 8-point "inching test" for idiopathic carpal tunnel syndrome: a correlation of nerve conduction study severity and duration of clinical symptoms. *BMC Med Imaging.* 2011;11:22.
45. Chen SF, Huang CR, Tsai NW, et al. Ultrasonographic assessment of carpal tunnel syndrome of mild and moderate severity in diabetic patients by using an 8-point measurement of median nerve cross-sectional areas. *BMC Med Imaging.* 2012;12:15.
46. Lee D, van Holsbeeck MT, Janevski PK, et al. Diagnosis of carpal tunnel syndrome. Ultrasound vs. electromyography. *Radiol Clin North Am.* 1999;37:859–872.
47. Fox J, Haig AJ, Todey B, et al. The effect of required physiatrist consultation on surgery rates of back pain. *Spine.* 2013;38(3):E178–E184.
48. Jensen MC, Brant-Zawadzki MN, Obuchowski N, et al. Magnetic resonance imaging of the lumbar spine in people without back pain. *N Engl J Med.* 1994;331:69–73.

30: Pediatric Traumatic Brain Injury

Rajashree Srinivasan

PATIENT CARE

GOALS

Evaluate and develop a comprehensive rehabilitative plan of care for the pediatric patient with traumatic brain injury (TBI) that is compassionate, appropriate, and effective for the treatment and management of TBI problems and the promotion of health.

OBJECTIVES

1. Describe the key elements of the history and pertinent physical examination of the child with TBI.
2. Describe the key impairments, functional and activity limitations, and participation restrictions in the child with TBI.
3. Describe the psychosocial and vocational implications in the child with TBI and strategies to address them.
4. Describe the impact of TBI on the school-age child in school and community activity.
5. Describe the long-term consequences of pediatric TBI.
6. Describe potential injuries associated with pediatric TBI.
7. Describe the key components of a rehabilitation or treatment plan for the child with TBI.

First, an evaluation is done by the medical team involved in the care of the child. The child's complete medical history—current and past—is obtained from the caregivers. Sometimes, the history may have to be obtained from the medical records as caregivers may not be available, as in the cases of nonaccidental TBI or associated fatalities. The detailed history is followed by a physical examination. The details of the history that the physician should focus on are included in Table 30.1.

Children in distress are naturally apprehensive of strangers. Therefore, it is important to initially observe the child before performing a hands-on examination. Newborns show spontaneous mass movement patterns. A child who is in pain or afraid may not demonstrate a normal movement pattern. Instead, he or she may just lie on the bed or show abnormal patterns of movement when compensating for pain (e.g., antalgic gait pattern when ambulating, guarding a limb when performing bimanual activities). A child in a coma will not interact with the environment. Reflex movements may sometimes be mistaken for purposeful responses to stimulus. It is important to distinguish this with a thorough and consistent examination. These children may need to be examined either on the bed or on the parent's lap. Initial observation is followed by a hands-on examination, performed at the end of the evaluation to minimize the distress associated with the procedure.

The physical examination should be thorough, complete, and cephalocaudal; the physician should have a set blueprint in performing it, so every aspect is addressed. The vitals are documented to ensure stability prior to starting therapies. Documentation of weight-bearing status and use of prophylaxis for deep vein thrombosis when applicable is important. It is also important to document if the child is in a coma, using the Ranchos Los Amigos Scale or the Rappaport Scale. The head and neck examination is followed by detailed examinations of the cardiorespiratory system, abdomen, and central nervous system. Skin examination should document any rashes, breakdown, or wounds/sutures/staples. It is important to document when the sutures/staples have to be removed. If a tracheostomy is present, the physician should note its size and take care to ensure that a spare is present at the patient's bedside. Gastrostomy sites should be examined to determine if there is any leakage, skin irritation, or signs of infection.

In the ICU setting, as the focus is on ensuring medical stability, range of motion can be performed; the physician should also monitor heart rate and note any signs of distress. The child can be placed in splints/positioning braces at the ankles and the wrists for proper positioning. Once in the rehabilitation setting, strength and sensory testing are performed, as well as evaluations for any early contracture formation. Also, it is important to evaluate for any occult fractures that may be missed or the presence of associated spinal cord injury. Associated amputations can complicate the rehabilitation process, particularly if the weight-bearing limb is the one that has non-weight-bearing restrictions.

Cognitive ability also plays an enormous role in the rehabilitative process. The child may not remember not to place any weight on the limb if there are any documented restrictions, and may require frequent cueing to maintain the non-weight-bearing status. The restrictions compound the impairments, both physically and cognitively, particularly if there are weight-bearing

TABLE 30.1 History Taking-Points to Focus On

History of present illness	Modality of injury, motor vehicle accident, nonaccidental traumatic brain injury, all-terrain vehicle rollover, gunshot injuries, injury with sports; was the child adequately restrained—seat belt, car seat with restraints, time needed to extract; presence of drugs or alcohol; Glasgow Coma Scale, loss of consciousness, seizures at the scene, presence of posturing, presence of dirty wounds, additional wounds
Medical and surgical history	Surgical procedures like intramedullary nailing, open reduction and internal fixation of fractures, wound debridements, sutures of lacerations, presence of any grafts, placement of any central lines, duration of placement of external ventricular drain, ventricular peritoneal drain, electrolyte abnormalities, presence of additional injuries, spinal cord injury, extremity fractures, liver and spleen lacerations, lung contusion
Past medical history	History of brain injury; history of ADHD; developmental history; history of any allergies to medications; list of medications
Social history/family history	Number of people in the family available to provide support to the family; any problems with behavioral issues in the family; any history of drug use in the family; the kind of house they live in; whether caregivers are physically capable of taking care of the child
Review of systems	Focus on spasticity, decerebrate and decorticate posturing, dysphagia, dysautonomia, seizures, and weakness. Was there a history of infection? How long was the child on the ventilator? Did the child need to have a tracheostomy and was a gastrostomy tube placed?

restrictions in an existing limb after amputation (depending on the level). Depending on the ability of the patient, he or she might sit up on the edge of the bed, or in a chair—if able to do so with adequate head and trunk control—providing assistance when necessary. Use of standing frames, tilt tables, wheelchairs for positioning and mobility, and development of skills is of paramount importance. Spasticity may interfere with these, requiring aggressive range of motion and providing splinting and orthoses, serial casting, and medications.

Autonomic dysfunction is an important complication of severe TBI. The incidence is 8% to 9.3%. The condition is caused by disruption of inhibitory activity from the brainstem. causing sympathetic outflow (1). It is usually triggered and exacerbated by any noxious stimuli like a full bladder, incomplete bowel evacuation, and spasticity, underlying infection, deep vein thrombosis, heterotopic ossification, or progressive hydrocephalus. Patients present with increased heart rate or blood pressure, tachypnea, hyperpyrexia, sweating episodes, and posturing. Addressing the underlying cause usually diminishes the symptoms. The presence of dysautonomia should be a cautious indicator when performing therapies.

Patients in a coma are usually evaluated based on their responsiveness to their surroundings. There are various scales used: Rappaport Scale, Ranchos Los Amigos Scale (Revised), Western Neuro Sensory Stimulation Profile, and the JFK Coma Recovery Scale (Revised), to name a few. The Glasgow Coma Scale (GCS) is unsuitable for use in the rehabilitation setting as it does not predict outcomes in brain injury or guide treatment.

Depending on the part of the brain injured, severity of the injury, and resulting complications, post-TBI effects are varied. The patients may continue in a persistent vegetative state, needing tracheostomy and gastrostomy support. They may continue to have tetraparesis, spasticity setting in, and contractures developing later. Improvements in physical conditions are varied, with complete physical recovery—including ability to ambulate to hemiparesis with a circumducted gait pattern—being seen. Spasticity may be persistent, affecting activities of daily living, positioning, and ambulation. These may be seen as long-term complications.

Associated dysfunctions in TBI include olfactory dysfunction (anosmia, a common consequence, seen with severe TBI). There is questionable association of anosmia with executive function. Hearing impairment may be due to central processing deficit, peripheral nerve damage, cochlear injury, or disruption of middle ear structures. Vertigo secondary to vestibular impairment resolves within 6 months of injury; however, electronystagmogram abnormalities can persist for years. Central auditory processing deficits are seen due to damage to tracts or cortical tissue. Normal pure tone audiometry is seen, but speech discrimination or late waveforms of brainstem auditory evoked potentials are abnormal. Conductive hearing loss is seen due to disruption of ossicles, or the presence of cerebrospinal fluid (CSF) or blood in the middle ear, which is associated with fractures of temporal bone. Conductive hearing loss resolves spontaneously in 3 weeks. If recovery is greater than 3 weeks (especially for 30 db), repeat audiogram and exploration of the middle ear are recommended. Fluid in the middle ear usually resolves spontaneously. Sensorineural hearing loss is noted at higher frequencies and associated with inner-ear pathology. Eighth cranial nerve pathology or injury to the labyrinthine capsule, or labyrinthine concussion, causes hearing loss because of transmission of high-energy vibrations and a pattern similar to hearing loss after prolonged exposure. Injuries to the labyrinthine capsule and eighth cranial nerve are associated with basilar skull fracture.

Visual impairments include visual acuity deficit as the most common deficit seen with frontal lobe injuries. Visual impairments may be associated with more severe neuropsychological impairments. Temporal lobe involvement causes visual memory impairment; parietal lobe involvement causes impairment of spatial awareness. Diplopia is due to extraocular muscle imbalance due to trochlear palsy, sixth nerve palsy, or difficulties with convergence seen due to supranuclear impairment (1). It is important to be vigilant about electrolyte imbalances and neuroendocrine dysfunctions like syndrome of inappropriate antidiuretic hormone secretion (SIADH), Diabetes Insipidus (DI), and cerebral salt wasting and address them as they arise.

Speech impediments may be seen in the form of dysarthria, word-finding problems, grammatical errors, or understanding social cues. This can complicate communication further, deepening the patient's gorge of social isolation.

Neuropharmacologic agents are frequently used in the acute rehabilitation setting. Medications typically used are dopamine agonists like amantadine, methylphenidate, gamma-amino butyric acid (GABA), agonists like baclofen, and anticonvulsants like phenytoin and lamotrigine, to name a few (2). It is important to be able to identify side effects and adverse reactions.

Spasticity is defined as velocity-dependent resistance to stretch. Treatment of spasticity is based on whether function is affected, caregiving including hygiene becomes difficult, and positioning in bed and wheelchair is very difficult. It is measured by the Ashworth and Modified Ashworth Scales, and the Tardieu Scale. Range-of-motion exercises, stretching, and placement of orthoses are noninvasive methods of managing spasticity. Use of oral medications like baclofen and diazepam (GABA receptors), tizanidine (α1 antagonist), or dantrolene (acts on sarcoplasmic reticulum) should be monitored for side effects like sedation, abnormalities of liver enzyme, hypotension, and liver and renal dysfunctions. Use of dantrolene in the pediatric patient should be circumspect, prompting the physician to monitor liver function tests regularly. Chemodenervation with botulinum toxin injections or phenol injections has been shown to be helpful in reducing spasticity. Intrathecal baclofen (ITB) pump placement has been found to be extremely helpful in the day-to-day activities by managing spasticity efficiently. It should, however, be noted that ITB in children should be managed with care as children are dependent on the adult caregivers for regular maintenance. It is also important to emphasize the criticality of not refilling the ITB use in a timely fashion, as the result is far more life threatening and can result in death, stressing the also importance of proper education and proper selection of candidates for the placement. Selective dorsal root rhizotomy is a permanent surgical procedure used more often in children with cerebral palsy that has been found to be helpful in managing spasticity.

Table 30.2 provides a list of areas to monitor after brain injury.

Physical therapists focus on range of motion, stretching, strengthening of lower extremities, transfer and mobility training, ambulation and assistive devices needed for ambulation, evaluation of splints and adaptive equipment, and family training. Occupational therapists focus on evaluating activities of daily living like eating, brushing one's teeth, toileting, bathing, dressing, and upper extremity range of motion, stretching, strengthening, evaluating for splints and assistive devices, cognitive screen, and family training. Occupational therapists also evaluate for visual, spatial, and perceptual deficits. Speech and language therapists evaluate swallow function, communication skills, thinking, and processing. If unsure of the swallow status of a patient, a bed swallow usually provides the answer until a modified barium swallow can be performed by the speech therapists. Neuropsychologists evaluate the patient's ability to think and process

TABLE 30.2 To Monitor After Brain Injury

AREAS TO MONITOR	INTERVENTIONS THAT CAN BE HELPFUL
Spasticity/contractures	Timely management of spasticity either with range of motion, bracing, serial casting, medications, chemodenervation, or surgical options; once contractures set in, recognition of surgical options is needed to maximize function
Aspiration pneumonia	Recognition of dysphagia to minimize risk of aspiration and educate families about the same; well-meaning families may feed their loved one under the mistaken impression of doing good
Endocrine problems	Monitor for hypothyroidism by following up on TSH, free T4; monitor urine output, oral intake output where concerns of diabetes exist; depending on the location and severity of injury, important to monitor for hypopituitarism, DI, and SIADH; precocious puberty can be seen 2–17 months after initial injury
Hydrocephalus	Change in neurological status, altered mental status, loss of bladder control; loss of balance should prompt a workup for hydrocephalus
Pressure sores/fractures	Frequent turning, as well as monitoring skin with skin checks, can decrease the incidence of pressure sores from forming. Once developed, care focus should be on early resolution to prevent the worsening complications of infections, sepsis, and osteomyelitis
Social isolation	Reintegration into school and community is important and should be achieved at the earliest moment possible. Return to school may depend upon the endurance level and may warrant starting off with half days and working up to full days. Community resources should be provided such as local brain injury chapters and so on. Physiatrists should familiarize themselves with the IDEA Act, ensuring education for all handicapped children (Pub law-94-142)

information, determine impulse control, and determine the best strategy to facilitate learning.

One of the key components to coordinated care for the patient is the ability to provide a continuum of care. This spans inpatient and outpatient programs. Typically, inpatient programs provide therapies on a daily basis 5 to 6 times a week, particularly during the acute phase of recovery. Once the recovery plateaus off, or slow progress is seen, then outpatient therapies are set up. It is important for the outpatient therapists to have access to documentation to the inpatient progress as this provides a basis for future care. For instance, if the patient had performed certain activities during the inpatient stay that he or she is unable to replicate, then it may indicate either that the recovery has slowed off or a worsening neurological status needing further evaluation is present.

Brain injury is a leading cause of morbidity and mortality in children. The range of severity varies from concussion to persistent vegetative state (3). Despite improvements in care and rehabilitation, the impact of brain injury on children and their families is enormous with regard to finances and caregiver burden, to name a few factors. Children may be left with residual hemiparesis, speech deficits including dysarthria, aphasia, or behavioral problems, all of which impact the patient's return to school and reintegration into the community. Schools can be preinformed about the limitations that a student has, so that they can be prepared for that child and make return to school as seamless as possible. An educational program can be provided to the patient, family, and school to help facilitate care and understand needs.

Children may recover with residual long-term complications of hemiparesis, vision deficits, spasticity, gait abnormality, behavioral problems, frontal disinhibition, attentional problems, problems with hearing, and cognitive delays.

Discharge disposition should be identified at the time of admission to ensure adequate training is complete by discharge. The process of discharging the patient begins at admission. Based on the recovery a patient makes, appropriate equipment is ordered. A wheelchair may need to be ordered on a rental basis for a child making rapid recovery. For a patient who is able to ambulate by the time of discharge, a wheelchair may be needed only for long distances for endurance. As spasticity evolves during the stay, it may be wiser to order orthoses closer to discharge as they may not fit well otherwise. The same principle also holds for ordering equipment for the patients.

MEDICAL KNOWLEDGE

GOALS

Demonstrate knowledge of differences in pediatric versus adult TBI, and established and evolving biomedical, clinical epidemiological, and sociobehavioral sciences pertaining to the field of pediatric TBI, as well as the application of this knowledge to guide patient-centered holistic care.

OBJECTIVES

1. Describe the pertinent anatomy, physiology, pathophysiology, and epidemiology relevant to pediatric TBI rehabilitation.
2. Identify developmental milestones that should be addressed to develop a successful rehabilitation program.
3. Describe the various diagnostic tests available in the care of children and adolescents with brain injury and their advantages and limitations.
4. Describe the fundamental principles that are relevant to the treatment of children and adolescents with brain injury.

Brain injury is the leading cause of death and disability in children and adolescents. In the United States, three TBIs occur every minute (4); 5.3 million people live with TBI-related disability. TBI costs Americans $76.5 billion in medical care, rehabilitation, and loss of work every year.

According to the CDC, the two age groups at greatest risk for TBI are ages 0 to 4 and 15 to 19 years. Among 0 to 19 years, 62,000 need hospitalization due to motor vehicle accidents, falls, sports injuries, physical abuse, and other causes; 564,000 children are seen in the emergency room for TBI and released. In children between 0 and 14 years, TBI causes 2,685 deaths, 37,000 hospitalizations, and 435,000 emergency department visits. Approximately 1,300. children in the United States experience severe or fatal head trauma from child abuse each year (5).

There are two age peaks for patients with TBI—one below age 5 and the other in mid to late adolescence. Incidence is higher in the males when compared to females (60%:40%). A history of preexisting attention deficit hyperactivity disorder is seen with a prevalence of 10% to 20%. Motor vehicle accidents are the commonest cause of TBI in adolescents at 66% and at 20% in children. Nonaccidental TBI is the cause of brain injury in 17% of infants and 5% of those between 1 and 4 years. Falls account for 39% of brain injury in children less than 14 years. Falls are the leading cause of injury in children less than 4 years. Association of other injuries, such as undetected fractures, is about 50% (1).

Brain injury differs in children when compared to adults. Brain development is a complex process starting in the third gestational week and continuing through early adulthood. Neurulation, proliferation, migration, dendritic development, synaptogenesis, differentiation, and apoptosis transform primitive neural tubes to a series of complex neural networks comprising the central nervous system (CNS) (6). The growing brain is more susceptible to insult and injury with long-lasting effects. Severity of injury, age at injury, and environment (social factors, family support, and interventions) impact recovery. Impact, as well as deceleration and rotational forces due to the large head, weak neck musculature, higher brain water content, and lack of myelination, contribute to the primary injury. The noted factors make it easier to transmit forces to deeper brain structures.

Primary injury includes blunt injury, gunshot wounds, contusions on the brain surface, and shear-type injury associated with deceleration and rotational forces. Primary injury is due to mechanical disruption of axons and membranes (1). Secondary injury occurs due to complications after the initial trauma (Table 30.3).

Diffuse swelling and second impact injury due to diffuse cerebral swelling occur more in children than adults. This is due to increased diffusion of excitotoxic neurotransmitters through the immature brain, with increased blood–brain barrier permeability after injury to the immature brain. Diffuse cerebral edema is associated with poor outcome. Cerebral blood flow varies with age—24 cm/s in healthy newborns, 97 cm/s in children 6 to 9 years, and then decreasing to adult value of 50 cm/s. Possible lower middle cerebral artery perfusion rate in children causes hypoperfusion. Second impact syndrome is due to repeated concussion in children and adolescents.

TABLE 30.3 Secondary Injury

Causes	Hypotension, vasospasm, infarction, prolonged seizure activity, diffuse edema resulting in increased intracranial pressure, and decreased cerebral perfusion pressure
Biochemical cascades involved	Cellular power failure, acidosis, overstimulation of excitatory neurotransmitter receptors, lipid membrane peroxidation, increase in intracellular calcium, and cellular damage by free radicals

Nonaccidental TBI is characterized by a triad of subdural hemorrhage, retinal hemorrhage, and encephalopathy with an incompatible history of mechanism of injury. The history of mechanism of injury does not match the actual injury.

The Glasgow Outcome Scale is a functional outcome scale rating patients into death through vegetative state to recovery (Table 30.4).

Given how common TBI is in the pediatric population, it is important to be able to pay attention to the developmental aspects of rehabilitation. Developmental milestones are critical factors in the development of any rehabilitation program. It is imperative to take growth and development into account while devising any rehabilitation program in children. Infants who suffer nonaccidental TBI do not have the repertoire that older children and adults have to fall back on. For children who have been able to sit, stand, and walk, the rehabilitation program should include developing these skills. It is important to remember that children who have prior developmental delay will have more to work on to reach their baselines.

Primitive reflexes may resurface after a brain injury, causing difficulty in positioning and in therapies. It is important to know what the child was capable of prior to the injury to ensure proper goals are established. Developmental assessment is dependent on parental history. It is important to note if the child had the opportunity to learn the said skill, such as knowing body parts and colors in a 2-year-old. The rehabilitation goals should be individualized to each child and not necessarily based on protocols as each child is different.

Growth and development play a key role in the ever-changing face of brain injury. Not only do children lack the rich experiential knowledge an adult has, but they also have to assimilate the process of development and maturation while striving to achieve altered milestones. Deficits may not be apparent initially and present later as the child grows. This is particularly seen in infants who have suffered brain injury and may initially do well physically but later show cognitive and functional deficits.

Table 30.5 provides a list of tests that can be performed in the care of children with brain injury. It should be noted that this is by no means exhaustive as research is ongoing.

It is important to discuss the extent of the injury with the family so that they understand the intricacies involved in the care of the patient.

Access to proper health care is a desirable goal. Physicians must remember to do no harm in medicine. It is easy to get carried away in our quest for "proper care" of the patient. It is, however, important to remember to take the wishes/beliefs of the patient/family into consideration while making a recommendation. All of the information should be provided to the patient/family. For instance, if a procedure is associated with risk of more harm than benefit, then it should be discussed with the family/patient before being performed. The concept of beneficence should be inbuilt in patient care to ensure that the welfare of the patient is foremost. For example, it would be important to discuss the risks and benefits of performing an ITB pump placement in a patient with severe spasticity. The procedure is not without complications and carries the risks of anesthesia reaction, blood loss during surgery, malfunction of the pump, infection, overdosage or underdosage/withdrawal, and lack of commitment to follow up regularly for maintenance of the pump. These issues have to be discussed, along with an evaluation of the social situation; this includes the family's ability (i.e., adequate transportation) and determination to keep appointments, as missing a refill can prove fatal.

Also, the limitations of the payer source should be taken into consideration, as the payer source may pay for the procedure and not for the ongoing maintenance of the pump, jeopardizing the patient's life. It is also important to provide the family/patient with all the information prior to the procedure to enable an informed decision to be made, understanding that what we may recommend may be incongruous with family and patient values. Hence, the recommendations may not be accepted. It is important to be supportive to the patient/family in their autonomous decision. It is crucial to recognize the autonomy of the adolescent patient while addressing family issues as these may differ.

TBI impacts and challenges success in the school system, also affecting the social realm. It is important to educate parents and caregivers about the deficits and provide them with information and strategies on how this can be addressed. Pediatric

TABLE 30.4 Rating of Brain Injury Severity

	MILD	MODERATE	SEVERE	PROFOUND
Initial GCS	13–15 with no deterioration	9–12 with no deterioration	3–8	
PTA Post Traumatic Amnesia	<1 hr	1–24 hr	>24 hr	
Duration of unconsciousness	<15–30 min	15 min to 24 hr	1–90 days	>90 d

TABLE 30.5 Benefits and Limitations of Procedures in Brain Injury

TEST	BENEFITS	LIMITATIONS
MRI of head and neck; Magnetic resonance angiography	Effective in obtaining information about structural damage to the brain, including evidence of diffuse axonal injury, hydrocephalus, encephalomalacia Lesser exposure to radiation Associated information regarding cervical ligamentous injury can be obtained Information about vascular structures obtainable	As obtaining an MRI requires a child to lay still, sedation may be required to complete the test, adding to its risks. Difficult to perform in a person with claustrophobia If being performed with contrast, there is a risk of the contrast dye causing an allergic or anaphylactic reaction Not helpful for evidence of molecular damage Need transfer to radiology in the main/acute care hospital as the services may not be available in a rehabilitation setting Difficult to perform on a patient on a ventilator
Computed axial tomography of head and neck	Effective in providing information about fractures, acute bleeds, and hydrocephalus Quick to perform	Risk of exposure to radiation; hence, cannot be done repeatedly Need to be transferred to radiology in the acute care hospital
Ultrasound of head	Provides immediate information regarding ventricular size and acute bleeds	Requires a patent fontanelle to perform the procedure Needs a skilled person to perform the procedure and interpret the results in a timely fashion
X-rays of chest, extremities	Can be obtained easily to follow up on the rehabilitation unit	Risk of radiation with repeated exposure
Transcranial magnetic stimulation	Used in measuring connection between primary motor cortex and muscle to evaluate extent of damage Generates electric current without physical contact	Risk of inducing seizures, fainting, pain, headache Electrode heating can cause skin burns
Functional MRI	MRI that measures brain activity by detecting associated changes in blood flow	Difficult in patients with claustrophobia. Loud-pitched noises are disruptive Malfunction of pacemakers may occur Close monitoring in patients with fever, diabetes, and circulatory problems seen due to heating of the coil Static magnetic field can pull nearby metal objects, converting them to projectile objects
Somatosensory evoked potentials	SEP from lower limbs can be helpful in monitoring postacute phase of TBI and in identifying patients needing further intensive rehabilitation	Pediatric values in brain injury not as standardized and may not be available everywhere, having more of a research implication
Tractography—3D modeling technique to visually represent neural tracts by diffusion tensor imaging	Results obtained in 2- and 3-dimensional images	Shows path of least resistance to water diffusion, which may not correspond to the actual fibers Unable to detect anterograde and retrograde pathways, synapses, presence of functional pathway
Doppler ultrasound	Useful for detecting deep vein thrombosis Carotid Dopplers are useful for detecting blood flow in cases of arterial damage	Need transfer to radiology as this may not be available in a rehabilitation setting
Triple-phase bone scan	Effective in detecting heterotopic ossification, occult fractures	Need repeated transfers to radiology to complete the test Risk of allergy or anaphylaxis to the contrast agent
Blood work—alkaline phosphatase	May be an early marker for heterotopic ossification	Nonspecific test

rehabilitation of brain injury focuses not only on the medical and rehabilitation aspect, but also on the integration into schools and the community.

It was initially erroneously thought that children recovered better from brain injury when compared to adults. This has been disproved with ongoing research showing that children have more of a functional impact due to brain injury. They do not have the same repertoire of information and experience available to them to utilize and fall back on. The relatively high plasticity of a developing brain could have a negative impact on overall outcome after diffuse TBI and be partially responsible for poorer outcomes seen in those injured at a very young age.

Many patients may recover well physically but are left with many cognitive, behavioral, and emotional problems. Language-related deficits seen in mild and severe TBI include verbal and learning memory, word finding, discourse, metalinguistic tasks, abstract and indirect language, complex lexical-semantic and morphosyntactic manipulation, effective reading of others, mental states, social communication, and behavioral self-regulation (7). Children injured before 8 years of age are more impaired than those injured later in life (8). Story retelling correlates with measures of executive functioning (9). Functional memory problems are seen in worsening academic growth curves over years after TBI.

General impulsivity, frontal disinhibition, increased aggressive behavior, and communication problems cause problems with social interaction. Language problems after TBI are due to cognitive and executive system impairments (7). Adolescents with TBI process social information less efficiently than typical normally developing peers (10). In practice based learning, sentence should read- The physiatrist should also be aware of community and school resources available for children with brain injuries.

Growing skull fracture occurs when a linear skull fracture in a child less than 3 years of age is accompanied by a dural tear and a leptomeningeal cyst develops. Fluid pulsations cause bone erosion and a palpable skull defect needing skull repair.

At 1 year after injury, 46% are able to ambulate independently without assistive device; 27% ambulate with an orthotic or assistive device; 79% have independent mobility according to one study. Children with TBI have marked reduction in gait velocity, stride length, cadence, and balance; hand function tests show deficits in fine motor skills, speed, and coordination. Hand function skills improve less than gait; degree of impairment increases with severity of injury. Younger age is not associated with better recovery. Absence of spasticity is a good predictor of ambulation recovery by discharge. Impaired fine motor skills, including slowing, are seen (1).

Twenty-five percent of pediatric concussions are associated with athletic activity (11); 9% of high-school athletic injuries are due to concussions, the highest rates being in contact and collision sports. Concussion is due to rotational acceleration of the brain, thought to be due to weaker cervical musculature versus greater force causing injury in a smaller individual. Children present with a period of lucidity followed by deterioration. This is thought to be due to diffuse brain swelling due to differences in glutamate expression, expression of aquaporin 4 by microglia, and brain water content.

Neuropsychological testing is sensitive in picking out the subtle differences that present. There is a relationship between age and outcome. Long-term sequelae are seen in younger children with brain injury. (The reader is referred to McCrory et al. "Consensus Statement on Concussion in Sport: The 3rd International Conference on Concussion in Sport, Zurich, Switzerland," Nov 2008, *Br J Sports Med.* 2009;43[Suppl]:76-90 for further details.)

Mild TBI can be followed in an outpatient setting. However, it is important to note that children with mild TBI are deceptively well functioning physically and may be able to mask their cognitive deficits, compounding the fact that they fall through the cracks in the system. Recognition of mild TBI, concussion, and return to play should be rigorously monitored. Patients can present with headache, dizziness, academic problems, and behavioral and personality changes. Having a working knowledge of these symptoms and ensuring a preparticipation physical may be helpful in decreasing the morbidity involved.

PRACTICE-BASED LEARNING AND IMPROVEMENT

GOALS

Demonstrate competence in continuously investigating and evaluating your own pediatric TBI patient care practices, appraising and assimilating scientific evidence, and continuously improving your patient care practices based on constant self-evaluation and lifelong learning.

OBJECTIVES

1. Identify areas of lifelong learning and self-assessment of strengths and deficiencies for physiatrists with respect to pediatric brain injury.
2. Identify evidence-based medicine resources and clinical practice guidelines that physiatrists can use in the area of pediatric brain injury.
3. Identify key points that physiatrists should emphasize in the education of patients and their families with respect to pediatric brain injury, its treatment, and impact on patient's life activities.

Physiatrists providing care for children with TBI should have a working knowledge of the key elements of the medical history and physical examination of the child who sustained such an injury. The physiatrist should be able to identify impairments, activity limitations, and participation restrictions and then, in conjunction with members of the rehabilitation team, develop rehabilitation programs to address them. The physiatrist should be able to recognize patient safety concerns in this population and implement strategies to minimize them from occurring. The physiatrist should be up-to-date on advances in the understanding of the pathophysiology of brain injury in children and its treatment. The physiatrist should also be aware of community and school resources available for children with brain injury who live in their communities. Lastly, it is equally important that physiatrists have the necessary interpersonal and communication skills to effectively provide care for their patients and advocate for their needs.

There are several strategies that physiatrists can use to identify gaps in their knowledge base about pediatric TBI and the medical and rehabilitative care of these patients. Self-reflection on their clinical practice, self-assessment examinations, and asking trusted colleagues to provide feedback to them on their practice are some examples. Seeking feedback from the families and caregivers of these children is another.

To offer best care, it is important to be able to provide the latest information regarding the care of the child with TBI. Hence it is valuable to be aware of resources like MD consult, Ovid searches, PubMed searches, and Cochrane reviews, to name a few. There are numerous journals on rehabilitation such as *PMR* (published by AAPMR), *Archives of PMR, Pediatric Rehabilitation, Brain, Neurorehabilitation, Pediatrics, Seminars in Pediatric Neurology,* and *Neuropsychological Journals,* all featuring the latest information. The AAPMR also has online educational tools with topics that are pertinent to pediatric rehabilitation such as Knowledge NOW (12). For physiatrists interested in this subspecialty of rehabilitation medicine, there are also advanced training opportunities through fellowships in pediatric rehabilitation.

Once the child is discharged home, the family becomes the primary caregiver, expert in that child's and in being the child's advocate. Hence, patient and family education should be addressed from day 1. There are various aspects that need to be covered. As the care of a child with special needs is very complex and families have had to deal with a catastrophic change, it is not uncommon for them to be overwhelmed with all the information being presented. The families need constant education, repeated multiple times, and the willingness of the staff to provide education as the need arises. They should be educated to ask questions and be their child's advocate.

Table 30.6 provides a checklist.

INTERPERSONAL AND COMMUNICATION SKILLS

GOALS

Demonstrate interpersonal and communication skills that result in the effective exchange of information and collaboration with pediatric TBI patients, their families, and the rest of the rehabilitation team.

OBJECTIVES

1. Identify key areas for physicians to counsel patients and families, across socioeconomic and cultural backgrounds, specific to pediatric TBI.
2. Identify key points to be documented in patient records to provide effective communication between team members with respect to pediatric TBI.

Families are under a lot of duress in the hospital setting. Siblings of patients also undergo a lot of stress and anger. They may feel neglected. Child life personnel and rehabilitation psychologists are trained in helping patients and their siblings learn about their impairments and how to help them. They are also able to provide both patients and families with coping strategies in the wake of the devastation faced by the families. It is very important to be able to clearly state what the ongoing needs are while being sympathetic and empathetic to the distress the family is undergoing. Families may need to be given the information time and again as they may not necessarily process all the information. The feelings of denial and anger being experienced by families may create barriers to assimilating information.

It may be necessary for more than one team member to discuss the information with the families. Members involved in the care of children with TBI include physiatrists, physical therapist, occupational therapist, speech therapist, neuropsychologist, dietician, teacher, child life therapist, and nurses. Depending on the setting—an acute care hospital, a rehabilitation hospital, or a subacute facility—access to specialists may be limited. It is important at such times for all team members to be consistent in providing information as difference in the nature of information creates confusion and lack of trust in the treating team. This creates a divide among team members and also among parents. It is important for health care providers to be able to provide accurate information to families not tainted by personal emotions and outlook. There may be dissension among the team members and the families. It is imperative to come to a working relationship despite the differences between the two to guarantee safe and adequate care for the patient. Information should be provided in a nonthreatening and nonjudgmental manner.

Teams can provide well-coordinated care. For instance, when a child has issues with blood pressure evident with any of the therapies, communication to the medical team can prompt workup for dysautonomia or hypertension, which can address the issues either with a CT of the head or by looking for inciting factors like infection, electrolyte disturbances, deep vein thrombosis (DVT), and so on.

When information is presented to families, they are under so much stress that the information is not assimilated and understood. It may be necessary to present the information frequently and in small amounts to help them understand various aspects of care. Families may be in denial about the extent of injuries and disabilities. It is important to assess the literacy of families to help provide better educating tools. It is also valuable in identifying barriers to learning.

Proper documentation of patient status is important from a medical and legal stance. Also, it is good care. It is necessary to document weight-bearing status, any associated injuries, social limitations, and so on, to be able to provide better care. In an inpatient setting, it is necessary to document the extent to which the patient and his or her family have been educated. Communication errors frequently happen at transition points when the patient is admitted from acute care, at the time of discharge, and at times of nursing and physician shift changes. Information being translated to another person can very easily be misunderstood; improper transcription of medications can occur; if families do not understand the proper application of orthotics, skin problems ensue. A lot of these issues can be addressed by the maintenance of electronic health records, adequate and safe handoffs, providing families with printed documentation of medications, and donning and doffing of orthoses. Documentation of patient and family education is helpful with addressing legal issues. Adequate documentation is also useful in helping the physiatrist be a better advocate for the patient.

Not only is it stressful to be in a hospital setting during the acute injury and recovery phase, but a new journey also begins

TABLE 30.6 Rehabilitation Checklist for Families

Technology training: Tracheostomy care	Families should be trained in the care of tracheostomies, their replacements, identification of mucous plugs, and ensuring adequate supplies at home. Ideally two caregivers should be trained. (This is per the American Thoracic Society recommendations, 2012.)
Nasogastric (NG) or gastrostomy (G) tube care	Gastrostomy tube or NG tube care should be suitable to ensure adequate nutrition. Families should be trained in the placement of NG tubes, checking their placement, and recognizing when the child is in trouble. They should also be trained in the actual feeding of the child via either a gastrostomy tube or NG tube
Ventilator care	If there is a chance that the child needs to be on a ventilator, transition should be made to appropriate home ventilators, and families should be trained in the management of the ventilator. Family training is becoming more of a norm. Children with complex medical conditions need nursing care. However, this may not be available to them, depending on the payor source. Hence, families are trained
Medications: Oral, NG, or administration via G tube	Families should be trained in the administration of the medicine either via a G tube, NG tube, or orally. Proficiency must be documented prior to discharge
Transfers, bed mobility, range of motion	It is important to teach families proper techniques for transfers from wheelchair to bed and vice versa, positioning the child in bed in a fashion to minimize contractures from forming and skin breakdown from happening. By the same token, it is important to teach families to perform transfers, position the child, and perform necessary home exercises in a safe fashion, to where they do not hurt themselves in the process
Transportation: Car seats/EZ-ON vests	It is important to evaluate the child for transportation and educate the family regarding safe processes. Car seats with appropriate restraints and supports should be evaluated with families. Children who are unable to sit up in a car may need to lie down in the back with an EZ-ON vest. This is helpful for children who do not have either adequate head and neck control or have spasticity interfering with positioning. The vest can be strapped on safely and the child is able to lie down and be safely transported
Community reintegration and return to school	Families should be educated to appreciate the cognitive and behavioral impairments that the child with TBI has. This impacts school, socialization, and relationships at school and home. Families should be equipped with techniques to defuse situations. Lack of safety awareness puts the child at risk for exploitation and risk of violence. Deficits due to TBI may put the child at physical risk: for instance, anosmia may put a child at risk when there is gas exposure or exposure to toxic fumes. Families should also be educated and trained in various aspects of care so they can be advocates for their children. They should be encouraged to be involved in the discussion of therapies to be provided, educational modifications at school, and counseling services. They should also be educated about working with the school to help the child get the best services. Children with mild TBI/concussion may fall through the cracks as they may not necessarily present with problems right away. Families should be educated about things to watch for to be able to address issues
Spasticity management	Families should be trained in the range-of-motion exercises, use of orthotics, watching for skin breakdown, and tolerance to braces. They should also be encouraged to participate in therapy sessions to identify any changes that spasticity may be causing. They should be educated about possible osteopenia seen post-TBI. Children with severe TBI are more at risk for osteopenia as their mobility is more limited

after discharge. Families realize the extent to which care is needed for their loved one. They have to relive the pain of having lost what once was, and face what is now. An adolescent who was an honor student prior to the TBI may be an average or below-average student now. This would be extremely distressing to families and to the patient particularly if the patient had insight into his or her deficits. This may cause the patient to get frustrated and act out. If the family does not comprehend the nature of TBI and its effects, they will not be in a position to help the patient. This only makes a bad situation worse. It is vital to teach families strategies to deal with patients with TBI once they reach home, to not exacerbate situations, and to face them in a mature fashion (Table 30.7). It is also important to suggest joining peer groups or local TBI chapters as they provide support for patients and for families.

Talking to the patient in a calm and comforting manner and providing a calm environment can help decrease the aggression and agitation that a patient may have. It also helps to repeat vital information in a calm fashion so that it is easier to accept it.

TABLE 30.7 Problems With Executive Function After Brain Injury

PROBLEMS	STRATEGIES TO HELP
Impulsivity	Constant cueing, remind families to be watchful about the activities of the patient
Aggression	Teach families to not allow situations to escalate to the point of uncontrollable rages with aggressive acting out; to learn to distract from the current inciting act/talk
Behavioral changes	Socialization becomes difficult due to poor memory or poor social skills. Recognition of these can help with addressing the issue. Using a calm voice while talking to the patient helps defuse the situation
Memory	Repetition of information can be helpful. Encouraging the patient to use a memory book can also be helpful

Talking to families in a nonthreatening manner and maintaining a compassionate attitude are supportive in the care.

PROFESSIONALISM

GOALS

Reflect a commitment to carrying out professional responsibilities and an adherence to ethical principles in pediatric TBI.

OBJECTIVES

1. Demonstrate humanistic qualities of integrity, respect, compassion, ethics, and courtesy in the care of the child and adolescent with a brain injury.
2. Exemplify patient-centered care, informed consent, and maintaining patient confidentiality with respect to pediatric brain injury.
3. Respect patient's beliefs and goals, privacy, and autonomy as it applies to pediatric brain injury.
4. Exhibit sensitivity to culture, diversity, gender, age, race, religion, disabilities, and sexual orientation as it may apply to pediatric brain injury.
5. Demonstrate responsibility, accountability, and commitment to excellence in quality care as it applies to pediatric brain injury.
6. Describe the role of the physiatrist as an advocate for patients with pediatric brain injury.

Post-TBI, the most common question asked by patients and families is whether they can return to their prior level of activity. More information is being obtained by ongoing research that demonstrates that once the brain has been injured, it is vulnerable to repeat injuries. The second impact syndrome is seen due to repeated concussion in children and adolescents. Typically, most rehabilitation physicians do not recommend return to competitive contact sports, or horse riding, post severe TBI. Unfortunately, due to lack of consensus among various specialties like neurology, neurosurgery, and physiatry, there is bewildering information provided to the public. However, studies are ongoing to reach a compromise regarding the same.

Families undergo a lot of stress and pain after such a devastating phase in life. It is very important to be sensitive to the needs of the families and patients. For a successful discharge and recovery, the importance of having a family working with the team cannot be stressed enough. Once the family is on board, it becomes easier to educate the patients. This is particularly important in caring for adolescents. Adolescents, especially if they are emancipated minors, may be able to make decisions regarding their care depending on their cognitive competence. Any information being shared with the families will have to conform to the Health Insurance Portability and Accountability Act (HIPAA) guidelines, keeping in mind their autonomy. For adolescents who are unable to assist in making decisions, because of either medical reasons (e.g., coma) or not being competent to make a decision after a TBI, it may be necessary for families to obtain a medical power of attorney. Assistance for this is usually provided by social workers who are knowledgeable in this regard. Without this, care may become complicated secondary to legal issues.

The field of health care and medicine is overwhelming. Health care providers need to be the voice of what is best for their patients. Physiatrists are in a position to articulate the needs of their patients and their impairments, activity limitations, and participation restrictions. Physiatrists can be helpful in ascertaining that their patient is receiving adequate care. Families need to be encouraged to face the daunting task of advocating for their loved one. Assistance is needed in navigating the various landmines of insurance limitations, therapy recommendations, school recommendations, legal situations, medical care postdischarge, vocational rehabilitation, and ongoing care. Care coordinators and social workers, in either an inpatient or an outpatient setting, provide yeoman service in this regard. Some insurance companies, particularly managed health care companies, may have people who can help in such situations. The coordination of all care helps in providing safe affordable care for the patients and their families.

The physiatrist is in a unique position to help advocate for patients and families by being involved in local chapters (e.g., Brain Injury Association of America), local rehabilitation councils, and pediatric chapters. Getting the community to rally around can help influence legislation. Thinkfirst National Injury Prevention Foundation is a platform that the physiatrists can associate with locally to reduce the number of injuries and fatalities.

It is important to note the accountability of the physiatrist for problems in the scope of rehabilitation medicine, including overall care of the child. It is up to the physiatrist as one of the caregivers involved to okay return to play; other responsibilities include driving, overall management of a child's needs, and coordination of the team members.

The physiatrist is able to direct the care of the child effectively while being an advocate for the child if the patient is at the center of the decision-making process. The physiatrist is critical in communicating with the other specialists and helping coordinate care. The family may have difficulty in comprehending that their loved one is not as before. Hence, expectations may still be that the patient will function at the same level as prior to the injury. This can cause a lot of angst and anger with the situation. Families have to be provided with information about the injury, interventions to manage the same, and the benefits versus risks of not following through with the recommendations. Sometimes, the family's wishes may not be congruent with the patient's welfare, when the importance of making recommendations that are patient centered rise to the occasion (Figure 30.1).

It is important to be sensitive to the various aspects of care including race, culture, or disability. In some cultures, it is considered acceptable for a certain family member to be the decision maker (e.g., the patriarch or matriarch). In some cultures it may be considered a sign of weakness to demonstrate one's emotions/tears in front of the treating team. This may sometimes be mistaken for either arrogance or not being sufficiently concerned by the medical team's standards. The family may also have difficulty in accepting the disability and may need a lot of compassionate care from the treating team. End-of-life issues or the finality of the TBI with its deficits may not be an acceptable topic for discussion in certain cultures based on this author's experiences. It is important for families to realize that even though they may have a source of funding to pay for the durable medical equipment, there is a cost to families as well. It can include copays for physician visits, for therapy sessions, and for the adaptive equipment. Each state has its version of funding sources based on income. Medicaid and managed Medicaid payments differ from state to state.

Physiatrists are usually asked about return to driving and return to play. Accountability rests on the physiatrist, who has to judiciously come to a decision regarding these issues. Education of the family is very important regarding impulsivity, behavioral changes, mood changes, aggressiveness, and how it can affect day-to-day living. The families also need to understand about the long-term effects of brain injury despite improving physically. They should be educated about the behavioral aspects of brain injury such as frontal disinhibition, impulsivity, perseveration, inattention, and poor memory and provided with strategies to help deal with these issues.

SYSTEMS-BASED PRACTICE

GOALS

Awareness and responsiveness to systems of care delivery, and the ability to recruit and coordinate effectively resources in the system to provide optimal continuum of care as it relates to pediatric TBI.

OBJECTIVES

1. Describe key components of rehabilitation continuum of care delivery, services, referral patterns, and resources for the child with brain injury.
2. Identify patient safety components as they apply to the child with brain injury.
3. Describe optimal follow-up care for the child with brain injury.
4. Describe markers of quality in the care of the child with brain injury.
5. Describe cost/risk–benefit analysis as it applies to the child with brain injury.
6. Participate in identifying and avoiding potential systems— and medical-related errors and strategies to minimize them— in the care of the child with brain injury.

Rehabilitation in TBI can be in an inpatient or outpatient setting, depending on the severity of brain injury. Inpatient units are staffed by rehabilitation physicians as the primary admitting service or with rehabilitation physicians in a consulting role to hospitalists, who are the admitting physicians. When there are more medical issues, it is wiser to take care of these patients in an inpatient setting, as management of blood pressure, potential infections, and possible thrombosis, to name a few, are better managed in an inpatient setting as long as the patient is able to tolerate the therapies.

In the acute phase, with daily improvements, it is important to be able to provide daily therapies. However, this becomes challenging when there are limitations based on the availability of funding. However, if the patient does not have the capability to participate in a daily therapy regimen due to endurance issues or if there is ongoing medical need (e.g., antibiotics for treatment of an infection), then it may be prudent to transition the patient to a subacute or skilled nursing facility. Therapies provided here are, however, not as intense as in an inpatient setting with medical supervision.

Once daily progress slows down, it may be time to transition the patient to an outpatient setting where he or she will receive therapies two to three times per week. If the patient is medically

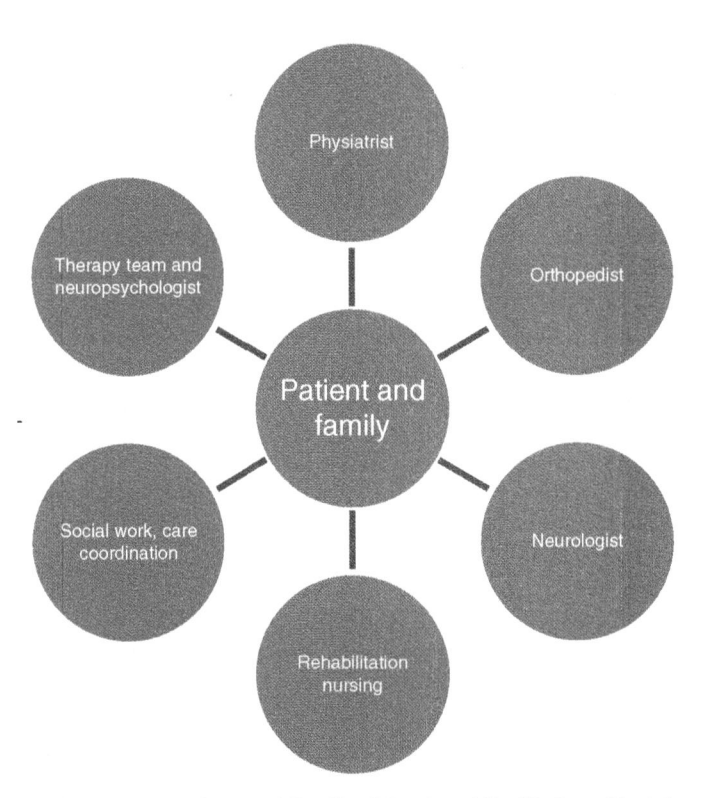

FIGURE 30.1 Patient and Family at Center of Health Care Model

stable but needs intensive therapies, this can be achieved with services in a day rehabilitation setting. Day rehabilitation settings provide consistent daily therapies, simulating an entire school or work day. Therapies provided usually include physical therapy, occupational therapy, speech therapy, and neuropsychological services. School services also are incorporated during the day, as the patient works on increasing endurance. Outpatient therapies, on the other hand, provide services two to three times per week. If families are unable to attend outpatient therapies due to problems with transportation, financial constraints, or problems with positioning, or medical issues like the presence of tracheostomies placing the patient at risk for infections or needing frequent suctioning, then the option may be to provide the therapies at home, utilizing home health agencies. This may be manageable in a comatose child; however, in a child able to interact, outpatient therapies are a better option. Depending on the geographical location, there are differences in the quality of services provided in various settings. It is important to know what is available in the area being practiced in to be able to recommend adequate services.

Effective rehabilitation can be provided only when the entire team of individuals involved in the care function as a well-oiled machine. Communication between team members is very important to facilitate ongoing care. If the acute care team does not communicate with the rehabilitation team about medical stability, weight-bearing status, prophylaxis for DVT, duration of infections treated, or management of autonomic dysfunction, then not only is the patient placed at risk due to inadequate information, but there is duplication of investigations leading to depletion of resources. This can be harmful not only due to exposure to unnecessary radiation, for instance, but also due to increased costs to the patient and the insurance companies.

Outpatient therapies or home health therapies will need to be set up after discharge depending on patient tolerance and on family ability to provide transportation safely.

Hospitals become a safe sanctuary for families, particularly after life-altering catastrophic injuries. Discharge signifies a time when families have to face the reality of the diagnosis and also realize that they have to take their loved one home, causing a lot of stress and angst. Families may not necessarily remember all of the information provided to them. Details of patient education and follow-ups need to be documented and provided to families. It is imperative to establish a relationship with a primary care physician and educate the families about the role of each specialty. They can be referred to agencies to help with obtaining extra assistance. Optimal follow-up care should be set up postdischarge. It is critical to recognize the importance of integrating care between specialists like orthopedists, neurologists, physiatrists, and so on. The primary care physician is in a position to provide this service; however, depending on the comfort level of the practitioner, many a physiatrist takes on this role to help coordinate care better.

Markers of quality would be identified by how well the child is integrated in school, how well seizures are controlled, how timely is the necessary orthopedic intervention, how effective is spasticity management, and how minimal has the child's hospitalization been postdischarge, to name a few. Given the complexity of these issues, the physiatrist, in addition to the primary care physician, can provide effective care.

TBI alters school performance. Hence, recommendations need to be provided to schools to assist the child with a brain injury. This can include recommendations about school work, wherein the child might need help with note taking, extra time for tests, and use of computers to help with course work, to name a few. It also includes therapies at school that are considered educationally necessary based on the Individuals With Disabilities Education Act (IDEA). Unfortunately, this leads to loopholes wherein the decision to determine what is educationally necessary is at the school's discretion. With limited resources at their behest, schools provide only so much.

Community integration is paramount so the child does not suffer social isolation. It is important to teach the families and patients coping strategies to ensure that they are integrated within the system and not living as social pariahs (Table 30.8).

Once the child is discharged from an inpatient setting, it is important to set up regular follow-up. This is to follow up on different aspects of complications, such as cognitive deficits, contractures, and spasticity, to name a few. Cognitive deficits are not evident until the child is placed in a challenging environment. These may manifest after returning to school and being tested by either the school counselor or the neuropsychologist. Neuropsychological tests should be performed whenever there is a change in the setting, for instance, transition from elementary to middle school or middle to high school, or high school to college. Dysphagia should be addressed on an ongoing basis in conjunction with speech therapists to identify and address the effects of aspiration. Equipment and braces may need to be modified when the child presents in the outpatient setting. This is to account for a change in status as the condition and capability may have improved, or there may be a worsening in the status with regard to spasticity and contracture formation. This is something that is monitored on an ongoing basis with regular outpatient follow-ups either virtually (if the family has to travel a long distance) or in person. Skin should be monitored for breakdown from the braces or ill-fitting wheelchairs. If the wheelchairs have not been adjusted and there is scoliosis, there is a risk of skin breakdown.

In the ideal world, the child would receive adequate inpatient rehabilitative care. After discharge from an inpatient setting, the child would either get day rehabilitative services or outpatient therapy services. Visits to primary care physicians and specialists should be based on ongoing need and continuity of care. Adequate provision of services is vital to maintain quality of life/care (e.g., therapy after chemodenervation is important in strengthening, maintaining range of motion, and preventing contractures).

There are various times in the care of the child with TBI when system errors can occur. Watchful monitoring can reduce the risk. The commonest times when these can happen are at times of handoffs, between transfer from an acute to a rehabilitation setting, transfer from a rehabilitation setting to subacute setting or discharge home, or at the time of setting up of outpatient therapies. Diligent care to detail can

TABLE 30.8 Safety Concerns After TBI

PATIENT SAFETY CONCERNS	STRATEGIES TO MINIMIZE THEM
Aspiration	Ensure safe swallow; proper positioning while feeding, chin tuck, frequent swallows, complete and slow chewing of food, supervision with feeds
Contractures	Range of motion, positioning, standing, management of spasticity, early detection of contractures and aggressive ranging, surgery when indicated
Seizures	Recognize aura if present, positioning during an active seizure with safe airway, rectal diazepam when needed
Falls	May occur due to impulsivity, lack of gait belt, help with toileting when needed to decrease patient getting up without supervision, family education regarding lack of insight
Risk of another brain injury	Adequate education of the patient and family about the risks of another brain injury with risk-taking behavior. It may be necessary to prevent/restrict return to playing contact sports. Return to driving should be addressed after a driver's evaluation, which is usually performed by an occupational therapist or any therapist trained in assessing reaction time, visual spatial, and visual perceptual deficits Education about the use of alcohol and drugs is important Education regarding gun safety with respect to the patient and other members of the family and patient's circle is important
Agitation	Frequent rest breaks may be needed; evaluate cause of agitation, whether environment related, or due to medical causes such as infection, electrolyte imbalance, and so on, and address each appropriately
Medication safety	Proper education of caregivers regarding administration of medications including recognizing signs and symptoms of under-and over-dosage

minimize these risks. At the time of transfers, written documentation of a list of medications, setting up of therapies, weight-bearing restrictions, type of feeds being given (via either a nasogastric tube or a gastrostomy tube), and documentation of home health companies and durable medical companies can be helpful in providing a checklist for the families. Having the nurse call from an acute care setting to the rehabilitation unit can be helpful in actual continuity of care to be maintained.

The SHARE acronym is useful and helps in decreasing errors (Table 30.9).

TABLE 30.9 SHARE Acronym

Standardize critical content	Including detailed history, compiling all data, ensuring availability of vital information
Hardwire within your system	Standardized forms, tools, methods, checklists, quiet workspace to share information, set expectations about successful handoffs using new and current techniques
Allow opportunities to ask questions	Utilize critical thinking skills, sharing information, exchanging contact information
Reinforce quality and measurement	Demonstrating leadership commitment to successful handoffs, ensuring accountability on all ends, and compliance by use of forms and methods as prescribed
Educate and coach	Teaching staff effective handoff strategies

This table was created from the chapter on handoff in rehabilitation medicine in *PMR Clinics of North America* (May 2012).

CASE STUDY

A 4-year-old boy is admitted to the inpatient pediatric rehabilitation unit 3 weeks after a TBI due to a motor vehicle crash. He was an unrestrained front-seat passenger. He also has an associated femur fracture, a tracheostomy placement for airway management, and a gastrostomy tube for nutrition. He is in a coma. He lives with his parents and a 6-year-old sister in a 2-storied home. He was a typically developing 4-year-old until the accident.

CASE STUDY DISCUSSION QUESTIONS

1. Identify the key medical and rehabilitative issues in the care of this child and describe a medical and rehabilitative treatment plan for his care.
2. What factors contribute to injury in a growing brain? Describe the long-term effects of pediatric TBI. What is the difference between secondary injury and second impact syndrome?
3. Identify key principles in pediatric brain injury rehabilitation. Discuss outcomes in pediatric brain injury. Discuss the rehabilitation process in pediatric brain injury.
4. What are the key factors to be addressed in the discharge planning of this child? What quality indicators can be measured to ensure adequate provision of care?
5. What are the different settings in which rehabilitative services can be provided? What are a few safety concerns that must be addressed with families?
6. Describe the importance of sensitivity with regard to patient care while maintaining patient confidentiality. Describe the importance of proper communication to families with documentation of the same.

SELF-EXAMINATION QUESTIONS
(Answers begin on p. 367)

1. Which of the following medications is used in the treatment of spasticity in pediatric brain injury?
   A. Amoxicillin
   B. Propranolol
   C. Carbolic acid 5%
   D. Amytryptiline
   E. Sertraline

2. Signs of autonomic dysfunction after TBI include
   A. Apnea
   B. Hypotension
   C. Decreased respirations
   D. Sweating and posturing
   E. Hypothermia

3. Which of the following assessment tools is most recommended to monitor patients in coma?
   A. Wechsler Memory Scale
   B. Tardieu Scale
   C. EEG
   D. CAT scan
   E. Western Neuro Sensory Stimulation Profile

4. Which of the following is true about pediatric TBI?
   A. Visual acuity deficit is seen with parietal lobe involvement
   B. Sensorineural hearing loss is seen with fluid in middle ear
   C. VIII cranial nerve injuries are seen with basilar skull fractures
   D. Diplopia is due to olfactory nerve involvement
   E. Spasticity can be treated with hypertonic saline

5. The most common cause of TBI in adolescents is
   A. Motor vehicle accidents
   B. Falls
   C. Gunshot wounds
   D. Abuse
   E. Sports injuries

REFERENCES

1. Krach LE, et al., eds. Traumatic brain injury. In: *Pediatric Rehabilitation: Principles and Practice.* 4th ed. New York, NY: Demos Medical Publishing; 2009:231–260.
2. Pangilinan PH, Argento AG, Shelhaas R, Hurvitz EA, Hornyak JE. Neuropharmacology in pediatric brain injury: a review. *PMR.* December 2010;2:1127–1140.
3. Byard K, et al. Taking a developmental and systemic perspective on neuropsychological rehabilitation with children with brain injury and their families. *Clin Psychol Psychiatr.* 2011: 16(2):165–184.
4. Cdc.gov website. Accessed November 26, 2011.
5. Biusa.org. Accessed November 26, 2012.
6. Anderson V, et al. Do children's brains recover better? *Brain.* 2011:134;2197–2221.
7. Ylvisaker M, et al. Pediatric brain injury–social, behavioral and communication disability. Physical Medicine and Rehabilitation Clinics of North America-2007, Feb; 18(1):133–144.
8. Chapman SB, et al. Discourse macrolevel processing after severe pediatric TBI. *Dev Neuropsychol.* 2001;25(1&2):37–60.
9. Chapman SB, et al. Discourse ability in head injured children: consideration of linguistic, psychosocial and cognitive factors. *J Head Trauma Rehabil.* 1995;10:36–54.
10. Turkstra LS, et al. Social information processing in adolescents and preliminary data from their peers with TBI. *J Head Trauma Rehabil.* 2001;16:469–483.
11. Meehan, WP, et al-Clinics in Sports Medicine, Jan 2011, Vol 30 Issue 1, p. 133–144.
12. http://now.aapmr.org/peds/Pages/default.aspx. Accessed February 9, 2014.

Rajashree Srinivasan
Callenda Hacker
Nora Cubillos

31: Juvenile Idiopathic Arthritis

PATIENT CARE

GOALS

Provide patient care that is compassionate, appropriate, and effective for the treatment of a child with juvenile idiopathic arthritis (JIA) and the promotion of good health.

OBJECTIVES

1. Describe the key components of the assessment of the child with JIA.
2. Discuss the long-term outcomes of JIA.
3. Assess the impairments, activity limitations, and participation restrictions associated with JIA.
4. Describe the psychosocial, vocational, and educational aspects of JIA.
5. Describe potential injuries associated with JIA.
6. Formulate the key components of a rehabilitation treatment plan for the child with JIA.

ASSESSMENT OF THE CHILD WITH JIA

In performing a thorough history and physical examination, a clinician must be aware that there is no single pathognomonic finding for JIA. It is therefore important to look for patterns of signs and symptoms that may lead to the appropriate diagnosis.

HISTORY OF PRESENT ILLNESS

The child suspected to have JIA may complain of pain with ambulation, morning stiffness, "gelling" sensation, joint swelling, decreased activity level, decreased use of an arm or leg, fevers, rash, and difficulty with buttons and writing (1). JIA is associated with uveitis, which can be asymptomatic and lead to blindness. Uveitis is usually asymptomatic, but can present with photophobia, pain, redness, headache, and visual change. Isolated musculoskeletal pain is generally *not* JIA (1).

Past Medical History

It is important to ask about conditions related to the child's specific type of JIA. These include psoriasis, uveitis, enthesitis, history of macrophage activating syndrome, pericarditis or myocarditis, splenomegaly, and history of lymphadenopathy. The clinician should also inquire about conditions associated with JIA in general, such as presence of osteopenia, micrognathia, leg-length discrepancy, growth impairment, and hearing loss, as well as specific treatments such as autologous stem cell transplantation for cases refractory to medications. Given the use of several medications for the treatment of JIA (see Current and Past Medications section), it is also important for physiatrists to inquire about conditions related to their use such as (a) nonsteroidal anti-inflammatory drugs (NSAIDs) (gastritis, hypertension, impaired renal function), (b) disease-modifying antirheumatic drugs (DMARDs) (leucopenia, thrombocytopenia, anemia, hepatotoxicity, nephrotoxicity, ulcerative stomatitis, nausea, diarrhea, hair thinning, pulmonary fibrosis, exfoliative dermatitis), and (c) biologics (serious infection, malignancy, myelosuppression, optic neuritis, photosensitivity, rash).

Past Surgical History

Although surgeries for JIA are less common with advanced medical treatments, the physiatrist should nevertheless inquire about them in the treatment of JIA. These include (a) soft-tissue releases, (b) contracture releases, (c) total joint replacement, (d) osteotomy for severe bony deformities, (e) epiphysiodesis for leg-length discrepancy, and (f) synovectomy or tenosynovectomy for uncontrolled inflammation.

Current and Past Medications

The clinician should inquire about current and past use of medications commonly used to treat JIA. These include (a) NSAIDs or glucocorticoids; (b) DMARDs such as sulfasalazine, methotrexate (taken with folic acid to reduce side effects), and leflunomide; (c) biologic agents such as etanercept, infliximab, and adalimumab; (d) selective costimulation pathway modulators such as abatacept, interleukin-1 (IL-1) antagonist anakinra, IL-1beta antagonist canakinumab, and IL-6 inhibitor tocilizumab; and (e) history of intraarticular steroid injections.

Current and Past Functional History

Physiatrists should obtain a thorough current and past functional history. Some pertinent questions include the following: (a) How long does it take the child to get out of bed? (b) Is the pain worse after sitting or lying a while? (c) Compared to prior visits, what is the child's activity level? (d) Is the child still able to keep up with peers, or has he or she become more of a reader or video game player? (e) Is the child doing well (academically and socially) at school and can the child carry needed supplies from class to class? (f) Has the child been attending physical and occupational therapies? (g) Is the child performing the exercises in his or her home exercise program?

Social history/level of family support: The following are important questions to ask: (a) Who lives with the child? (b) Does the family encourage activity within limits of pain and does the family include the child in activities? (c) Is the child part of a social group at school and outside of school? (d) Is the child given his or her medications as written and is he or she willing to take them? (e) Are there any environmental factors contributing to noncompliance? (f) Are the child's treatments covered by insurance?

Review of Systems Related to JIA

Pain and other specific complaints can occur with each subtype of JIA in different patterns and should be reviewed at each visit. Important questions to ask include the following: (a) Is sleep interrupted by pain? (b) Does the child have pain on awakening or later in the day after activities? (c) Which joints are affected by pain? (d) Have any joints been swollen? (e) How much and what type of pain medicine does the child take? (f) Is the child growing and gaining weight appropriately?

Oligoarticular JIA generally causes pain in the large joints. Polyarticular JIA tends to cause pain in the small joints of the hands and feet. The cervical spine and temporomandibular joint can also be involved. Children with systemic JIA may complain of fevers twice daily and evanescent rash possibly with Keener phenomenon (skin lesions along line of trauma). Uveitis is also associated with JIA and the child may have symptoms of a red, painful, photophobic eye that can be insidious in presentation.

PHYSICAL EXAMINATION

JIA presentation may be subtle. The most common presentation is a single swollen knee. Other small and/or large joints may have synovitis that is not always symmetric. Polyarticular JIA usually involves knees, wrists, and ankles. Children may have subcutaneous nodules. Boutonniere and swan neck deformities can also be seen. Range of motion (ROM) and flexibility may be decreased. Axial joints can also be affected. Later in the disease, asymmetric growth can be seen and patients may develop torticollis due to cervical spine involvement, decreased oral opening, and micrognathia due to temporomandibular joint involvement, conductive hearing loss due to middle ear involvement, hoarseness due to cricoarytenoid cartilage involvement, rheumatoid nodules, nail pitting, rash, and gait disturbance. Enthesitis-related JIA may have point tenderness over tendon insertion sites (tibial tuberosity and posterior heel) and mildly decreased ROM (ROM 0). Systemic JIA may also have pericarditis or myocarditis, splenomegaly, and lymphadenopathy (2). Children with enthesitis-related JIA might complain of pain, stiffness, and decreased mobility in the lower back, as well as red, painful, photophobic eyes (uveitis). Children with psoriatic-type JIA demonstrate involvement of the hands and feet such as protruding sausage digits and nail bed changes.

Laboratory studies: There may be evidence of leukocytosis, thrombocytosis, elevated liver enzymes, and increased acute-phase reactants. The clinician should not miss the potentially life-threatening macrophage activation syndrome (MAS) that is associated with systemic JIA. A common sign of MAS is a low erythrocyte sedimentation rate (ESR) (in contrast with a high sedimentation rate in systemic JIA exacerbation).

LONG-TERM OUTCOMES OF JIA

Systemic, rheumatoid factor (RF)-negative and -positive polyarthritis have the highest incidence of advanced joint damage and prospects for long-term disability. Radiologic joint damage occurs over time even in the absence of clinical symptoms. A prolonged active disease course leads to increased joint damage (3). Extraarticular damage (eye damage, growth retardation, pubertal delay), subcutaneous atrophy due to intraarticular glucocorticoids, leg-length discrepancies, avascular necrosis, striae rubrae, and abnormal vertebral curve occur often in systemic and enthesitis-related JIA. Pain is common early in the disease course but diminishes as patients complete puberty. Pain frequently keeps patients awake at night and causes daytime fatigue, which affects school, work, and hobbies (4).

IMPAIRMENTS, ACTIVITY LIMITATIONS, AND PARTICIPATION RESTRICTIONS ASSOCIATED WITH JIA

Activity limitations and participation restrictions are frequent in all subtypes of JIA but can improve over time, despite worsening radiologic joint damage (3). Approximately 20% of patients will continue to have activity limitations, especially in dressing and activities that require reaching. Of all subtypes of JIA, systemic JIA and children with wrist and hip involvement have the most activity limitations and participation restrictions over time that are most likely to persist into adulthood (3). The Childhood Health Assessment Questionnaire (CHAQ) for disability highly correlates with parent's/patient's assessment of pain, well-being, level of disease, and functional status. It is inversely correlated with remission (3,5). Historically, decreased activity was recommended, but studies have shown that muscle atrophy occurs rapidly secondary to local arthritis. Weight-bearing exercise increases bone mass, and increased bone mass improves muscle strength. Evidence shows that structured low-intensity programs can lead to improved physical fitness, quality of life, and functional abilities in kids with JIA (6). Moderate adherence to an exercise program has shown improved parental CHAQ scores. Exercise therapy has also been shown to assist preschool children in reaching and maintaining milestones. Weight-bearing exercise is not ideal for patients with large joint disease, and alternative exercise therapies that can be tried include yoga and tai chi. The goal is not only to increase activity in the present but to also make healthy habits for a lifetime (6).

PSYCHOSOCIAL, VOCATIONAL, AND EDUCATIONAL ASPECTS OF JIA

Most kids with JIA can expect to lead normal lives (7). However, at some point in the course of disease, JIA does affect relationships between family members as well as intimate relationships. Many patients express fear of becoming pregnant and having children (4). JIA can cause patients to feel different from others, and negatively affect their self-esteem and body image. Good friendships and a sense of belonging to a social group are essential (4). Pain is a major factor during childhood and adolescence of patients with JIA, which can lead to absenteeism and decreased participation in activities. Patients with JIA have more anxiety and depression than healthy peers, which correlate with disability and active disease (8). Recent studies have reported that improvements in medications have been associated with decreased pain. However, patients often complain of the complicated and chronic medication regimen, the side effects, and the perceived lack of education regarding the medications. Individuals with JIA have expressed concern that JIA affected their relationships with siblings and worry that their parents do not receive enough outside support. Patients are also afraid of the future and how the disease will evolve (4).

A recent systematic review of qualitative studies revealed very invaluable insights into how children with JIA are coping and dealing with their chronic disease. One important insight was that children do not feel normal when they compare themselves to their peers. Children with JIA have to ask for help with certain tasks and feel that they are treated differently due to their disease if others around them are aware of it. They also feel that no one quite understands their disease or can even empathize with the unremitting pain that they suffer from on a regular basis. Physiatrists are adept at treating chronic pain and chronic diseases, which provides them ample experience that can be utilized in relating to children with JIA. Therefore, they can gain rapport with patients and their families by offering compassion and understanding of what the child with JIA has to endure (9).

Quality of life can be hindered in children with JIA. It was found that children with JIA desire to be active participants in their care and feel that health care professionals do not adequately explain the JIA disease process or even relay the reasoning behind why certain treatments were selected. Children with JIA are interested in being continually educated about all aspects of JIA including activity restrictions and therapy programs. Patients with JIA in general do not fully understand the benefits of exercise; therefore, it is vital to relay to patients and families that a therapy program as an outpatient or one instituted at home is necessary to alleviate joint stiffening and keeping joints at their optimum functioning. Physiatrists have the unique ability to work collaboratively with patients in designing an individualized strengthening and stretching therapy regimen that will lead to less pain, participation in more activities, and provide them with a sense that they have some control over certain aspects of their disease and bodies. It will also foster confidence and establish a strong patient and physician dynamic. Physiatrists and therapists can integrate child-friendly activities with a wide assortment of physical games into the patients' therapy programs, so that patients are more likely to be compliant with their physical and occupational therapy plans (9).

It is important to be aware that JIA can decrease patients' participation in school activities, hobbies, and jobs (4). Weiss et al. found that 30% of patients with JIA do not graduate from high school, and 30% are unemployed (8). Federal and state programs may provide assistance to children with JIA with school accommodations or services (Federal Act 504). The Juvenile Arthritis Alliance has resources related to education and vocation (7).

INJURIES ASSOCIATED WITH JIA

Patients with JIA have a higher fracture risk due to lower bone mass. Factors such as disease process, medication side effects, and physical inactivity combine to disrupt bone development and homeostasis. Long bones and vertebra are most at risk (10). Joint replacement surgeries may be needed in up to 72% of JIA patients, primarily those with the oligoarticular, polyarticular, and systemic subtypes. RF-positive patients have the greatest number of joint surgeries (8).

REHABILITATION OF THE PATIENT WITH JIA

JIA involves a cycle of symptoms that decrease physical activity, which in turn worsens the symptoms. Localized arthritis, decreased joint use, and glucocorticoid use all contribute to muscle atrophy. Children with JIA have reduced strength when compared to peers (11). Physical and occupational therapy can help maintain or increase joint ROM, reduce pain, and increase function strength and endurance. Gentle ROM, cold packs, heat, and appropriate rest during flares are key. ROM with passive extension more than flexion two to three times a day helps preserve joint ROM. Gentle relative rest helps decrease fatigue; resting in prone position helps decrease contractures from forming at the hip and knees.

Splinting can help with aligning during a flare-up. It provides local joint rest, supports weakened structures, and assists function. Heat helps in decreasing stiffness, increasing tissue elasticity, and decreasing pain and muscle spasm. Caution should be used while applying heat to insensate areas. Avoid heat during acute flare-ups. Avoid cold over insensate areas in patients with Raynaud phenomenon. Showers, heating pads, and paraffin baths are recommended, but ultrasound is avoided due to lack of evidence regarding growth plates. Custom splints may be needed to help prevent or slow joint tightening and/or deformities. School-based therapists can provide input on issues at school (7). Rehabilitation of JIA includes relative rest, splinting of joints as appropriate, maintaining ROM, use of modalities as tolerated, and socialization. Strengthening activities are important; swimming is a safe activity for children. Care has to be taken to minimize side effects like burns while using moist heat. Surgical correction of deformities or for conditions like avascular necrosis of the femoral neck should be followed by early rehabilitation with adequate pain control. Provision of assistive devices like a long-handled sponge and long-handled hairbrushes can make independence in day-to-day activities more manageable. Occupational therapists can help with school modifications like frequent rest breaks, having two sets of textbooks (one at home and one at school), reduced amount of writing, extra time to move between classes, note taker, and extra time to complete assignments. Vocational counseling after high school and college is critical for independence, education, and employment plans. Social work is valuable in ensuring coping strategies for patients and families in providing emotional and financial resources and helping transition of adolescents to adult status.

Exercise and Sports

Regular exercise ranging from low to high intensity has been shown to improve joint ROM, increase muscle strength, improve clinical symptoms, and improve health-related quality of life (11). In fact, studies show that exercise is a vital part of treatment in children with JIA. Inactivity decreases both aerobic and anaerobic capacities, and in combination with the disease can lead to deconditioning and further disability (6). Tai chi and yoga are recommended (6). Sports are not contraindicated, and participation in sports will not exacerbate the disease. Children with JIA can participate in any sport of interest, including impact activities and competitive contact sports, if their disease is well controlled and they have adequate physical capacity. Children with neck arthritis should have radiographic screening of atlantoaxial joints, with abnormal films needing further evaluation. Participation should be limited based on pain. As in the general population, children with JIA should wear appropriate protective equipment, including mouth guards and eye protection (12). Exercises in water showed benefits similar to those of land-based programs (13). It is very important to note that multiple studies have reported no adverse events related to exercise training (11).

MEDICAL KNOWLEDGE

GOALS

Demonstrate knowledge of established and evolving biomedical, clinical epidemiological, and sociobehavioral sciences pertaining to JIA, as well as the application of this knowledge to guide holistic patient care.

OBJECTIVES

1. Describe the epidemiology, anatomy, physiology, and pathophysiology of JIA.
2. Discuss the seven subtypes of JIA and their characteristics.
3. Identify the pertinent laboratory and imaging studies important in JIA.
4. Review the treatment of JIA.
5. Recognize the complications and red flags associated with JIA.
6. Examine the ethical issues in JIA.

JIA is the most common rheumatic disease of childhood; 50% to 75% of patients seen in pediatric rheumatology referral clinics are due to JIA (1); 1 in 1,000 children is affected with JIA. Epidemiologic studies report the incidence of JIA from 1 to 22 per 100,000 with a prevalence of 8 to 150 per 100,000. European descent appeared to be an important predisposing factor for oligoarticular JIA; in addition, psoriatic JIA is also more common in patients of European descent. Black and Native American patients are more likely to have RF-positive polyarthritis. In general, girls are more often affected than boys. Females are more affected with oligoarticular and polyarticular JIA, and males are more affected with enthesitis-related JIA. Systemic subtype is relatively equal between the sexes. Age ranges of JIA development are median 5 to 8 years of onset, earliest with oligoarthritis and latest with seropositive polyarthritis (14).

JIA involves infiltration of the synovium by lymphocytes and macrophages with production of fibroblasts and macrophage-like synoviocytes. The anatomy of a growing child's joint differs from that of adults. Children have thicker cartilage than adults due to ossification still being in progress; in addition, cartilage in children is able to renew itself better than in adults. Patients with JIA have been shown to improve radiographically with or even without treatment. Joint space narrowing is the most common form of radiographic damage in JIA (15).

The cause of JIA continues to remain inexact. JIA is hypothesized to be due to multifaceted genetic traits involved in immunity and inflammation that predispose one to develop JIA. When these genes are triggered by environmental factors such as stress, joint trauma, infection, or imbalanced hormones, then disease arises (8).

Particular human leukocyte antigen (HLA) class I and class II alleles have been found to be linked to an increased risk of JIA. Inflammation also is involved. Serum levels of circulating immune complexes have been found in JIA, as have antinuclear antibodies (ANAs), C-reactive protein (CRP), and RF. Synovial fluid of JIA patients has revealed T cells and increased amounts of interleukins (15).

JIA, previously called juvenile rheumatoid arthritis, refers to a complex collection of rheumatologic disorders characterized by chronic arthritis and prolonged synovial inflammation that causes joint deterioration, thereby leading to diminished function and worsening of quality of life (15).

JIA is characterized by (1):

- Arthritis for 6 weeks or longer in any one joint
- Onset age 16 years or less
- Diagnosis of exclusion

Patients have a similar set of complaints such as joint heat, joint pain, morning stiffness that improves throughout the day, "gelling phenomenon," decreased ROM of a joint, and difficulty performing activities of daily living (ADLs) (1). The International League of Associations for Rheumatology (ILAR) has set specific criteria for classification of JIA subtypes. There are 7 subtypes of juvenile arthritis: oligoarticular, polyarticular RF-positive, polyarticular RF-negative, systemic, enthesitis related, psoriatic, and "other" (15).

Oligoarticular JIA, the most common subtype of JIA, is characterized by arthritis in less than 5 large joints of the lower extremities during the first 6 months of disease. It is also possible for only one joint to be involved, which is most often the knee (1). Approximately 50% of patients with oligoarthritis JIA proceed to develop extended disease, and within a few years are afflicted with polyarticular JIA. Oligoarthritis JIA is the most common subtype associated with chronic uveitis (1,9–11). Other differential diagnoses should be considered if the patient displays a red and painful joint, hip involvement, systemic symptoms, refusal to bear weight, or if small joints are involved (1).

In *polyarticular JIA*, patients have five or more affected joints within the first 6 months of disease. Patients can have RF-negative and RF-positive diseases, and girls are more affected in general than boys. This subtype has no strong HLA association. The seronegative patients develop polyarticular JIA in early childhood. The seropositive polyarticular JIA patients are usually girls who develop severe erosive disease in late childhood and adolescence in symmetric pattern in small joints (14).

In *systemic JIA*, patients develop systemic extraarticular manifestations such as salmon-pink macular rash, 2 weeks of high-spiking twice-daily fever, lymphadenopathy, hepatosplenomegaly, pericardial effusions, and serositis. Patients then usually develop polyarticular joint involvement within 6 months of systemic symptoms. Uveitis is a very rare occurrence (8).

Enthesitis-related arthritis commonly involves the lower limbs, especially the hip. It is characterized by inflammation at the insertion of tendons, ligaments, or joint capsules such as bone iliac crest, posterior and anterior superior iliac spine, femoral greater trochanter, ischial tuberosity, patella, tibial tuberosity, Achilles, and plantar fascia insertion sites. It can also involve the sacroiliac joints (14).

In *psoriatic JIA*, psoriasis and arthritis may not occur at the same time. Positive laboratory markers include ANA and HLA-B27. Psoriatic arthritic JIA patients have asymmetric arthritis that can affect both large and small joints. If the rash is absent, then the diagnosis can be made if the patient has a family history of psoriasis in a first-degree relative, dactylitis, and nail pitting. These patients are at risk for iritis and need frequent ocular evaluations (14).

"*Other*" subtype includes children with symptoms that do not fall into any specific subtype or who have characteristics of more than one subtype of JIA (8). The characteristics of JIA subtypes are given in Table 31.1.

Diagnosis of JIA is based on patterns of clinical information and not solely on one particular imaging modality or diagnostic study. JIA is a diagnosis of exclusion and other possible causes need to be fully investigated. There is no specific laboratory test to definitively diagnose JIA. ESR is a nonspecific marker of inflammation and can be normal in patients with JIA. The majority of JIA patients are RF negative (95%) (1). RF can be positive in a number of conditions such as malignancy and is positive most commonly in viral infections. ANA can be positive in normal children. When ANA is positive in oligoarticular JIA, then the patient is at risk for ocular involvement. A very high ANA titer can indicate rheumatologic disease other than JIA, such as systemic lupus erythematosus (SLE). Serial trending of inflammatory markers like CRP and ESR can help guide the effectiveness of medical management. Patients can also display hematologic abnormalities such as anemia of chronic disease and leukocytosis. Joint aspiration can be helpful in ruling out septic arthritis (15).

TABLE 31.1 Characteristics of JIA Subtypes

	OLIGOARTICULAR	POLYARTICULAR RF NEGATIVE	POLYARTICULAR RF POSITIVE	SYSTEMIC	ENTHESITIS	PSORIATIC
Frequency of cases	60%	20%–25%	3%	10%	5%–19%	5%–10%
Joint involvement	<5	>5	>5	Variable	Weight-bearing joint, especially hip and intertarsal joints. History of inflammatory back pain or sacroiliac joint tenderness	Asymmetric or symmetric small or large joints
Age at onset	1–4 yr	1–4 yr	9–16 yr	1–5 yr	9–12 yr	1–3, 9–11 yr
Sex ratio (F:M)	3:1	3:1	4:1	F = M	4:1	F > M
Ethnicity		White	Hispanic, Black	White	Native American	White
Chronic uveitis	20%	15%	Rare	Rare	7%	10%
Systemic involvement/ Extraarticular	Not present	Moderate involvement	Moderate involvement	Yes	Yes	Yes

In the past, in order to evaluate the degree of joint inflammation and erosion, plain radiography was frequently employed. However, joint erosion is not made apparent on plain radiographs until there is substantial damage to the joint. There are joint scoring systems in place for adults suffering from chronic arthritis that are able to monitor joint destruction. These include the simple erosion narrowing score (SENS) and Sharp/van der Heijde score (16). Most recently, these scoring systems are being used in children. It is difficult to progressively follow joint destruction due to the structural variability in the joints of growing children and changes brought about by chronic arthritis (e.g., growth disturbances). MRI is now being utilized more due to its capacity to detect early changes of joint destruction and instability and to better visualize certain joints like the temporomandibular joint. Drawbacks include increased cost, possible allergy to dye, and possible need for sedation in younger patients. Studies have shown that bone depressions in normal individuals can imitate erosions in JIA, making the ability to discern actual joint deterioration in JIA patients difficult (17).

Ultrasonography is now being used more to evaluate joints in JIA. Advantages include noninvasiveness, capability to evaluate multiple joints, safety, and high tolerability among patients. It can be difficult to assess joints if the operator is not knowledgeable about ultrasound and certain joints cannot be visualized accurately. Ultrasonography may be used for identifying synovitis, subclinical synovitis, and cartilage; however, it may be avoided in children due to concern of damaging growth plates (18). It may not be as useful for enthesitis-related JIA, as ossification centers were incorrectly recognized as enthesitis on ultrasound. Continued research into MRI and ultrasonography is promising and will likely lead to earlier recognition of joint damage and prevention of disability (17) (Table 31.2).

Treatment involves a strategic approach that is centered on early intervention. Nonpharmacologic therapy such as occupational and physical therapy is essential to effectively treat JIA. Therapy programs focus on strength and stretching exercises, serial casting, splints, and orthotics, which are important tools in enhancing mobility, increasing ROM of joints, and avoiding joint contractures (19). Resting splints should be used at night only, because if used longer they can worsen joint stiffness. Splints should be evaluated by physiatrists at least twice a year as children grow frequently. Assistive devices like reachers and raised toilet seats are essential for JIA patients who have difficulty with ADLs. Modalities such as heat and cold are also used to help decrease pain and inflammation. Exercise has been shown to be helpful in achieving better function and aiding in quality of life for JIA patients (18). Adaptive strengthening exercises are important in play and day-to-day recreational activities. Isometric strengthening activities are allowed in acute flare-ups, with vigorous activities being embarked upon after the acute flare. Activities like swimming, dancing, noncontact karate, and Tai Chi are good options. Hydrotherapy with land-based therapies is helpful.

Ambulation should be promoted. Use of a posterior walker and a standing program are essential to the rehabilitation in JIA. A presurgical joint rehabilitation program focuses on strengthening muscles, training for future ambulation, and identifying other joints that may influence the rehabilitation process (Table 31.3).

Exercise prescription should include the type of exercise being recommended such as isometric versus isotonic; use of modalities (i.e., heat versus cold); precautions regarding falls, presence of contracture, atlantoaxial instability; duration of therapy (i.e., frequency and how many times a week); and evaluation for splints and adaptive equipments.

TABLE 31.2 Pertinent Laboratory and Imaging Findings in JIA Subtypes

	OLIGOARTICULAR	POLYARTICULAR RF NEGATIVE	POLYARTICULAR RF POSITIVE	SYSTEMIC	ENTHESITIS	PSORIATIC
CBC	Normal	Normal or with anemia, thrombocytosis	Anemia, thrombocytosis	WBC > 15,000—left shift, anemia, thrombocytosis	Possible anemia, thrombocytosis	Anemia of chronic disease, and thrombocytosis
ESR	Normal to mildly elevated	Elevated, may be normal	Elevated	Markedly elevated	Elevated	May be elevated
Urine analysis (UA)	Negative	Normal	Normal	Normal	Normal	Normal
ANA	Positive in 80%	Sometimes positive	Positive	Normal	Negative	May be positive
Rheumatoid factor	Negative	Negative	Positive	Normal	Negative	Negative
Radiographic findings	Normal	Normal	Joint erosions	Negative	Sacroiliac films abnormal over time	Dactylitis, joint erosions
HLA association	Yes	Yes	Yes	Yes	HLA-B27 positive in >80%	HLA-B27 Yes

Sources: Rotte (1); Eyckmans et al (4); Long et al (6).

TABLE 31.3 Joint Care in JIA

JOINTS	WHAT TO ADDRESS
Cervical (C) spine	More involved in children than adults; soft cervical collar helps remind of proper alignment and provides warmth; helpful in acute pain with muscle spasm. Minimize flexion time as weakened transverse ligament leads to atlantoaxial subluxation. Firm cervical collar should be worn with transport in presence of subluxation
Temporomandibular joint (TMJ)	Affected in two-thirds of children with JIA. Causes pain with chewing, opening mouth, stiffness, and micrognathia. Younger children modify diet to avoid pain. Mandibular and facial growth disturbances seen more in polyarticular types of JIA
Upper extremities	Shoulder involvement in polyarticular and psoriatic disease causes loss of adduction and abduction, internal rotation of shoulder affecting midline ADLs like grooming and toileting. Loss of >45° elbow extension limits feeding, grooming, and reaching. Nighttime wrist splint in 15°–20° of extension with fingers in few degrees of flexion; ulnar deviation built in if needed. Strengthening wrist extensors and radial deviators is important. Moist heat to reduce spasm and improve tissue elasticity followed by serial casting for 48–72 hours as tolerated helps decrease contractures
Lower extremities	Flexion contractures seen at hip and knees. Lying prone >20 min/d helpful. Strengthen hip extensors, external rotators, abductors, and quadriceps, with ROM exercises to stretch hip flexors, internal rotators, adductors, and hamstrings. Hip extensors and quadriceps can be strengthened via swimming, aquatic therapy, and bicycling

One of the most common initial medications used in JIA treatment is NSAIDs (e.g., Naproxen, diclofenac, and ibuprofen). Prescribers should be careful in prescribing Naproxen in fair-skinned children, as they are at risk for developing pseudoporphyria cutanea tarda, a photodermatitis that may cause skin scarring. If patients require long-term NSAID use, then kidney and liver function tests must be followed carefully (20).

JIA patients, specifically systemic JIA, are treated with corticosteroids, both oral and intraarticular. Corticosteroids are not used for disease remission due to possible side effects from extended steroid use. For severe polyarticular JIA, oral steroids are used in the interim until other medications become effective. Intraarticular steroid injections have been shown to achieve sustained remission. Intraarticular steroid injections are tolerated well; however, small children often necessitate general anesthetic or sedation. A particular steroid, triamcinolone hexacetonide, is believed to be more efficacious compared to triamcinolone acetonide (20).

DMARDs such as sulfasalazine, methotrexate, and etanercept are commonly used to effectively control disease activity. In the past, there was reluctance to prescribe these medications to children with JIA due to possible toxicity. Now, DMARDs have been proven safe for use in children. In addition, DMARDs have been revealed to be integral to preventing permanent destruction. Methotrexate, administered either orally or by subcutaneous injections, is the most commonly used DMARD in the treatment of JIA. Studies have shown that methotrexate is most effective in treating extended oligoarticular JIA. The most common side effect of methotrexate is gastrointestinal upset, specifically nausea and vomiting, which can lead to noncompliance with medication ingestion. Subcutaneous administration may be helpful in avoiding this unpleasant side effect. Otherwise, methotrexate is typically well tolerated in children. Other less frequent side effects include hepatic fibrosis, oral ulceration, alopecia, hematologic abnormalities, mood changes, rash, diarrhea, and headache. Liver function and complete blood count should be followed up regularly if methotrexate is taken long term (15).

Biologic agents are directed at particular inflammatory substances such as cytokines (tumor necrosis factor [TNF]-α), IL-1, and IL-6 and signaling molecules involved in the regulation of B-cell and T-cell lymphocyte responses. TNF-α inhibitors that are utilized in JIA (like etanercept, infliximab, and adalimumab) help reduce disease flare-up. Side effects include rash and headache. TNF-α inhibitors also have the risk of developing more serious complications like severe infections and demyelinating diseases. IL-1 receptor antagonists like anakinra are used in systemic JIA, which is resistant to methotrexate and TNF-α antagonists. Studies revealed disease remission; however, these results are not always reproducible with all systemic JIA patients. Side effects of anakinra include local injection site reactions and pain; more serious side effects are infection and anaphylaxis (20).

The chronic nature of the disease process prompts families to seek complementary and alternative (CAM) treatment modalities. Also, fear of side effects of conventional medications and a perception of no improvement in the child's condition is a factor in choosing CAM therapies (Box 31.1). The 5 domains per the National Center for Complementary and Alternative Medicine (NCCAM) are given in Table 31.4.

BOX 31.1 Factors Associated With CAM Use in Children

- Longer disease duration
- Presence of more than one illness
- Previous CAM use by parents
- Parent perception of medication not helping

TABLE 31.4 Examples of Complementary and Alternative Medicine (CAM)

TYPE OF CAM	EXAMPLES
Alternative medical system	Homeopathy, naturopathy, traditional Chinese medicine
Mind–body intervention	Hypnosis, biofeedback
Biologically based therapies	Herbal supplements, aromatherapy
Manipulative and body-based methods	Chiropractic, massage therapy
Energy therapies	Therapeutic touch

Common therapies used include copper bracelets, diet modifications, natural health products, and chiropractic. Popular types of interventions include prayer, massage therapy, and meditation/relaxation.

Pain is the common symptom for which CAM is chosen. Health care providers should be able to help the patient and family make a correct choice with regard to CAM and about its potential benefits and harm. An open dialogue should be maintained with the patient's family (21).

COMPLICATIONS AND RED FLAGS ASSOCIATED WITH JUVENILE ARTHRITIS

One of the more common and destructive complications associated with JIA is a form of chronic anterior nongranulomatous uveitis, specifically iridocyclitis. It is usually *asymptomatic* and can present *bilaterally*. Patients may also have conjunctivitis, unequal pupils, photophobia, eye pain, eye redness, headache, or visual disturbances. If not diagnosed in a timely fashion, patients can develop posterior synechiae, cataract, band keratopathy, glaucoma, and even permanent blindness. Therefore, patients with JIA require early vision evaluations with slit lamp examinations conducted by an ophthalmologist. Chronic anterior uveitis is more common in females affected with oligoarticular arthritis and in patients less than 6 years of age with a positive ANA. Systemic JIA has very little risk of uveitis and does not require vision screening. Treatment of uveitis involves topical steroids and ophthalmic glucocorticoids. If the patient is not responsive to topical steroids, then oral steroids are used (15).

Surveillance for growth disturbances such as growth retardation and accelerated growth is also essential. JIA patients can develop leg-length discrepancy due to protracted arthritis to the knee triggering accelerated growth of the affected leg. On the other hand, protracted arthritis in ankles, feet, wrists, or hands can cause growth retardation. Alternating days of steroid intake and even growth hormone has been shown to be helpful in decreasing growth retardation. Micrognathia is also a possibility if temporomandibular joint arthritis disturbs the nearby growth plate. Patients are at risk for osteopenia and osteoporosis due to persistent arthritis and joint destruction and also treatment with corticosteroids. With osteopenia and osteoporosis comes the threat of fractures (14). In order to help avert these complications, it is important to manage the arthritis well, add calcium and vitamin D supplementation, and encourage physical activity (8).

MAS is a complication that occurs in about 5% to 8% of patients with systemic JIA that involves life-threatening persistent fever, pancytopenia, hepatosplenomegaly, and coagulopathy. It can be associated with viral infections, changes in medications, or it can even be spontaneous and without an obvious cause. It is important to differentiate it from systemic JIA flares. Diagnosis is made by bone marrow aspirate, and treatment involves steroids (1,14) (Box 31.2).

BOX 31.2 Complications in JIA and in Treatments

- JIA: Blindness due to iridocyclitis, increased atlantoaxial distance causing instability, joint destruction, and renal diseases. Atlantoaxial instability puts patients at risk for spinal cord injury.
- DMARDs: Suppress immune system; hence, one is at risk for infection and malignancies.
- Steroids: Osteoporosis/osteopenia, avascular necrosis of femoral neck, gastritis, mood disturbances, and cataract.
- Bisphosphonates: Affect bone metabolism, cost, convenience of medication administration, and toxicity.
- Abnormalities in skeletal growth can be seen due to disease process.

ETHICAL ISSUES IN THE CARE OF JIA

The newest biologic agents that are now used to treat JIA do not have substantial research to demonstrate their safety in children. This raises the ethical question of whether these treatments should be used at all in children. It is a common practice to determine pediatric dosing on adjustment of adult dosage extrapolated to the weight of the child. Moreover, since 50% of children with JIA can progress to adults, these patients will be exposed to medications for long periods of time. The long-term effects of these medications to treat arthritis from childhood to adulthood have not been well studied. Research that is necessary to adequately assess the safety profile of various medications requires a large, multicenter trial that is often difficult and time consuming to undertake. Various legislations have been enacted, such as the Best Pharmaceuticals for Children Act, which has helped foster more pediatric research and even set mandatory research in place to better understand medication adverse events (22).

PRACTICE-BASED LEARNING AND IMPROVEMENT

GOALS

Demonstrate competence in continuously investigating and evaluating your own JIA patient care practices, appraising and assimilating scientific evidence, and continuously improving your patient care practices based on constant self-evaluation and lifelong learning.

OBJECTIVES

1. Describe key components of self-assessment and lifelong learning for the physiatrist with respect to continuing medical education (CME) and continuing professional development (CPD) as related to JIA.
2. Teach patients, families, residents, students, and other health professionals regarding JIA.
3. Identify benchmarks/best practices, and describe key practice-related systematic quality improvement (QI) markers and practice performance improvement (PI) for JIA.
4. Identify sources of evidence-based practice guidelines and information technology useful in the treatment of JIA.

CME and CPD are the hallmarks of practice-based learning and improvement. Physiatrists should keep up-to-date with respect to the medical, surgical, and rehabilitation aspects of JIA. This includes resources such as the Pediatric and Rheumatology Clinics of North America, web-based resources such as Knowledge NOW, eMedicine, and the American College of Rheumatology. Attendance at the Pediatric Rheumatology Symposium organized by the American College of Rheumatology can also be helpful.

It is important that physiatrists educate their patients and their families about the underlying disease process of JIA, as well as its treatment, prognosis, and strategies to minimize long-term complications such as long bone fractures, contractures, and uveitis. Physiatrists should also provide education about exercise programs, pain management, and strategies that can help their patients achieve their educational, personal, and vocational aspirations.

Juvenile arthritis does not yet have specific published quality measurement and improvement initiatives (23). However, some areas of interest in QI and quality assurance with respect to JIA include the following: (a) incidence of fractures, (b) incidence of falls, (c) incidence of joint contractures, (d) pain severity level, (e) quality of life measures, and (d) prevalence of participation in exercise program. An online resource for PI is www.rheumatology.org via the Practice Management menu (24).

INTERPERSONAL AND COMMUNICATION SKILLS

GOALS

Demonstrate interpersonal and communication skills that result in the effective exchange of information and collaboration with JIA patients, their families, and other health professionals.

OBJECTIVES

1. Demonstrate skills used in effective communication and collaboration with patients with JIA and their caregivers across socioeconomic and cultural backgrounds.
2. Delineate the importance of the role of the physiatrist as the team leader and consultant pertinent to JIA.
3. Demonstrate proper documentation and effective communication between health care professional team members in patient care as it applies to JIA.

JIA is an entity that affects all aspects of a child's life: physical, social, emotional, intellectual, and economic. It not only affects the child but the family as a whole. It is important to be able to communicate with patients and families about a complete picture of the health condition, impact on socioeconomic status, functional aspects, and overall quality of life (25). It is not only the disease process that affects the lifestyle but also the treatments used.

In a pediatric setting, the parent is the decision maker for the child. It is important for the parents to be fully informed about the disease, its course with and without medications, use of medications, and their associated risks and benefits. Complete information helps them make an informed decision with a framework of comprehension of the risks versus benefits. It is important to involve the family in the decision-making process. Families may not necessarily comprehend all the information presented the first time. They should be provided with opportunities to ask questions relating to the disease process and its treatment options. They should be informed and not persuaded. Persuasion implies communication that is focused on influencing the acts of the decision maker; for example, getting families and patients to agree to treatment with the subtle unintended use of threat of progression of disease, forcing the caregiver to evaluate the health threat and capacity to cope with the side effects, count as persuasion. On the other hand, medication guides that are provided with medications are able to provide families with more information. Informed decision making implies provision of all information to enable patients and their families to make an equitable, reasonable decision (26). When the benefits and risks are equal, the decision should be by patient/parent/family choice.

At the time the diagnosis is made, there is a lot of angst and anxiety regarding the disease process, use of medications, growth and development, and side effects of medications. Counseling regarding these issues is important at that time. Depending on the type of JIA, education should be provided regarding vision involvement and the reason to monitor it. Health literacy, independent of low educational achievement or other demographic, is a common predictor of risk perception and willingness to take a proposed DMARD. Risk perception of the gravity of the disease is altered by negative rheumatoid arthritis disease and treatment, while willingness to take a proposed DMARD is reduced as perception of current RA control improves. This shows the influence of patient disease experiences on decision-making processes.

Documentation is an important communication tool between providers with respect to the medical, psychosocial concerns, and treatment plan for the patient with JIA. Excellent documentation is essential at times of transition in the patient's care, including (a) transition between institutions, (b) transition between wards within a medical center, (c) handoffs at change of shifts within a medical center, (d) discharge from medical center to community, and (e) follow-up between outpatient providers. Key elements in the medical documentation are (a) type of JIA and presence of ocular involvement; (b) patient's current and past medical, surgical, and rehabilitative history including risk of injury (e.g., atlantoaxial instability); (c) current and past medications and side effects; (d) key components of physical examination; (e) key providers in the patient's care; and (f) recommended treatment plan including any precautions (e.g., weight-bearing restrictions). The documentation should be dated, timed, and written in legible handwriting with an easily recognizable signature for the provider if electronic medical records are not available.

It is important to also document patient and family education. The patient's key family members should be educated about (a) weight-bearing status; (b) recommended medical, surgical, and rehabilitative treatments; and (c) duration of treatment.

Without adequate communication between team members, it is not easy to coordinate care. Information regarding patient status as previously mentioned should be shared between the rheumatologist, physiatrist, orthopedist, physical therapist, occupational therapist, social worker, psychologist, and rehabilitation nurse as available and needed.

PROFESSIONALISM

GOALS

Reflect a commitment to carrying out professional responsibilities and an adherence to ethical principles in caring for patients with JIA.

OBJECTIVE

1. Describe the importance of integrity, respect, compassion, ethics, and courtesy in the care of patients with JIA.
2. Describe the importance of patient-centered care, informed consent, and maintaining patient confidentiality in JIA.
3. Describe the importance of patient's beliefs and goals, privacy, and autonomy as it applies to JIA.
4. Describe sensitivity to culture, diversity, gender, age, race, religion, disabilities, and sexual orientation as it may apply to JIA.
5. Describe responsibility and accountability of physiatry as it applies to JIA.
6. Describe the role of the physiatrist as an advocate for the patient with JIA.

Integrity, respect, compassion, ethics, and courtesy are integral aspects in the provision of rehabilitative care to children living with JIA and their families. The physiatrist needs to place the child and his or her well-being at the center of the treatment plan to ensure that patient-centered care is being provided.

Physiatrists by training concentrate on functional goals to help their patients achieve the highest level of function and quality of life possible. They need to advocate for patients with JIA in the medical, school, home, and community settings as well as with medical care payers whenever the need arises. If a patient develops severe contractures that are not amenable to conservative measures, the physiatrist plays a role in directing patients and their families to seek orthopedic surgical expertise for surgical evaluation (9). Physiatrists can also advocate for children with JIA in schools, communities, and local and national organizations, as well as government. They can use such forums to educate teachers and community leaders about JIA and its activity limitations and participation restrictions. Other examples of advocacy include working with schools and community officials to improve access to care and reduce architectural barriers.

Involvement of nurses in monitoring the status of patients with JIA helps maintain continuity. Utilization of elevators in schools, building of ramps, and use of grab bars in bathrooms are a few ways that barriers can be reduced.

In relation to privacy, informed consent, and confidentiality children with JIA are accustomed to those physicians with whom they have already established a connection. Outside health professionals, such as medical students who are present during consultations, can hinder the patient's ability to adequately communicate with his or her physician. It is necessary to seek consent from patients and families before any unknown health care professional is introduced to patients. Effectively communicating the reason why other health professionals may be present helps alleviate the fear of being judged or misunderstood that children with JIA may experience and also reassures patients that no outside health professional will breech confidentiality. This emphasizes the importance of a good physician–patient relationship in order to achieve optimal care for patients with JIA (9). Other considerations include HIPAA rules as they apply to children/adolescents with JIA as well as the principle of informed consent as applicable to children with JIA.

The physiatrist needs to take the time to listen and get to know his or her patients with JIA in order to understand their beliefs and goals as individuals. The physiatrist should be sensitive to the patient's cultural background, ethnicity, gender, age, religious beliefs, and sexual orientation as it may apply to the treatment plan for his or her patients with JIA. Shared decision making between the patient and the physiatrist should be a fundamental principle and cornerstone guiding medical care. The physiatrist has a responsibility to provide the highest level of compassionate care to the child with JIA within the scope and practice of rehabilitation medicine. Within that context, he or she is accountable for the provision of appropriate care. Some examples of accountability include (a) minimizing medical errors, (b) maximizing patient safety, and (c) providing high quality of rehabilitative care for the patient with JIA.

SYSTEMS-BASED PRACTICE

GOALS

Awareness and responsiveness to systems of care delivery, and the ability to recruit and coordinate effectively resources in the system to provide optimal care as it relates to JIA.

Understand the components of the rehabilitation continuum of care for the individual with JIA as well as his or her strengths, limitations, and potential for system errors.

OBJECTIVES

1. Describe key components and available services in the rehabilitation continuum of care and community rehabilitation facilities.
2. Discuss how to work effectively in various systems of care.
3. Identify patient safety components or checklist.
4. Review proper medical record keeping and documentation as the patient moves along the continuum of care.
5. Participate in identifying and avoiding potential systems- and medical-related errors for JIA and strategies to minimize them.

The rehabilitation of a child with JIA can be achieved in an inpatient rehabilitation setting, subacute setting, outpatient therapy setting, or home health setting. Once the child has been stabilized from an acute inpatient medical setting, the appropriateness of determining the rehabilitation process sets in. In the acute medical setting, the rheumatologist and the hospitalist are more of the key members of the team. Once the child is transferred to the rehabilitation setting, the physiatrist takes on a primary role. Depending on the needs of the child, the other team members can include physical, occupational, and speech therapists. Psychologists can help with coping strategies. Social workers and care coordinators can help with discharge planning and setting up therapies after discharge. Nurses and various team members are involved in teaching the patient and family members.

Inpatient rehabilitation is useful in helping build endurance and strength, and also in managing acute medical problems that are not life threatening. However, when the stamina is low, it may be wise to enroll the patients with JIA in subacute rehabilitation. This setting helps in monitoring any associated residual medical issues also. Once the patient is medically stable, outpatient therapies can be set up. It is important to ensure that the family has the ability to transport the child to and from therapies. If the child is medically stable, but not able to participate in therapies, home health may be an option. This is invaluable in maintaining the child/patient in a safe, familiar setting, which is more conducive to give the child ample time to recuperate.

Various specialists and members of the interdisciplinary team involved in the care of the child need to be able to communicate with each other to ensure continuity of care. This is to ensure safe transition of care from one stage to the other. Some instances may require inpatient admission; for instance, deconditioning due to renal disease needs twofold management of the disease process and functional rehabilitation. Upon discharge, information should be conveyed to the primary care physician and to the treating therapists. A summary of the inpatient therapy progress should be made available to the therapists.

Errors can be minimized by providing written documentation regarding medications, their side effects, complications that can arise, and therapy limitations including precautions and use of various therapy modalities. It is important to recognize that errors can occur at the time of transfer from an acute setting to the rehabilitation setting, handoff between nursing and therapists, at the time of discharge to home, and at the time of follow-up with the primary care physician.

Educating families regarding the importance of follow-up is vital in the care of the patient with JIA. Families need to understand that lack of proper ROM can lead to contractures and fractures. Patients and families need to understand the gravity of not taking medications. Proper follow-up can decrease hospitalizations, address comorbidities early, and decrease complications.

Patients/families should be provided with information regarding complications of the disease and its various treatments. This is vital to empower them with information of medical complications (such as MAS) associated with it. Atlantoaxial involvement (evidenced by atlantoaxial space 2.5–3 mm) precludes involvement with contact sports, involvement in gymnastics, and jumping on trampolines. It is important to educate families about the risk of atlantoaxial subluxation/dislocation causing spinal cord injury.

BOX 31.3 Safety Issues

- Accurate diagnosis of condition
- Education of patient and families about disease progress with or without treatment
- Side effects of medications
- Complications of disease (e.g., joint destruction)
- Psychosocial impact of disease and treatment
- Appropriate access to services: therapy, medications, counseling, social work/care coordination
- Contraindication of modalities with acute flares

Pediatric providers usually care for patients long after they become adults. This is usually because transition to adult providers, based on acceptance by funding source, is difficult. Also, not every provider is comfortable with the idea of caring for patients with childhood onset disease. This is seen more in providing primary care. It should be stressed to families that routine health maintenance is essential in bettering outcomes. This involves immunizations, eye examinations, osteoporosis, cardiovascular factors, cognitive impairment screen, and discussion of reproductive health and contraception (Box 31.3).

Per Institute of Medicine (27), health care quality is defined as the "degree to which health services for individuals and populations increase the likelihood of desired health outcomes and are consistent with current professional outcomes." Children are at risk for psychological and physical delays in development leading to disability and unemployment as adults. Per the CDC (28), people with RA have worse functional status than those with osteoarthritis and those without arthritis. People with RA have more functional losses than people without arthritis.

The cost of medications, therapies, hospitalizations, ambulatory care, and treatment of complications add up to the financial burden on a family, not to mention the cost of lost wages that families incur by missing work while caring for the child with JIA.

CASE STUDY

A 4-year-old White girl presents to your clinic with her parents for evaluation. The parents state that she had been well until a few days ago, when she started being increasingly fussy. She was refusing to walk and wanted to be carried all the time. She also had an occasional limp. She has been increasingly sleepy after playing.

When asked, she complains of her eyes hurting and squints as she tries to color a book. When asked she points to her head and states "it hurts." Parents state that she has become a picky eater and seems to have lost weight over the past few months. She has a history of a macular rash in association with her symptoms.

CASE STUDY DISCUSSION QUESTIONS

PATIENT CARE. Describe the key elements of the medical history and physical examination of this child with suspected JIA.

Describe the key elements of the rehabilitation treatment plan for this child if she is diagnosed with JIA.

MEDICAL KNOWLEDGE. What are the different types of JIA? Describe the epidemiology and the important laboratory parameters in JIA.

PRACTICE-BASED LEARNING AND IMPROVEMENT. What are the important areas to educate patients and families about JIA?

INTERPERSONAL AND COMMUNICATION SKILLS. Describe the importance of communicating with families. Identify the difference between persuasion and informed consent.

PROFESSIONALISM. Describe the importance of providing efficacious care in the context of maintaining patient privacy.

SYSTEMS-BASED PRACTICE. Describe patient safety concerns in the care of patients with JIA and strategies to minimize their occurrence.

SELF-EXAMINATION QUESTIONS
(Answers begin on p. 367)

1. JIA can present with all of the following *except*
   A. Asymmetric limb use
   B. Blurred vision
   C. Problems with fine motor skills
   D. Isolated musculoskeletal pain
   E. Joint swelling

2. CHAQ correlates inversely with
   A. Remission
   B. Bone mass
   C. Joint swelling
   D. Kidney disease
   E. Hypertension

3. All of the following are recommended in the treatment of JIA *except*
   A. Heating pads
   B. Showers
   C. Ultrasound
   D. Splints
   E. Therapy

4. Children with JIA can participate in all the following sports *except*
   A. Soccer
   B. Tai Chi
   C. Swimming
   D. Aerobic exercise
   E. Running

5. A 9-year-old girl with systemic JIA presents with persistent fever, pancytopenia, coagulopathy, and hepatosplenomegaly. Index of suspicion should be high for which of the following?
   A. SLE
   B. Flare of systemic JIA
   C. Viral infection/sepsis
   D. MAS
   E. Brucellosis

REFERENCES

1. Gotte A. *Pediatric Rheumatology: An Overview of JIA and SLA*. PowerPoint presentation. Dallas, TX: Baylor University Medical Center, Rehabilitation Residency Lecture Series; 2012.
2. Marzan KA, Shaham B. Early juvenile idiopathic arthritis. *Rheum Dis North Am*. 2012;38:355–372.
3. Susic GZ, Stojanovic NN, Pejnovic. Analysis of disease activity, functional disability and articular damage in patients with juvenile idiopathic arthritis: A prospective outcome study. *Clin Exp Rheum*. 2011;29:337–344.
4. Eyckmans L, Hilderson D, Westhovens, et al. What does it mean to grow up with juvenile idiopathic arthritis? A qualitative study on the perspectives of patients. *Clin Rheumatol*. 2011;30:459–465.
5. Singh G, Athreya BH, Fries JF, et al. Measurement of health status in children with juvenile rheumatoid arthritis. *Arthritis Rheum*. 1994;37:1761–1769.
6. Long AR, Rouster-Stevens KA. The role of exercise therapy in the management of juvenile idiopathic arthritis. *Curr Opin Rheumatol*. 2010;22:213–217.
7. Patient education fact sheet written by Dr LS Abramson and reviewed by American College of Rheumatology in 2013 and updated in 2013.
8. Weiss JE, Ilowite NT. Juvenile idiopathic arthritis. *Pediatr Clin North Am*. 2005;52:413–442.
9. Tong A, et al. Children's experiences of living with juvenile idiopathic arthritis: a thematic synthesis of qualitative studies. *Arthritis Care Res*. 2012;64(9):1392–1404.
10. Burnham JM. Inflammatory diseases and bone health in children. *Curr Opin Rheumatol*. 2012;24:548–553.
11. Gualano B, Sa Pinto AL, Perondi M, et al. Evidence for prescribing exercise as treatment in pediatric rheumatic diseases. *Autoimmun Rev*. 2010;9 (8):569–573.
12. Philpott JF, Houghton K, Luke A. Position statement: physical activity recommendations for children with specific chronic health conditions: juvenile idiopathic arthritis, hemophilia, asthma and cystic fibrosis. *Clin J Sports Med*. 2010;20:167–172.
13. Gualano B, Sa Pinto AL, Perondi MB, et al. Therapeutic effects of exercise training in patients with pediatric rheumatic diseases. *Brazilian J Rheumatol*. 2011;51(5):484–496.
14. Espinosa M, Gottleib BS. Juvenile idiopathic arthritis. *Pediatr Rev*. 2012;33(7):303–313.
15. Gowdie PJ. Juvenile idiopathic arthritis. *Pediatr Clin North Am*. 2012;59:301–327.
16. Barnabe C, Hazlewood G, Barr S, Martin L. Comparison of radiographic scoring methods in a cohort of RA patients treated with anti-TNF therapy. *Rheumatology (Oxford)*. 2012;51(5):878–881. Epub January 5, 2012.
17. Magni-Manzoni S, et al. Advances and challenges in imaging in juvenile idiopathic arthritis. *Nat Rev Rheumatol*. 2012;8:329–336.
18. JIA-AAPMR Knowledge NOW http://now.aapmr.org/peds/musculoskeletal/Pages/Juvenile-Idiopathic-Arthritis.aspx.
19. Critical elements of care for juvenile arthritis, Arthritis Foundation Handout http://www.arthritis.org/.

20. Huang J-L. New advances in JIA. *Chang Gung Med J.* 2012;35(1):1–14.
21. April KT, Walji R. The state of research on complementary and alternative medicine in pediatric rheumatology. *Rheum Dis Clin North Am.* 2011;37:85–94.
22. DeWitt EM. Medication safety in children with arthritis. *NC Med J.*2007;68(6):427–429.
23. Saag KG, et al.; on behalf of American College of Rheumatology Quality Measurement White Paper Development Workgroup. Defining quality of care in rheumatology: The American College of Rheumatology white paper on quality measurement. *Arthritis Care Res.* 2011;63:2–9.
24. http://www.rheumatology.org/ACR/practice/-Re- Accessed on 6-19-14
25. Duffy CM. Measurement of health status, functional status, and quality of life in children with JRA: clinical science for the pediatrician. *Rheum Dis Clin North Am.* 2007;33:389–402.
26. Martin RW. Communicating the risk of side effects to rheumatic patients. *Rheum Dis Clin North Am.* 2012;38:653–662.
27. Crossing the Quality Chasm; 2001.
28. http://www.cdc.gov/arthritis/basics/childhood.htm. Accessed February 13, 2013.

Answers

CHAPTER 2: THE USE OF NARRATIVE MEDICINE AND REFLECTION FOR PRACTICE-BASED LEARNING AND IMPROVEMENT

1. **Correct answer: D.** All levels of learners (students, residents, fellows, and professionals) can benefit from deliberately focusing on their clinical experiences and using narrative as a tool to both begin the reflective process and to enhance it as they process their own learning during a clinical encounter.
2. **Correct answer: A.** To promote "reflection on action," which Donald Schon promotes as a balance to "reflection in action," the prompt should not be restrictive or suggestive as this would narrow the expansion of the learning process during moments of reflection. This is a time for the learner to move beyond the usual structured thinking and be able to think openly.
3. **Correct answer: C.** Small groups participating in a reflective process focused on thinking and learning from previous experiences must have rules of conduct for all group members. The focus is respectful group dynamics that allow each group member to engage in a comfortable interaction.
4. **Correct answer: C.** A piece of prose or poetry is a "prompt" to support reflection and must be thoughtfully selected to support the purpose of the group's learning through a reflective process. As this is only one step in a three-step process (reading the poem or prose, writing about it, and then group sharing of written thoughts), time must be sufficient to allow all three-steps to occur in a defined time period so attention to length of the written piece is imperative.
5. Communal viewing of artistic paintings as a modality to increase sensitivity, team building, and collaboration among medical trainees. VTS appears to increase team building as medical interns work together, challenging each other to form a cohesive idea about the art form studied. This may later prove useful as they strategize differential diagnoses and treatment plans for patients on the wards. It appears to increase listening skills, as each intern patiently and respectfully listens to their colleagues' viewpoints prior to responding. In a profession where physicians are quick to "give the answers," perhaps this is a strategy that can increase physician trainees' listening skills both for colleagues and for patients. The process also appears to increase analytical thinking as students "decode" the images seen in the paintings. Perhaps this can extend to an increased ability to find multiple solutions to complex problems as noted in the younger students who have been studied through the VTS process. The increased visual literacy observed through this process may be useful as the interns begin analyzing x-rays, increasing their awareness about the lights and shadows that may obscure disease processes, and in the analysis of EKG patterns. To reflect means to look back and consider something. While such thoughtfulness can result in insight and learning, it does not automatically lead to the high-level analysis, questioning, and reframing required for transformative learning. Critical reflection is the process of analyzing, questioning, and reframing an experience in order to make an assessment of it for the purposes of learning (reflective learning) and/or to improve practice (reflective practice).
   —From Reilly JM, MD; Ring J, PhD; Duke L. Visual thinking strategies: A new role for art in medical education. *Fam Med* 2005; 37(4):250–2.

   One potential solution is the teaching of "visual literacy," i.e., the ability to find meaning in imagery, which in medical parlance translates into the ability to reason physiology and pathophysiology from visual clues. Educators have confirmed that visual literacy can be developed, and limited efforts to introduce similar teaching methods into clinical training have been promising. Clinical habits are formed early in training, and therefore we designed a novel preclinical course to enhance medical students' diagnostic acumen by expanding their visual skills through the (1) close observation and guided discussion of visual art, (2) exploration of core artistic concepts, and (3) opportunity to apply these skills to the clinical assessment of patients with a broad range of disorders.
   —From Naghshineh, S, et al. Formal art observation training improves medical students' visual diagnostic skills. *J Gen Intern Med* 23(7):991–7.
6. If we take the example of a medical mistake, a superficial, educationally ineffective reflection will consist of a description of the events or a description accompanied by reasons such as the team/clinic was busy and other people failed in

their responsibilities. A more useful and deeper reflection would include consideration of how and why decisions were made, underlying beliefs and values of both individuals and institutions, assumptions about roles, abilities and responsibilities, personal behavioral triggers, and similar past experiences ("when pressed for time, I . . . "), contributing hospital/clinic circumstances and policies, other perspectives on the events (frank discussion with team members, consultation of the literature or other people who might provide alternative insights and interpretations), explicit notation of lessons learned and creation of a specific, timely, and measurable plan for personal and/or system change to avoid future similar errors. Effective reflection, then, requires time, effort and a willingness to question actions, underlying beliefs and values and to solicit different viewpoints.

—From Aronson, L. Twelve tips for teaching reflection at all levels of medical education. *Med Teach* 2011; 33: 200–205.

7. Reflection artifacts (writings, pictures, diagrams) can be produced in class or as homework. In class reflection will be shorter but assures timely compliance and can sometimes be explicitly linked to other educational activities. Assignments completed outside of formal sessions offer the advantages of allowing learners more time to choose an appropriate experience upon which to reflect and opportunities to look things up and seek the feedback necessary to help them reframe their experience. Educators should consider their learning objectives when deciding which instructional methods to use for a given reflection exercise.

—From Aronson, L. Twelve tips for teaching reflection at all levels of medical education. *Med Teach* 2011; 33: 200–205.

8. Self-assessment (an ability), self-directed assessment seeking and reflection (pedagogical strategies), and self-monitoring (immediate contextually relevant responses to environmental stimuli) in an attempt to clarify the rhetoric pertaining to each activity. Equally important, internal factors or capacities influence one's ability to self-assess and self-monitor, such as reflection, mindfulness, openness, curiosity. Central challenges to informing self-assessment are the dynamic interrelationships and underlying tensions among the components comprising self-assessment. Therefore reflective practice can be a strategy to help professionals work through and untangle the interrelationships and tensions and foster the development of self-assessment as a life-long learning skill.

—From Sargeant J, et al. The processes and dimensions of informed self-assessment: a conceptual model. *Acad Med*. 2010 Jul;85(7):1212–20; Sargeant J. Toward a common understanding of self-assessment. *J Contin Educ Health Prof*. 2008 Winter; 28(1):1-4. Eva KW, Regehr G. "I'll never play professional football" and other fallacies of self-assessment space. *J Contin Educ Health Prof*. 2008 Winter;28(1):14–19.

9. In selecting learning goals, educators should answer the following questions: Are there key competencies, attitudes, content areas, or skills in need of greater attention or assessment? How can the exercise be used to help learners integrate (1) new learning with existing knowledge; (2) affective with cognitive experience; and/or (3) past with present or present with future practice? Will reflective learning or reflective skill building be an explicit focus of the exercise? Is one of the goals to identify learning or practice needs and strategies to address them?

—From Aronson, L. Twelve tips for teaching reflection at all levels of medical education. *Med Teach* 2011; 33: 200–205. The effective practice of medicine requires narrative competence, that is, the ability to acknowledge, absorb, interpret, and act on the stories and plights of others. Medicine practiced with narrative competence, called narrative medicine, is proposed as a model for humane and effective medical practice. Adopting methods such as close reading of literature and reflective writing allows narrative medicine to examine and illuminate four of medicine's central narrative situations: physician and patient, physician and self, physician and colleagues, and physicians and society.

—From Charon R. Narrative medicine: A model for empathy, reflection, profession, and trust. *JAMA*. 2001;286: 1897–1902.

CHAPTER 3: CONSCIOUS, COMPASSIONATE COMMUNICATION IN REHABILITATION MEDICINE

1. **Correct answer: C.** The DESC communication model uses four statements. Each one typically opens with the capitalized words in this example, where a doctor talks to his secretary: DESCRIBE the situation – "When you are late to work which has been often recently, and we've already discussed it," EXPLAIN impact – "I feel frustrated because the office becomes chaotic." STATE need – "I need you to be on time from now on." CONSEQUENCE (to be only used if necessary) – "If not, I'll have to write you up."

2. **Correct answer: D.** Open-ended questions ask for full sentence responses, vs. closed-ended questions which seek limited, one word answers. When asked respectfully, they elicit important information, emotions, needs, and so forth, and make the person feel valued and cared about. Examples to a patient: "What situations trigger your pain?" vs. "Does it hurt when you walk?" The latter elicits "Yes" or "No." The former might elicit, "It hurts when I walk, bend, stand too long – anything I do makes it hurt. I'm so frustrated, Doc, because I can't move without being in awful pain!" Then the patient starts to cry. This response provides a much clearer picture of the patient's situation and allows a needed release of pent up feelings.

3. **Correct answer: C.** It's very important in resolving conflicts for each party to look honestly at him- or herself and what he or she did to worsen the situation and to humbly express this to the other(s), with an apology if needed. Though one might be correct about what someone else did wrong, and it may even be appropriate to express that with neutral language in a non-derogatory way, more of the focus should be on individuals owning up to their side of the problem. This calms the tone of the situation, causes less defensiveness in the others, and creates space for problem solving.

4. **Correct answer: C.** Reflective listening means "reflecting back" to a person or paraphrasing (not verbatim) their content, plus emotions or needs they didn't state but that seem present.

This makes the speaker feel heard, keeps the focus on them, and lets the listener hear accurately. Say a resident says to his peer, "I can't believe that the chairman, Dr. Marks, corrected and criticized me in front of the nurses. The nerve of him!" A reflective response is, "Wow, I hear how angry you are that Dr. Marks called you out on a mistake in public like that." Other responses like sharing a similar story of one's own or giving advice may be common and even appropriate at times, but they don't have quite the same effect as reflective listening.

5. **Correct answer: B.** Using "I" statements to express emotions, needs and opinions create honesty, vulnerability and humility in the speaker – as they may be saying things that are hard to say – and less defensiveness in the listener. It's hard to argue with someone's feelings. For example if a resident says to a nurse, "I felt embarrassed and humiliated when you yelled at me in front of my patient," or "You are incredibly rude for yelling at me in front of my patient," the nurse will more likely feel badly and apologize after hearing the former statement.

CHAPTER 4: APPLICATION OF PRINCIPLES OF PROFESSIONAL EDUCATION FOR PHYSICIANS

1. **Correct answer: C.** The other options require understanding of NAS's five levels according to the Dreyfus Competencies Model, Stages of Learning Model from Unconscious Incompetence to Unconscious Competence, and the RIME model.
2. **Correct answer: D.** Practice-based learning and improvement (PBLI) is the ability to investigate and evaluate patient care practices, appraise and assimilate scientific evidence, and improve their patient care practices. Some qualities of PBLI include: quality improvement (QI) and performance improvement (PI); evidence-based practice; guidelines/best practices/benchmarks; continuous professional development (CPD)/continuing medical education (CME); teaching skills; lifelong learning and practice self-assessment; and utilization of medical informatics and information technology to improve patient care (acgme.org).
3. **Correct answer: E.** Adults are predominantly self-directed and learner-centered. Reflection is a source for learning and improvement. Learner's past experience, knowledge, skills, values, and motives impact their need for learning. Adults prefer immediate feedback after their performance. Learning is relevant, meaningful, practical, and relates to current task and application.
4. **Correct answer: D.** This is a learning contract between the resident and the faculty supervisor and outlines what should happen when rotation begins. B (background assessment of resident competency), O (opportunities offered during rotation, and seek resident need for opportunities), G (goals/objectives/competencies of rotation), E (when, how, and by whom will resident be evaluated?), R (rescue plan, consequences, remediation plan if milestones not being met), D (mutual understanding of deal).
5. **Correct answer: A.** Wolpaw's SNAPPS six-step model is an ideal learner-centered process for conducting case presentations where the resident presenting the case takes the active lead. Shewhart Deming's PDSA (plan/do/study-check/act) cycle is a process for conducting quality and continuous practice improvement. Kern's six-step approach is one of the best tools to use when developing a curriculum. Kirkpatrick is well known for articulating four levels of evaluation (perceived reaction change, learning change, translation to behavior change, and results or learning outcomes). Moore, Cervero, and Fox contributed to a conceptual model for continuing medical education (CME).
6. **Correct answer: E.** All the methods included for PBL&I are rated as most desirable. In all the other choices for A to D, one or more methods are not suggested as most desirable. (See Chapter 4, Appendix 2, ACGME Competencies: Suggested Best Methods for Evaluation).
7. **Correct answer: C.** According to Panagaro's RIME model, a PGY 2 fits into the top right-hand quadrant of Peel's table: Interpreter of information, Dreyfus' Advanced Beginner, ACGME Indirect (with Direct immediately available) supervision level, Disillusioned Beginner, and Conscious Incompetence.
8. **Correct answer: E.** SAFETY refers to the resident guide for attending input. SUPERB refers to the guide for attending supervision. The "S" in SAFETY refers to the resident seeking attending input early. The "S" in SUPERB is setting resident expectations for when the attending should be notified.

CHAPTER 5: ETHICAL CONSIDERATIONS IN THE PRACTICE OF REHABILITATION MEDICINE

1. **Correct answer: C.** The essential ingredients of the Nuremburg Code are as follows: (a) voluntary consent of the human subject is essential; (b) there must be no coercion, no deceit, and a full explanation of risks and benefits by the investigator(s); (c) there must be an expectation of gaining useful knowledge; (d) thorough preliminary studies must be conducted before human studies; (e) avoidance of unnecessary suffering or injury is mandatory; (f) there must be no expectation of death or injury as an outcome; (g) risks must not exceed benefits; (h) proper facilities are required; (i) only qualified investigators should be allowed; (j) subject(s) can withdraw at any time; (k) investigator must terminate the study if harm seems likely.
2. **Correct answer: A.** The primacy of patient welfare helps provide a moral compass for the physician, in that the physician's altruism must not be affected by economic, bureaucratic, and political challenges that are faced by the physician and the patient. The principle of patient autonomy asserts that physicians make the recommendations but patients make the final decisions. Autonomy is the idea that people should have the right and freedom to choose, pursue, and revise their own life plans. The principle of social justice symbolizes that a patient–physician interaction exists in a community or society. The physician has a responsibility to the individual patient and a broader society to promote access and to eliminate the disparities in health and the health care system. This calls upon the profession to promote a fair distribution of health care resources.
3. **Correct answer: C.** The principle of social justice symbolizes that a patient–physician interaction exists in a community

or society. The physician has a responsibility to the individual patient and a broader society to promote access and to eliminate the disparities in health and the health care system. This calls upon the profession to promote a fair distribution of health care resources.

4. **Correct answer: B.** The principle of patient autonomy asserts that physicians make the recommendations but patients make the final decisions. The physician is an expert advisor who must inform and empower the patient to base a decision on scientific data and how this information can and should be integrated with the patient's preferences. The patient's decision about his or her care must be paramount, as long as those decisions are in keeping with ethical practice and do not lead to demands for inappropriate care. The patient's family can make decisions only in the event when the patient lacks decision-making capacity based on the medical recommendation as well as the patient's prior expressed preferences, if any.

5. **Correct answer: D.** The 10 professional commitments in the Charter of Medical Professionalism are (a) professional competence, (b) honesty with patients, (c) patient confidentiality, (d) maintaining appropriate relations with patients, (e) improving the quality of care, (f) improving access to care, (g) just distribution of finite resources, (h) scientific knowledge, (i) maintaining trust by managing conflicts of interest, and (j) professional responsibilities.

6. **Correct answer: C.** The principle of Double effect is an important ethical principle designed to ensure safe and adequate patient care and to protect health care providers who treat these patients. It validates the use of treatments that are aimed at relieving suffering even in the event that these interventions may inadvertently shorten a patient's life. The intent of treatment must be to relieve symptoms, not to end life. The four elements of the doctrine are as follows: (a) the good effect has to be intended (pain or dyspnea relief with opioids); (b) the bad effect can be foreseen but not intended (awareness of possible shortening of life); (c) the bad effect cannot be the means to good effect (cannot end life to relieve dyspnea); (d) the symptoms must be severe enough to warrant taking risks. (This is proportionality.)

CHAPTER 6: PROFESSIONALISM

1. **Correct answer: A.** Impaired physicians can have a significant negative impact on patient care as well as on the effectiveness of the team providing care to the patient. According to the Federation of State Medical Boards, the definition of an impairment is "the inability of a physician to practice medicine with reasonable skill and safety as a result of a mental disorder or physical illness or condition, including but not limited to those illnesses or conditions that would adversely affect cognitive, motor or perceptive skills or substance-related disorders including abuse and dependency of drugs and alcohol."

2. **Correct answer: A.** The Ethical Issues Subcommittee of the Medical Practice Committee of the American Academy of Physical Medicine and Rehabilitation (AAPM&R) has developed a Code of Conduct for the practice of rehabilitation medicine. This code is meant to "serve as a guideline for professional and personal behavior and to promote the highest quality of physiatric care." The code is meant to outline ethical practice for physiatrists. The code addresses relationships between physiatrists and their patients and families, members of the rehabilitation team, other physicians, and the community and government. It also addresses research and scholarly activities.

3. **Correct answer: C.** The Code addresses conflicts of interest that can impact patient care by stating: "Conflicts of interest must be resolved in the best interest of the patient." Physicians must identify potential conflicts of interest and disclose them to their patients.

4. **Correct answer: D.** The physician should ask clinical questions designed to elicit information from patients about their ideas about what they think might be wrong with them and their feelings and fears about their illness.

5. **Correct answer: C.** The 10 professional responsibilities from the Physician Charter published by the American Board of Internal Medicine Foundation and the American College of Physicians Foundation are as follows: (a) commitment to professional competence, (b) commitment to honesty with patients, (c) commitment to patient confidentiality, (d) commitment to maintaining appropriate relations with patients, (e) commitment to improving quality of care, (f) commitment to improving access to care, (g) commitment to a just distribution of finite resources, (h) commitment to scientific knowledge, (i) commitment to maintaining trust by managing conflicts of interest, and (j) commitment to professional responsibilities.

CHAPTER 7: SYSTEMS-BASED PRACTICE

1. **Correct answer: A.** According to the IHI, the purpose of performing an RCA is to understand the systems failures that led to the adverse event in order to prevent it from happening again in the future. A root cause analysis seeks to learn what happened and why, and what can be done that both prevents recurrence and maintains confidence in patient safety measures in the future.

2. **Correct answer: C.** The patient admitted to the IRF following a recent serious illness or exacerbation of a serious illness has a decreased ability to perform activities of daily living or ambulate safely. He or she needs close medical monitoring of his or her illness or comorbidities, needs rehabilitation nursing services 24 hours per day and 7 days per week, can actively participate in a rehabilitation program of 3 hours per day for 5 days per week, can achieve realistic goals in a reasonable period of time, and can safely be discharged to home or a community setting.

3. **Correct answer: A.** Ottenbacher and Graham described four types of barriers to access for rehabilitation services: financial, personal, structural, and attitudinal. Financial barriers include insurance coverage and out-of-pocket expenses for treatments. Personal barriers include lack of understanding of rehabilitative resources available, lack of knowledge about

how to access these services by patients, and socioeconomic factors. Examples of structural barriers include referral patterns restricted to specific providers and institutions, and the 3-hour rule, which limits access to certain types of rehabilitation facilities. Attitudinal barriers are based on individual beliefs and preferences about rehabilitation services and their outcomes.

4. **Correct answer: D.** In order for an IRF to be paid under the prospective payment system instead of the acute care hospital inpatient prospective payment system, the facility must treat patients with 1 of 13 medical conditions for a minimum of 60% of its total inpatient population. This compliance threshold is known as the "60 percent rule." These medical conditions are stroke, spinal cord injury, congenital deformity, amputation, major multiple trauma, hip fracture, brain injury, and neurological disorders (multiple sclerosis, motor neuron disease, polyneuropathy, muscular dystrophy, Parkinson's disease, and burns).

5. **Correct answer: A.** A course of outpatient rehabilitation commonly includes services provided by physical therapists, occupational therapists, speech pathologists, and physiatrists. Medicare pays for services provided by skilled professionals, which are appropriate, effective for a patient's condition, and reasonable in terms of frequency and duration. The beneficiary must be under the care of a physician, have a treatable condition, and be improving. Medicare does not cover maintenance-level outpatient therapy services.

6. **Correct answer: B.** Medicare covers costs of an admission in a skilled nursing facility for patients following a hospital stay of at least 3 days that requires specialized nursing and/or rehabilitative care. Medicare pays the SNF on a predetermined per diem rate for up to 100 days through a prospective payment system. The base payment rate takes into account geographic differences in labor costs and case mix. Case mixes enable the Resource Utilization Groups (RUGs), which have nursing and rehabilitative therapy weights that are applied to the base payment rate.

7. **Correct answer: C.** According to Peter Senge, systems thinking is the practice of seeing wholes. It is a framework for identifying significant relationships between the influences of macrocosmic forces and structures rather than within them. It is seeing patterns of change, rather than static snapshots. It is a focus on "circles of causality" and interrelationships, rather than linear cause-and-effect chains, and underscores the maxim that "every influence is both cause and effect. Nothing is ever influenced in just one direction."

CHAPTER 9: UPPER EXTREMITY AMPUTEE

1. **Correct answer: B.** The ideal shape of a transhumeral amputee should be cylindrical to allow optimal fit of the socket.
2. **Correct answer: B.** Phantom limb pain is reduced from immediate placement in a compressive rigid dressing. The most common type of compressive dressing used has been an IPOP.
3. **Correct answer: C.** Joint Commission and the Accreditation have stressed the holistic and spiritual approach to all patients.
4. **Correct answer: D.** The most important person on any health care team is the patient. Patient-centric models are now being adopted across the health care industry as evidenced in Patient Aligned Care Teams (PACTs) in the VA.
5. **Correct answer: B.** Hand transplants are a major undertaking and are not the answer for everyone. They are considered when there are multiple amputations, particularly in military-related injuries. The screening for hand transplants is complex and needs to include a functional assessment and mainly a psychological assessment for candidacy. As in all transplants, this will involve a commitment to a lifetime of immunosuppressive therapy as well as almost 2 years of intensive occupational therapy in order to perform basic hand functions.
6. **Correct answer: A.** Errors most commonly occur in hand-offs between services, changes in shifts, and change of health care teams. The communication during these transitions is key to avoiding errors. The Joint Commission realizes this and looks for system applications in facilities and via tracer rounds on all who are involved in a particular patient's care.

CHAPTER 10: LOWER EXTREMITY AMPUTATION

1. **Correct answer: D.** While all of these issues are important in a physiatric history, an issue often overlooked and important for donning and doffing prosthesis is hand dexterity. This should be a consideration for deciding the type of suspension and prosthesis that may be used in each individual patient.
2. **Correct answer: C.** Choke syndrome is an important issue to note and correct in a new amputee for both functional and safety issues. The first step in correcting choke syndrome, before making major modifications to the socket, is that a distal socket pad should be used to see whether this alleviates the issue. This is both the most efficient and cost-effective means of correcting the situation and often fixes the situation without major fabrication or changes.
3. **Correct answer: C.** CARF accreditation has become a system standard in defining a program that is focused on effective and efficient rehabilitation and outcome-based measures. The Commission in the recent years has emphasized a holistic approach as evidence-based medicine has demonstrated that a holistic approach in rehabilitation is more beneficial to patients in both functional outcome and psychosocial well-being.
4. **Correct answer: E.** Clear and efficient communication with a patient should be a goal for the physician in communicating with the patient. A slow-to-moderate pace, varying tone demonstrating conversational appearance, appropriate time, and vocabulary are all integral to effective communication with a patient. It is not, however, the physician's duty to convey treatment plan information to all who visit the patient, as this can be both time-consuming and possibly a HIPAA-related issue.
5. **Correct answer: B.** Complex regional pain syndrome can be devastating, but is not an indication for elective amputation. Instead, the most appropriate next step would be to have this patient see a counselor who specializes in pain to help with coping strategies and to remove focus on a surgery that would more likely limit function rather than improve function.

6. **Correct answer: A.** Multiple studies have demonstrated transition periods are the most common time for a medical error to occur. This can be seen in deletion of allergies, accidental changes in medications or dosing, or miscommunication of precautions. While it is always important to follow systems processes and communication protocols, transition times are the most important time to recheck and review for these errors.

CHAPTER 11: CARDIOPULMONARY REHABILITATION

1. **Correct answer: D.** This is the measured physiological efficiency of oxygen extraction by cardiac myocytes. It is important to know this as it reflects a high degree of extraction of oxygen at all levels of activity and reflects that any reduction of blood flow will cause ischemia to the heart tissue.
2. **Correct answer: A.** This is a measured value from experimental physiology. The reason it is important for physiatrists and those who work with patients with disability to know this is that many of our patients perform exercise in a non-erect position—either seated or sometimes in recumbent positions. Exercise in these other positions and with arms increases the myocardial oxygen consumption relative to the same level of activity in nondisabled individuals and places patients with disability at greater risk of myocardial ischemia.
3. **Correct answer: C.** This is an established and measured value form of exercise physiology. It appears that the more intensive the exercise the greater the effect, so there is a dose–response curve. The latest investigations are looking into the efficacy and safety of high-intensity interval training, which may be most effective of all, but has possible adverse side effects in some populations. This is a dynamic area of exercise physiology that may have new recommendations in coming years.
4. **Correct answer: D.** This is the benefit of exercise training. With exercise, the heart muscle (unless the patient has severely decreased ejection fraction below 25%) with hypertrophy can be able to have a higher ejection fraction at all stages of activity. Along with a higher ejection fraction, the heart will also have enhanced relaxation so that end diastolic volume will increase and end systolic volume will decrease. This yields a higher volume with each heartbeat (increased stroke volume). An increased stroke volume is beneficial as it will allow a lower heart rate for any level of activity. Since heart rate is the major determinant of mVO_2, this will lower the incidence of angina or ischemia at a given workload.
5. **Correct answer: D.** This is the effect of cardiac denervation in the transplanted heart. Patients post transplant will have no vagal or sympathetic innervation of their heart as those nerves are not reconnected as a part of the normal transplant surgery. The result is a lack of parasympathetic inhibition at rest (higher heart rate at rest) and a blunted heart rate at exercise due to a lack of sympathetic innervation. There is also a delayed onset of increase in heart rate in response to exercise since only circulating catecholamines can increase heart rate, and a prolonged recovery to baseline due to the lack of parasympathetic innervation. Patient education about this is important to reassure a patient that the altered responses are normal post transplant and to allow them to incorporate longer warm-up and cool-down periods for exercise.

CHAPTER 12: CANCER REHABILITATION

1. **Correct answer: B.** Cisplatin is a platinum-based compound that is used to treat metastatic testicular and ovarian cancers and advanced bladder cancer. It has been linked with dose-related and cumulative nephrotoxicity, ototoxicity, myelosuppression, nausea, vomiting, and peripheral neuropathy. The neuropathy usually occurs after several months of therapy; however, it can be seen even after one treatment or after the treatment has been discontinued. Elderly patients may be more susceptible to developing the peripheral neuropathy. Dorsal column myelopathy and autonomic neuropathy have also been reported.
2. **Correct answer: A.** Breast, lung, prostate, renal, and thyroid cancers have been linked with metastasis to bone. Metastatic lesions can increase the risk of pathological fracture. Factors such as size of lesion, type of lesion, site of lesion, and pain can be used to characterize the risk of a pathological fracture. Weight-bearing precautions should be established prior to inception of a rehabilitation program in patients with metastatic disease to bone.
3. **Correct answer: D.** Cancer staging describes the extent or severity of a patient's malignancy and is based on the TNM system, which stands for T = tumor (size of the primary tumor); N = nodes (whether the cancer has spread to regional lymph nodes); M = metastasis (distant spread). The TNM classification system is specific to the cancer type.
4. **Correct answer: B.** Prehabilitation is really the beginning of the cancer rehabilitation care continuum and has been defined as "a process on the cancer continuum of care that occurs between the time of cancer diagnosis and the beginning of acute treatment and includes physical and psychological assessments that establish a baseline functional level, identify impairments, and provide interventions that promote physical and psychological health to reduce the incidence and/or severity of future impairments."
5. **Correct answer: C.** This is multifactorial in nature: (a) reluctance on the part of patients to tell their oncologists about their problems with ambulation, generalized weakness, impaired balance, and cognition; (b) lack of awareness and inquiring about these problems on the part of the ontological team; and (c) lack of referral for appropriate rehabilitation services.

CHAPTER 13: STROKE

1. **Correct answer: E.** Age, gender, race, and heredity have been identified as nonmodifiable risk markers for stroke. Although these factors cannot be modified, their presence helps identify those at greatest risk, allowing treatment of those risk factors that can be modified, such as hypertension, diabetes mellitus, and cigarette smoking.
2. **Correct answer: B.** Atrial fibrillation is an arrhythmia in which blood does not flow quickly through the heart, which

makes it more likely for a clot to form. The source of embolic strokes is most often cardiac in nature as up to 75% of all cardiac emboli travel up to the brain, causing an ischemic stroke.
3. **Correct answer: A**. As much as 85% of strokes are ischemic in nature; they can be divided into embolic and thrombotic.
4. **Correct answer: C**. Heterotopic ossification is the presence of bone tissue growth in an area outside the skeleton. It is a complication most frequently noted in musculoskeletal trauma, spinal cord injury, and brain injury.
5. **Correct answer: C**. As many as 15% of stroke patients suffer from urinary incontinence 1 year post stroke.

CHAPTER 14: MODERATE AND SEVERE TRAUMATIC BRAIN INJURY

1. **Correct answer: B**. Severity of TBI is graded based upon GCS, PTA, and LOC. Using Table 14.1, GCS places the patient in the moderate severity category, LOC in the mild severity category, and PTA in the moderate severity category. When grading severity, use the worst severity indicated by the three measures. In this patient's case, it is moderate.
2. **Correct answer: D**. Autonomic dysfunction or dysautonomia is characterized by hypertension, tachycardia, and diaphoresis due to increased sympathetic tone.
3. **Correct answer: D**. Beta-blockers (propranolol), SSRIs (sertraline), antiepileptics (valproic acid), and antipsychotics (olanzapine) are effective in treating agitation after TBI. Acetaminophen has not been evaluated in the treatment of agitation after TBI.
4. **Correct answer: A**. Baclofen, tizanidine, diazepam, and clonazepam all are active on the central nervous system at different receptors. By acting upon the central nervous system, they will cause sedation. Dantrolene acts within the muscle and does not cause sedation.
5. **Correct answer: B**. The Centers for Disease Control and Prevention (CDC) calculates the lifetime costs of a person severely injured by TBI as between $600K and $1.875M.

CHAPTER 15: MILD TRAUMATIC BRAIN INJURY

1. **Correct answer: D**. This marine sustained a head trauma that induced a physiological disruption of brain function manifested as 10-minute alteration in mental state (dazed and confused). The other options are incorrect. Option A is incorrect because the LOC was longer than 30 minutes; option B is incorrect because the GCS was lower than 13; in options C and E the persons do not fulfill any of the ACRM criteria for MTBI.

   In order to meet the ACRM criteria for mild TBI, a traumatically induced physiological disruption of brain function must be manifested by at least one of the following: (a) LOC, (b) any alteration in mental state at the time of the accident, (c) any loss of memory immediately before or after the accident, and (d) focal neurological deficit that may or may not be transient. The limit included in this definition is that the loss of consciousness cannot exceed 30 minutes; the initial GCS after 30 minutes cannot be lower than 13; and the period of posttraumatic amnesia (PTA) cannot exceed 24 hours.

2. **Correct answer: C**. This patient has chronic daily posttraumatic migraine headache that is interfering with his function. At this point, he requires not only an abortive but also a prophylactic treatment because his headaches are daily.
3. **Correct answer: D**. Obstructive sleep apnea is often seen after a traumatic brain injury. Headache upon awakening from sleep and unrefreshed sleep are some of the symptoms that may raise suspicion of sleep apnea. In addition to treatment of her headache, she also should be referred for a sleep study.
4. **Correct answer: B**. Although this 70-year-old man appeared to be back to his baseline, he may be in a lucid interval. It is imperative to rule out intracranial bleed and a CT scan is indicated in this case.

   Non contrast head CT is *indicated* (level A recommendations) when the patient has loss of consciousness or posttraumatic amnesia plus one or more of the following: age >60 years, GCS <15, headache, vomiting, evidence of trauma above the clavicle, posttraumatic seizure, drug or alcohol intoxication, short-term memory impairment, coagulopathy, or focal neurological deficit.
5. **Correct answer: A**. Early education of patients and their families is the best available treatment for mild TBI and for preventing or reducing the development of persistent symptoms.

CHAPTER 16: SPINAL CORD INJURY

1. **Correct answer: B**. Per ISNCSCI convention, each key muscle is thought to be innervated by two nerve roots. If the muscle strength is normal or 5/5 in a particular key muscle, both its nerve roots are thought to be intact. If the muscle strength is 3/5 or 4/5, one root is thought to be intact and the other impaired, while if strength is less than 3/5, neither root is thought to be intact. As the elbow flexors are innervated by the C5 and C6 nerve roots and the wrist extensors by the C6 and C7 nerve roots, the motor level on the right is by definition C6, while on the left it is C5.
2. **Correct answer: A**. After SCI, HO is most commonly found around the hip.
3. **Correct answer: E**. Injury to the spinal cord at a discrete location results in LMN injury at the level of injury and UMN injury at levels below. A cauda equina syndrome by definition is an injury to nerve roots within the canal distal to the termination of the cord and is an LMN-type injury. As sacral reflexes usually are not present after cauda equina injury, reflex evacuation of the rectum cannot take place.
4. **Correct answer: B**. A constellation of weakness greater in the arms than the legs and variable bowel and bladder involvement combined with a mechanism of injury that includes hyperextension of the cervical spine in the setting of underlying cervical spondylosis is pathognomic of a central cord syndrome.
5. **Correct answer: D**. Approximately 20% of deaths after SCI are related to respiratory causes; of these, nearly 80% are pneumonia.

CHAPTER 17: PARKINSON DISEASE

1. **Correct answer: C**. PD is a neurological disease that affects the motor system. It is a result of the loss of dopaminergic brain cells that control motor function. PD is a clinical

diagnosis that consists of primary motor signs of bradykinesia, resting tremor, rigidity, and gait/postural instability.

2. **Correct answer: C.** PD affects roughly 1% of the population over the age of 60, with the average onset at 60 years of age. About 10% of the PD population is below the age of 40. PD has been estimated to cause an additional $20 billion in societal cost.

3. **Correct answer: B.** PD is a neurological disease that affects the motor system. It is a result of the loss of dopaminergic brain cells that control motor function. These cells are primarily located in the substantia nigra.

4. **Correct answer: A.** While there are many types of treatment for PD targeting the symptoms of the disease, the gold standard medical treatment for PD is L-dopa. This directly correlates with the fact that the disease is caused by a loss of dopaminergic cells in the brain, and L-dopa increases the amount of dopamine available for neurons to use.

5. **Correct answer: A.** There are several common side effects of taking L-dopa, including nausea, vomiting, loss of appetite, lightheadedness, low blood pressure, and confusion. One side effect that can be of particular concern is dyskinesia, which is involuntary movement of the limbs or trunk. Apraxia, hemiballismus, dementia, and urinary incontinence are not known side effects with the treatment of L-dopa.

6. **Correct answer: A.** Rehabilitation has been extremely effective in helping patients suffering from PD. With focused exercises and rehabilitation, many of the symptoms of PD can be alleviated, such as problems with gait, voice disorders, tremors, rigidity, cognitive decline, and depression.

CHAPTER 18: NEUROMUSCULAR DISEASES

1. **Correct answer: C.** The American Academy of Neurology recommends the placement of gastrostomy tubes for individuals with ALS while they can still tolerate oral intake and before the forced vital capacity (FVC) falls below 50% of predicted to reduce the complications associated with the procedure compared with patients without severe respiratory compromise.

2. **Correct answer: A.** Amyotrophic lateral sclerosis (ALS) is the most common adult-onset motor neuron disease affecting 1.8 per 100,000 with the average age of onset around 60 years of age.

3. **Correct answer: D.** Acute inflammatory demyelinating neuropathy (AIDP), also known as Guillain-Barré syndrome, causes an acute generalized weakness with initial symptoms of distal numbness and areflexia/hyporeflexia. Cerebral spinal fluid (CSF) of AIDP patients shows increased proteins and low white blood cell counts (cytoalbumino-disassociation). Nerve conduction studies may show prolonged or absent F reflexes. *Campylobacter jejuni* enteritis has been implicated as a trigger for AIDP. Treatment includes medical stabilization and then treatment with plasmapheresis or IVIG.

4. **Correct answer: D.** Myotonic dystrophy type I (DM1) is an autosomal dominant disease that is linked to chromosome 19. The neck flexors are affected early, and atrophy and weakness of the facial and jaw muscles results in a "hatchet face" appearance. Many patients are not aware of their myotonia but it usually can be seen on examination when there is delayed relaxation of the fingers after forceful hand grip. Percussion of muscle groups gives rise to a delayed relaxation. Associated manifestations include cataracts, mild mental retardation, infertility, and cardiac arrhythmias/cardiomyopathy.

5. **Correct answer: D.** Acetylcholine receptor at the postsynaptic neuromuscular junction causes destruction of the receptors. Early symptoms of myasthenia include ptosis and double vision secondary to ocular muscle weakness. Approximately 10% of patients will have a thymoma; thus, imaging with chest x-ray (CXR) or computed tomography (CT) scan are often indicated. Specialized EMG testing with increased jitter on single-fiber EMG or a decremental response on repetitive stimulation at slow rates help confirm myasthenia gravis.

CHAPTER 19: MULTIPLE SCLEROSIS

1. **Correct answer: A.** The sine qua non of MS is that symptomatic episodes are "separated in time and space"—that is, episodes occur months or years apart and affect different neuroanatomic locations. As an example, a patient may present with paresthesias of a hand that resolves, followed a few months later by weakness in a leg or visual disturbances. In addition, the duration of the attack should be longer than 24 hours. Presentation of MS often varies among patients. Some patients have a predominance of cognitive changes, while others present with prominent ataxia, hemiparesis or paraparesis, depression, or visual symptoms. Additionally, it is important to recognize that the progression of physical and cognitive disability in MS may occur in the absence of clinical exacerbations.

2. **Correct answer: C.** The location where the patient spent the first 15 years of his or her life is valuable information since migration studies indicate that the likelihood of developing the disease depends on where a person spent the first 15 years of life.

3. **Correct answer: C.** MS is the most common cause of nontraumatic disability affecting young people in the Northern Hemisphere. There are about 400,000 persons in the United States living with MS, and the prevalence ranges from 40 to 220 per 100,000 people. The incidence of MS is 171/100,000 persons, with females accounting for approximately 70% of cases.

4. **Correct answer: D.** Falls are the most important consequences of gait and balance disturbances in patients with MS. Studies reveal that about 50% to 60% of patients report at least one fall in the community within the past 2 to 6 months. Common activities in which falls occur are transfers and ambulation.

5. **Correct answer: D.** Whereas the use of disease-modifying therapies has been shown to reduce relapses and slow down the disease process, they come at a very high cost that prohibits some patients from receiving them. This is especially problematic for low-income patients, whom may not have even received adequate education, particularly about immunomodulating drugs. This is important in light of the fact that starting disease-modifying treatment earlier in the disease

process before signs of disability start result in less cost per quality-adjusted year and improvements in long-term effects of MS.

CHAPTER 20: OSTEOARTHRITIS

1. **Correct answer: C.** Obesity is a strong and modifiable risk factor for osteoarthritis, both locally and systemically. Weight reduction has been proven to reduce both the development and progression of osteoarthritis. Therefore, prevention efforts and education aimed at weight management or weight reduction are likely to reduce the prevalence and slow the progression of osteoarthritis at a population level.
2. **Correct answer: E.** The initial diagnosis of osteoarthritis is often based on the clinical findings, and routine imaging is not recommended for most cases. The signs and symptoms of osteoarthritis are often apparent before the development of plain radiographic changes; therefore, plain radiographs are insensitive for early osteoarthritis and normal radiographs do not rule out the diagnosis. Musculoskeletal ultrasound, MRI, and CT scanning are not recommended for routine evaluation, but are often done to rule out other potential causes of pain. The choice of modality will depend on the differential diagnosis.
3. **Correct answer: B.** Medications available for the treatment of osteoarthritis are prescribed for the relief of pain. There are currently no available agents that prevent or reduce the progression of osteoarthritis. The first-line agent for pain relief is acetaminophen. NSAIDs are second-line agents and the choice of NSAID should be based on risk factors, as both nonselective and COX-2-selective NSAIDs have similar efficacy. Opioids of any type are considered only for patients who have contraindications to or treatment failure with acetaminophen or NSAIDs.
4. **Correct answer: D.** Exercise has been shown in clinical studies to assist with weight management and has resulted in greater weight loss when combined with reduced caloric intake. Regular exercise maintains muscle strength, which protects the articular cartilage from the effect of forces across the joint. Additionally, it protects against functional decline and reduces pain over time.
5. **Correct answer: A.** ACL injury prevention programs have resulted in declines in injury rates and consist of eccentric training programs, not concentric exercise programs. In addition, the prevention programs utilize a variety of strategies that include avoidance of high-risk behaviors, balance and proprioceptive training, standardized warm-ups and practices, and training in sports-specific agility skills.

CHAPTER 21: REHABILITATION FOLLOWING TOTAL KNEE ARTHROPLASTY AND TOTAL HIP ARTHROPLASTY

1. **Correct answer: C.** There are several complications to be aware of after joint arthroplasty surgery. These include, but are not limited to, infections, blood clots, joint dislocation, nerve injuries, and contractures. Increased muscle tone is not a known common complication of joint arthroplasty.
2. **Correct answer: C.** The common life span of the majority of joint replacements is approximately 10 to 20 years in 90% of patients.
3. **Correct answer: C.** Antibiotics serve to both protect and treat bacterial infections associated with surgery. Antibiotics do not directly affect the other complications of bone fractures, joint dislocations, contractures, and joint pain.
4. **Correct answer: E.** All of these diseases can cause joint pain in adults, including the hip joint.
5. **Correct answer: D.** According to recent studies, over the years of 1990 and 2002, there has been an increase of approximately 50%.

CHAPTER 22: SPASTICITY

1. **Correct answer: D.** Using "open-ended" questions is the correct answer. All of the other choices are not correct examples of effectively communicating between physicians and patients when dealing with spasticity. Using "open-ended" questions showing empathy and listening promote effective communication.
2. **Correct answer: C.** Baclofen binds to GABA receptors in the spinal cord to inhibit the reflexes that lead to increased tone. Baclofen is typically started at a lower dose to avoid the side-effect profile of sedation. It should not be immediately withdrawn, as doing so may cause possible seizures. Tizanidine and clonidine are both alpha 2 agonists. Dantrolene works in the striated muscle at the level of the sarcoplasmic reticulum. Botulinum toxin irreversibly binds neuromuscular junction transmission by inhibiting presynaptic acetylcholine release. Clinical efficacy of botulinum toxin is typically up to 3 to 4 months and recovery is due to axonal sprouting.
3. **Correct answer: B.** One of the key roles that the physiatrist plays in caring for a patient with spasticity is to be their advocate. There are few, if any, other fields in medicine that truly understand spasticity, its impact on function, and the treatment options available. Treatment should not be guided solely by patient presentation but rather should be guided on goals set by the patient and their caregivers. Goals set will be specific to each patient. Although the physiatrist is an important part of the patient's care team, goals are set by patients and/or their caregivers, not by the physician. Another responsibility of the physiatrist is to ensure patients have all options available to them, regardless of economic status or insurance plan.
4. **Correct answer: C.** Although cost, side effects, and insurance coverage are all important factors to consider, ultimately it is the patient's decision as to which treatment option he or she would like to pursue. Physiatrists are responsible for ensuring the patient is equipped with all the information he or she needs to make an informed consent, which includes information about cost and insurance coverage, as well as risk vs. benefit analysis. Physician preference should not be a factor when presenting options to patients.
5. **Correct answer: C.** The MAS is scored from 0 to 4 with a 1+. A MAS of 0 indicates no increase in muscle tone, a 1 is

a slight increase in muscle tone manifested by a catch and release or by minimal resistance at the end of the range of motion when the affected part(s) is moved in flexion or extension, a 1+ is a slight increase in muscle tone manifested by a catch and followed by minimal resistance throughout the remainder (less than half) of the ROM, a 2 is a more marked increase in muscle tone through most of the ROM but affected part(s) are easily moved, a 3 is a considerable increase in muscle tone making passive movement difficult, and a 4 indicates that affected parts are rigid.

CHAPTER 23: MUSCULOSKELETAL DISORDERS: UPPER EXTREMITY

1. **Correct answer: C.** de Quervain tenosynovitis is a tenosynovitis of the sheath that surrounds the two tendons that control movement of the thumb, the extensor pollicis brevis and abductor pollicis longus tendons. Finkelstein's test, which was described in 1930 by Harry Finkelstein, an American surgeon, is used to diagnose de Quervain syndrome in people who have wrist pain. The patient, either sitting or standing, forms a fist around the thumb. The examiner stabilizes the forearm while holding the patient's fist with his or her other hand. The examiner then moves the wrist into ulnar deviation. If there is an increased pain in the radial styloid process and along the length of the extensor pollicis brevis and abductor pollicis longus tendons, then the test is positive. Neer's and Hawkins' tests are used to help localize pathology to the rotator cuff and not the wrist. Green test is not an actual test at the time of chapter publication. Phalen test is a test of the wrist and hand, but it is used to help diagnose carpal tunnel syndrome, not de Quervain syndrome. Phalen's maneuver pinches the median nerve between the transverse carpal ligament and the anterior border of the distal end of the radius, causing compression of the median nerve within the carpal tunnel, leading to burning, tingling, or a numb sensation over the thumb, index, middle, and ring fingers.

2. **Correct answer: D.** Manual muscle testing (MMT), an important part of the physical examination, is used to determine the extent and degree of muscular weakness resulting from disease, injury, or disuse. A consistent method of manually testing muscle strength is essential to assess accurately a patient's present status, progress, and the effectiveness of the treatment program. Manual muscle testing is graded on a scale of 0 to 5, with a score of 5 out of 5 for normal strength and a score of 0 out of 5 when no contraction is palpable in the muscle. If a patient is able to resist only against moderate pressure throughout ROM, he or she is graded a 4 out of 5.

3. **Correct answer: D.** The normal range of motion (ROM) for elbow flexion and extension is from 0° to 145°. The normal range of motion for pronation and supination of the forearm would be 0° to 90°. The shoulder is the only joint of the upper extremity that is able to move 180°. Shoulder flexion and abduction both have normal ROM values of 0° to 180°. After a serious elbow injury, many patients will not regain their full range and an ROM of 5° to 115° would be found on examination.

4. **Correct answer: C.** Corticosteroid injections for tendonitis can have both short- and long-term complications. Short-term complications include shrinkage (atrophy) and lightening of the color (depigmentation) of the skin at the injection site, introduction of bacterial infection into the body, local bleeding from broken blood vessels in the skin or muscle, and aggravation of inflammation in the area injected because of reactions to the corticosteroid medication (postinjection flare). In people who have diabetes, cortisone injections can elevate their blood sugar. Tendons can be weakened by corticosteroid injections in or near tendons, and tendon ruptures as a result have been reported, thus making tendon rupture a feared complication of corticosteroid injection for tendonitis.

   Long-term risks of corticosteroid injections depend on the dose and frequency of the injections. With higher doses and frequent administration, potential side effects include thinning of the skin, easy bruising, weight gain, puffiness of the face, acne (steroid acne), elevation of blood pressure, cataract formation, osteoporosis, and avascular necrosis.

   Pain and soreness at the injection site can occur but is not a feared complication of injection.

   Urinary retention, risk of cancer, and risk of bone fractures are not direct complications of corticosteroid injections.

5. **Correct answer: B.** The rotator cuff muscles are made up of a group of four muscles that are important in shoulder movements and in maintaining glenohumeral joint stability. These muscles arise from the scapula and connect to the head of the humerus, forming a cuff at the shoulder joint. They hold the head of the humerus in the small and shallow glenoid fossa of the scapula. The names of these four muscles can be remembered by the acronym SITS, which stands for the supraspinatus muscle, infraspinatus muscle, teres minor muscle, and subscapularis muscle. The teres minor muscle originates from the middle half of the lateral border of the scapula and inserts on the inferior facet of the greater tuberosity of the humerus to externally rotate the arm.

   The teres major muscle, although helping stabilize the humeral head in the glenoid cavity, is not considered one of the four rotator cuff muscles. It functions as a medial rotator and adductor of the humerus and assists the latissimus dorsi in drawing the previously raised humerus downward and backward (extension, but not hyperextension).

   The deltoid muscle originates from the lateral third of the clavicle, acromion, and spine of the scapula and inserts into the middle of the lateral surface of the humerus (deltoid tuberosity) acting to abduct the arm. It is not part of the rotator cuff muscles.

   The rhomboid major muscle originates from the thoracic spine (T2–T5) and inserts into the scapula to retract the scapula.

   The long head of the triceps muscle does stabilize the shoulder joint, but the main action of the muscle is elbow extension. It is not part of the rotator cuff muscles.

CHAPTER 24: LUMBAR SPINE DISORDERS

1. **Correct answer: D.** Numbness of the bilateral feet is not considered a "red flag" in the clinical evaluation of the lumbar spine. The other choices are all "red flags."
2. **Correct answer: D.** 70% to 90% of patients will recover from "acute" low back pain.
3. **Correct answer: A.** 70% to 90% of patients will recover from low back pain. Imaging or diagnostic studies are not necessary at 2 weeks. Current recommendations from the American College of Physicians regarding imaging for low back pain are that (a) imaging is only indicated for severe progressive neurological deficits or when red flags are suspected, and (b) routine imaging does not result in clinical benefit and may lead to harm.
4. **Correct answer: E.** All of the above are ethical issues related to chronic pain.
5. **Correct answer: D.** The likelihood of return to work for an individual who has been out of work for 6 months is 50%. If the individual has been out of work for 1 year, the likelihood drops to 25%.

CHAPTER 25: RHEUMATOID ARTHRITIS

1. **Correct answer: C.** "Gait imbalance," "diffuse symmetric upper extremity weakness and paraesthesias," and "bowel and bladder incontinence" are all symptoms of myelopathy, a later finding in atlanto-axial instability. Musculoskeletal nociceptive pain complaints are the most common and earliest symptoms. Rashes are not common signs of atlanto-axial instability.
2. **Correct answer: D.** Smoking is the strongest known risk RA. Viral infections are not well-known risk factors for RA, but antibodies to the bacteria *Porphyromonas gingivalis*, often associated with periodontitis, were found to be associated with ACPAs in patients with RA and their relatives. There is conflicting evidence for alcohol as a risk factor, and it is clearly not as strong as smoking. Silica exposure is not a known risk factor.
3. **Correct answer: E.** "Extraarticular disease," "erosions within 2 years of disease onset," "education level <11th grade," and "persistently elevated CRP" are all markers of a poor prognosis. "Morning stiffness for 15 minutes or less" is a feature of remission, as outlined in the 2011 ACR criteria.
4. **Correct answer: B.** During a flare, exercise intensity should be reduced, but ROM exercises should be continued. Therefore, "Reduce exercise intensity, splinting, and limited ROM to affected joints" is correct. "Eliminate all ROM exercises" is the opposite of the correct answer, and "Progress isometrics to isotonics" is incorrect because this would increase intensity. "Add ultrasound to treatment regimen" is incorrect because deep heat is indicated for patients with chronic inflammation and contractures, whereas cold therapy is ideal for acute flares, especially in joints with effusions. Patients in a flare can still participate in gentle ROM exercises.
5. **Correct answer: B.** Anakinra (Kineret®) is the only IL-1 inhibitor. Etanercept (Enbrel®), Infliximab (Remicade®), and Adalimumab (Humira®) are TNF-alpha blockers. Gabapentin (Neurontin®) is a GABA analog used to treat neuropathic pain and epilepsy.

CHAPTER 26: FIBROMYALGIA

1. **Correct answer: D.** Chronic widespread pain is characterized as pain for a minimum of 3 months' duration in all four quadrants of the body, including the axial skeleton. The pain must be present on both sides of the body, both above and below the waistline.
2. **Correct answer: A.** Aerobic training with low-intensity exercise improves fatigue and depression, and participants were found to tolerate increased levels of pressure over their tender points. Aerobic training has also been shown to reduce muscle and cognitive fatigue and to decrease symptoms of depression.
3. **Correct answer: D.** Both EULAR and APS recommend a multidisciplinary approach emphasizing both pharmacological and nonpharmacological treatment modalities. The treatment should be tailored individually based on presenting symptoms and comorbid conditions. Moreover, the APS gave its highest level of recommendation to aerobic exercise, cognitive-behavioral therapy (CBT), amitriptyline, and multicomponent therapy.
4. **Correct answer: A.** With regard to fibromyalgia, there is perhaps no other disease entity that requires more comprehensive patient communication in combination with best diagnostic practices. The initial and most important step in effective patient communication is an acknowledgment that FMS is real and has a medical explanation. The physician should assure the patient that the condition is not life-threatening, and that even though no cure currently exists, treatment strategies are available to lessen pain and improve function.
5. **Correct answer: B.** The fibromyalgia patient should be treated with respect and compassion, particularly given that he or she is often misdiagnosed with rheumatologic conditions or psychiatric disorders prior to the arrival at a diagnosis of fibromyalgia. Patients suffering from FMS have seen on average four physicians and have waited 2.3 years prior to receiving their correct diagnosis.

CHAPTER 27: CERVICAL RADICULOPATHY

1. **Correct answer: C.** Hoffman's sign is a sign of upper motor neuron lesion, which is seen in cervical myelopathy. Peripheral neuropathy, cervical radiculopathy, and brachial plexopathies are lower motor neuron lesions. Cervical myofascial pain syndrome is a myofascial entity and not an upper motor lesion hence, you would not expect Hoffman's sign.
2. **Correct answer: C.** The wrist extensors are supplied by radial nerve with primarily C6 roots. The C7 and the C8 mainly supply the intrinsic muscles of the hand.

3. **Correct answer: A.** The shoulder region is supplied by the C5 dermatome. The thumb is supplied by the C6 dermatome, the little finger is supplied by the C8 dermatome, the middle finger by the C7 dermatome, and the inner arm by the T2 dermatome.
4. **Correct answer: C.** The triceps reflex is primarily indicative of a C7 root lesion; the biceps and the brachioradialis reflex loss is due to C5/C6 root lesions.
5. **Correct answer: B.** Cerebrovascular accidents during spinal injection occur due to intravascular embolization of the vertebral artery with particulate steroid. This is seen most likely in transforaminal epidural steroid injections. The other sites of injections such as interlaminar epidural injection, facet blocks, medial branch blocks, and trigger point injections are not close to the vertebral artery and hence are unlikely choices.

CHAPTER 28: SPORTS MEDICINE: PREPARTICIPATION EVALUATION

1. **Correct answer: A.** Conditional clearance allows participation with activity restrictions based on the suspected medical condition; for example, an athlete with a recent concussion may be granted conditional clearance for noncontact sports. It can also be given with the requirement of completing further evaluation or rehabilitative/conditioning programs prior to participation; for example, a newly found cardiac murmur requiring cardiology evaluation and clearance.
2. **Correct answer: C.** Football combines aggressive body contact with sudden changes in position and momentum. It is not surprising that it carries the highest injury rate. Total and partial contact sports are generally riskier than noncontact sports.
3. **Correct answer: D.** A history of concussion is a big red flag when it comes to participation in contact sports. Second impact syndrome is a potentially catastrophic event that can occur when an athlete suffers a second injury while a first concussion has not yet resolved. It can result in diffuse cerebral edema, herniation, and death. Aerobic endurance is more related to the sporting activity, rather than whether there is contact during play. Laboratory work is not part of routine screening, but can be required at the discretion of the evaluating physician.
4. **Correct answer: A.** The history is the most detail-oriented component of the screening process, and is where most potential issues are identified. The physical examination is relatively quick and used to identify major limitations that could affect safety and performance. Laboratory work, EKG, and x-rays are not part of routine screening.
5. **Correct answer: B.** When an athlete is granted conditional clearance with instructions to have further evaluation by a specialist, or to undergo rehabilitation, it is up to the screening physician to follow up with the referred services and ensure that the patient is evaluated and treated prior to participation. It is not sufficient to document findings and pass the burden off to any other.

CHAPTER 29: ENTRAPMENT NEUROPATHIES

1. **Correct answer: B.** Anterior or anterolateral approaches to total hip replacements are a rare but likely underreported cause of femoral neuropathies. The femoral nerve enters the thigh lateral to the femoral vessels approximately 1 to 4 cm distal to the inguinal ligament, where it is vulnerable to compression, traction, and stretch injuries. Injuries to the tensor fascia lata muscle and lateral femoral cutaneous nerve may, in fact, be more common than femoral nerve injuries in cases of direct anterior hip replacements. Sciatic neuropathies, causing foot drop, are more common after posterior or posterolateral approaches to hip replacement. Pudendal neuropathies have not been reported after anterior hip replacements.
2. **Correct answer: C.** The short head of the biceps femoris muscle is the only peroneal-innervated muscle above the knee. The adductor magnus muscle is dually innervated by the tibial portion of the sciatic nerve and the obturator nerve. The long head of the biceps femoris muscle and the semimembranous muscle are tibially innervated. The rectus femoris muscle receives its innervation from the posterior division of the femoral nerve.
3. **Correct answer: C.** Robinson's Combined Sensory Index has a sensitivity of 83% and a specificity of 95% for diagnosing CTS when the summated latency difference is greater than 0.9 ms. The median-ulnar sensory latency difference to digit 4, median-radial sensory latency difference to digit 1, and mixed sensorimotor mid-palm median-ulnar latency difference studies can be helpful in cases where the diagnosis of CTS is equivocal.
4. **Correct answer: A.** The medial half of the flexor digitorum profundus muscle may be of higher diagnostic yield than sampling the FCU muscle in patients with CuTS, as the branch of the ulnar nerve to the FCU traverses the cubital tunnel in only 50% of individuals in one published study. The superficial head of the flexor pollicis brevis muscle is innervated by the median nerve and is part of the thenar muscle group. The pronator teres muscle is also median innervated.
5. **Correct answer: D.** The most likely site of median nerve entrapment in patients undergoing ultrasonographic evaluation for idiopathic CTS was shown to be approximately 2 cm distal to the distal wrist crease. The Chen et al. 8-point ultrasonographic "inching test" measuring the median nerve's CSA has been shown to positively correlate with NCS severity and duration of CTS symptoms.

CHAPTER 30: PEDIATRIC TRAUMATIC BRAIN INJURY

1. **Correct answer: C.** Carbolic acid or phenol is a chemodenervating agent used in spasticity management. Phenol is injected into motor points. Its effects in relaxing the muscles can last for up to 6 months.

2. **Correct answer: D.** Autonomic dysfunction after TBI is due to disruption of inhibitory activity from the brainstem causing sympathetic outflow. Tachypnea, hypertension, and hyperthermia are seen in autonomic dysfunction due to brain injury. Treating the cause, like a full bladder, bowel, and so on, decreases the symptoms.
3. **Correct answer: E.** Wechsler Memory Scale is a neuropsychological test to measure memory function. WMS-IV is made up of seven subtests, which look at spatial addition, symbol span, design memory, general cognitive screener, logical memory, verbal paired associated reproduction, and visual reproduction. The Tardieu scale is used to quantify spasticity. EEG is used to evaluate for seizures. A CAT scan is a computer-processed x-ray used to produce virtual slices of a scanned object. Western neurosensory stimulation profile is used to monitor coma.
4. **Correct answer: C.** Visual acuity deficits are seen with frontal lobe injuries. Sensorineural hearing loss is seen with inner ear pathology. Olfactory nerve involvement causes anosmia. Hypertonic saline is used to treat hyponatremia and not spasticity. Diplopia is due to dysfunction of extraocular muscles.
5. **Correct answer: C.** Falls are the leading cause of TBI in children younger than 4 years. As per CDC, assault is the leading cause of head injury in children 0 to 4 years. Falls are more common in people 65 years and older. Blunt trauma is the second most common cause of TBI-related ED visits in children aged between 5 and 14 years.

CHAPTER 31: JUVENILE INFLAMMATORY ARTHRITIS

1. **Correct answer: D.** Asymmetric limb use, blurred vision suggesting uveitis, fine motor skill problem, and joint swelling are all seen with JIA. Isolated musculoskeletal pain is nonspecific and does not signify JIA, as it can be seen with viral infections, fatigue, and generalized malaise.
2. **Correct answer: A.** CHAQ correlates with the patient's/parent's perception of pain, well-being, level of disease, and functional status. It inversely correlates with remission. The other parameters listed are monitored in the presence of disease and medications.
3. **Correct answer: C.** Ultrasound is avoided due to lack of evidence around growth plates. Showers, heating pads, and paraffin baths are recommended. Heat and cold should be used with caution in insensate areas. Splinting and therapy promoting range of motion are recommended in treatment of JIA.
4. **Correct answer: A.** Exercise is vital in the treatment of JIA. Contact sports are not generally advisable during acute flare-ups. Participation is based on extent of pain. All others aforementioned sports are recommended in the treatment of JIA.
5. **Correct answer: D.** MAS is a complication of systemic JIA involving life-threatening, persistent fever; pancytopenia; hepatosplenomegaly; and coagulopathy. Brucellosis is caused by ingestion of unsterilized milk or meat, or contact with its secretions, due to a Gram-negative, nonmotile, nonspore-forming, rod-shaped bacteria.

Index

AAN. *See* American Academy of Neurology
AAPMR. *See* American Academy of Physical Medicine and Rehabilitation
"ABC" approach, cervical radiculopathy, 316
abductor pollicis longus (APL), 269
ACA syndrome. *See* anterior cerebral artery syndrome
Accreditation Council for Graduate Medical Education (ACGME), 3, 16, 317
    competency of professionalism, 9
    competency protocols, 71
    NAS and educational milestones, 32–33
    program requirements, 7
    residency programs, 3
    supervision levels, 44–46
ace wrapping, 101
ACGME. *See* Accreditation Council for Graduate Medical Education
ACS. *See* anterior cord syndrome
ACT. *See* Amputation Care Team
active listening, 22–23
activities of daily living (ADLs), 90, 200–204, 260
    occupational therapy for, 168
AD. *See* autonomic dysreflexia
ADLs. *See* activities of daily living
adult learning, principles and practice, 36
aerobic capacity, 116
aerobic training, cardiopulmonary rehabilitation, 117–125
American Academy of Neurology (AAN), 231
American Academy of Physical Medicine and Rehabilitation (AAPMR), 229
American Board of Medical Specialties, 220
American Parkinson Disease Association (APDA), 206
amputation
    energy demands by level of, 92–94, 101
    rehabilitation, stages of, 90
    types of, 102
Amputation Care Team (ACT), 110

Amputation Points of Contact (APOC), 110
Amputation System of Care, 96
amputee care, 102
anterior cerebral artery (ACA) syndrome, 154
anterior cord syndrome (ACS), 193
anticonvulsants, 306
APDA. *See* American Parkinson Disease Association
APL. *See* abductor pollicis longus
APOC. *See* Amputation Points of Contact
arm ergometry, 105
arteries, variation of, 115
aspiration, 149–150
autonomic dysreflexia (AD), 192
autonomy, ethical principle of, 96

bedside teaching, 40
beliefs, ingrained, 17
Belmont Report, 55
biomarkers, 182
blame-free approach, 79
Bobath method, 258, 260
body language, 21–22
BOGERD process, 38
brain injury
    benefits and limitations of procedures in, 344
    in children, 342–344
    severity, rating of, 343
Brain Trauma Foundation (BTF), 170
Brown-Séquard syndrome (BSS), 193
Brunnstrom method, 258, 260
Brunnstrom stages, 150
BSS. *See* Brown-Séquard syndrome
BTF. *See* Brain Trauma Foundation

cancer rehabilitation
    care, improving, 135
    case study, 141

interpersonal and communication skills (ICS), 137–138
medical histories and data gathering, 130–131
oncology review, 133–134
patient care, 130
patient-centered care, 136
patient safety and system errors, 140–141
physical examination, 131–132
practice-based learning and improvement (PBLI), 136–137
professionalism, 138
prospective surveillance model (PSM), 134
and rehabilitation care continuum, 134
risk-benefit analysis and cost awareness, 140
safety concerns in cancer survivors, 135
screening cancer survivors, 134–135
socioeconomic issues in, 136
systems-based practice (SBP), 138–141
treatment plan, 132–133
cancer-related fatigue (CRF), 135–136
cancer survivors
  examples of rehabilitation in, 135–136
  improving quality of care, 139–140
  safety concerns in, 135
  screening, 134–135
cardiac output, 116
cardiac precautions, 150
cardiopulmonary rehabilitation
  abnormal physiology, 119–120
  aerobic training, 117–125
  assessment of cardiopulmonary function, 112–113
  cardiac anatomy, 114–115
  cardiac arrhythmias, 123
  cardiac physiology, 115
  cardiac rehabilitation, 120–123
  cardiomyopathy, 123
  case study, 128
  interpersonal and communication skills (ICS), 126
  physical examination, 113–114
  in physically disabled, 124–125
  practice-based learning and improvement (PBLI), 125–126
  professionalism, 127
  pulmonary anatomy, 115–116
  pulmonary physiology, 116
  pulmonary rehabilitation, 121
  systems-based practice, 127–128
  valvular heart disease, 123
Carotid Revascularization Endarterectomy versus Stenting Trial (CREST), 156
case presentations with feedback, 40–42
case study
  cancer rehabilitation, 141
  cardiopulmonary rehabilitation, 128
  cervical radiculopathy, 320
  entrapment neuropathies, 336
  fibromyalgia, 311
  lumbar spine disorders, 286
  mild traumatic brain injury (MTBI), 187
  multiple sclerosis (MS), 232
  neuromuscular diseases (NMDs), 221
  osteoarthritis, 245–246
  Parkinson diseases, 207
  preparticipation evaluation (PPE), 327

rheumatoid arthritis (RA), 300
spasticity, 266
spinal cord injury (SCI), 198–199
stroke, 162
total hip arthroplasty (THA), 254–255
total knee arthroplasty (TKA), 254–255
traumatic brain injury (TBI), 175, 351–352
upper extremity limb loss, 97
upper extremity musculoskeletal injuries (UEMIs), 275–276
cauda equina syndrome (CES), 193
CBT. *See* cognitive behavioral therapy
CCC. *See* clinical competency committee
CCS. *See* central cord syndrome
CDT. *See* complex decongestive therapy
Center for Disease Control, suggestions and resources for clinicians, 77
Center for Studying Health System Change (HSC) study, 318
Centers for Medicare and Medicaid Services (CMS), 194
central cord syndrome (CCS), 193
central nervous system (CNS), 342
cerebrospinal fluid (CSF), 340
cervical radiculopathy
  "ABC" approach, 316
  case study, 320
  comprehensive assessment of, 314
  electrodiagnosis, 316
  impairments, activity limitations, and participation restrictions associated with, 315
  interpersonal and communication skills (ICS), 317–319
  medical knowledge, 315–316
  patient care, 314–315
  physical examination, 314–315
  practice-based learning and improvement (PBLI), 316–317
  professionalism, 319–320
  system-based practice, 320
  treatment plan for neck pain, 315
cervical spine
  range of motion, 315
  soft-tissue structures within, 316
cervical steroid injections, 316
CES. *See* cauda equina syndrome
chemo brain, 136
chemodenervation, 170
chemotherapy-induced peripheral neuropathy (CIPN), 130–132, 135
children, brain injury in, 342–344
choke syndrome, 104
chronic cervical neck pain, 319
chronic widespread pain, 303
cineplasty, 92
CIPN. *See* chemotherapy-induced peripheral neuropathy
clinical competency committee (CCC), 7
clinical practice guidelines (CPGs), 262
clinical supervision, 44
clinical teaching, microskills for, 41
clonidine (Catapres), 261
Clostridium botulinum bacteria, 261
CMS. *See* Centers for Medicare and Medicaid Services; conus medullaris syndrome
CNS. *See* central nervous system
Code of Conduct, 68–69
Cognitive and Emotional Preparedness Model, 319
cognitive behavioral therapy (CBT), 281

fibromyalgia, 305
cognitive deficits, 350
coiling aneurysms, 155
collective reflection, 10
coma, evaluation scales of, 340
Commission on Accreditation of Rehabilitation Facilities (CARF), 91, 139, 198, 220
    holistic approach to care of lower limb amputee, 109
communication
    case study, 29
    challenges to, 16–18
    components of, 18–29
    conscious, compassionate, 19–29
    objectives, 16
    patterns, 17
    preferences, 21
    styles, 20–21
    team, 18
community
    and government relationships, 69
    integration, 350
compassion, 84
compassionate care, 66
competency, 31–32, 83
    types of, 3
competency-based evaluations, 43–44
competency-based journal club, 38
competency-based medical education, 3
complementary and alternative medicine (CAM), examples of, 360
complex decongestive therapy (CDT), 135
conductive hearing loss, 340
constipation, 149, 167
constraint-induced therapy, 150
continuous passive motion (CPM), 252
continuum of care
    MTBI, 187
    rehabilitation, 186
    rheumatoid arthritis (RA), 298–299
continuum of rehabilitative care for PD, 207
contractures, 250
conus medullaris syndrome (CMS), 193
coronary artery anatomy, 115
coronary artery disease, 105
corticosteroids, 227
cost awareness, 140
Cozen test, 269
CPGs. *See* clinical practice guidelines
CPM. *See* continuous passive motion
CREST. *See* Carotid Revascularization Endarterectomy versus Stenting Trial
CRF. *See* cancer-related fatigue
cryotherapy, 252
CSF. *See* cerebrospinal fluid

dantrolene, 170, 260
DARPA. *See* Defense Advanced Research Projects Agency
decision-making process, 56–57
Defense Advanced Research Projects Agency (DARPA), 94
degeneration of lumbar spine, 281
delivering bad news, 27–28
depression, 149

de Quervain tenosynovitis, 269
DESC Communication Model, 24–25
detail complexity, 72
diazepam (Valium), 260
didactic lecture presentations, 38–39
diffusion of the lung for carbon monoxide (DLCO), 116
disruptive behavior, 69
distraction tests, 280
DNR/DNI. *See* do not resuscitate/do not intubate
doctor-patient visit, issues during, 18
do not resuscitate/do not intubate (DNR/DNI), 204
double swallow technique, 207
dynamic complexity, 72
dysfunctional listening behavior, 23
dysfunctional speaking behavior, 26
dysphagia, 148, 350

EAAs. *See* excitatory amino acids
educational components for patient, family, and caregivers, 107
EDX testing, 336
effective communication, 58, 126, 137, 335
    challenges to, 16–18
    documentation and, 173
    key points for conducting, 185
    in medicine, 318
    principles of, 196
effective rehabilitation, 350
effective teaching, 36–37
elbow disorders
    medical knowledge, 270–271
    patient care, 269
electrodiagnosis, cervical radiculopathy, 316
electronic communication, 18
electronic medical records (EMRs), 220, 318–230
emotions, 19
empathy, 20
empty can test, 269
EMRs. *See* electronic medical records
endurance, 83
energy, 83
entrapment neuropathies
    case study, 336
    ethical principles in, 335
    interpersonal and communication skills (ICS), 335
    medical knowledge, 331–334
    patient care, 329–331
    practice-based learning and improvement (PBLI), 334–335
    professionalism, 335–336
    systems-based practice (SBP), 335
EPB. *See* extensor pollicis brevis
epidural hematomas, 169
ethical conflicts, addressing and resolving, 62–64
    analysis, 63–64
    biographical data, 63, 64
    clinical data, 63, 64
    cultural data, 63, 64
    practice of physical medicine and rehabilitation, 62–63
ethical decision making
    decision-making process, 56–57
    principles, 61–62
    steps in process for, 57–62
ethical frameworks, 56

ethical issues
    in care of juvenile idiopathic arthritis (JIA), 360
    in care of multiple sclerosis (MS), 228
    in MTBI, 183
    osteoarthritis, 238
    during rehabilitation and treatment, 133
    in rehabilitation medicine
        addressing and resolving ethical conflicts, 62–64
        ethical decision making, 56–62
        frameworks, 56
        research, 55–56
evaluation, 42–44
    competency-based, 43–44
    formative and summative, 43
evidence-based practices
    guidelines, 184
    resources for, 171
    useful websites for, 171
excitatory amino acids (EAAs), 168
exercise, self-reflective, 17
exercise therapy, 281
extensor pollicis brevis (EPB), 269

Failure Mode and Effects Analysis (FMEA), components of, 79
falls, 148
    injuries associated with, 250
family education points, key patient and, 184
family meeting, indications for, 195
FCE. See functional capacity evaluation
feedback, 39–40
    case presentations with, 40–42
    and educational contract, 37–38
    teaching and, 34–39
FEES. See fiberoptic endoscopic evaluation of swallow studies
FERNE. See Foundation for Education in Research in Neurological Emergencies
fiberoptic endoscopic evaluation of swallow studies (FEES), 204
fibromyalgia
    case study, 311
    cognitive behavioral therapy (CBT), 305
    diagnosis of, 303
    interpersonal and communication skills (ICS), 308–310
    medical knowledge, 305–307
    nonpharmacological treatment of, 307
    pain diagram, 309
    patient care, 303–305
    pharmacological treatment of, 306–307
    practice-based learning and improvement (PBLI), 307–308
    professionalism, 310
    questionnaires, 309
    sample rehabilitation program, 304–305
    systems-based practice (SBP), 310–311
fibromyalgia syndrome (FMS), 303
    psychosocial aspects associated with, 304
Finkelstein test, 269
FMEA. See Failure Mode and Effects Analysis
FMS. See fibromyalgia syndrome
footdrop, 250–251
forced expired vital capacity (FVC), 116
forearm disorders
    medical knowledge, 270–271
    patient care, 269

formal physical therapy, 280
formative evaluation, 43
Foundation for Education in Research in Neurological Emergencies (FERNE), 171
four-box model, 57
functional capacity evaluation (FCE), 280

GARS. See Groningen Activity Restriction Scale
GCS. See Glasgow Coma Score
Glasgow Coma Score (GCS), 155
glucocorticoids, 293
government relationships, community and, 69
graduate medical education, 71–73
Groningen Activity Restriction Scale (GARS), 106

hand disorders
    medical knowledge, 271
    patient care, 269
hand transplants, 92
Hawkins tests for impingement, 268
health care quality, 77–78
health care safety, 78–79
health care systems, defined, 71–72
Health Insurance Portability and Accountability Act (HIPAA)
    guidelines, 348
    regulations, 162
heart rate (HR), 116
Helsinki Declaration, 55
hemiplegic shoulder pain, 149
hemorrhagic stroke, 155–156
heterotopic ossification (HO), 167
    of joints, 104
HHA. See home health agency
HIPAA. See Health Insurance Portability and Accountability Act
hip dislocation, 250
hip fracture, 250
HO. See heterotopic ossification
home health agency (HHA), 74
hydrocephalus, 167

IADLs. See instrumental ADLs
ICA syndrome. See internal carotid artery syndrome
ICH. See intracerebral hemorrhage
ICS. See interpersonal and communication skills
immobility, 148
immunomodulator agents, 227
immunosuppressive agents, 227
infections, 250
information to patients, 27
ingrained beliefs, 17
inpatient rehabilitation facilities (IRFs), 73, 207
    organizational characteristics of, 76

Institute for Healthcare Improvement (IHI), 317
instrumental ADLs (IADLs), 204
integrity, 83
internal carotid artery (ICA) syndrome, 154–155
International Spinal Cord Injury Pain (ISCIP) Classification, 192
International Spine Intervention Society (ISIS), 317
International Standards for Neurological Classification of SCI (ISNCSCI), 190, 191
interpersonal and communication skills (ICS), 5

cancer rehabilitation, 137–138
cardiopulmonary rehabilitation, 126
cervical radiculopathy, 317–319
entrapment neuropathies, 335
fibromyalgia, 308–310
juvenile idiopathic arthritis (JIA), 361–362
leadership, 84–85
lumbar spine disorders, 283–284
mild traumatic brain injury (MTBI), 185
multiple sclerosis (MS), 229–230
neuromuscular diseases (NMDs), 218
osteoarthritis, 243–244
Parkinson disease, 205–206
preparticipation evaluation (PPE), 324–325
rheumatoid arthritis (RA), 296–297
spasticity, 262–263
spinal cord injury (SCI), 195–196
stroke, 158–159
total hip arthroplasty (THA), 252–253
total knee arthroplasty (TKA), 252–253
traumatic brain injury (TBI), 346–348
moderate and severe, 173
upper extremity limb loss, 95
upper extremity musculoskeletal injuries (UEMIs), 272–273
intracerebral hemorrhage (ICH), 155
intrathecal baclofen (ITB) pumps, 261
placement, 341
IRFs. *See* inpatient rehabilitation facilities
ischemic stroke syndromes, 152–154
ISNCSCI. *See* International Standards for Neurological Classification of SCI
ITB pumps. *See* Intrathecal baclofen pumps

juvenile idiopathic arthritis (JIA)
assessment of child with, 355
case study, 363
complications in, 360
ethical issues in care of, 360
history of present illness, 355–356
impairments, activity limitations, and participation restrictions, 356–357
injuries associated with, 357
interpersonal and communication skills (ICS), 361–362
joint care in, 359
long-term outcomes of, 356
physical examination, 356
practice-based learning and improvement (PBLI), 360–361
professionalism, 362
psychosocial, vocational, and educational aspects of, 357
rehabilitation of patient with, 355–356
subtypes, characteristics of, 357, 358
systems-based practice (SBP), 363–364
treatments, 360

Krukenberg procedure, 94

lacunar infarcts, 151–152, 155
lateral epicondylitis, 269
LEA. *See* lower extremity amputee
leadership
ability to build team, 85–86
decisiveness and ability to implement, 86

interpersonal and communication skills (ICS), 84–85
qualities, 83–84
vision and foresight, 84
learning
continuum over life span, 36
principles and practice, adult, 36
retention pyramid, 37
rules for, 39
styles, 37
levels of needs, 19–20
levels of questioning, 41
listening, 22–23
behaviors, 23
LMN. *See* lower motor neuron
LMWH. *See* low-molecularweight heparin
lower extremity amputee (LEA), 91
case study, 110
interpersonal and communication skills (ICS), 106–108
K-level rating with description, 100
medical knowledge, 100–103
patient care, 99–100
physical examination components, 100
postamputation complications, 102–104
practice-based learning and improvement (PBLI), 105–106
professionalism, 108–109
stance phase problems, 104
swing phase problems, 104
systems-based practice (SBP), 109–110
lower motor neuron (LMN), 191
low-molecularweight heparin (LMWH), 148
lumbar spine disorders
case study, 286
cost-related and return to work considerations, 285
effective communication and listening skills, 284
ethical considerations, 282
imaging, laboratory studies, and electrodiagnosis, 282
impairments, activity limitations, and participation restrictions, 279–280
incidence and prevalence, 281
interpersonal and communication skills (ICS), 283–284
markers of quality, 285
medical documentation, 283
medical knowledge, 280–282
patient advocacy, 285
patient assessment, 278
patient care, 278–280
patient education, 283
patient safety, 285
practice-based learning and improvement (PBLI), 282–283
practice-related quality improvement activity, 283
professionalism, 284
"Red Flags", 279
system-related errors, 286
systems-based practice (SBP), 285–287
treatment, 281–282
lymphedema, 135

manual lymphatic drainage (MLD), 135
manual muscle testing, grading for, 268
MAS. *See* Modified Ashworth Scale
MBS. *See* modified barium swallow

MCA syndrome. *See* middle cerebral artery syndrome
MCI. *See* mild cognitive impairment
McKenzie exercises, 280, 281
MCL. *See* medial collateral ligament
medial collateral ligament (MCL), 269
Medicaid, 349
medical ethics, 56
medical knowledge, 5
    cervical radiculopathy, 315–316
    entrapment neuropathies, 331–334
    fibromyalgia, 305–307
    lumbar spine disorders, 280–282
    multiple sclerosis (MS), 225–228
    neuromuscular diseases (NMDs), 213–214
    osteoarthritis, 238–242
    Parkinson disease, 202–204
    preparticipation evaluation (PPE), 323–324
    rheumatoid arthritis (RA), 290–294
    spasticity, 258–261
    stroke, 151–157
    total hip arthroplasty (THA), 251–252
    total knee arthroplasty (TKA), 251–252
    traumatic brain injury (TBI), 342–345
        moderate and severe, 168–171
    upper extremity limb loss, 91–94
    upper extremity musculoskeletal injuries (UEMIs), 269–271
medicine, changing culture in, 17
medullary lateral reticular formation (MLRF), 260
mentorship, 46–47
    pyramid hierarchy, 46
microskills
    for clinical teaching, 41
    models, 40–42
middle cerebral artery (MCA) syndrome, 152
mild cognitive impairment (MCI), 136
mild traumatic brain injury (MTBI)
    case study, 187
    diagnostic criteria for, 182
    diagnostic test and imaging, 182
    epidemiology, 181, 182–183
    ethical issues in, 183
    functional impairments and activity limitations associated with, 178
    interpersonal and communication skills (ICS), 185
    management of common symptoms in, 180–181
    pathophysiology, 182
    patient care, 177–178
    patient safety components/checklist applicable to, 186
    pharmacological treatment approach to, 179
    practice-based learning and improvement (PBLI), 183–184
    professionalism, 185–186
    psychosocial aspects associated with, 178–179
    sample rehabilitation program, management, 179
    in sports, 183
    systems-based practice (SBP), 186–187
    treatment approach to, 183
    treatment plan, 179–180
military population, epidemiology in, 182–183
MLD. *See* manual lymphatic drainage
MLRF. *See* medullary lateral reticular formation
Modified Ashworth Scale (MAS), 166, 224, 257, 341
modified barium swallow (MBS), 204

motor neuron disease, 214
MS. *See* multiple sclerosis
MSAA. *See* Multiple Sclerosis Association of America
MTBI. *See* mild traumatic brain injury
multigenerational workforce, 34
    attributes, 35
multiple sclerosis (MS)
    case study, 232
    cost-benefit considerations in, 232
    diagnostic testing in, 226–227
    ethical issues in care of, 228
    impairments, activity limitations, and participation restrictions in, 224–225
    interpersonal and communication skills (ICS), 229–230
    medical knowledge, 225–228
    patient and family counseling, 229–230
    patient care, 223–225
    patient counseling and resources in, 231
    patient safety in rehabilitation of, 231–232
    physical examination, 224
    practice-based learning and improvement (PBLI), 229
    professionalism, 230–231
    psychosocial, vocational, and educational issues affecting, 225
    rehabilitation continuum of care for, 231
    rehabilitation treatment plan for, 225
    systems-based practice (SBP), 231–232
    treatment, 227–228
Multiple Sclerosis Association of America (MSAA), 231
muscle reinnervation, targeted, 92
muscles, diseases of, 215–216
muscle spindle, nuclear bag and chain fibers of, 259
mutual support, 273
myocardial oxygen consumption, 116
myodesis, 92
myoplasty, 92

narrative medicine
    practical approaches for implementation of, 11–14
    steps in establishing, 14
NAS. *See* National Academy of Sciences; new accreditation system
National Academy of Sciences (NAS), 56
National Family Caregivers Association (NFCA), 231
National Institute of Neurological Disorders and Stroke (NINDS), 171
National Multiple Sclerosis Society, 231
National Network of Libraries of Medicine (NNLM), 317
National Parkinson Foundation (NPF), 206
National Patient Safety Foundation, 317
neck pain
    differential diagnosis of, 315
    treatment plan for, 315
needs, levels of, 19–20
Neer sign, 268
neurofacilitation technique, 150
neurologic level of injury, functional outcomes by, 194
neuromuscular diseases (NMDs)
    case study, 221
    diseases of muscles, 215–216
    interpersonal and communication skills (ICS), 218
    long-term goal of medical care for patients with, 221
    medical knowledge, 213–214
    motor neuron disease, 214
    neuromuscular junction disorders, 215

neuropathies, 214–215
patient care, 211–213
practice-based learning and improvement (PBLI), 217–218
professionalism, 218–219
rehabilitation, 216–217, 220
systems-based practice (SBP), 219–221
neuromuscular junction disorders, 215
neuropathies, 214–215
new accreditation system (NAS), 32–33
NFCA. *See* National Family Caregivers Association
NIPPV. *See* noninvasive positive pressure ventilation
NMDA receptors, 103
NMDs. *See* neuromuscular diseases
noninvasive positive pressure ventilation (NIPPV), 220
nonmaleficence, principle of, 58
nonsteroidal antiinflammatory drugs (NSAIDs), 316
nonverbal communication, 318
NSAIDs. *See* nonsteroidal antiinflammatory drugs

1-minute preceptor, 41
optimal follow-up care, MTBI, 187
orthostatic hypotension, 148–149
orthostatic medications, 149
Orthotics and Prosthetics User's Survey (OPUS), 106
osseointegration, 92
osteoarthritis
case study, 245–246
diagnostic testing, 239–240
epidemiology, 238–239
interpersonal and communication skills (ICS), 243–244
medical knowledge, 238–242
patient care, 235–238
practice-based learning and improvement (PBLI), 242–243
professionalism, 244
relevant anatomy and pathophysiology, 239
rheumatoid arthritis (RA) versus, 292
systems-based practice (SBP), 244–245
treatment options, 240–242
Outcome and Assessment Information Set (OASIS), 74
outpatient rehabilitation services, 73
overreaction, 280

pain mnemonics, 267, 268
pain syndromes, 90
PAIs. *See* patient assessment instruments
Pangaro's RIME model, 45
Parkinson disease
case study, 207
interpersonal and communication skills (ICS), 205–206
medical knowledge, 202–204
patient care, 200–202
practice-based learning and improvement (PBLI), 205
professionalism, 206
systems-based practice (SBP), 206–207
Parkinson's Action Network (PAN), 206
Parkinson's Disease Foundation (PDF), 206
Parkinson Study Group (PSG), 206
passion, 84
patient assessment instruments (PAIs), 73
patient autonomy, principle of, 56
patient care (PC), 4
advocacy for quality and optimal, 140

cervical radiculopathy, 314–315
coordination, 74
entrapment neuropathies, 229–331
fibromyalgia, 303–305
lumbar spine disorders, 278–280
multiple sclerosis (MS), 223–225
neuromuscular diseases (NMDs), 211–213
osteoarthritis, 235–238
Parkinson disease, 200–202
preparticipation evaluation (PPE), 322–323
rheumatoid arthritis (RA), 288–290
spasticity, 257–258
stroke, 144–151
total hip arthroplasty (THA), 248–251
total knee arthroplasty (TKA), 248–251
traumatic brain injury (TBI), 341–342
moderate and severe, 165–168
upper extremity limb loss, 89–91
upper extremity musculoskeletal injuries (UEMIs), 267–269
patient-centered care, 66
patient-controlled analgesia (PCA) system, 90
Patient Reported Impact of Spasticity Measure (PRISM), 258
patients
calming, 28–29
constructive feedback, 25–26
information to, 27
interview, 26–27
patient safety, 77–79
components, MTBI, 186
and rehabilitation treatment plan, 133
and system errors, 140–141
PBLI. *See* practice-based learning and improvement
PC. *See* patient care
percutaneous endoscopic gastrostomy (PEG), 220
peripheral entrapment neuropathies, 336
personal resistance in profession, 17
pharmacological treatment approach to MTBI, 179
Physiatric Association for Spine, Sports, and Occupational Rehabilitation (PASSOR), 317
physiatrist
as resource manager, 74–78
as systems consultant in rehabilitation health care delivery systems, 73–74
as team leader, 185
physical examination, juvenile idiopathic arthritis (JIA), 356
physically disabled, cardiopulmonary rehabilitation in, 124–125
Physical Medicine and Rehabilitation (PM&R), 3–4, 14, 82, 220
criteria for good assessment, 4–5
methods to assess, 4–6
NAS for, 34
research, 55–56
Physician Charter, professional responsibilities from, 67–68
physician to physician relationships, 69
Plan, Do, Study, and Act (PDSA) cycle, 79
PM&R Review Committee of ACGME, 7
polypharmacy, 104
Polytrauma Amputation Network Sites (PANS), 110
posterior cerebral artery (PCA) syndrome, 155
posterior cord syndrome (PCS), 193
posttraumatic headaches, 167
posttraumatic seizures (PTSs), 167–168
PPE. *See* preparticipation evaluation

PPS. *See* prospective payment system
practice-based learning and improvement (PBLI)
    cancer rehabilitation, 136–137
    cardiopulmonary rehabilitation, 125–126
    cervical radiculopathy, 316–317
    entrapment neuropathies, 334–335
    fibromyalgia, 307–308
    juvenile idiopathic arthritis (JIA), 360–361
    lumbar spine disorders, 282–283
    mild traumatic brain injury (MTBI), 183–184
    multiple sclerosis (MS), 229
    neuromuscular diseases (NMDs), 217–218
    osteoarthritis, 242–243
    practical approaches for implementation of narrative medicine, 11–14
    preparticipation evaluation (PPE), 324
    rheumatoid arthritis (RA), 294–296
    spasticity, 261–262
    stroke, 157–158
    theoretical framework for, 9–11
    total hip arthroplasty (THA), 252
    total knee arthroplasty (TKA), 252
    traumatic brain injury (TBI), 345–346
        moderate and severe, 171–173
    upper extremity limb loss, 94–95
    upper extremity musculoskeletal injuries (UEMIs), 271–272
prehabilitation, cancer, 134
preparticipation evaluation (PPE)
    case study, 327
    interpersonal communication and skills (ICS), 324–325
    key elements of physical examination, 323
    medical knowledge, 323–324
    patient care, 322–323
    practice-based learning and improvement (PBLI), 324
    professionalism, 325–326
    systems-based practice (SBP), 326–327
pressure ulcers, 250
problem-based learning and improvement (PBLI), 5
procedural skills teaching, 41–42
professionalism, 68–69
    ACGME competencies of, 9, 67
    cancer rehabilitation, 138
    cardiopulmonary rehabilitation, 127
    cervical radiculopathy, 319–320
    definition of, 66
    entrapment neuropathies, 335–336
    fibromyalgia, 310
    goals, 66
    juvenile idiopathic arthritis (JIA), 362
    lumbar spine disorders, 284
    mild traumatic brain injury (MTBI), 185–186
    multiple sclerosis (MS), 230–231
    neuromuscular diseases (NMDs), 218–219
    osteoarthritis, 244
    Parkinson disease, 206
    preparticipation evaluation (PPE), 325–326
    research and scholarly activity, 69
    responsibilities from Physician Charter, 67–68
    rheumatoid arthritis (RA), 297–298
    spasticity, 263–264
    spinal cord injury (SCI), 196–197
    stroke, 159–160

    total hip arthroplasty (THA), 253
    total knee arthroplasty (TKA), 253
    traumatic brain injury (TBI), 348–349
        moderate and severe, 173–174
    upper extremity limb loss, 95–96
    upper extremity musculoskeletal injuries (UEMIs), 273–274
proprioceptive technique, 150
prospective payment system (PPS), 73
prospective surveillance model (PSM), 134
PSM. *See* prospective surveillance model
psychomotor skills, 41–42
pulmonary anatomy, cardiopulmonary rehabilitation, 115–116
pulmonary physiology, cardiopulmonary rehabilitation, 116
pulmonary rehabilitation, 121
    cardiopulmonary rehabilitation, 121
    goals and methods of, 118–119
    programs in specific conditions, 124
pulmonary testing, interpretation of, 116–117

quality and optimal care, patient advocacy for, 76–77
quality improvement project, 79
quality of care
    markers of, 299
    for patients with MTBI, 187
quality of rehabilitative care systems, 78, 79
quality supervision, 44
questioning levels, 41

RA. *See* rheumatoid arthritis
radiation fibrosis syndrome (RFS), 136
range of motion (ROM), 258
RCA. *See* root cause analysis
reflection
    definition of, 9–10
    elements of, 10
    tips for teaching, 11
    understanding of, 11
reflection-in-action, 9
reflective listening, 22–23
reflective practice strategies, 10
Regional Amputee Center (RAC), 110
regional disturbances, 280
rehabilitation
    continuum of care, 186, 231, 336
    effective, 350
    lower extremity amputee (LEA), 101
    neuromuscular diseases (NMDs), 216–217, 220
    patient safety in multiple sclerosis (MS), 231–232
    of patient with juvenile idiopathic arthritis (JIA), 355–356
    program in MS, 227–228
    stages of, 90
    stroke, 144–145
    in TBI, 170, 349
    team relationships, 69
    treatment plan, 133
rehabilitative care systems, quality of, 78, 79
rehabilitative process, cognitive ability in, 339
renal disease and amputation, 105
Renshaw cells, 260
reporting, milestone expectations and, 33–34
residual volume (RV), 116
RFS. *See* radiation fibrosis syndrome

rheumatoid arthritis (RA)
    atlantoaxial instability, 289
    case study, 300
    Cochrane reviews, 295–296
    continuum of care, 298–299
    cost considerations, 299–300
    diagnosis, 291
    disease activity index, 289
    epidemiology and pathophysiology, 290–291
    ethical issues, 298
    exercise precautions, 290
    exercise prescription modification, 290
    flares, 294
    functional assessment, 289
    functional classification, 289
    history and physical examination, 288–289
    interpersonal and communication skills (ICS), 296–297
    laboratory tests, 291–292
    medical record, 297
    medical treatment, 293–294
    mortality, 297
    natural history, 291
    versus osteoarthritis, 292
    pain management, 290
    patient care, 288–290
    patient-centered communication, 296–297
    patient education, 297
    patient safety issues, 299
    practice-based learning and improvement (PBLI), 294–296
    privacy issues, 298
    professionalism, 297–298
    prognosis, 294
    quality improvement/performance improvement, 294–296
    radiology, 292
    rehabilitation-centered treatment of, 294
    rehabilitation goals, 299
    rehabilitation program, 289–290
    remission, 293
    sample rehabilitation prescription, 290
    sociocultural factors, 298
    systems-based practice (SBP), 298–300
RIME model, 43–46
risk-benefit analysis, 109, 140, 320
    in practice of rehabilitation medicine, 75–76
ROM. *See* range of motion
root cause analysis (RCA), steps in performing, 79
rotator cuff (RTC) tears/syndromes, 267
safe health care, defined, 78–79
SAFETY models, 45–46
SBAR methodology, 252, 254
SCI/D. *See* spinal cord injury and disease
selective serotonin reuptake inhibitors (SSRIs), 170, 306
self-assessment
    defined, 9
    learning, components of, 184
self-reflective exercise, 17
sensitive information, 27
serotonin-norepinephrine reuptake inhibitors (SNRIs), 306
shared decision making model, 56–57
SHARE, 351
shoulder disorders
    medical knowledge, 270
    patient care, 267–269
sign-out/transition of care, 161
simple erosion narrowing score (SENS), 358
simulation tests, 280
situation monitoring, 273
skilled nursing facilities (SNFs), 73–74
    IRF versus, 76
skills checklist, 38–39
SNAPPS, 40–42
    six-steps, 40
social justice, 56
socioeconomic issues in cancer rehabilitation, 136
somatosensory evoked potential (SSEP), 170
spasticity, 149, 340
    case study, 266
    defined, 260, 341
    interpersonal and communication skills (ICS), 262–263
    management team, 263
    medical documentation, 263
    medical knowledge, 258–261
    patient care, 257–258
    patient education, 263
    practice-based learning and improvement (PBLI), 261–262
    professionalism, 263–264
    system-based practice, 265–266
    treatments, 260–261
speaking behaviors, 26
spinal cord injuries and amputations, 105
spinal cord injury and disease (SCI/D)
    case study, 198–199
    causes of death, 191
    interpersonal and communication skills (ICS), 195–196
    medical knowledge, 192–193
    patient care, 190–192
    practice-based learning and improvement (PBLI), 193–194
    professionalism, 196–197
    syndromes, 193
    systems-based practice (SBP), 197–198
spurling test, 315
stroke
    Brunnstrom stages, 150
    case study, 162
    hemorrhagic, 155–156
    interpersonal and communication skills (ICS), 158–159
    medical knowledge, 151–157
    patient care, 144–151
    practice-based learning and improvement (PBLI), 157–158
    professionalism, 159–160
    rehabilitation, 144–145
    risk factors, 151
    syndromes, 152–154
    systems-based practice (SBP), 160–162
    workup, 156–157
stroke volume (SV), 116
styles, communication, 20
summative evaluation, 43
SUPERB models, 45–46
supervision, 44
    models of, 44–46
    types of, 45
supraspinatus test, 269

symptom severity (SS) scale, 303–304
syndrome of inappropriate antidiuretic hormone secretion (SIADH), 340–341
system-based medicine, 310–311
system errors, 78–79
    for MTBI, 187
    patient safety and, 140–141
system evaluator, 79
systems-based practice (SBP), 5
    cancer rehabilitation, 138–141
    cardiopulmonary rehabilitation, 127–128
    cervical radiculopathy, 320
    entrapment neuropathies, 336
    fibromyalgia, 310–311
    health care systems, 71–72
    juvenile idiopathic arthritis (JIA), 363–364
    lumbar spine disorders, 285–287
    mild traumatic brain injury (MTBI), 186–187
    multiple sclerosis (MS), 231–232
    neuromuscular diseases (NMDs), 219–221
    osteoarthritis, 244–245
    Parkinson disease, 206–207
    patient care coordination in practice of rehabilitation medicine, 74
    patient safety, systems errors, and quality, 78–79
    physiatrist as resource manager, 74–78
    physiatrist as systems consultant, 73–74
    preparticipation evaluation (PPE), 326–327
    rheumatoid arthritis (RA), 298–300
    spasticity, 265–266
    spinal cord injury (SCI), 197–198
    stroke, 160–162
    system evaluator, 79
    systems thinking, 72–73
    and teams, 77
    total hip arthroplasty (THA), 253–254
    total knee arthroplasty (TKA), 253–254
    traumatic brain injury (TBI), 349–351
        moderate and severe, 174–175
    upper extremity limb loss, 96–97
    upper extremity musculoskeletal injuries (UEMIs), 274–275
systems thinking, 72–73
systolic blood pressure (SBP), 116

Tardieu scale, 257, 341
TBI. *See* traumatic brain injury
TCAs. *See* tricyclic antidepressants
teaching
    bedside, 40
    competencies strategies, 36–37
    description, 34–36
    and feedback, 34–37
    rules for, 39
team communication, 18
Team STEPPS, 272–273
temporal lobe involvement, 340
tenderness tests, 280
THA. *See* total hip arthroplasty
thoracolumbar sacral orthosis (TLSO), 281
tidal volume (TV), 116
tizanidine (Zanaflex), 261
TKA. *See* total knee arthroplasty

total hip arthroplasty (THA)
    case study, 254–255
    interpersonal and communication skills (ICS), 252–253
    medical knowledge, 251–252
    patient care, 248–251
    practice-based learning and improvement (PBLI), 252
    professionalism, 253
    systems-based practice (SBP), 253–254
total joint arthroplasty in lower extremities, injuries following, 250–251
total knee arthroplasty (TKA)
    case study, 254–255
    interpersonal and communication skills (ICS), 252–253
    medical knowledge, 251–252
    patient care, 248–251
    practice-based learning and improvement (PBLI), 252
    professionalism, 253
    systems-based practice (SBP), 253–254
total lung capacity (TLC), 116
traditional culture in medicine, 17
tramadol, 307
transcutaneous electrical nerve stimulation (TENS), 103, 316
transfemoral residual limb length, 102
transformative action, 10
transhumeral amputation (TH), 93–94
transradial amputation (TR), 92–93
transtibial prosthetic sockets and suspension, 103
traumatic brain injury (TBI), 182–183
    autonomic dysfunction in, 340
    case study, 351–352
    history, 340
    interpersonal and communication skills (ICS), 346–348
    medical knowledge, 342–345
    monitor after, 341
    patient care, 341–342
    practice-based learning and improvement (PBLI), 345–346
    problems with executive function after, 348
    professionalism, 348–349
    rehabilitation checklist for families, 347
    safety concerns after, 351
    systems-based practice (SBP), 349–351
traumatic brain injury (TBI), moderate and severe
    anatomy, 168
    biomechanics, 169
    case study, 175
    complications of, 167–168
    counseling patients and families, 173
    diagnostic testing, 170
    documentation and effective communication, 173
    education, 171–172
    epidemiology, 169
    ethical issues, 170–171
    history of present illness, 165–166
    impairments, activity limitations, and participation restrictions, 167
    leadership skills, 173
    pathophysiology, 168
    patient assessment, 171
    patient safety checklist, 175
    physical examination, 166–167
    physiology, 168
    professionalism, 173–174

quality improvement/practice improvement activity, 172–173
sample rehabilitation program, 168
severity grading of, 165
systems-based practice (SBP), 174–175
treatment, 169–170, 171
tricyclic antidepressants (TCAs), 306

UEMIs. *See* upper extremity musculoskeletal injuries
UMNDs. *See* upper motor neuron disorders
Uniform Data System for Medical Rehabilitation, 74
upper extremity (UE) amputations, 91
upper extremity limb loss
    case study, 97
    etiology of, 91
    interpersonal and communication skills (ICS), 95
    levels of amputation, 92–94
    medical knowledge, 91–94
    patient care, 89–91
    practice-based learning and improvement (PBLI), 94–95
    professionalism, 95–96
    surgical techniques, 92
    systems-based practice (SBP), 96–97
upper extremity musculoskeletal injuries (UEMIs)
    case study, 275–276
    interpersonal and communication skills (ICS), 272–273
    medical knowledge, 269–271
    patient care, 267–269
    practice-based learning and improvement (PBLI), 271–272
    professionalism, 273–274
    systems-based practice (SBP), 274–275
upper motor neuron disorders (UMNDs), 258
urinary incontinence, 149

VA/DoD clinical guidelines, 106
venous thromboembolism (VTE), 250
    prophylaxis, 168
ventilatory failure, assessment of, 125
ventilatory support, indications for, 125
verbal read-back procedures, 23
vertebrobasilar system, 155
Veterans Affairs Amputee System of Care, 110
Visual Teaching Strategies (VTS), 10
vital capacity (VC), 116
VTE prophylaxis. *See* venous thromboembolism prophylaxis
VTS. *See* Visual Teaching Strategies

Waddell signs, 280
widespread pain index (WPI), 303
Williams exercises, 280
Wolff-Parkinson-White (WPW) syndrome, 115
workplace-based assessments, 6
WPI. *See* widespread pain index
WPW syndrome. *See* Wolff-Parkinson-White syndrome
wrist disorders
    medical knowledge, 271
    patient care, 269